Comparative Animal N̶ ̶ ̶ ̶ ̶ n̶

Comparative Animal Nutrition and Metabolism

Peter R. Cheeke

Professor Emeritus
Department of Animal Sciences
Oregon State University, USA

and

Ellen S. Dierenfeld

Novus International
St Louis, Missouri, USA

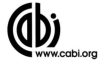

www.cabi.org

CABI is a trading name of CAB International

CABI Head Office
Nosworthy Way
Wallingford
Oxfordshire OX10 8DE
UK

CABI North American Office
875 Massachusetts Avenue
7th Floor
Cambridge, MA 02139
USA

Tel: +44 (0)1491 832111
Fax: +44 (0)1491 833508
E-mail: cabi@cabi.org
Website: www.cabi.org

Tel: +1 617 395 4056
Fax: +1 617 354 6875
E-mail: cabi-nao@cabi.org

A catalogue record for this book is available from the British Library, London, UK.

Library of Congress Cataloging-in-Publication Data

Cheeke, Peter R.
Comparative animal nutrition and metabolism / Peter R. Cheeke and Ellen S. Dierenfeld.
       p. cm.
   Includes bibliographical references and index.
   ISBN 978-1-84593-631-0 (alk. paper)
   1. Animal nutrition. 2. Metabolism. I. Dierenfeld, Ellen Sue, 1956- II. Title.

SF95.C4634 2010
636.089'32--dc22

2009051950

ISBN-13: 978 1 84593 631 0

Commissioning editor: Sarah Hulbert
Production editor: Kate Hill

Typeset by SPi, Pondicherry, India.
Printed and bound in the UK by Cambridge University Press, Cambridge.

Contents

Contributors

Guest Contributors for Chapter 23

J.A. Carroll, *USDA-ARS, Livestock Issues Research Unit, Lubbock, Texas, USA; jeff.carroll@ars.usda.gov*

N.E. Forsberg, *OmniGen Research, Corvallis, Oregon, USA; nforsberg@omnigenresearch.com*

S.B. Puntenney, *OmniGen Research, Corvallis, Oregon, USA; punten@msn.com*

Y. Wang, *OmniGen Research, Corvallis, Oregon, USA; yqwang72@gmail.com*

Preface

This book has had a long gestation period. In 1969, I began my teaching career at Oregon State University with a class called 'Comparative Nutrition'. I concentrated on comparative aspects of domestic animals: ruminants, 'monogastrics' and non-ruminant herbivores. Several students suggested that my notes could be organized into a book quite readily. I made a small effort to do this in the early 1970s, but other pressures on a young faculty member resulted in this project falling by the wayside. In the mid-1980s I started again, but got sidetracked writing another book. Finally, in the late 1990s, I decided to get serious and tackle a book on comparative nutrition. By this time, it had become apparent to me that there were many interesting nutritional strategies of wild as well as domestic animals. To assist in the area of wild animal nutrition, I sought the collaboration of Dr Ellen Dierenfeld, one of the world's leading authorities on this subject. I wanted to take a 'systems approach' to this subject. Virtually all animal nutrition texts deal with each nutrient in order, one after another. Typically, there will be a major section on vitamins, starting with vitamin A, then vitamin D, followed by vitamin E, and so on, with the process repeated for minerals. I wanted to consider the nutrients in the context of how they function. For example, minerals and vitamins involved in regulation of energy metabolism are discussed in the context of their roles in metabolic processes. My perception is that it may be more interesting to students to encounter nutrients in their functioning roles, rather than just going down a list. This approach has some advantages, but, I've discovered, also has some disadvantages. In some cases, diverse functions of a nutrient make it difficult to decide where the major discussion of it should be. Hopefully, my decisions on subject placement make sense, and will facilitate 'whole animal' integration of nutritional principles by students.

Nutrition is basically applied biochemistry. Paradoxically, throughout my career, I've noted that many students interested in majoring in animal nutrition have a profound dislike of biochemistry. I've endeavoured to provide a strong biochemical basis for nutritional principles, and hope that by showing the relevance of biochemistry to the full understanding of nutrition, it will be somewhat more palatable to animal science and veterinary students than traditional biochemistry courses. Application of biochemical principles to domestic and wild animals should lead to a greater student appreciation of the discipline of biochemistry, which sometimes leaves the impression that life consists only of giant rat liver cells. I'm not intending to produce a 'watered-down' biochemistry course, but hope that by stressing the relevance of biochemistry to animal nutrition, students will find traditional biochemistry courses more palatable. Some things are discussed in more detail than the average reader might need. It is intended that the book can serve as a primary source of nutritional information. For example, if in the feed industry one encounters a form of vitamin E called RRR-α-tocopherol, and hasn't a clue what that means, the answer can be found herein.

I have jettisoned certain 'nutrition classics'; just because we learned certain things in nutrition classes years ago does not mean that current students need to. For example, a pantothenic acid deficiency causes 'goose-stepping' in pigs. Do 21st century students really need to be able to answer 'What nutrient deficiency causes goose-stepping in pigs?' Pantothenic acid literally means 'an acid found everywhere'. When was the last time that there were goose-stepping pigs in a commercial pig operation? As Scott *et al.* (1982) indicate for poultry, 'Pantothenic acid deficiency in sufficient severity to cause characteristic symptoms has not been demonstrated to occur under field conditions.' So I have resisted the temptation of assuming that everything that was taught when I was a student must be included.

In his book, *Wildlife Feeding and Nutrition*, Charles Robbins (1993) noted in his Preface, 'Unfortunately, although many of the principles of nutrition could be learned by wildlife students taking the standard animal nutrition course taught in the animal science department, most of these departments have chosen virtually to ignore the nondomesticated and nonlaboratory species.' Our book is an effort to address this need.

Large numbers of animal science students are in pre-veterinary programmes. Exotic animal and wildlife medicine are of increasing importance in the veterinary field. Many zoos and animal parks now employ animal nutritionists, such as co-author Dr Ellen Dierenfeld who has coordinated the nutrition programmes at the St Louis Zoo and the Bronx Zoo. Thus there are many employment options involving 'non-traditional species' for animal science and veterinary graduates, and these opportunities are steadily increasing. Global climate change, increasing human populations in developing countries, habitat loss, and numerous other factors are putting many animals on an endangered status. Professionals with an adequate background in comparative animal nutrition will play vital roles in preservation of endangered species, especially in wildlife conservation parks and preserves involving captive animals. Loss of a single animal from a nutritional disorder could mean irreparable damage to an extremely narrow gene pool.

For the past several years, I have taught a course on comparative nutrition using the manuscript as the text. I thank the students for their perceptive and useful comments and contributions. Several anonymous reviewers also contributed very useful comments.

Finally, I gratefully acknowledge two people who have made particularly valuable contributions to the preparation of this manuscript. Helen Chesbrough has worked long, hard and cheerfully on numerous renditions of the manuscript. Her competence, enthusiasm and grammatical skills are greatly appreciated. I also acknowledge with pleasure the work of Dr Jianya Huan, who prepared the figures of chemical structures and metabolic pathways. He has undertaken this project with enthusiasm, and has been of tremendous help.

Peter R. Cheeke
Corvallis, Oregon

References

Robbins, C.T. (1993) *Wildlife Feeding and Nutrition*, 2nd edn. Academic Press, San Diego.
Scott, M.L., Nesheim, M.C. and Young, R.J. (1982) *Nutrition of the Chicken*. M.L. Scott and Associates, Ithaca, New York.

Acknowledgements

The authors sincerely appreciate the support of Novus International, Inc. for sponsoring printing of the colour plates on the following pages. They would also like to thank E. Koutsos for the photograph of carotenoids in chicken legs supplied for the colour plates.

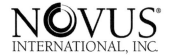

www.novusint.com

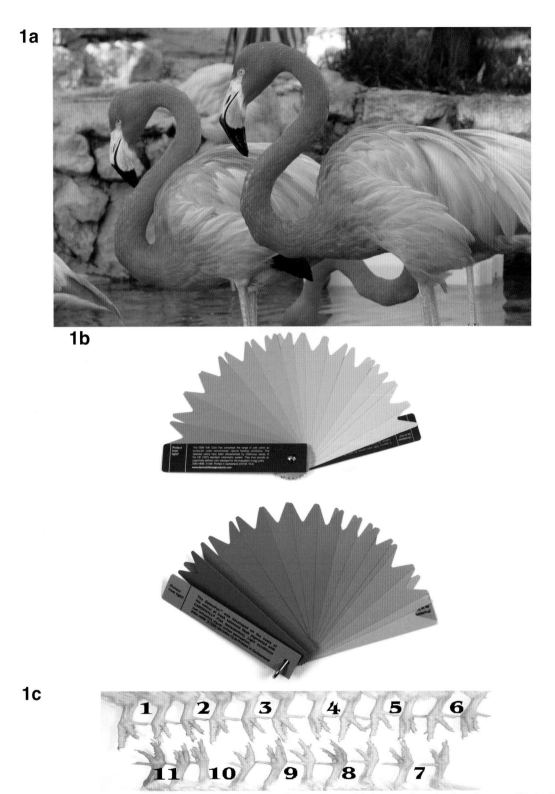

Plate 1. (a) Many colourful birds, like the flamingo, rely on dietary carotenoid pigments for colouring plumage. (Photo: E. Dierenfeld.) (b) Colour scoring tools (e.g. egg yolk (top fan) and salmon meat (bottom fan)) have been developed for quantifying pigmentation in agricultural products. (Photo: J. Mahoney.) (c) Pigment variation in broiler chicken legs from birds fed 0–60 ppm total carotenoids (lutein and canthaxanthin). (Photo: E. Koutsos.)

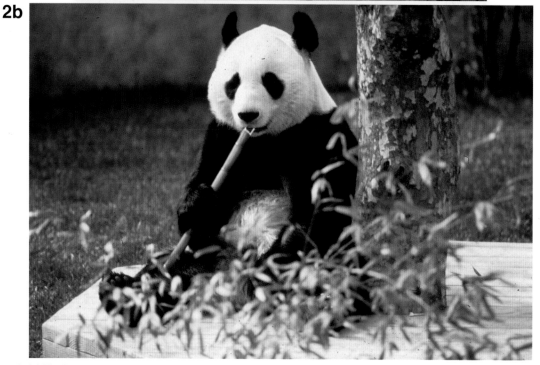

Plate 2. (a) The koala (*Phacolarctos cinereus*) and (b) giant panda (*Ailuropoda melanoleuca*) represent well-known examples of specialist herbivores, preferentially consuming various species of eucalyptus and bamboo, respectively. This behaviour notably limits captive feeding options.

PART I
Introduction and Digestive Tract Physiology

This part is intended to introduce the general subject of animal nutrition, and to categorize domestic and wild animals according to their digestive physiology.

Part Objectives

1. To introduce the nutrients that animals require in their diets.
2. To describe the major types of animal digestive tracts and to indicate the significance of particular digestive functions relative to nutritional requirements.

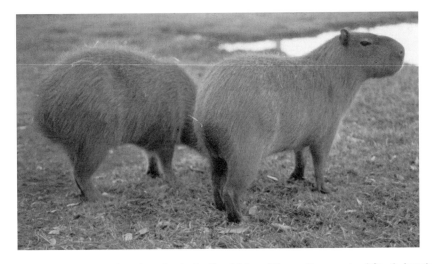

The capybara, the world's largest rodent, is native to the floodplains of the northern parts of South America. It is a nonruminant herbivore with cecal fermentation.

1 Introduction

Nutrition is a very broad discipline, encompassing various aspects of biochemistry, physiology, endocrinology, immunology, microbiology and pathology. Discussion of virtually any aspect of nutrition draws upon some prior knowledge of these disciplines. Nutrition can be defined as applied biochemistry, and is commonly referred to as **nutritional science**. Animal nutrition has conventionally meant the study of nutritional needs of domestic animals, in contrast to human nutrition, which specifically targets humans. **Dietetics** refers to the formulation and preparation of diets to meet the needs of humans. The comparable activity with domestic animals is **diet formulation**. Nutritional science deals with the principles of nutrition, while dietetics and diet formulation deal with their application.

Animal and poultry nutritionists have played key roles in the development of the nutritional sciences. Many of the nutrients were discovered by animal nutritionists using chicks or rats as experimental animals. Human nutrition developed more slowly as a scientific discipline, emerging in most cases from the discipline of Home Economics.

The objectives of this book are to clearly explain principles of animal nutrition. A comparative approach is taken, recognizing that there are considerable differences in nutrient digestion, metabolism and requirements among various mammalian and avian species. On a molecular level, the similarities in metabolic processes among animals are far greater than the differences, reflecting their common evolutionary history. However, the passage of nutrients from the environment to the molecular level of the animal cell involves great species differences, largely because of differences in food selection and food-seeking strategy, and in digestive tract physiology and digestive strategies. These comparative differences will be explained and their significance to nutritional needs discussed. Within categories of animals, there are similarities in the nutrition of domestic and wild species. For example, there are similarities among wild avian species (i.e. birds) to domestic poultry, as well as numerous differences. Digestive processes in hindgut digester wild animals, such as elephants, share some similarities with domestic species such as horses, whereas the koala resembles the rabbit in hindgut function. The basic nutritional requirements and digestive physiology of wild ruminants such as deer, antelope and giraffes resemble to some extent those of domestic ruminants such as cattle, sheep and goats. It is intended that this text will be relevant and useful to those interested in wildlife nutrition as well as to those primarily interested in domestic animals. The principles involved are similar. While it is true that more nutritional research has been conducted with domestic livestock species than with wild animals, animal scientists are perhaps not generally appreciative of the degree to which findings with non-domestic species can influence the understanding of nutritional principles. For example, a greater understanding of the variations in rumen anatomy and physiology of wild ruminants could lead to greater recognition by animal scientists that it is simplistic to view sheep, goats and cattle as functionally equivalent in terms of digestive functions and processes. Thus, it is anticipated that the comparative approach developed in this text will enhance the appreciation of nutritional principles by students having either domestic animal or wildlife orientations.

The Nutrients

Nutrients may be defined as dietary essentials for one or more species of animal, implying that not all animals require all nutrients. For example, few species besides primates and the guinea pig have a dietary requirement for vitamin C. Ruminant animals do not normally have a dietary requirement for B-complex vitamins and amino acids.

Other nutrients can in fact be omitted from the diet if appropriate dietary adjustments are made. There is no dietary requirement for carbohydrates per se, either individually or collectively. While glucose is an essential metabolite in mammalian metabolism, it is not a dietary essential. Nevertheless, glucose and other sugars are commonly considered to be nutrients. This ambiguity about what is and what is not a nutrient exists primarily with energy-yielding substances, for which there is not a specific requirement for individual sugars and fatty acids, but rather there is a collective requirement for carbohydrates, fats and amino acids which can be metabolized to provide energy. For minerals and vitamins, the requirements are unequivocal; they have specific metabolic roles which cannot be replaced by other nutrients.

Those substances that can be considered nutrients fit into one of the following six categories:

- proteins;
- carbohydrates;
- lipids;
- minerals;
- vitamins; and
- water.

Water is considered to be a nutrient, although for domestic animals it does not totally fit the definition of a nutrient because it is not generally required in the diet (food) but is usually consumed separately as drinking water. Some desert animals (e.g. pack rat) never drink, but survive on metabolic water (see Chapter 20). Marine mammals (e.g. seals, sea lions) never drink, but obtain their water from their diet (fish tissue), while fruit-eating animals (frugivores) obtain a major portion of their water from the diet (fruit). Thus water is truly a nutrient for these species.

A brief description of each of these major nutrient categories will be given for introductory purposes; they will be discussed in detail in later chapters.

Proteins

Proteins are large molecules composed of amino acids joined together by peptide bonds (see Chapter 4). Plant and animal proteins are composed of about 20 amino acids, arranged in various sequences to form specific proteins. A few other amino acids (e.g. citrulline) do not occur in protein tissue but have other specific functions, and are known as **non-protein amino acids**. Over 300 individual amino acids are known; most of them are non-protein amino acids in plant tissue, with no role in animal nutrition (except a negative one if they are toxic). Some sources indicate even greater numbers of known amino acids in plants, as high as over 900 (Wink, 1997). The genetic control of protein synthesis involving DNA and RNA metabolism is one of the marvels of life. Each cell (except non-avian erythrocytes) contains a genetic code, programming the cell to synthesize particular proteins. Proteins are an integral part of animal structure and metabolism. They constitute a major part of the body structure, as components of muscle, connective tissue and cell membranes. All metabolic reactions are dependent on proteinaceous enzymes.

A major concern of animal nutritionists is the provision of adequate dietary protein and amino acids. From a comparative standpoint, there are great differences in protein utilization, with ruminant animals largely insulated from specific dietary amino acid requirements because of the activities of rumen microbes, whereas carnivores have some distinct differences from omnivores in amino acid needs.

All amino acids contain nitrogen; therefore, all proteins contain nitrogen. Protein utilization by animals is often studied by measuring nitrogen in nitrogen balance trials. Protein digestibility, for example, is determined by measuring the nitrogen content of feed and faeces to determine the amount of absorbed (hence digested) nitrogen, reflective of amino acid absorption. In general, proteins contain about 16% nitrogen. The protein content of feeds is usually measured by determining the nitrogen content and multiplying it by the factor of 6.25. Crude protein is defined as $N \times 6.25$ (16 g of nitrogen (N) come from 100 g protein; therefore, 1 g of nitrogen is associated with $100/16 = 6.25$ g of protein). Nitrogen is measured by the **Kjeldahl** procedure, which is named after the Danish chemist who developed it. The feed sample is boiled in concentrated sulfuric acid, resulting in the complete oxidation of all organic material. The proteins and amino acids are completely degraded; their nitrogen is released as ammonium ion (NH_4^+). The solution is then made alkaline, converting NH_4^+ to ammonia (NH_3). Steam is passed through the solution (steam distillation), driving off the NH_3, which is trapped in a boric acid solution. The concentration of NH_3 is measured by titration. It is important to recognize that the crude protein procedure measures nitrogen. Thus, it does not distinguish between high-quality and poor-quality protein, or protein and non-protein nitrogen.[1]

Carbohydrates

Besides containing carbon, **carbohydrates** $(CH_2O)_n$ contain hydrogen and oxygen in the proportions found in water; hence the name (hydrates of carbon). Carbohydrates are the basic energy source of almost all animal life. They are produced as the end products of photosynthesis by green plant tissue. Photosynthesis is a very complicated process, but in simple terms, consists of the reduction (gain of hydrogen) of carbon dioxide in plants to produce carbohydrate. An in-put of energy is required. Plant tissues contain pigments, including chlorophyll and carotenoids (vitamin A precursors) that trap solar energy to provide electrons to accomplish the reduction of carbon dioxide. The overall reaction is:

$$\text{Solar energy} + 6CO_2 + 6H_2O \rightarrow C_6H_{12}O_6 + 6O_2$$

Plants use the compounds formed in photosynthesis to synthesize all their other organic components such as amino acids, sugars, starch, cellulose, lignin, lipids and so on. When animals eat plants, the energy contained in the carbohydrates and other organic compounds synthesized from carbohydrate (amino acids and lipids) is made available by metabolic processes. Animal metabolism is in essence the reverse of photosynthesis:

$$C_6H_{12}O_6 + 6O_2 \rightarrow 6CO_2 + 6H_2O + ATP$$
$$+ \text{ Heat energy}$$

Adenosine triphosphate (ATP) is the compound used in animal metabolism as the energy source for biochemical reactions. Animals are not capable of converting all of the available energy in carbohydrates to ATP, with a large part of the energy lost as heat.

As these reactions indicate, plant and animal metabolisms are symbiotically intertwined. Plants require the carbon dioxide and water excreted as metabolic wastes by animals and animals require the oxygen excreted by plants and the organic compounds they synthesize. The whole process is sustained by a constant infusion of solar energy.

Plants are categorized in terms of their photosynthesis reactions as either C3 or C4 plants. In **C3 plants**, the first products of photosynthesis are three-carbon compounds such as phosphoglyceric acid, while in **C4 plants** the first photosynthetic products (oxaloacetic, malic and aspartic acids)

have four carbon atoms. This is agriculturally significant because C4 plants are photosynthetically more efficient than C3 plants, and thus are more productive. Most C4 plants are tropical (e.g. sugarcane) or have a tropical origin (e.g. maize). Tropical grasses, being C4 plants, can be highly productive, yielding large amounts of biomass per unit of land. However, they have a leaf anatomy characterized by a high content of poorly digested vascular tissue and a low content of the more readily digested mesophyll cells. Thus they have 12–15% lower dry matter digestibility in ruminants than temperate grasses. Low digestibility is a major reason that accounts for the low productivity of ruminants in the tropics.

Carbohydrates are the major dietary energy source for most animals, with the exception of obligate carnivores. They consist of two major types: (i) the starches, sugars and other readily available carbohydrates; and (ii) cellulosic compounds which are more resistant to digestion. The readily available carbohydrates are associated with the plant cell contents, while the cellulosic compounds are constituents of the fibrous cell walls of plant tissue.

Lipids

Lipids are defined as those constituents of plant and animal tissue that are soluble in organic solvents like diethyl ether. The lipid content of feeds is usually referred to as the **ether extract (EE)**. The EE is determined by extracting a feed sample with diethyl ether; the loss of weight of the extracted sample is the EE. Dietary lipids of importance in animal nutrition are mainly fats and oils, which are energy-rich compared to carbohydrates, having about 225% the energy content of carbohydrate on an equal weight basis. The properties of a particular fat or oil are determined by the fatty acids they contain. **Fatty acids** differ in the number of carbon atoms and in the amount of hydrogen they contain. Those which are fully saturated with hydrogen are called saturated fatty acids, while the unsaturated fatty acids contain one or more carbon–carbon double bonds that are not saturated with hydrogen. Fatty acids contain a carboxyl group (–COOH) at the end of a carbon chain. Fats contain mainly saturated fatty acids and are solids at room temperature, while oils contain unsaturated fatty acids and are liquids at room temperature.

Other lipids include the fat-soluble vitamins and cholesterol. Cholesterol is an important metabolite necessary for the synthesis of steroid hormones and bile acids and is an essential component of cell membranes. In plants, other important lipids include the photosynthetic pigments (chlorophyll and carotenoids), and waxes and cutin which form the water-shedding waxy surface of leaves.

Minerals

Mineral elements are the inorganic components of plant and animal tissue. In animal nutrition, they are classified in two categories: (i) macro-minerals; and (ii) micro (trace) minerals (elements). The **macro-elements** are required in relatively large quantities; **trace elements** are required in very small amounts. The macro-elements calcium, phosphorus and magnesium are major components of the skeletal system, and thus function in a structural role. The other minerals function primarily in regulatory roles. For example, sodium, potassium and chlorine are involved as electrolytes in regulating fluid balance between the gut, blood, cells, tissue spaces and body cavities. Sulfur as such is not a dietary essential, but is a component of many organic constituents of tissues such as the sulfur-containing amino acids, the vitamins biotin and thiamin, mucopolysaccharides such as chondroitin sulfate, and the metabolically essential coenzyme A (CoA). Other elements regulate enzyme activity, either as integral components of enzymes or as cofactors. Examples include selenium as an integral component of the enzyme glutathione peroxidase and copper as a cofactor of cytochrome oxidase. The following are the generally recognized nutritionally essential elements:

- Macro-elements – calcium, phosphorus, sodium, potassium, chlorine, magnesium, sulfur.
- Trace elements – manganese, zinc, iron, copper, molybdenum, selenium, iodine, cobalt, chromium.

There are a few other minerals, such as vanadium, silicon, tin, boron and nickel, for which dietary need has been demonstrated only with laboratory animals fed highly purified diets. They are unlikely to be of practical importance for animals consuming diets composed of naturally occurring constituents.

Vitamins

The term 'vitamin' was coined in 1912 by a Polish chemist, Casimir Funk, who discovered that the antipolyneuritis factor in rice husks was nitrogenous in nature. He called it a 'vital amine', and proposed the term 'vitamine' for accessory food factors. Vitamins can, like minerals, also be classified into two groups: (i) the fat-soluble; and (ii) water-soluble vitamins. The **fat-soluble vitamins** are vitamin A (retinol), vitamin D (cholecalciferol), vitamin E (α-tocopherol) and vitamin K (phylloquinone). The **water-soluble vitamins** are vitamin C (ascorbic acid) and the members of the vitamin B-complex group. These include vitamin B_1 (thiamin), vitamin B_2 (riboflavin), vitamin B_6 (pyridoxine), vitamin B_{12} (cyanocobalamin), niacin (nicotinic acid), folacin (folic acid), biotin, choline and pantothenic acid. It is preferable to refer to vitamins by their accepted names (e.g. thiamin) rather than by the B-designation (e.g. vitamin B_1).

Vitamins are organic compounds other than proteins, carbohydrates and lipids that have specific roles in metabolism and are required in the diet in very small amounts.[2] Deficiency causes a specific disease, which is cured or prevented only by restoring the vitamin to the diet. In most cases, these roles are in the regulation of enzyme function. In vitamin deficiencies, the loss of particular enzyme activities results in specific deficiency symptoms. Thus in vitamin K deficiency, as an example, impaired blood clotting occurs because of the enzymatic role of vitamin K in the clotting process. Vitamin A has a role in vision; hence vitamin A deficiency can result in blindness.

The dietary requirements for vitamins are very low in quantitative terms. Once the metabolic need has been satisfied, there is no further response from additional quantities. In spite of this, there is a huge commercial industry, based on an unlikely alliance of multinational drug companies that manufacture vitamins and 'anti-establishment' concerns such as 'health food' stores that sell them, involved in megadosing of vitamins by the human population of the USA! (The excess vitamins wind up in wastewater treatment plants.)

There are a number of 'bogus' vitamins (e.g. vitamin H, vitamin P) that do not exist. In some cases, they are names coined by entrepreneurs selling dietary supplements. In other cases, they were named by scientists who believed they had isolated a new vitamin, but subsequent work revealed it was either a previously named vitamin or it was a substance that did not meet the criteria for vitamin status (e.g. vitamin B_4). The B-complex group does not have all the numbers from 1 to 12, because some of them (e.g. vitamin B_4) proved to be invalid.

The last vitamin to be discovered was vitamin B_{12}, in 1948. Before its chemical identification, extracts with the enzyme activity were called the 'cow manure factor' and the 'animal protein factor'.

Dietary supplements (nutraceuticals)

A number of dietary supplements are often used in animal feeding, particularly in the horse industry. The term 'supplements' in this context refers to non-nutritive substances, in contrast to the known nutrients. Those with perceived medicinal properties are sometimes called nutraceuticals. Commonly, a number of herbal products are used. Some herbal products, such as yucca, are known to have anti-inflammatory properties. In general, dietary supplements are unproven scientifically, and their use is promoted by anecdotal 'evidence'. Lack of scientific proof is a reflection of a lack of financial incentive for research support, because most herbal products are not patentable. The problem with 'anecdotal evidence' is that it is often due to the placebo effect (Kienzle *et al.*, 2006). The only acceptable proof is a double-blind study (in which neither the investigator nor the subject knows the identity of which subjects are on which treatment). Subjective types of responses, particularly in equine studies, are also a problem. With dressage horses, for example, the responses are the evaluations of the rider, such as unresponsiveness or stiff back, horse 'too hot', and so on. The more subjective the criteria, the more likely that the rider's imagination comes into play (Kienzle *et al.*, 2006).

Animal Cellular Metabolism

Enzymes and hormones

Enzymes and hormones have important roles in regulation of metabolism. Some general comments of an introductory nature will be made here, and specific roles of various enzymes and hormones will be discussed later as appropriate.

Enzymes are organic catalysts. Catalysts are substances that accelerate chemical reactions. They undergo chemical changes during the reaction, but revert to their original state when the reaction is completed, and can be reused. Virtually every chemical reaction that takes place in living tissues requires an enzyme catalyst. With some exceptions (e.g. drug metabolizing enzymes), enzymes are very substrate-specific, having an active site that is very specific in its binding capabilities. All enzymes are proteins. Enzymes can be extracted from tissues and purified, and utilized in research, medicine and for industrial purposes.

Enzymes have traditionally been named for the substrate upon which they act, with the addition of the ending 'ase'. Some of the enzymes encountered in nutrition, such as trypsin, chymotrypsin, pepsin and rhodanese, were named before a unifying system of nomenclature was developed. The current system includes information on the type of chemical reaction catalysed and cofactors required. For example, oxidoreductases catalyse oxidation–reduction reactions, transferases catalyse transfer of a group (e.g. glutathione-S-transferase), hydrolases act to hydrolyse ester bonds, isomerases catalyse interconversions of isomers (e.g. *trans*-vitamin A to *cis*-vitamin A), etc. Essential cofactors, such as nicotinamide adenine dinucleotide (NAD) and NAD phosphate (NADP), are included in the name. The result can be some real tongue-twisters, such as UDP-N-acetylglucosamine:dolicholphosphate N-acetylglucosamine phosphate transferase! This enzyme is essential for formation of glycoproteins, and is inhibited by the mycotoxins responsible for annual ryegrass toxicity of sheep.

Cofactors associate reversibly with enzymes or substrates; they are often metal ions. Enzymes that require a metal ion cofactor are called metal-activated enzymes, in contrast to metalloenzymes that contain a metal ion as a prosthetic group. Copper, iron and zinc frequently function as cofactors. Organic cofactors are called **coenzymes**. Coenzymes act as reusable shuttles that can transport substrates from their point of generation to their point of utilization. Several B-vitamins function as constituents of coenzymes, including pantothenic acid (coenzyme A, CoA), niacin (NAD, NADP), riboflavin (flavin mononucleotide, FMN; flavin adenine dinucleotide, FAD), thiamin, folic acid and vitamin B_{12}. Many coenzymes are derivatives of adenosine monophosphate (e.g. CoA, NAD, NADP, FAD).

The distribution of enzymes in living tissues is highly ordered, with enzymes located so that the product(s) of one enzymatic reaction are substrates for the next reaction. They are compartmentalized in subcellular fractions; the enzymes of glycolysis, for example, are in the cell cytosol while the citric acid cycle enzymes are in the mitochondria.

Enzymes have an 'active site' or 'catalytic site' where the interactions between enzyme, substrate and coenzymes occur.

Many enzymes are produced and secreted as **proenzymes** or zymogens, which must be activated to the active enzyme form. This process is physiologically necessary in many cases, such as when the enzyme is needed intermittently, but when it is needed, it is needed immediately. Prothrombin is a proenzyme in the blood; when blood clotting is required, prothrombin is activated to the enzyme thrombin. Pepsinogen is secreted from the gastric mucosa, and activated by hydrochloric acid (HCl) in the stomach to pepsin. Other proteolytic enzymes are secreted as zymogens (e.g. trypsinogen, chymotrypsinogen). It would be physiologically difficult for a cell to store an active proteolytic enzyme without digesting itself.

Many enzymes require metal ions for their activity. **Metalloenzymes** contain a mineral as an integral part of their structure, while **metal-activated enzymes** require the presence of a less tightly bound mineral (cofactors). There are many zinc and copper metalloenzymes, such as thymidine kinase (Zn) and cytochrome oxidase (Cu).

The activity of enzymes is regulated in various ways in order to direct metabolic activity to maintain homeostasis. **Homeostasis** refers to the constancy of the internal environment, whereby cellular metabolism is regulated to attempt to maintain a steady-state condition. An example is blood glucose. Homeostatic hormones such as insulin and glucagon function to maintain a fairly constant blood glucose concentration. Marked deviations from normal are pathological (e.g. diabetes). Another example is serum calcium, which in most species is homeostatically maintained within a narrow concentration range. Enzyme concentration can be increased by **inducers**. For example, many drugs and natural toxins are detoxified by drug-metabolizing enzymes (mixed function oxidases) in the liver. Many of these toxins act as inducing agents, inducing increased concentration of the enzymes required to detoxify them. Conversely, enzymes involved in nutrient metabolism may be 'turned off' by feedback inhibition. When adequate quantities of a product have been produced and begin to accumulate, one or more of the enzymes involved in its production may be inhibited. The metabolism of glucose and directing it to either ATP production or energy storage as glycogen is regulated by feedback inhibition.

Many enzymes are regulated by hormones such as thyroxine which regulates the metabolism of glucose and fat.

Hormones, along with enzymes, are intimately involved in animal metabolism. Classically, **hormones** have been defined as substances that are produced in one tissue (a gland) and transported to a target tissue, with their production or release regulated by positive or negative feedback inhibition. It is now recognized that, in addition to target tissues, hormones can also act in non-target adjacent tissues as well as in the cells in which they are produced. Many hormones are nutritionally important. These include thyroid hormones (thyroxine and calcitonin), pancreatic hormones (insulin and glucagon), parathyroid hormone, growth hormone, and a number of gastrointestinal hormones. Many hormones are proteinaceous in nature, being derived from single amino acids (e.g. thyroxine and adrenalin are derivatives of tyrosine; serotonin is derived from tryptophan) or consisting of one or more polypeptide chains (e.g. insulin, glucagon, parathyroid hormone, growth hormone). Others are lipids, derived from cholesterol (e.g. androgens, oestrogens and 1,25 dihydroxycholecalciferol) and fatty acids (e.g. prostaglandins).

To exert their physiological effects, hormones react with receptor molecules. These may be within the cell (e.g. thyroid hormones bind to intracellular receptors) or at the cell surface. In the latter case, the cell surface receptor releases a second messenger, which mediates the intracellular effects of the hormone. For example, a common second messenger is cyclic adenosine monophosphate (cAMP). Hormones and enzymes are thus intimately co-involved in regulating animal metabolism. Receptor activity can be modified to regulate cellular uptake according to need. Activity is **up-regulated** to increase inflow of a substance, and **down-regulated** to decrease its uptake.

Metabolism and metabolomics

Metabolism refers to the summation of biochemical processes in living tissue. **Catabolism** refers to the breakdown or oxidation of fuels, while **anabolism** refers to the synthetic reactions that build up tissues (e.g. protein synthesis). The combined catabolic and anabolic processes constitute metabolism. Metabolomics is an emerging discipline, similar in concept to other 'omics' such as genomics and proteomics. **Metabolomics** is the 'big-picture' study of all metabolites – all molecules smaller than proteins and polynucleotides – in an individual. This concept recognizes 'biochemical individuality', in that each individual has a unique internal chemistry (the **metabolome**). Hopefully the ultimate result of the understanding of an individual's metabolome will be a recognition of metabolic 'choke points' and the ability to modify nutritional status to optimize internal chemistry. The discipline is in its infancy. The concept was first advanced in a classic book, *Biochemical Individuality*, by Roger J. Williams (first published 1956; reprinted 1998). Williams proposed that each individual is biochemically unique, and has unique nutritional requirements. He recognized that nutritional status can influence the expression of genetic characteristics. It is only recently that advances in instrumentation and analytical techniques have permitted determination of unique metabolic characteristics (the metabolome).

Metabolites (metabolic intermediates) are substances formed during the catabolism or anabolism of nutrients. They are generally small molecules.

For example, pyruvic acid is a metabolite of glucose; it is an intermediate formed during the catabolism of glucose by a metabolic pathway (glycolysis). A **metabolic pathway** is a series of biochemical reactions catalysed by enzymes, and generally proceeds from a state of higher energy to lower energy.

In 1942, a German biochemist, R. Schoenheimer, published a book entitled *The Dynamic State of Body Constituents*. By the use of radioactive isotopes, he had discovered that many tissues are in a constant state of catabolism–anabolism, or being mobilized and replaced by newly formed tissue. For example, adipose tissue is not an inert deposit of lipid; it is continually being mobilized and replaced by new lipid (see Chapter 15). Muscle tissue undergoes degradation and re-formation. Humans turn over 1–2% of their total body protein daily. Liver proteins have half-lives of 30 min to several hours. Bone is a dynamic structure that undergoes continuing remodelling, with mobilization of bone mineral followed by deposition of new bone tissue (see Chapter 18).

Questions and Study Guide

1. What is dietetics? What comparable term is used in animal nutrition?
2. What is a nutrient? Is water a nutrient? Why or why not?
3. What classes of nutrients are organic (in the chemical sense)? Which nutrient category consists only of inorganic substances?
4. What is the basic unit of (a) protein structure and (b) carbohydrate structure?
5. What does the name 'carbohydrate' mean?
6. What is measured by the Kjeldahl procedure?
7. How is the crude protein content of feeds measured?
8. Why is maize (*Zea mays*) more productive than barley (*Hordeum vulgare*)?
9. What is the difference between saturated and unsaturated fatty acids?
10. What is the main chemical difference between animal fats (e.g. beef tallow) and vegetable oils (e.g. maize (corn) oil)?
11. What is a vitamin? What was the last vitamin to be discovered?
12. What are nutraceuticals?
13. How is a 'double-blind' study conducted? What is the main advantage of this type of study?
14. How do enzymes function? How do cofactors and coenzymes affect enzyme function? What are metalloenzymes?
15. Blood glucose and blood calcium are said to be homeostatically regulated. What does this mean?
16. What is a hormone? Name some examples of nutritionally important hormones.
17. Define catabolism and anabolism.
18. What is meant by the term 'biochemical individuality'?

Notes

[1] This relationship was thrust in the public eye in 2007–2008. First, pet food manufactured in China resulted in animal deaths in the USA; the toxic industrial chemical **melamine** was added to ingredients to increase their nitrogen content, to make it appear that they met crude protein specifications. In 2008, melamine was deliberately added to dairy products, to increase their apparent crude protein contents. This resulted in widespread poisoning, including the deaths, of Chinese children.

[2] Some vitamins do not need to be consumed directly in the diet. For example, the B vitamin niacin can be synthesized by animals from the amino acid tryptophan.

Vitamin D can be obtained by the non-dietary route of exposure to sunlight.

References

Kienzle, E., Freismuth, A. and Reusch, A. (2006) Double-blind placebo-controlled vitamin E or selenium supplementation of sport horses with unspecified muscle problems. An example of the potential of placebos. *Journal of Nutrition* 136, 2045S–2047S.

Schoenheimer, R. (1942) *The Dynamic State of Body Constituents*. Harvard University Press, Cambridge, Massachusetts.

Williams, R.J. (1998) *Biochemical Individuality: the Key to Understanding What Shapes Your Health*. Keats Publishing, New Canaan, Connecticut.

Wink, M. (1997) Special nitrogen metabolism. In: Dey, P.M. and Harborne, J.B. (eds) *Plant Biochemistry*. Academic Press, San Diego, California, pp. 439–486.

2 Digestive Physiology: Autoenzymatic Digesters

The nutritional requirements of animals are greatly influenced by the nature of their **gastrointestinal tracts**. This influence is at least twofold as digestive physiology is closely linked to: (i) food selection and dietary strategies; and (ii) the ability of the animal to derive nutritional benefit from particular types of feedstuffs.

Animals have evolved to occupy virtually all ecological niches, and in many cases have developed specialized feeding strategies. A summary of some of the most important feeding strategies is given in Table 2.1. Domestic animal types include carnivores (cats), omnivores (pigs, chickens) and herbivores (cattle, sheep, horses, rabbits). These **feeding strategies** can influence nutrient metabolism and requirements. For example, members of the cat family have an almost exclusively meat-based diet, and as a result have a substantially different protein and amino acid metabolism than other animals. Frugivores (fruit eaters) generally have a dietary requirement for vitamin C (e.g. fruit-eating bat). They have lost the ability to synthesize vitamin C because it is normally present in adequate amounts in their diets. Some animals are **specialist feeders**, and have coevolved with particular plant species. Koalas and several other Australian arboreal folivores have evolved dietary preferences for eucalyptus foliage. It is difficult to raise koalas on any other diet except eucalyptus leaves, making their exhibition in zoos a challenge (although synthetic diets containing eucalyptus oil have been used successfully). Giant pandas are specialist feeders, consuming mainly bamboo foliage (the panda is a vegetarian carnivore; it is a member of the order Carnivora and has the dentition and digestive tract of a true carnivore but is vegetarian by feeding strategy). Other animals are very cosmopolitan in their dietary habits, such as pigs and other omnivorous species, and consume a very wide variety of foods.

Digestive tract physiology has a profound effect on nutrient digestion and metabolism. Differences in digestive strategies will be discussed in some detail here, and will also be considered when digestion and metabolism of specific nutrient categories are discussed. A classification of animals based on digestive physiology is given in Table 2.2, while Table 2.3 provides a classification combining both feeding strategy and digestive tract physiology. These categories will be described and discussed.

Autoenzymatic Digesters

Autoenzymatic digestion refers to digestive processes carried out by enzymes that the animal secretes into the digestive tract (auto = self), in contrast to **alloenzymatic digestion** (allo = other), in which digestion is accomplished in large part by enzymes produced by microbes inhabiting the gut. These terms have been introduced by Langer (1986). Animal scientists have traditionally referred to autoenzymatic digesters as **monogastrics** or non-ruminants. These terms are unsatisfactory in some respects. All animals are monogastric (i.e. have one gastric stomach). Many animals such as the ruminants have a complex, compartmentalized stomach, but technically speaking, they are monogastric. Thus, the term monogastric animal is physiologically incorrect when used to differentiate pigs from cows, for example. The term **non-ruminant** carries negative overtones, in that it connotes that ruminants are somehow superior to other animals. Despite this, the term non-ruminant will sometimes be used in this book (to differentiate types of foregut fermenters, for example), for want of a better term.

The general features and functions of the digestive tract of the autoenzymatic digesters will be described. Mammalian species of this type, such as humans, pigs, dogs, cats, rats, mink and so on, have a pouch-like, non-compartmentalized stomach. The general features of their digestive tract are shown in Fig. 2.1. Food is consumed, chewed and

Table 2.1. Classification of animals by feeding strategy.

Feeding strategy	Examples
Carnivores (meat eaters)	Cats, sharks
Omnivores (mixed, opportunistic feeders)	Dogs, humans, pigs, chickens
Insectivores (insect eaters)	Bats, swallows, anteaters
Granivores (seed and nut eaters)	Sparrows, quail
Frugivores (fruit eaters)	New World monkeys, fruit bats
Herbivores (forage, foliage eaters)	
A. Arboreal folivores (tree-dwelling tree-leaf eaters)	Primates (New World monkeys), hoatzin, marsupials (koala)
B. Terrestrial folivores	Rock wallaby
C. Terrestrial herbivores	
i. Bulk and roughage eaters (grazers)	Ruminants (cattle) and non-ruminants (horse, hippopotamus, kangaroo)
ii. Concentrate selectors (browsers)	Ruminants (deer, giraffes) and non-ruminants (rabbits)
iii. Intermediate feeders	Ruminants (sheep, goats)
D. Aquatic	Manatee
E. Avian graminivores (birds that eat the blades and rhizomes of grasses)	Geese

Table 2.2. Classification of animals by digestive tract physiology.

Digestive tract physiology	Examples
Autoenzymatic digesters	
A. Mammalian species	Pigs, human
B. Avian species	Chicken
Alloenzymatic digesters	
A. Foregut fermenters	
i. Ruminants	Sheep, cattle, deer
ii. Non-ruminants	Hyrax, peccary, hippopotamus, kangaroo
B. Hindgut fermenters	
i. Caecal fermenters	
Mammalian species	Rabbit
Avian species	Ostrich
ii. Colonic fermenters	Horse
iii. Caeco-colonic fermenters	Elephant, manatee

swallowed, moving down the oesophagus into the stomach. Functions of the stomach include digestion and absorption, food storage and mixing, and secretion. The stomach of most autoenzymatic digesters consists of four functionally distinct zones (Fig. 2.2). The **oesophageal region** is basically an extension of the oesophagus. There are no glandular secretions in this region; there is some limited bacterial growth. The **cardiac region**, adjacent to the oesophageal region, contains glands which exude mucus. The mucus, consisting of glycoproteins, has an alkaline reaction and serves to protect the stomach lining from being digested by the proteolytic enzymes and strong acid secreted into the stomach. The **fundus gland** and **pyloric regions** are the sites of other gastric secretions, including mucus, HCl and pepsin, a proteolytic enzyme. The HCl is not secreted preformed, but as hydrogen (H^+) (derived from carbonic acid) and chloride (Cl^-) ions which are secreted separately, forming HCl at the membrane surface of the secretory glands. The concentration of H^+ ions in the stomach acid is about a million times greater than that of the blood. The energy required to secrete H^+ ions across such a huge concentration gradient is derived from ATP. The **HCl secretion** is responsible for the low pH of the stomach, which varies from pH 1 to 3, depending upon the animal species.

Table 2.3. Classification of animals by feeding strategy and digestive tract physiology.

Digestive tract physiology	Feeding strategy	Examples
Autoenzymatic digesters	A. Simple non-ruminants (mammalian species)	
	i. Carnivores	Cats, mink
	ii. Omnivores	Pigs, humans
	iii. Herbivores	Giant panda
	iv. Granivores (seed and nut eaters)	Harvest mice
	v. Frugivores	Fruit-eating bats
	vi. Insectivores	Insectivorous bats
	B. Simple non-ruminants (avian species)	
	i. Carnivores (raptors)	Hawks, owls
	ii. Omnivores	Chickens
	iii. Herbivores	Geese, emu
	iv. Granivores (seed-eating birds)	Sparrow
	v. Frugivores (fruit-eating birds)	Toucans
	vi. Insectivores (insect-eating birds)	Swallow
Alloenzymatic digesters	A. Foregut fermenters	
	i. Ruminants	
	a. Bulk and roughage eaters (grazers)	
	Fresh grass grazers	Cattle, buffalo
	Roughage grazers	Hartebeest, topi
	Dry region grazers	Camel, oryx
	b. Concentrate selectors (browsers)	Deer, giraffe
	c. Intermediate (mixed feeders)	Sheep, goats
	ii. Non-ruminants	
	a. Carnivores	Probably none
	b. Omnivores	Peccary
	c. Herbivores	Hyrax, hippopotamus, kangaroo
	B. Hindgut fermenters	
	i. Caecal fermenters	Rabbit, guinea pig, ostrich
	ii. Colon fermenters	Horse, donkey, zebra
	iii. Caeco-colon fermenters	Elephant

The high acidity sterilizes the stomach contents, killing virtually all bacteria consumed by way of the diet. The low pH also has some digestive functions, causing some hydrolysis of proteins and polysaccharides, and denaturation of proteins, exposing the bonds of the amino acid polymer to further enzymatic digestion in the stomach and small intestine. It also activates the proenzyme pepsinogen, secreted by the gastric glands, forming the active proteolytic enzyme **pepsin**. Ingesta exit the stomach from the pyloric region, entering the duodenum of the small intestine. Release of food from the stomach is controlled by the pyloric sphincter; it is regulated hormonally so as not to overload the digestive capacities of the small intestine.

Gastric secretions are controlled by gastrointestinal-tract hormones, with the process initiated by the nervous system. A large number of gastrointestinal-tract hormones have been discovered. Perception of food by visual or taste senses causes stimulation of the vagus nerve, resulting in the release of the hormone gastrin from specialized secretory cells in the cardiac region. **Gastrin** is actually a family of polypeptides (big gastrin, little gastrin and mini-gastrin contain 34, 17 and 14 amino acids, respectively). Gastrin acts by regulating histamine production in gastric mucosal cells. Histamine in turn attaches to membrane receptors on the oxyntic cells of the gastric glands, activating cAMP. The cAMP activates carbonic anhydrase, producing H^+ ions, and ATPase, causing secretion of Cl^- in exchange for potassium (K^+) ions. Gastrin secretion is also regulated by the intestine. Gastric inhibitory polypeptides (GIP) secreted from the small intestine mucosa initiate neural responses to inhibit gastrin secretion.

Young animals (e.g. piglets) do not secrete pepsinogen, but rather secrete chymosin (**rennin**) which

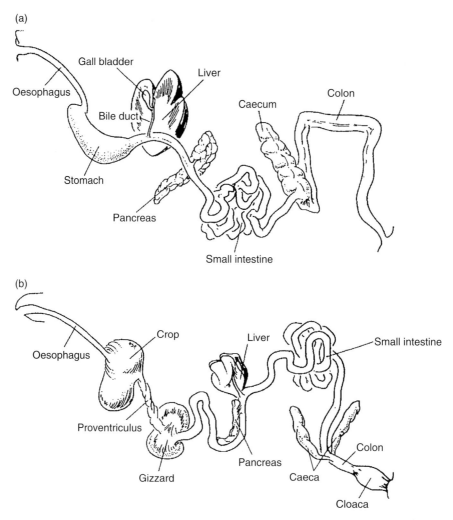

(a)

Gall bladder

Liver

Oesophagus

Caecum

Colon

Bile duct

Stomach

Pancreas

Small intestine

(b)

Crop

Liver

Small intestine

Oesophagus

Proventriculus

Colon

Pancreas

Gizzard

Caeca

Cloaca

Fig. 2.1. The general features of the simple non-ruminant digestive tract. Note the simple, non-compartmentalized stomach and the differences in the foregut of (a) the mammalian type (pigs) and (b) avian species (chicken).

clots milk. Formation of a milk clot is necessary to keep the immature small intestine from being overloaded. The HCl secretion is lower in the young animal; as a result, the stomach pH is higher (pH 3–5), allowing colonization of the intestine with bacteria. **Acidifiers** (organic acids such as citric and fumaric acids) are sometimes used in diets for baby pigs, in an effort to avoid colonization of the gut with pathogens. Besides lowering gut acidity, organic acids can disrupt the internal physiology of pH-sensitive bacteria. Non-dissociated (non-ionized) organic acids can penetrate the bacterial cell wall and dissociate inside the bacterial cell. The H^+ ion lowers the cell's internal pH, while the organic anion

accumulates and disrupts metabolic functions leading to an increase in osmotic pressure and cell death (Presser *et al.*, 1997). The pH-sensitive bacteria include such well-known pathogens as *Escherichia coli*, *Salmonella* spp., *Clostridium perfringens*, *Listeria monocytogenes* and *Campylobacter* spp.

Stomach motility is necessary for mixing gastric juice with the ingested feed and for moving the digesta into the small intestine. In spite of these stomach movements, there are differences between regions of the stomach and mixing of the food is not complete. If meals of different coloured food are given at intervals, distinct layers of different colours exist for several hours. Acidity is highest in

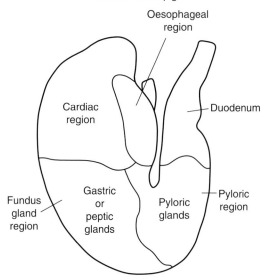

Stomach of the pig

Fig. 2.2. The regions of the pig stomach (courtesy of E.T. Moran, Jr, Auburn University, Auburn, Alabama, USA).

the pyloric region, while in the oesophageal region there is little gastric acid, allowing microbial survival and growth in this area. Stomach motility is largely controlled by events in the small intestine which regulate gastric emptying according to the capacity of the intestine to receive ingesta. This regulation appears to be largely accomplished by osmotic pressure; osmotic control of gastric emptying coordinates entry of material into the intestine with intestinal absorptive capacity. The presence of unabsorbed lipid in the intestine also influences stomach emptying, mediated through the hormone **cholecystokinin**. If the rate of stomach emptying were not reduced when high amounts of fat are fed, much of the fat would pass through the intestine unabsorbed, decreasing digestive efficiency.

Pigs are susceptible to the development of **ulcers** in the oesophageal region of the stomach. Ulcer development seems to be a consequence of carbohydrate fermentation by bacteria in the oesophageal region, producing acids that have a corrosive effect. This problem is most acute in pigs fed high-energy, low-fibre diets with a high fermentation capacity. It can be controlled by reducing the dietary energy density by increasing the fibre content with oat hulls or other fibre sources. Gastric ulcers are also a problem in horses. Hay (roughage) diets have a protective effect, in part because chewing stimulates

salivary secretion, which neutralizes stomach acid. Lucerne hay has a high buffering capacity and may decrease the risk of ulcers. Horses continuously secrete stomach acid; in grazing horses, the stomach contents are always partially filled and buffered with fibrous feeds. Stabled animals fed high carbohydrate (grain) diets twice a day often have empty stomachs, and are susceptible to tissue damage caused by the continuously-secreted acid.

Stomach ulcers are common in humans. A peptic ulcer is a sore or lesion on the lining of the stomach or duodenum. Most cases of peptic ulcers are caused by a bacterial infection, specifically by *Helicobacter pylori*. *H. pylori* weakens the mucous coating of the stomach, allowing invasion by other bacteria. *H. pylori* is able to survive in the highly acid stomach because it secretes urease, which converts urea (which is normally secreted into the stomach) into carbon dioxide and ammonia. Ammonia is alkaline, and neutralizes the stomach acid in the immediate environment of the bacterial cell. Although *H. pylori* was first recognized in 1875, its role as a cause of ulcers was not appreciated until Australian researchers Warren and Marshall isolated the organism from human gastric mucous (Marshall and Warren, 1984). To convince the medical community that *H. pylori* is the cause of ulcers, Marshall consumed a dose of the organism, developed gastritis, and recovered the bacteria from his stomach lining. In 2005, Warren and Marshall were awarded the Nobel Prize in medicine for their work on *H. pylori*.

Digestion is the preparation of ingested nutrients for absorption. Normally, only small molecules are absorbed. Thus proteins are hydrolysed into small units (peptides and amino acids), complex carbohydrates into simple sugars (monosaccharides) and fats into monoacylglycerides and fatty acids. (Hydrolysis is the cleavage of a chemical bond accompanied by the splitting off of water.) Minerals and vitamins generally do not undergo digestion, and are absorbed as such. In some cases (e.g. niacin), vitamins exist in plants in a bound form that must be degraded to facilitate absorption. Minerals may be complexed as phytates, which may undergo digestion to release the bound minerals. In newborn animals of many species, large intact protein molecules are absorbed, permitting the absorption of antibodies from colostrum (passive immunization). After a period of time, from several hours to several days (depending upon species), the intestinal mucosa is altered (closure) to prevent absorption of large molecules. For example, **closure** occurs at 1 day of age in the guinea pig, around 5 days of age for the hamster, and at 23 days of age for the rabbit (Lecce and Broughton, 1973). The fetal enterocytes are capable of engulfing (pinocytosis) large molecules such as immunoglobulins. Enterocytes formed post-natally are unable to take up large molecules by pinocytosis. Thus as the fetal enterocytes are replaced, the ability to absorb large molecules is lost (Rooke and Bland, 2002).

The major site of digestion and absorption in autoenzymatic digester animals is the small intestine. It is comprised of three distinct regions: the duodenum, jejunum and ileum. The **duodenum** is attached by mesentary tissue to the wall of the abdominal cavity, whereas the remainder of the intestine is freely moveable. To fit into the small volume of the body cavity, the small intestine is highly coiled. **Immune function** is another very important characteristic of the intestine that is not related to the digestive or absorptive functions. The mucosal membranes of the gut are the largest interface of an animal with its environment, and are the major sites of entry of foreign antigens. The gut has the body's major immunologic defences, the **gut-associated lymphoid tissue (GALT)**, including the Peyer's patches and the Bursa of Fabricius in chickens (see Chapter 24).

Both digestive and absorptive functions of the intestine are facilitated by a large surface area. In larger mammals, the first order of surface area enhancement is the presence of circular folds in the duodenum, increasing the surface area by a factor of about three. Small mammals lack these folds. In all animals the main increase in surface area is achieved by small projections called **villi** lining the intestinal mucosa and giving it a velvety appearance. The villi are very dynamic structures. Each villus (Fig. 2.3) is lined with a single layer of cells called **enterocytes** which are continually formed in generative areas called the crypts of Lieberkuhn at the base of the villus. The enterocytes are immature when formed in the **crypts**, and mature as they move up the villus, acquiring full complements of digestive enzymes. As they reach the tip of the villus, they have become 'worn out' by physical and chemical attrition, and are extruded into the intestinal lumen. It is estimated that about 17 billion cells/day are lost in this way in the human intestine (Moog, 1981). These sloughed off cells constitute a large part of the **metabolic faecal nitrogen** or

endogenous nitrogen, often referred to as resulting from 'wear and tear'. Diets high in fibre, having an abrasive effect, tend to increase the loss of enterocytes.

Each villus contains an arteriole, venule and lacteal, providing access to the circulatory and lymph systems. Absorption of nutrients takes place across the surface of the villi, with the nutrients entering the circulatory system, or lymph in the case of lipids. Besides the enterocytes, the villi have **goblet cells** which produce and secrete mucus. Mucus protects the intestinal lining and provides lubrication to facilitate movement of digesta through the gut.

The surface area of the villi is greatly enhanced by minute projections called **microvilli** (Fig. 2.3). The microvilli in turn have filamentous fuzzy projections called the **glycocalyx**. These filamentous appendages, rich in carbohydrate (as a component of glycoproteins), function in trapping nutrients for completion of digestion. Digestion in the intestine begins in the intestinal lumen with the action of pancreatic enzymes which break large molecules (proteins, polysaccharides) into smaller molecules (polypeptides, oligosaccharides). These smaller molecules become trapped in the glycocalyx, which contains the enzymes that complete the digestive process. The enzymes protrude out from the microvilli, and in the process of their action, the end products (amino acids, sugars) are released into the microvilli and ultimately transported to the circulatory system in the villi. Thus considerable digestion takes place within the microstructure of the **brush border** (microvilli plus glycocalyx). The brush border is also known as the **unstirred water layer**. This designation derives from the resemblance of the intestine to a water pipe. Water in a pipe moves at different speeds depending on where it is. It moves fastest in the centre of the pipe (the lumen of the intestine) and slowest against the wall of the pipe (the intestinal mucosa) because of friction or drag.

As alluded to above, the **pancreas gland** secretes enzymes into the duodenum, initiating digestive processes. Pancreatic enzymes such as trypsin function in hydrolysing large molecules into smaller molecules, which are then subjected to further breakdown in the brush border. Pancreatic enzymes are important in the digestion of proteins, carbohydrates and lipids, with enzymes such as trypsin, amylase and lipase involved.

The **liver** is closely associated with digestive processes. Blood from the gastrointestinal tract goes first to the liver, before entering the general

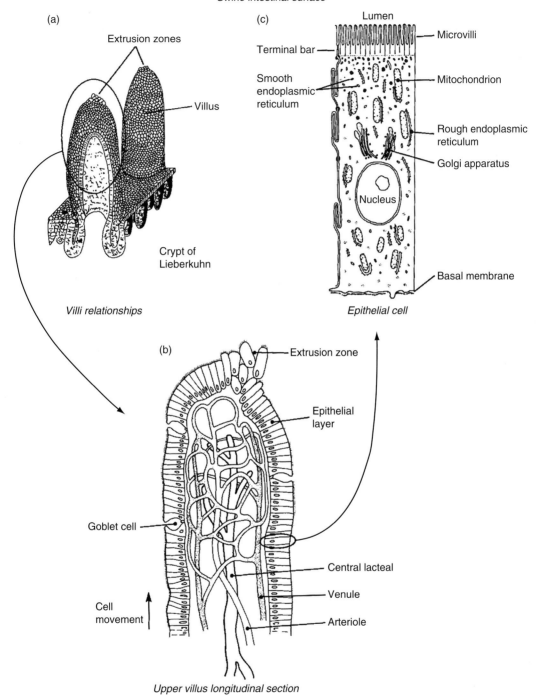

Fig. 2.3. Intestinal villi of pigs. The illustration shows a three-dimensional appearance (a), a longitudinal section of a villus with enterocytes (epithelial cells) (b), and an expanded view of an enterocyte (c). The glycocalyx is not illustrated; it is a filamentous web connected to the microvilli (courtesy of E.T. Moran, Jr, Auburn University, Auburn, Alabama, USA).

circulation. Many nutrients are removed from the blood by the liver and modified before being released to the general circulation. Numerous toxins such as ammonia are taken up by the liver before they can reach the other tissues. The liver produces bile which is secreted through the bile duct into the intestine. Bile contains bile salts which have an essential function in lipid digestion.

Motility of the intestine is important in mixing the contents and in propelling them down the tract. **Segmentation** is a process that mixes material by dividing the food mass into several pieces by constrictions, and then churning it up by a series of contractions. **Peristalsis** is the process of muscular contractions by which the contents are moved along the intestine by a moving ring of contraction, pushing material ahead of it. **Antiperistalsis** occurs when the material is moved 'backwards' or in a retrograde manner; this occurs primarily in the hindgut as a means of moving material from the colon into the caecum. This action is important in small herbivores such as the rabbit, as discussed in Chapter 3. In chickens, antiperistalsis occurs in the colon; digesta mixed with urine from the cloaca refluxes small particles (fines) and fluids into the caeca (Moran, 2006).

In typical autoenzymatic digesters, the bulk of digestion and absorption takes place in the small intestine, with the **jejunum** the principal area of absorption. Digesta pass from the ileum into the hindgut, consisting of the caecum and colon (large intestine). In autoenzymatic digesters, the caecum is relatively small. The main digestive functions of the hindgut are the absorption of water and electrolytes. As a result, the faeces are normally quite dry in comparison to the intestinal contents. The hindgut is also an area of anaerobic microbial growth, which is of some nutritional importance in autoenzymatic digesters, and of much greater importance in animals with hindgut fermentation.

Avian (bird) species with autoenzymatic digestion have some modifications from the mammalian digestive system. The stomach is divided into two compartments, the **proventriculus** (gastric stomach) and the **gizzard** (ventriculus). In addition, between the beak and proventriculus is a diverticulum of the oesophagus called the **crop**. In domestic avian species, the crop functions mainly as a food storage area, although some microbial digestion may occur here. Mucus glands in the upper oesophagus secrete mucus, which aids in the movement of ingested feed to the crop, where further moistening with consumed water occurs. In some birds, such as pigeons, doves, parrots, penguins, flamingos and pelicans, the crop produces 'milk' which is regurgitated into the crops of the young. The milk consists largely of lipid-rich epithelial cells plus ingested feed. The production of crop milk is stimulated by the hormone prolactin.

The proventriculus elaborates HCl and pepsinogen in much the same manner as the mammalian stomach. The ingesta then move to the **gizzard**, where grinding of the material occurs. There is some refluxing of ingesta from the gizzard back to the proventriculus. The gizzard performs the functions of mammalian teeth in grinding ingested material into small particles. It is a thick-walled, highly muscular organ with an extremely tough lining. The lining contains 'gizzard teeth' which are rods of a hard protein–polysaccharide complex somewhat akin to keratin in feathers (Fig. 2.4). Grinding is accomplished by coordinated contractions of the gizzard musculature, and is facilitated by grit (small particles of rock). **Grit** is unnecessary for poultry when commercial diets of ground ingredients are used, but is required when birds are fed whole grains, and by plant- or seed-eating wild birds. Carnivorous birds do not require grit. Grit feeding may also improve the utilization of high fibre diets. Pathology of the gizzard sometimes occurs such as with gizzard erosion caused by high dietary copper concentrations and gizzard degeneration in vitamin E-selenium deficiency. A toxic dipeptide in fish meal, called gizzerozine, causes gizzard myopathy (Masumura *et al.*, 1985).

Although birds do not have true teeth (scarce as hen's teeth), their early reptilian ancestors had teeth; avian teeth were lost 70–80 million years ago. A mutant chicken has been identified with rudimentary embryonic teeth (Harris *et al.*, 2006). These authors postulate that while birds lost teeth, they retained tooth development potential. The presence of embryonic teeth in birds is actually not a new finding. In his famous book, *On the Origin of Species*, Charles Darwin (1859) observed, 'It has been stated on good authority that rudiments of teeth can be detected in the beaks of certain embryonic birds.'

Digestive processes in the small intestine of the fowl are similar to those in mammals. The hindgut, however, is quite different. The colon is very short, and birds have two long caeca (Fig. 2.1).

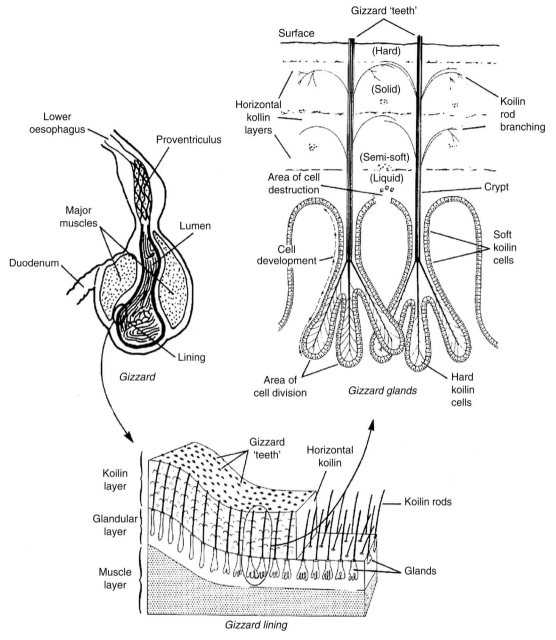

Fig. 2.4. Structure of the avian gizzard, showing the 'gizzard teeth' (courtesy of E.T. Moran, Jr, Auburn University, Auburn, Alabama, USA).

The colon has very little digestive activity. Some fermentation in the caeca occurs; reverse peristaltic contractions move fluids and fine particles from the colon into the caecum. Some bacterial vitamin synthesis occurs, which is of nutritional benefit to birds that have access to their excreta and consume them (coprophagy). The caeca may also serve as the site for several functions, including digestion of small food particles, nutrient absorption, production of immunoglobulins and antibodies, microbial action, absorption of water and conversion of uric acid into amino acids (Clench, 1999). In chickens, the main significance of the caeca is that they are a site of infection with coccidia, the protozoa that cause **coccidiosis**. This disorder is characterized by damage to the caecal lining, bleeding of the mucosa, and often death. In birds, the gastrointestinal tract terminates in the **cloaca**, into which the urine is also excreted, so that faeces and urine are voided together in all avian species except the ostrich, which excretes faeces and urine separately (Duke, 1999). Some 'back flow' of urine into the hindgut may occur by antiperistaltic contractions which can lead to enhanced conservation of nutrients (Moran, 2006). For example, on low protein diets urinary nitrogen is conserved and recycled by this mechanism (Karasawa, 1999).

The intestinal tract of **terrestrial carnivores** such as mink is generally shorter than for omnivores and herbivores. In contrast, carnivorous marine mammals (dolphins, seals) tend to have comparatively large alimentary tracts (Williams *et al.*, 2001). **Marine carnivores** have high metabolic rates, and the exceptional lengths of their small intestines is probably a consequence of their high energy demands.

For a detailed consideration and comparison of the digestive tracts of pigs and poultry, Moran (1982) should be consulted. For poultry and other avian species, Klasing (1998) is recommended. Duke (1997) provided an excellent review of gastrointestinal physiology and nutrition in wild birds.

Questions and Study Guide

1. Give two examples of specialist feeders.
2. Why is the giant panda referred to as a vegetarian carnivore?
3. How does autoenzymatic digestion differ from alloenzymatic digestion?
4. It can be said that all animals are monogastrics. Why?
5. The gastric stomach secretes hydrochloric acid. How does this acid function in digestive processes?
6. What causes stomach ulcers in (a) humans and (b) pigs?
7. What is the difference between digestion and absorption? Do vitamins and minerals require digestion?
8. What is the difference between villi and microvilli?
9. What is the function of goblet cells?
10. How does the glycocalyx function?
11. What is the unstirred water layer?
12. Compare peristalsis and antiperistalsis.
13. How does the digestive tract of birds (e.g. chickens) differ from that of mammalian autoenzymatic digesters (e.g. pigs)?
14. Do birds have teeth? If not, how do they 'chew' food?

References

Clench, M.H. (1999) The avian cecum: update and motility review. *Journal of Experimental Zoology* 283, 441–447.

Darwin, C. (1859) *On the Origin of Species by Natural Selection, or the Preservation of Favoured Races in the Struggle for Life*. John Murray, London.

Duke, G.E. (1997) Gastrointestinal physiology and nutrition in wild birds. *Proceedings of the Nutrition Society* 86, 1049–1056.

Duke, G.E. (1999) Mechanisms of excreta formation and elimination in turkeys and ostriches. *Journal of Experimental Zoology* 283, 478–479.

Harris, M.P., Hasso, S.M., Ferguson, M.W.J. and Fallon, J.F. (2006) The development of Archosaurian first-generation teeth in a chicken mutant. *Current Biology* 16, 371–377.

Karasawa, Y. (1999) Significant role of the nitrogen recycling system through the ceca occurs in protein-depleted chickens. *Journal of Experimental Zoology* 283, 418–425.

Klasing, K. (1998) *Comparative Avian Nutrition*. CAB International, Wallingford, Oxon, UK.

Langer, P. (1986) Large mammalian herbivores in tropical forests with either hindgut- or forestomach-fermentation. *Zeitschrift fur Saugetierkunde* 51, 173–187.

Lecce, J.G. and Broughton, C.W. (1973) Cessation of uptake of macromolecules by neonatal guinea pig, hamster and rabbit intestinal epithelium (closure) and transport into blood. *Journal of Nutrition* 103, 744–750.

Marshall, B.J. and Warren, J.R. (1984) Unidentified curved bacilli in the stomach of patients with gastritis and peptic ulceration. *Lancet* 1(8390), 1311–1315.

Masumura, T., Sugahara, M., Noguchi, T., Mori, K. and Naito, H. (1985) The effect of gizzerosine, a recently discovered compound in overheated fish meal, on the gastric acid secretion in the chicken. *Poultry Science* 64, 356–361.

Moog, F. (1981) The lining of the small intestine. *Scientific American* 245, 154–176.

Moran, E., Jr (1982) *Comparative Nutrition of Fowl and Swine. The Gastrointestinal Systems*. University of Guelph, Guelph, Canada.

Moran, E.T., Jr (2006) Anatomy, microbes, and fiber: small versus large intestine. *Journal of Applied Poultry Research* 15, 154–160.

Presser, K.A., Ratkowsky, D.A. and Ross, T. (1997) Modelling the growth rate of *Escherichia coli* as a function of pH and lactic acid concentration. *Applied Environmental Microbiology* 63, 2355–2360.

Rooke, J.A. and Bland, I.M. (2002) The acquisition of passive immunity in the new-born piglet. *Livestock Production Science* 78, 13–23.

Williams, T.M., Haun, J., Davis, R.W., Fuiman, L.A. and Kohin, S. (2001) A killer appetite: metabolic consequences of carnivory in marine mammals. *Comparative Biochemistry and Physiology Part A* 129, 785–796.

3 Digestive Physiology: Alloenzymatic Digesters

Alloenzymatic digesters are those animals in which digestion is accomplished in part by enzymes produced by microbes inhabiting the gut. The site of microbial activity may be the foregut (e.g. ruminants) or the hindgut (e.g. horses and other non-ruminant herbivores).

Foregut Fermenters

Ruminants

The foregut has probably achieved its highest complexity in anatomy and function in the ruminant animals. Ruminants have a complex, compartmentalized stomach, characterized by one large compartment, the rumen, in which microbial fermentation of ingested feed occurs in an anaerobic environment (fermentation is defined as anaerobic respiration). Ruminants are classified in the order Artiodactyla, suborder Ruminantia. They are even-toed, hooved animals. The term ruminant is derived from *ruminare*, a Latin word meaning to chew again. Thus ruminants are animals which ruminate or 'chew their cud' by regurgitation of ingested material (**rumination**).

According to Simpson (1945) there are 86 living and 333 extinct genera of the order Artiodactyla, with 68 living and 180 extinct genera of ruminants. Only a few primitive species survive. Ruminants range in size from the tiny (1 kg) lesser mouse deer to the 1000 kg giraffe (Kay *et al.*, 1980). An abbreviated classification of ruminants is provided in Table 3.1.

General features of the ruminant stomach are shown in Fig. 3.1. The four compartments are the rumen, reticulum, omasum and abomasum. In the adult, and young animal with a functioning **rumen**, the rumen is the largest compartment. It functions as a fermentation vat. Rumen microbes, primarily many species of anaerobic bacteria, and to a lesser extent protozoa, secrete enzymes which digest the consumed feed. Because the rumen is an anaerobic environment, microbial fermentation cannot result in complete oxidation of carbohydrates to carbon dioxide and water. Anaerobic fermentation is basically the glycolysis pathway (see Chapter 9) by which glucose is broken down into pyruvic acid. In the rumen, the microbes convert pyruvic acid to several short-chain organic acids called **volatile fatty acids** (**VFAs**). They were originally called steam-volatile fatty acids (and still are in some countries) because they can be distilled from rumen fluid by the passage of steam. The VFAs are the main end product of rumen fermentation, and are the primary absorbed energy sources of ruminants. Of major significance is the production of the enzyme cellulase by rumen microbes, permitting the digestion of fibrous feeds containing cellulose. Rumen fermentation and VFA production are discussed in more detail in Chapter 8. Other benefits of rumen fermentation include the synthesis of amino acids and water-soluble vitamins by rumen bacteria. As a result, ruminants are largely independent of dietary sources of amino acids and water-soluble vitamins. The rumen is lined with projections called **papillae** (Fig. 3.2). The VFAs are absorbed into the papillae, in a similar manner as the absorption of nutrients into the villi of the small intestine.

The rumen is continuous with the **reticulum**; they are often considered together as the reticulorumen. The reticulum is lined with honeycomb-shaped projections (Fig. 3.3). One of the functions of the reticulum is the trapping of foreign material such as stones, nails, wire and so on, to prevent puncturing of the digestive tract (hardware disease). This is especially important in cattle, which by their indiscriminate grazing behaviour frequently consume foreign objects.

Material exits the reticulorumen via the **omasum**. The omasum is a small compartment containing membranous divisions called omasal leaves (*omasum* is Latin for book). The omasal leaves

Table 3.1. Classification of ruminants.

Suborder	Family	Examples
Tylopoda	Camelidae	Camelid species – alpaca, llama, vicuna, camel
Ruminantia	Tragulidae	Most primitive living ruminants – chevrotain, mouse deer
	Giraffidae	Giraffe, okapi
	Antilocapridae	Pronghorn
	Cervidae	Deer (caribou, deer, elk, moose)
	Bovidae	Hollow-horned animals – antelope, bison, buffalo, cattle, gazelle, eland, goat, sheep, yak

function as a sieve, retaining material in the rumen until it has been degraded into small particle sizes. Fluids and small particles flow through the omasum to the **abomasum**, or true gastric stomach. The abomasum contains large spiral folds in the fundus gland region. Gastric secretions, such as pepsinogen and HCl, are secreted in the abomasum. The acidity kills rumen microbes in the digesta; they are then subject to digestion in the small intestine.

There has been a tendency to regard all ruminant animals as being very similar in digestive physiology and rumen metabolism. This belief may be a fallacy, as pointed out by Hofmann (1973) in a classic treatise on the stomach structure and feeding habits of East African wild ruminants. Hofmann considered both feeding strategy and stomach anatomy as important determinants of nutritional requirements and digestive capabilities, and classified ruminants into three groups based on feeding strategy: (i) concentrate selectors; (ii) bulk and roughage feeders; and (iii) intermediate feeders. In general, concentrate selectors are small animals,

while roughage feeders are large. Small animals have a high metabolic rate, and thus must consume a readily digested diet or be capable of a high feed intake and fast rate of passage. Large animals, with a lower metabolic rate per unit of body size, can survive on bulky feeds that are retained for a

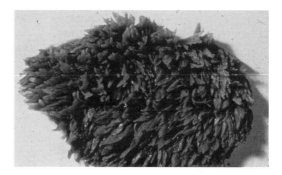

Fig. 3.2. The papillae are projections of the rumen wall that function in absorption of nutrients from the rumen.

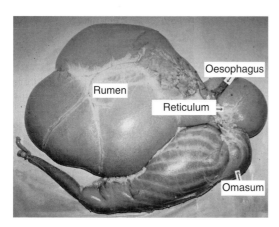

Fig. 3.1. A dried preparation of a ruminant stomach that shows the locations of each of the compartments.

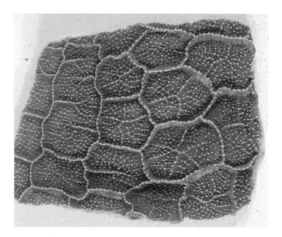

Fig. 3.3. The reticulum lining has a honeycomb appearance.

prolonged period to allow for microbial digestion of fibre.

Hofmann's ruminant classification system

Concentrate selectors (browsers)

Concentrate selectors consume the less lignified (more soluble fibre) parts of herbage, including tree and shrub leaves, herbs, fruit and other soft, succulent plant parts. This herbage, with a high concentration of cell contents and a low cell-wall content, is more readily digested than diets with similar total fibre but with more lignified and less soluble fibre. A considerable portion of the material, such as starches and sugars, does not require fermentation but can be digested by the animal itself. Although many concentrate selectors are small animals, such as the dik-dik and duiker, others such as deer, moose and giraffes are large. They tend to nibble on a wide variety of plants and plant parts, rather than feeding intensively on one type of vegetation. The larger concentrate selectors, such as deer and giraffes, consume the leaves and succulent foliage of trees, utilizing an ecological niche unavailable to grazing ruminants.

Concentrate selectors have a stomach anatomy adapted to the use of low fibre forage. They have a relatively small rumen and reticulum, so cannot consume a large quantity of feed at one time. The architecture of the rumen of concentrate selectors is simple, lacking the highly developed sacculations and muscular pillars seen in the roughage eaters. The rumen papillae are elongated and highly developed, facilitating absorption of the high concentration of fermentation end products produced from their high quality diet. Rumination is less important than in the roughage eaters. The omasum is small and its leaves are less well developed than in the grazers. The omasum can readily become impacted with coarse fibrous material. Thus, concentrate selectors are intolerant of a high fibre diet. Winter feeding of deer with lucerne hay often results in mass mortalities from rumen and omasal impaction. The feeding of captive ruminants in zoos requires knowledge of their feeding strategy; feeding a high fibre diet or the wrong type of diet to concentrate selectors sometimes results in mortality from impaction (more often, however, these animals develop acidosis from too much concentrate and too little fibre). Thus, the concentrate selectors have a digestive system attuned to their

feeding behaviour, maximizing the efficiency of utilization of low-fibre plant material.

Very small ruminants include a number of Asian and African forest dwellers of 1–3 kg body weight, such as duikers and mouse deer. They feed mainly on fruits and succulent leaves. In what Van Soest (1996) refers to as 'the naive purpose of evaluating forages more cheaply', Cowan (1986, cited by Shipley and Felicetti, 2002; Dehority and Varga, 1991) at Pennsylvania State University attempted to establish a colony of blue duikers to use as a 'ruminant laboratory rat' for evaluating forages. The attempt failed because of high mortality from impaction due to the inability of 'concentrate selector' browsers to digest coarse forage.

The giraffe and moose are the two largest concentrate-selector ruminants. They are difficult to exhibit in zoos because of health problems of nutritional origin. Clauss *et al.* (2002) summed it up succinctly: 'Moose are notoriously difficult to keep in captivity.' Wasting disease is a common problem in captive giraffe (Kearney, 2005). Problems include high neonatal mortality, wasting syndrome, rumen hypomotility syndrome, bloat and rumenitis. Moose wasting syndrome is a major cause of death in captive moose. They are rarely exhibited in zoos because of premature mortality. These problems are related to the difficulty of providing concentrate-selector ruminants diets similar to their natural ones of non-grass forage. Clauss *et al.* (2003c) suggest, 'Attention within the zoo community should focus on providing browsers with a fibre source that corresponds to the physical characteristics of their natural forage'.

In zoo environments, grazing ruminants have a lower incidence of gastrointestinal-tract disorders in general and of lactic acidosis damage to ruminal mucosa in particular (Clauss *et al.*, 2003c). Grazers, regardless of their size, seem better adapted to the conventional zoo diet of hay. Clauss *et al.* (2003c) point out an unresolved inconsistency:

> The extremely high incidence of acidotic changes in the ruminal mucosa of browers/concentrate selectors indicates a fact of semantic irony, namely that the so-called 'concentrate selectors' seem to have digestive problems when selecting too much concentrate feeds.

The **ventricular groove** (also referred to as reticular or oesophageal groove) is a muscular tube that functions to transport liquids from the base of the oesophagus to the omasum, thus bypassing rumen fermentation. This action occurs in suckling animals, so that the digestion of milk occurs post-ruminally. Hofmann (1984) noted that in concentrate selectors, the ventricular groove may function, in conjunction with copious salivary secretion in these species, in the washing of the soluble cell contents of succulent plant material directly to the omasum, avoiding rumen fermentation of soluble sugars and galactolipids, which the animal can digest more efficiently itself. This process would allow concentrate selectors to use plant material high in cell contents with a high efficiency. A flow-through of soluble sugars to the small intestine in browsers suggests the presence of mucosal glucose transporters, which are absent in grazers (Rowell et al., 1996, cited by Clauss et al., 2003c). Hofmann (1984) summarized a number of other adaptations of concentrate selectors that aid in efficient use of forages. They have a three to fourfold greater salivary gland mass than roughage eaters, facilitating the functioning of the ventricular groove, and also buffering the high concentration of rumen VFAs and by a 'wash-through' effect, reducing ruminal retention times. The glandular tissue of the small intestine is up to 100% greater than in roughage eaters and the liver weight is larger. The hind gut is relatively larger in concentrate selectors. Thus, as Hofmann (1984) states, 'These significant structural differences in post-ruminal anatomy suggest that more unfermented food escapes from the rumen and its digestion and absorption may be more important for many ruminant species than data from cattle and sheep only suggest.'

Bulk and roughage eaters (grazers)

Roughage eaters or grazers have a feeding and digestive strategy based on the utilization of high-fibre, low-solubles diets. Their stomach facilitates maximal digestibility of fibre. The capacity of the reticulorumen is high, and their grazing behaviour permits a rapid intake of a large quantity of fibrous feed. Rumination is pronounced, resulting in physical maceration of ingested forage. The omasum is highly developed with many omasal leaves, thus retaining fibrous feed in the rumen until microbial enzymes have degraded it. The papillae are less prominent than in concentrate selectors because there is a slower production of fermentation end products requiring absorption. Examples of roughage eaters include cattle, buffalo, camels and a variety of African antelope species (eg. wildebeest, topi, waterbuck, oryx antelope). A summary of some of the major differences in stomach anatomy and function between the roughage eaters and concentrate selectors is shown in Fig. 3.4.

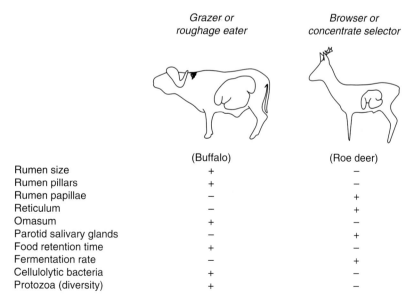

	Grazer or roughage eater (Buffalo)	Browser or concentrate selector (Roe deer)
Rumen size	+	–
Rumen pillars	+	–
Rumen papillae	–	+
Reticulum	–	+
Omasum	+	–
Parotid salivary glands	–	+
Food retention time	+	–
Fermentation rate	–	+
Cellulolytic bacteria	+	–
Protozoa (diversity)	+	–

Fig. 3.4. Some of the major differences in stomach anatomy and function between roughage eaters and concentrate selectors. +, relatively bigger or more developed; –, relatively smaller or less developed (adapted from Kay et al., 1980).

Intermediate feeders

Intermediate feeders have feeding and digestive strategies that share properties of both concentrate selectors and grazers. Thus, these animals tend to be highly adaptable to varying environments and changing habitats. Sheep and goats are domestic animals of this type; they graze on grass but also feed extensively on shrubs and forbs. Wild intermediate feeders include reindeer, elk, pronghorns, impala, gazelles and eland.

Other ruminants

The camels and other camelids (llama, alpaca, guanaco and vicuna) are considered to be ruminants, but have a substantially different stomach anatomy than other ruminants. The stomach has three compartments, roughly comparable to the rumen, reticulum and abomasum.

Summary and critiques of Hofmann's ruminant categories

While the three anatomical categories (concentrate selectors, bulk and roughage eaters, intermediate feeders) of ruminants described by Hofmann (1973, 1989) correlate well with feeding behaviour, it appears that diet selection may be more important than stomach anatomy in the nutritional ecology of ruminants (Gordon and Illius, 1994, 1996; Robbins *et al.*, 1995). Attempts to test and validate Hofmann's categories have nevertheless led to much greater understanding of ruminant evolution, behaviour, and ecology of herbivore communities (Robbins *et al.*, 1995). Ditchkoff (2000) maintains that the studies of Gordon, Illius and Robbins have failed to adequately test Hofmann's predictions. Specifically, the role of solubles bypassing the rumen via the reticular groove in concentrate selectors has not been tested under physiological conditions. Robbins *et al.* (1995) compared ruminal liquid flow rates, but only under resting (non-feeding) conditions. However, Robbins *et al.* (1995) maintain that immature browse is not equivalent to a 'concentrate' diet; thus they argue that physiological and ecological interpretations based on that premise are unfounded (Illius and Gordon, 1992). More recently, Rowell-Schafer *et al.* (2001) tested the rumen bypass potential of carbohydrates in roe deer (concentrate selectors). As metabolic evidence of incomplete fermentation in the forestomach, they reported an abundance of sodium-dependent glucose co-transporter in the duodenum, high activity of maltase, saccharase and α-amylase in duodenal and pancreatic tissue, and a high concentration of polyunsaturated fatty acids in the body fat. They concluded that these results supported Hofmann's predictions of rumen bypass in concentrate selectors. McArthur *et al.* (1991, 1993), Cork and Foley (1991) and Foley *et al.* (1995) suggested that differences in feeding behaviours by herbivores with different gut anatomy may reflect the response to toxins (secondary compounds) in plants, such as tannins. McArthur *et al.* (1991) conclude 'the various capacities of animals along a grazer to browser continuum to deal with a variety of plant secondary compounds should be examined'.

Clauss *et al.* (2003a) proposed another hypothesis as a refinement of Hofmann's classification of ruminants. Rather than focusing on the chemical characteristics of forages (grasses, browse), they proposed that the **physicomechanical characteristics** of forages are the main driving force of ruminant diversification. In contrast to browse, grass tends to be 'stringy' and stratifies to form a fibrous raft or mat in the rumen (Fig. 3.5). Stratification of rumen contents is more pronounced in grazing species than in browsers (Clauss *et al.*, 2009a, b). The greater rumen capacity of grazers, and the thicker rumen pillars (indicative of rumen musculature capacity) may be specific adaptations for a diet based on the grazing of grass. Grazers have larger, heavier chewing muscles than browsers, indicating an increased requirement to overcome the physical resistance of grass forage (Clauss and Hofmann, 2008). The small forestomach capacity and lack of strong reticulorumen muscles in browsers would explain their tendency to avoid grass forage (Clauss *et al.* prefer the term 'browsers' over Hofmann's 'concentrate selectors'). Grazers have less viscous rumen fluid than browsers, facilitating stratification and raft formation (Clauss *et al.*, 2005). The low viscosity allows particles to move in the liquid phase – either float or sink (Fig. 3.5). Ruminant species (grazers) that consume a diet high in grass have a smaller salivary gland mass than browsers, possibly indicating a smaller requirement for the production of salivary tannin-binding proteins (Hofmann *et al.*, 2008). Browsers tend to have a more proteinaceous, viscous saliva than grazers (Clauss *et al.*, 2005). A larger omasum in grazers

(a)

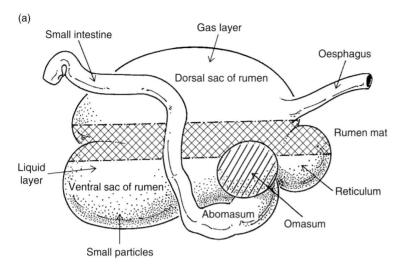

(b)

Browser

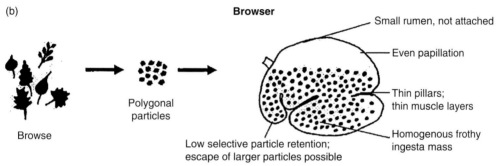

Grazer

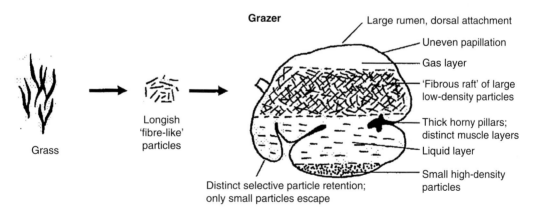

Fig. 3.5. (a) The rumen contents are stratified with a mat or raft of fibrous material floating on liquid. During rumination, a bolus is formed at the base of the oesophagus and regurgitated. As forage is digested, the particle size is reduced, and the small particles drop to the bottom of the rumen and flow through the omasum. (b) Hypothesized evolutionary adaptation of browsing and grazing ruminants to the physiomechanical characteristics of their respective forages. The structure that a forage is broken down into determines its potential behaviour in the forestomach. The tendency of grass particles to form a fibrous raft and a stratification of rumen contents is met by particular adaptations of grazing ruminants to handle, exploit and reinforce this tendency. Browsing ruminants are hypothesized to be unable to handle higher proportions of stratification-inducing forage in their forestomach (courtesy of M. Clauss, University of Zurich, Switzerland).

may function in reabsorption of water from the high outflow of fluids from the rumen. Perez-Barberia *et al.* (2004) note that ruminant feeding styles occur over a browser–grazer continuum, related to the grass:browse proportions in their natural diets. Fibre digestibility increases with increased dietary grass and decreased proportion of browse. Clauss *et al.* (2005) caution that nearly all the conclusions on the digestive physiology of large ruminant grazers are based on data with cattle, which may not be truly representative of grazers in general. Cattle retain particles in the rumen for very long retention times compared to their retention of fluids (Clauss *et al.*, 2005).

Knott *et al.* (2004) hypothesized that the digestive anatomy of neonatal ruminants should reflect the feeding strategy at adulthood. In other words, if differences in gut anatomy of intermediate feeders and grazers are innate, rather than determined by diet, the neonates should show evidence of these differences. Changes in digestive morphology of young animals should anticipate changes in diet. Knott *et al.* (2004) compared intermediate feeders (reindeer) with musk oxen (grazers). Digestive morphology of reindeer and musk oxen differed from birth, even with consumption of similar diets. Ruminal morphology of musk oxen exhibited early development of thick muscle walls and cornified epithelium that is consistent with the feeding strategy of grazers. Thick muscle walls allow better mixing of bulky, fibrous material. The larger rumen volume of musk oxen was evident from 60 days of age, and musk oxen had larger omasa than reindeer at birth. Young reindeer had specialized digestive morphology consistent with increased absorption rates that accrue from consumption of low fibre diets by intermediate feeders. For example, neonatal reindeer have greater surface area of papillae that are associated with high rates of VFA production in adults. Duodenal villi were also more complex, inferring greater post-ruminal absorption in the intermediate feeder. Abomasal parietal cells are greater in reindeer, which result in more acid production, facilitating the digestion of the higher protein levels of forbs and browse compared to grass. Thus the work of Knott *et al.* (2004) supports Hofmann's categories of intermediate feeders and grazers as innate anatomical types.

In summary, Hofmann's categories of ruminants (Fig. 3.6 and Fig. 3.7; Table 3.2) seem to be basically valid, with some controversy over details.

Digestive processes in ruminants

Digestion of the various nutrient categories will be considered in more detail later. The most fundamental aspect of alloenzymatic digestion is the fermentation process. Proteins are fermented in the rumen by microbial enzymes, and may be completely degraded to inorganic nitrogen (ammonia). Microbes synthesize the amino acids they require from ammonia and simple carbon compounds. Thus, much of the dietary protein is unavailable directly to the host animal. The ruminant derives a high proportion of its amino acids from digestion of microbes in the small intestine. Similarly, much of the ingested carbohydrate is unavailable directly to the animal. It is fermented by microbes in the rumen. Waste products of bacterial digestion, a variety of short-chain organic acids (VFAs), are the primary absorbed energy source. Thus, metabolism in ruminants is intimately associated with microbial digestion.

The rumen microbes

The rumen microbial population is responsible for much of the total digestive activity in ruminants, particularly in roughage eaters. The main microbes are bacteria and protozoa, although yeasts, fungi and phages are also found in small numbers. Rumen bacteria can be broadly considered as **starch digesters** (amylolytic) and **cellulose digesters** (cellulolytic). Examples of some of the main genera of rumen bacteria are *Bacteroides*, *Ruminococcus*, *Butyrivibrio*, *Selenomonas* and *Methanobacterium*. An example of an amylolytic organism is *Bacteroides amylophilus* while *Bacteroides succinogenes* is cellulolytic. Rumen bacteria accomplish their work of digestion primarily by attachment to feed particles, and digestion occurs at the point of attachment. Cellulase, for example, is not secreted into the rumen fluid, but rather is active at the point of attachment of cellulolytic bacteria to roughage particles. Comparative studies indicate that the rumen microbes are similar among different species of ruminants, and between wild and domestic animals. Some specialization may occur, particularly in isolated populations consuming unusual diets. Musk oxen and reindeer feeding on lichens in an Arctic environment are an example. Lichens contain specialized carbohydrates such as lichenin, a type of β-glucan. Digestibility of lichenin is about 15% in rumen fluid from non-adapted ruminants,

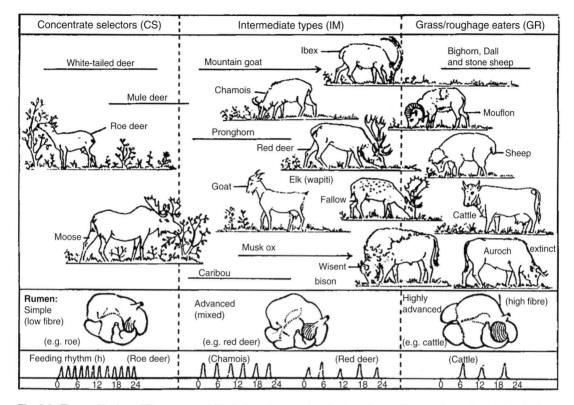

Fig. 3.6. The positioning of European and North American ruminants along the continuum of morphophysiological feeding types. The further the baseline of a species extends to the right, the greater its ability to digest fibre in the rumen, which has concurrently advanced. Selection for plant cell content implies shorter feeding intervals as the simple rumen of CS has fewer food passage delay structures than that of GR (courtesy of R.R. Hofmann, Justus-Liebig University, Giessen, Germany).

whereas digestibility trials with adapted rumen fluid and caribou indicate about 80% digestibility (Van Soest, 1994).

Coevolution between rumen microbes and secondary compounds in plants may occur. For example, ruminants in Hawaii and Indonesia are not affected by mimosine, a toxic amino acid in the tropical legume forage *Leucaena leucocephala*. Cattle in Australia, however, show alopecia (hairlessness), dermatitis, poor growth and goitre when consuming leucaena. Jones and Lowry (1984) demonstrated that Hawaiian and Indonesian ruminants have rumen bacteria that degrade mimosine, and when these bacteria are introduced into Australian cattle, they no longer are adversely affected by leucaena. It is likely that other examples of this type exist, such as with certain alkaloids (Cheeke, 1998).

Biotechnology may result in the 'domestication' of rumen microbes, with genetic modifications to alter their metabolism to the benefit of the host animal. It may be possible to develop rumen bacteria with a better balance of amino acids, to improve the protein nutrition of ruminants. It might be that bacteria specific for wool-producing sheep and for lactating dairy cattle might be developed, recognizing the differences in amino acid requirements for these two functions. Efforts along these lines have not been successful to date because of lack of competitiveness of engineered bacteria with the resident populations.

The **rumen protozoa** make up a substantial (about 40%) part of the total microbial mass of the rumen. However, their metabolic contribution appears to be much lower than their mass would suggest. Most of the rumen protozoa are ciliated, although there are a few flagellated types. The ciliated protozoa are mainly holotrichs and entodiniomorphs. The **holotrichs** (e.g. *Isotricha*) are ciliated

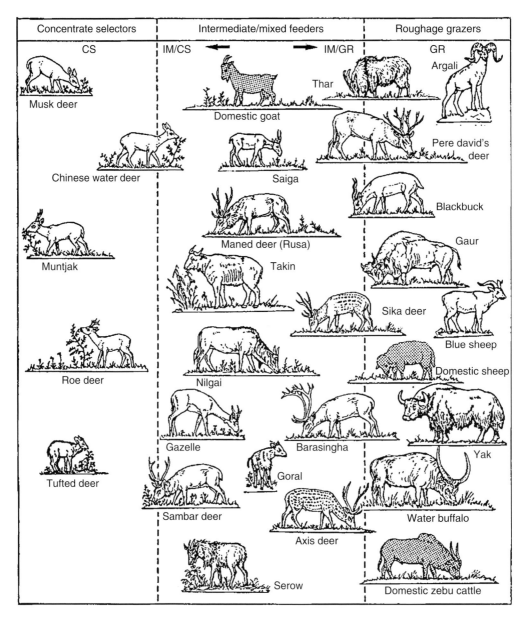

Fig. 3.7. The positioning of Asian ruminants according to morphophysiological feeding types. The baseline of a species indicates its potential adaptive range. The further to the right in general and within a feeding column, the greater the ability to digest cell wall components (dietary fibre) in the rumen. Overlap positions indicate seasonal adaptability, most pronounced in IM species (courtesy of R.R. Hofmann, Justus-Liebig University, Giessen, Germany).

over the entire body surface, while in the **entodiniomorphs** (e.g. *Entodinia*) the cilia are restricted to a band encircling the mouth.

The numbers and types of rumen protozoa are considerably influenced by the type of diet. Concentrate selectors tend to have a simple protozoal population, while mixed feeders have a more diversified fauna. For example, protozoal concentrations in African wild ruminants tend to be higher in concentrate selectors (giraffe, dik-dik) followed by intermediate feeders (impala, eland, Grant's gazelle) and lowest in grass and roughage

Table 3.2. Hofmann's categories of ruminants (adapted from Kay et al., 1980).

Common name	Scientific name	Body weight (kg)	Common name	Scientific name	Body weight (kg)
Grazers or roughage eaters			Fallow deer	Dama dama	70
American bison	Bison bison	800	Grant's gazelle	Gazella granti	60
African buffalo	Syncerus caffer	700	Impala	Aepyceros melampus	60
Ox	Bos taurus	600	Pronghorn	Antilocapra americana	50
Zebu	Bos indicus	400	Goat	Capra hircus	40
Roan antelope	Hippotragus equinus	250	Springbok	Antidorcas marsupialis	35
Waterbuck	Kobus ellipsiprymnus	220	Chamois	Rupicapra rupicapra	30
Wildebeest	Connochaetes taurinus	220	Maasai sheep	Ovis aries	30
Sable antelope	Hippotragus niger	200	Thomson's gazelle	Gaxella thomsoni	20
Oryx	Oryx gazelle	180	Chinese water deer	Hydropotes inermis	12
Hartebeest	Alcelaphus buselaphus	150	Steinbok	Raphicerus campestris	10
Topi	Damalisus lunatus	120			
Uganda kob	Adenota kob	90	**Browsers or concentrate selectors**		
Nile lechwe	Kobus megaceros	80	Giraffe	Giraffa camelopardalis	800
European sheep	Ovis aries	50	Moose	Alces alces	400
Reedbucks	Redunca spp.	40	Greater kudu	Tragelaphus strepsiceros	250
Mouflon	Ovis musimon	30	Bongo	Taurotragus eurycerus	200
Oribi	Ourebia ourebi	16	Lesser kudu	Tragelaphus imberbis	90
			Bushbuck	Tragelaphus scriptu	60
Intermediate or adaptable mixed feeders			Gerenuk	Litocranius walleri	40
European bison	Bison bonasus	800	Roe deer	Capreolus capreolus	20
Eland	Taurotragus oryx	700	Muntjacs	Muntiacus spp.	20
Musk ox	Ovibos moschatus	350	Red duiker	Cephalophus harveyi	16
Wapiti	Cervus canadensis	300	Grey duiker	Sylvicapra grimmia	14
Red deer	Cervus elaphus	150	Klipspringer	Oreotragus oreotragus	12
Mule deer	Odocoileus hemionus	120	Dik-diks	Madoqua spp.	5
Caribou	Rangifer tarandus articus	120	Suni	Nesotragus moschatus	4
Reindeer	Rangifer tarandus tarandus	100	Larger mouse deer	Tragulus napu	4
White-tail deer	Odocoileus virginianus	100	Lesser mouse deer	Tragulus javanicus	1.5
White sheep	Ovis dalli	80			

eaters (hartebeest, wildebeest) (Dehority and Odenyo, 2003). Diets that produce a fast passage rate through the rumen (eg. high concentrate diets) tend to result in a washing out of the protozoa, reducing their numbers. Protozoa feed on rumen bacteria as well as feed particles. Holotrichs tend to utilize soluble carbohydrates while entodiniomorphs engulf starch granules and bacteria. The efficiency of rumen protein utilization is reduced by protozoal digestion of bacteria. Some evidence indicates that defaunation of ruminants, by killing the protozoa with various chemical treatments (e.g. surfactants), improves metabolic efficiency. The practical benefits, if any, of defaunation are unclear.

A recent concern with protozoa, including those in the rumen, is that they may harbour pathogenic bacteria (Harb *et al.*, 2000). Pathogenic bacteria may be engulfed by rumen protozoa, and be retained as a reservoir of pathogens. For example, rumen protozoa may harbour strains of *Salmonella*, and equally significantly, may facilitate an increase in their virulence (Rasmussen *et al.*, 2005). Protozoa may play a key role as an intermediate in the transition of bacteria from the environment into mammals (Harb *et al.*, 2000). Retention of pathogens such as *Salmonella* and *E. coli* in rumen protozoa may help explain why it is difficult to remove these pathogens from the meat supply during animal slaughter and processing. Contamination of carcasses with gut contents containing pathogen-harbouring protozoa would serve to protect the bacteria from antibacterial treatments. Thus rumen defaunation prior to slaughter might be a useful means of reducing food poisoning from pathogenic bacteria, by causing a pre-slaughter 'flushing' of the microbes from the animal (Harb *et al*, 2000).

Anaerobic fungi are a component of the rumen microflora (Fig. 3.8). They were discovered fairly recently by Orpin (1975), who determined that some of what seemed to be flagellated protozoa were in fact fungal zoospores. Fungal zoospores invade fibrous plant material in the rumen, and begin the degradation of structural components of forage tissue (Fig. 3.9). They pave the way for colonization by cellulolytic bacteria. Rumen fungi break down lignin–cellulose complexes and solubilize the lignin (Gordon and Phillips, 1998), making the cellulose more accessible to bacteria. Rumen fungi have received relatively little attention by ruminant nutritionists.

(a)

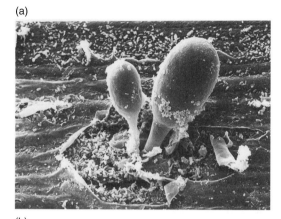

(b)

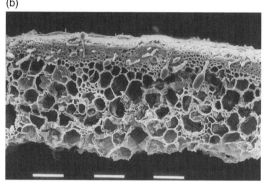

Fig. 3.8. Rumen fungi have an important role in digestion of low quality roughages. (a) Sporangia or fruiting body of a rumen fungus. The sporangia produce zoospores that infect other feed particles in the rumen (courtesy of K. Joblin, Department of Industrial and Scientific Research, Palmerston North, New Zealand). (b) Fungi growing on the cell walls of wheat straw in the rumen. Breakdown of the lignified cell wall by the rumen fungi renders the remainder of the plant cell more accessible to bacteria (courtesy of E. Grenet, P. Barry and the National Institute for Agricultural Research (INRA), France).

Salivation, eructation and rumination

Compared with non-ruminants, ruminant animals secrete copious quantities of saliva. The saliva is rich in sodium, potassium, phosphate and bicarbonate ions, serving to buffer the rumen VFAs. It is also high in mucin content, serving as an antifoaming agent in the rumen to aid in prevention of bloat. Urea is a component of ruminant saliva, functioning in urea recycling (see Chapter 5). Salivary flow is influenced by the amount of time spent eating and ruminating.

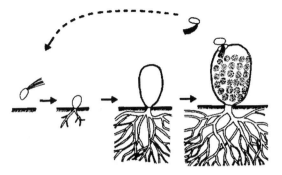

Fig. 3.9. Life cycle of the anaerobic fungi in the rumen showing the release of zoospores from the sporangia and the re-infection of fibre in the digesta.

Feeding of high concentrate diets decreases salivary flow, which in conjunction with the high rate of fermentation of a high starch diet, can lead to rumen acidosis. Interestingly, a natural toxin, slaframine, may have value as an additive to increase salivary flow with high concentrate diets (Froetschel *et al.*, 1995). Slaframine is an alkaloid produced in mouldy red clover hay, and causes profuse salivation.

Rumination is the process whereby consumed feed is regurgitated and chewed to break it up into smaller particles. Muscles at the base of the oesophagus form a bolus of fibrous material, which is then propelled by muscular action to the mouth. Mastication extracts the soluble cell contents, and mixes the remaining fibrous material with saliva. Rumination time is greatest with high fibre diets, and is more important in roughage eaters than in concentrate selectors. Rumen gases collect in a 'gas dome' at the top of the rumen. **Eructation** is the process by which rumen gases are expelled. The presence of foam in the rumen inhibits the eructation mechanism, resulting in the accumulation of rumen gases and bloat.

Rumen motility

Mixing of rumen contents is accomplished by contractions of the musculature of the rumen pillars and the rumen wall. The rumen contents, although well mixed, are not a homogeneous mass. Forage diets usually produce contents with a floating mat of coarse matter, below a gas dome and above a liquid layer of fluids and suspended particles (Fig. 3.5). As fibrous material in the mat is digested, it becomes more dense and sinks.

Particles towards the floor of the rumen are those most likely to move through the omasum.

Non-ruminant foregut fermenters

A variety of non-ruminant animals have a compartmentalized or chambered stomach, with microbial fermentation. Langer (1984a, b, 1986) has reviewed digestion in a number of forestomach fermenters. Some representative examples will be briefly discussed. A number of Australian marsupials, such as the kangaroo and wallaby, have a segmented forestomach and microbial digestion with significant VFA production (Hume, 1999). Other foregut fermenters include the hippopotamus, peccary, colobus monkey, tree sloth, and some whales (e.g. bowhead, minke and small, toothed whales) (Stevens and Hume, 1998). The colobus monkey and tree sloth are arboreal folivores, whose diet consists primarily of tree leaves. Their stomachs are sufficiently compartmentalized to have a separation of the ingesta into fermentative and the acid pyloric regions, so that the fermentation chamber remains at an optimal pH for microbial growth (Bauchop, 1978). The colobus monkey has a four-chambered stomach, with cellulolytic activity and VFA production similar to those of ruminants (Ullrey, 1986). A nutritional problem with captive colobines is the development of **phytobezoars** or masses of undigested fibre that obstruct the digestive tract, resulting in mortality. Phytobezoars are primarily a problem when highly lignified leaves such as those of *Acacia* species are fed (Ensley *et al.*, 1982). The fruit bat is a folivorous herbivore that has a fruit-based diet supplemented with leafy foliage. The gut is specialized for a largely liquid diet and a rapid rate of passage (Lowry, 1989). The animal consumes leaves of tree legumes, relatively high in protein content, to supplement the low protein concentrations in fruit. It has a unique strategy of chewing the leaves to a bolus, swallowing the liquid fraction, and expelling the pellet of fibrous residue from the mouth (Lowry, 1989).

An example of an avian foregut fermenter is a neotropical bird, the **hoatzin** (Grajal *et al.*, 1989; Dominguez-Bello *et al.*, 1993a, b). It feeds on tree leaves in the tropical rainforest canopies of Central America. The hoatzin (pronounced 'watson') has numerous adaptations for its aboreal folivorous life, including functional wing claws for climbing through trees, and a modified sternum to accommodate the enlarged foregut (Fig. 3.10). Its ability

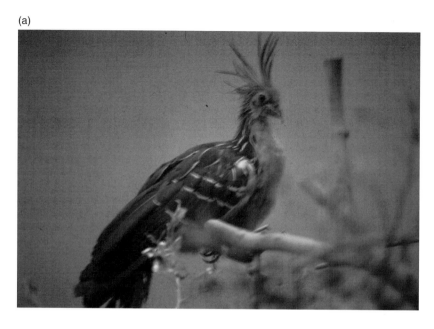

(a)

(b)

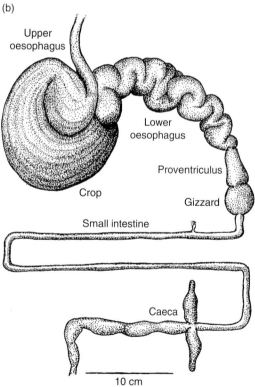

Upper oesophagus

Lower oesophagus

Proventriculus

Crop

Gizzard

Small intestine

Caeca

10 cm

Fig. 3.10. An adult hoatzin (a) and its digestive tract (b) (courtesy of S.D. Strahl and the Chicago Zoological Society, Chicago, USA).

to fly allows it to exploit patches of vegetation not accessible to other herbivorous vertebrates. The hoatzin has a microbial population of bacteria and protozoa in its crop that resembles the microflora of the rumen. Jones *et al.* (2000) compared the digestibility of six tropical tannin-containing shrub legumes and the tropical grass *Panicum maximum* in hoatzin crop fluid versus bovine rumen fluid. *In vitro* dry matter digestibility (IVDMD) was markedly lower with hoatzin crop fluid (mean = 40.5%) than with bovine rumen fluid (mean = 62.6%). The addition of polyethylene glycol (PEG), a tannin-binding substance, increased IVDMD in hoatzin crop fluid, suggesting that the hoatzin does not have a tannin-degrading microbial population. The low tannin content in the hoatzin crop contents indicated that the bird avoids tanniniferous leaves, and supports other findings that the hoatzin is very selective of a high quality leafy diet (Jones *et al.*, 2000). On the other hand, hoatzin crop fluid has a greater capacity than rumen fluid to detoxify saponins, another common type of toxin in tropical tree foliage (Dominguez-Bello *et al.*, 1999).

Hindgut Fermenters

In many non-ruminant herbivores, the hindgut or large intestine (caecum plus colon) is enlarged and has a microbial population performing many of the same digestive functions that take place in the rumen. Compared to the rumen, there are several nutritional disadvantages to the hindgut as a fermentation site. Soluble nutrients, such as sugars, amino acids, vitamins and minerals, are absorbed in the small intestine. Thus the composition of material entering the hindgut is less favourable for maximal microbial growth than is the case in the rumen, where the microbes have all the nutrients in the ingested feed as available substrate. The hindgut is a less efficient area for nutrient absorption. Products of rumen fermentation, including the microbes, are digested and/or absorbed in the rumen or small intestine. Microbes in the hindgut are not subject to digestion (unless the faeces are consumed). The passage rate through the hindgut is more rapid than through the rumen, leading to a lower efficiency of fibre digestion. There are, however, a number of significant advantages of hindgut fermentation, which will be discussed in the section 'Evolutionary Aspects of Digestive Physiology'.

Caecal fermenters

The rabbit is probably the best-known example of a caecal fermenter, and will be discussed in the most detail here. The hindgut of the rabbit functions to selectively excrete fibre, and retain the non-fibre components of forage for fermentation in the caecum. This separation is accomplished by muscular activity of the proximal colon. Fibre particles, being larger and less dense than non-fibre components, tend to be concentrated in the lumen of the colon. Fluids and material of small particle size tend to concentrate at the periphery of the colon. Peristaltic action propels the fibre particles through the colon rapidly, whereas antiperistaltic contractions of the haustrae of the proximal colon move the soluble nutrients and fluids 'backwards' into the caecum (Fig. 3.11). The digestive strategy of the rabbit and other small herbivores is to minimize the digestion of fibre, and to concentrate digestive action on the more nutritionally valuable non-fibre constituents. Thus the digestibility of fibre in the rabbit is very low. An additional refinement of this digestive strategy is that at intervals the caecal contents are ingested by the animal. After the colon is emptied of hard faecal pellets, consisting primarily of fibre, the caecum contracts and the caecal contents are squeezed into the proximal colon. Mucin is secreted by goblet cells, producing caecal material covered with a mucilaginous membrane. This material, known as **caecotropes** or 'soft faeces', is consumed by the animal directly from the anus. Consumption of caecotropes (**caecotrophy**) provides the animal with a means of more efficiently digesting the products of caecal fermentation, digesting the microbial protein, and obtaining microbially synthesized B vitamins. Thus this process of caecal fermentation allows the animal to utilize forage without the encumbrance of carrying around internally a large mass of slowly digested fibre.

Many other small herbivores besides rabbits have a similar process of caecal fermentation, with a mechanism for the selective retention of non-fibre components. Guinea pigs, for example, have a longitudinal furrow between two mucosal folds in the proximal colon which functions in moving fluids from the colon into the caecum (Holtenius and Bjornhag, 1985).

Because caecal fermentation is an adaptation for utilizing fibrous diets without the encumbrance of an overly large gut, most caecal fermenters are

---

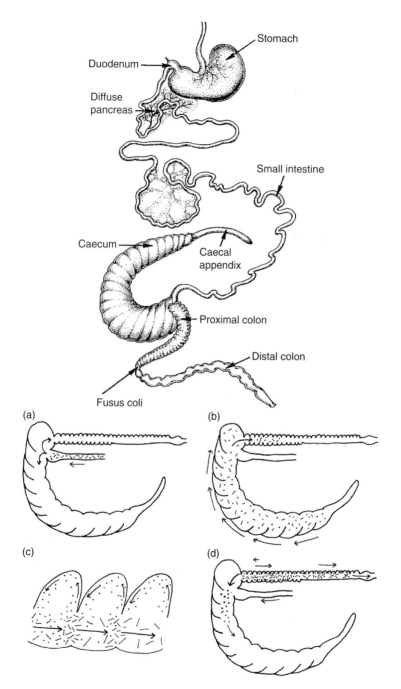

Fig. 3.11. Schematic view of the parts of the rabbit digestive tract (top) and mechanisms for the selective excretion of fibre and retention of small particles and solubles for fermentation in the caecum (bottom). (a) Intestinal contents enter the hindgut of the ileocaecal-colonic junction and uniformly disperse in the caecum and colon. Dashes represent large fibre particles, and dots represent non-fibre particles. (b) Contraction of the caecum moves material into the proximal colon. (c) Peristaltic action moves large fibre particles (dashes) down the colon for excretion as hard faeces. Contractions of the haustrae of the colon move small particles (dots) and fluids backwards into the caecum. (d) Small particles and fluids are thus separated from fibre (courtesy of M.A. Grobner, Oregon State University, Corvallis, Oregon, USA).

small animals. The largest include the koala (about 10 kg) and the capybara (about 50 kg). Small animals have a much greater relative metabolic rate and energy requirements than do large animals (see Chapter 17).

Some avian species, such as the ostrich, have enlarged caeca (Fig. 3.12) and caecal fermentation. While retrograde movement of fluid from the colon to the caeca occurs in the goose (Clemens *et al.*, 1975), the primary reason why this avian species can consume a high forage diet is simply a very high rate of passage and a high forage intake, allowing the bird to meet its energy requirements from the digestion of plant cell contents. The fibrous cell-wall material is excreted largely undigested.

Colonic and caeco-colonic fermenters

In all large (over 50 kg) hindgut fermenters, the enlarged proximal colon is the primary site of fermentation. Examples include the horse and other equids (zebra, donkey), the elephant and rhinoceros. The caecum is often enlarged as well, but performs as an extension of the colon as a fermentation site, rather than functioning in selective retention of small particles as in the caecal fermenters. Caeco-colonic fermenters also include a number of New World monkeys, lemurs and rodents such as the porcupine and beaver. The digestive strategy of colon fermenters is similar to that of ruminants:

hindgut fermentation functions in digestion of plant cell-wall constituents. The percentage of digestibility of fibre fractions is generally lower in colon fermenters than in ruminants, due primarily to the greater rate of passage and less optimal environment for microbial growth (Janis, 1976; Duncan *et al.*, 1990).

Some caeco-colonic fermenters engage in **coprophagy**, which is the consumption of faeces. Coprophagy is different than caecotrophy, which involves the consumption of caecal contents rather than faeces. On low protein diets, horses will consume their faeces, presumably as a means of conserving nitrogen. Wild horses on North American rangelands often practise coprophagy, probably as a nitrogen conservation measure when consuming mature weathered forage in the winter.

Fermentation in the ruminant hindgut

The words of Van Soest (1994) are relevant: 'The lower part of the ruminant gastrointestinal tract receives much less attention than the reticulorumen. Judging from the emphasis, one would think that ruminants have no lower tract.'

The hindgut of ruminants is enlarged, and has a microbial population resembling that of the rumen. Ruminant species adapted to arid environments tend to have a long colon, facilitating the resorption and retention of water (Clauss *et al.*, 2003b, 2004).

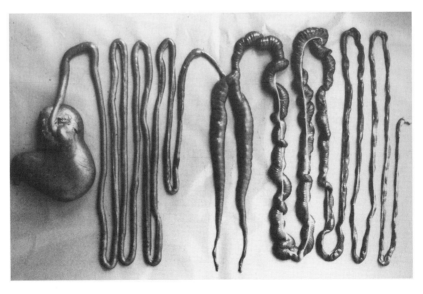

Fig. 3.12. Digestive tract of the ostrich, showing the two enlarged caeca.

Concentrate selectors have a larger lower tract and small intestine than grazers. Even more than in the non-ruminant herbivores, the hindgut of ruminants receives digesta from which most of the readily fermentable substances have already been digested and absorbed. Thus fermentation in the colon is limited to digestion of slowly digested residues from the reticulorumen, and the reabsorption of electrolytes and water. Water resorption tends to inhibit fermentation processes by way of a dehydration effect.

Foregut Versus Hindgut Fermentation and Body Size

The relative efficiencies of ruminant and non-ruminant digestion are influenced by body size and the abundance and quality of plant material. Among herbivores in general, the ruminants dominate in numbers in the intermediate body-size range. Very small (e.g. rabbits) and very large (e.g. elephants) herbivores are mainly non-ruminant herbivores (Fig. 3.13). Demment and Van Soest (1985) and Clauss *et al.* (2003b) considered this subject in detail. Gut volume among herbivores varies directly with body weight, whereas metabolic rate varies with a fractional power of body weight (Van Soest, 1996). Thus, small herbivores have a high metabolic requirement for energy and must consume high quality diets to be able to meet their energy requirements. For this reason, the smallest ruminants are concentrate selectors. Small non-ruminant herbivores are better able to utilize high quality forage than small ruminants because of direct digestion without fermentation, combined with coprophagy. As the body size of ruminants decreases, fermentation of forages can no longer meet the increasing (per unit of weight) energy requirements. With very large ruminants, however, insufficient fibrous feed can be ingested to meet the energy requirements of a large body mass through fermentation by-products. Large animals in the wild generally are not able to select sufficient amounts of the rapidly digested foods used by the smaller concentrate selectors because these foods are comparatively rare. Thus, large body size favours non-ruminant herbivores, such as the elephant and rhinoceros, because intake of low-quality, high-fibre forage is not limited by retention time in the gut.

Browsing ruminants are mainly represented by smaller species and grazing ruminants by larger species (Clauss *et al.*, 2003b). This difference is attributed not to physiological limitations but to forage abundance. Large species cannot be as selective as small species, and the large amounts of forage necessary to supply large species are available

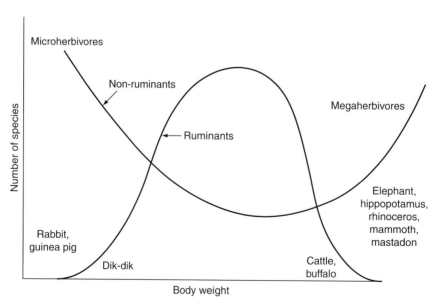

Fig. 3.13. Ruminants dominate the intermediate body weight ranges of herbivores, while non-ruminant herbivores are predominant at very small and very large body weights.

mainly as grasses. If there is an abundant food source for specific browsers, they also can attain large body sizes (for example, moose and giraffe).

Clauss *et al.* (2003b, 2004) speculate that the maximal reticulorumen capacity of grazers is limited by the available space in the abdominal cavity, for which all internal organs compete. As the relative size of the forestomach increases, there is a decrease in the abdominal space available for the colon, which tends to decrease in relative size. Decreased length of the descending colon reduces the capacity for water reabsorption (Clauss *et al.*, 2004). Thus in grazers, there is a general tendency for faecal water content to increase as body size increases. As noted by Clauss *et al.* (2003b), 'All large grazers defecate "pies", not "pellets".' For example, the African buffalo is the only ruminant species in its habitat that does not produce a faecal pellet. Clauss *et al.* (2003b) suggest that the largest existing grazers represent the largest possible increase in reticulorumen capacity that can be achieved without risking the integrity of colonic function.

Van Soest (1996) provides an extensive compilation of comparative fibre fraction digestibilities for a wide array of domestic and wild ruminant and non-ruminant herbivores.

Small Animals as Nutritional Models for Larger Ones

Primarily for cost savings in feed, animal facilities and other expenses, it is often desirable to utilize small laboratory animals as models for larger ones, particularly in preliminary or pilot trials. With new or unusual feedstuffs, there initially may not be sufficient quantities available to evaluate them with large animals. This is often true with plant breeding programmes. In the agricultural area, rats and mice have for many years been used in this way as models for pigs. In poultry research, Japanese quail are extensively used in preliminary studies. For forage utilizing animals, the choices are not so clear cut. Equine nutritionists often consider the rabbit or the guinea pig as 'laboratory rats' in horse nutrition studies. However, as described earlier, rabbits are caecal fermenters and horses are caecal-colonic fermenters. The digestive tract of the rabbit is quite efficient in the separation and rapid excretion of fibre, whereas in the horse, fibre is retained in the hindgut for microbial fermentation. The rabbit has caecal fermentation of low fibre constituents, and

Table 3.3. Comparative digestibility of whole maize plant pellets in rabbits and horses (from Schurg *et al.*, 1977).

Item	Digestibility (%)	
	Rabbits	Horses
Dry matter	47.4[a]	70.0[b]
Crude protein	80.2[a]	53.0[b]
Acid detergent fibre	25.0[a]	47.5[b]
Neutral detergent fibre	36.7[a]	68.9[b]
Ether extract	93.9[a]	99.2[b]
Ash	36.4	31.0
Energy (kcal)	49.3[a]	79.9[b]

[a,b]Different at $P < 0.05$.

engages in caecotrophy. The result is that digestibility data for rabbits bear little resemblance to those in horses (Table 3.3). The hindgut digestion in the horse is actually somewhat similar to rumen digestion, so sheep would probably be a better model than rabbits for horses.

As previously mentioned, an effort was made at Pennsylvania State University to develop a small concentrate-selector ruminant, the blue duiker, as a laboratory animal for ruminant nutrition studies. The effort failed, in large part because concentrate-selector small ruminants are unable to subsist on coarse forages typical of cattle and sheep diets. An attempt was made, also at Pennsylvania State University, to develop the meadow vole (*Microtus pennsylvanicus*) as a small animal for evaluation of forages (Shenk *et al.*, 1971; Russo *et al.*, 1981). Like the rabbit, the meadow vole digestive tract functions so as to rapidly eliminate dietary fibre, and the meadow vole proved to be unsatisfactory for evaluating forage quality for ruminants. Sheep function well as smaller animals for preliminary studies aimed eventually at cattle.

Evolutionary Aspects of Digestive Physiology

Current scientific evidence suggests the age of the universe to be about 15 billion years, and the age of the Earth about 4.6 billion years. The earth was born as a result of immense explosions, with the solar system formed by the condensation of clouds of gallactic dust and gas, collapsing under intense gravitational forces. Under the reducing conditions of the Earth's early atmosphere, rich in water, carbon dioxide and nitrogen and lacking free oxygen, chemical reactions could occur to produce simple organic molecules such as methane, ammonia, amino acids, simple carbohydrates and nucleotides. These reactions have been experimentally produced under conditions believed to closely simulate those early in the Earth's history. Over a period of about 300 million years, these simple organic compounds accumulated in warm, shallow seas, forming a **primordial soup**. Self-replicating molecules, probably formed on templates of clay minerals, developed and gave rise to simple prokaryote cells (single cells with no membrane-bound organelles; all bacteria are **prokaryotes**). The oldest known fossils, dated at about 3.5 billion years, are of prokaryote cells in tidal mudflats. Over the next 2 billion years, **eukaryotes** (cells with membrane-bound organelles) evolved, such as red and green algae and fungi. By 700 million years ago, multicellular green algae appear in the fossil record, while 600 million years ago, the first multicellular animals appeared. At the dawn of the Cambrian epoch, about 570 million years ago, animals with mineralized skeletons were abundant. The Mesozoic Era (240–195 million years ago) was the age of the dinosaurs. The first mammals appeared at this time, and after the abrupt extinction of the dinosaurs about 65 million years ago, became the dominant fauna of Earth.

Digestion began in a primitive manner with the first eukaryotes. With the evolution of vertebrates, microbial habitats were abundant in all regions of the gut (Ley *et al.*, 2008). Microbial involvement in digestion became critical to animals consuming plant foods containing appreciable fibre. The cellulase enzyme, necessary for cellulose (and fibre) digestion, is produced only by microbes. Surprisingly, and perhaps because of the evolution of symbiotic relationships between microbes and herbivores, no vertebrates evolved the ability to produce cellulase.

The earliest mammals were probably small nocturnal insectivores. The digestive system of early mammals would no doubt contain the same components as found in their reptilian ancestors: stomach, small intestine, caecum and colon. Hume and Warner (1980) have discussed the evolution of the digestive tracts of modern mammals. Because the fossil record provides no information on the morphology, physiology, biochemistry or microbiology of the gut, their deductions are unquestionably speculative. An intriguing question concerns the development of microbial digestion. Which

came first, foregut or hindgut digestion? Hume and Warner (1980) suggest it is likely that early insectivorous mammals began to ingest seeds, fruits and succulent vegetation, perhaps during periods of low prey availability. An increased intake of indigestible bulk would stimulate greater secretions of saliva and mucus, and greater sloughing of epithelial cells from the mechanical effects of fibre. These effects could lead to development of a mechanism to reabsorb fluid, electrolytes and metabolites from the lower tract, providing a selective advantage for prolonged transit time, to permit reabsorption to occur. The hindgut would enlarge, because of the presence of indigestible fibre. (Hindgut enlargement is readily demonstrated in pigs and rats, when a diet high in indigestible fibre is fed.) The presence of fibre, fluids and nutrients in the hindgut would provide an environment favourable to microbial growth. Thus, Hume and Warner (1980) believe that microbial digestion probably began in the hindgut, although the initial impetus for its development was the selective nutritional advantage of conservation of electrolytes and endogenous nutrients. Continued intake of a high fibre diet would place selection pressure on high salivary secretion, mucus secretion and hindgut enlargement. Coprophagy might develop from the habit of many omnivores of eating virtually every accessible edible item (as readily appreciated by observing the eating habits of dogs). The habit could be reinforced if a nutritional benefit accrued.

Foregut fermentation could arise from enlargement of the stomach or formation of diverticula to provide pouches where mixing of acid with the ingesta would be impeded. With the effects of stomach acid minimized, the foregut is an ideal site for microbial growth. Enlargement, elongation or sacculation of the stomach is very common in mammals, and appears to have independently evolved in diverse lines, including the marsupials (e.g. kangaroo), ruminants, rodents (e.g. hamster) and primates (e.g. colobus monkey). A primitive rodent-like animal, the rock hyrax of Africa, has a stomach with three fermentation chambers.

The large modern herbivores, ruminants and equids, evolved in the Miocene and Pliocene epochs in association with climatic changes which led to extensive development of grasslands. Ruminants and equids represent different evolutionary strategies for dealing with low-energy, high-fibre roughage. The ruminant is well adapted for achieving maximum digestive efficiency of high fibre diets. The reticulo-omasal orifice retains fibrous feed in the fermentation chamber until it has been digested. This maximal efficiency of fibre digestion would be of adaptive significance if the quantity of feed were limiting, and if the food were of low digestibility. Thus ruminant digestive strategy probably evolved in regions where quality or quantity of forage was at least periodically limiting, such as deserts or deciduous forests (Hume and Warner, 1980). Under conditions of a high availability of poor quality forage, hindgut digestion may be a superior adaptation (Janis, 1976), because intake is not limited by rate of digestion. Thus on the Serengeti plains of Africa, the zebra can survive on low quality roughages, selecting the most fibrous plant parts (Janis, 1976), on which wildebeest, ante-lope and other ruminants cannot survive. The equids are able to meet their protein requirements on high-fibre, low-protein forage because feed intake is not dependent on the rate of fibre digestion, whereas in ruminants fibrous material cannot exit the rumen until the fibre has been digested.

Clauss *et al.* (2003b) discussed fossil evidence of digestive type of extremely large mammals. The fossil record suggests that all extinct giant mammals (e.g. mammoths, mastadons, giant rhinos, giant ground sloths) were hindgut fermenters. The same is likely true of dinosaurs (Farlow, 1987).

Further information on the evolution of herbivory and microbial digestion is presented by Janis (1976), Hume and Warner (1980), Langer (1984b) and Stevens and Hume (1995).

Questions and Study Guide

1. Define fermentation.
2. Name the four compartments of the ruminant stomach, and describe their functions.
3. Describe Hofmann's system of classifying ruminant animals. Is the Hofmann system valid?
4. What are some of the problems in feeding very small ruminants (e.g. mouse deer) in captivity?
5. Moose and giraffes can be difficult to maintain in zoos. Why? What nutritional problems do they have?
6. What is the ventricular groove?
7. Cattle are specifically well adapted to consuming grass (grazing). Why?
8. In the free-ranging wild ruminant, much of the animal's protein and energy needs are met by microbial fermentation. Explain.
9. Explain the difference between rumination and eructation.
10. Name the major types of rumen microbes.
11. Give an example of a mammalian and an avian arboreal folivore.
12. What are phytobezoars? What kinds of animals develop them?
13. Name some unique characteristics of hoatzins.
14. Is the rabbit a good 'pilot animal' for horse nutrition studies, particularly those involving forages?
15. What is the difference between coprophagy and caecotrophy?
16. Why are very small and very large herbivores not usually ruminants?
17. Why do cows excrete 'cow pies' while sheep excrete pellets?
18. On the plains of Africa, zebras can often survive during droughts under conditions that result in heavy mortalities of ruminants such as wildebeest and antelope. Why are zebras more likely to survive when forage quality is very poor?
19. Cattle evolved as grazing animals, very well suited for consuming and digesting grass. In North America, beef (in feedlots) and dairy cattle are fed high concentrate diets based on grain (e.g. maize) with as little forage as possible. Why are we feeding a grazing animal as if it were a non-ruminant granivore?

References

Bauchop, T. (1978) Digestion of leaves in vertebrate arboreal folivores. In: Montgomery, G.G. (ed.) *The Ecology of Arboreal Folivores.* Smithsonian Institution Press, Washington, DC, pp. 193–204.

Cheeke, P.R. (1998) *Natural Toxicants in Feeds, Forages, and Poisonous Plants.* Prentice Hall, Upper Saddle River, New Jersey.

Clauss, M. and Hofmann, R.R. (2008) Higher masseter muscle mass in grazing than in browsing ruminants. *Oecologia* 157, 377–385.

Clauss, M., Kienzle, E. and Wiesner, H. (2002) Importance of the wasting syndrome complex in captive moose (*Alces alces*). *Zoo Biology* 21, 499–506.

Clauss, M., Lechner-Doll, M. and Streich, W.J. (2003a) Ruminant diversification as an adaptation to the physicomechanical characteristics of forage. A reevaluation

---

of an old debate and a new hypothesis. *Oikos* 102, 253–262.

Clauss, M., Frey, R., Kiefer, B., Lechner-Doll, M., Lochlein, W., Polster, C., Rossner, G.E. and Streich, W.J. (2003b) The maximum attainable body size of herbivorous mammals: morphophysiological constraints on foregut, and adaptations of hindgut fermenters. *Oecologia* 136, 14–27.

Clauss, M., Kienzle, E. and Hatt, J.-M. (2003c) Feeding practice in captive wild ruminants: peculiarities in the nutrition of browsers/concentrate selectors and intermediate feeders. A review. In: Fidgett, A., Clauss, M., Ganslosser, U., Hatt, J.-M. and Nijboer, J. (eds) *Zoo Animal Nutrition*, Vol. 2. Filander Verlag, Fürth, Germany, pp. 27–52.

Clauss, M., Lechner-Doll, M. and Streich, W.J. (2004) Differences in the range of faecal dry matter content between feeding types of captive wild ruminants. *Acta Theriologica* 49, 259–267.

Clauss, M., Hummel, J. and Streich, W.J. (2005) The dissociation of the fluid and particle phase in the forestomach as a physiological characteristic of large grazing ruminants: an evaluation of available, comparable ruminant passage data. *European Journal of Wildlife Research* 36, 14–27.

Clauss, M., Fritz, J., Bayer, D., Nygren, K., Hammer, S., Hatt, J.-M., Sudekum, K.-H. and Hummel, J. (2009a) Physical characteristics of rumen contents in four large ruminants of different feeding type, the addax (*Addax nasomaculatus*), bison (*Bison bison*), red deer (*Cervus elaphus*) and moose (*Alces alces*). *Comparative Biochemistry and Physiology* 152, 398–406.

Clauss, M., Hofmann, R.R., Fickel, J., Streich, W.J. and Hummel, J. (2009b) The intraruminal papillation gradient in wild ruminants of different feeding types; implications for rumen physiology. *Journal of Morphology* 270, 929–942.

Clemens, E.T., Stevens, C.E. and Southworth, M. (1975) Sites of organic acid production and pattern of digesta movement in the gastrointestinal tract of geese. *Journal of Nutrition* 105, 1341–1350.

Cork, S.J. and Foley, W.J. (1991) Digestive and metabolic strategies of arboreal mammalian folivores in relation to chemical defenses in temperate and tropical forests. In: Palo, R.T. and Robbins, C.T. (eds) *Plant Defenses Against Mammalian Herbivory*. CRC Press, Boca Raton, Florida, pp. 133–166.

Dehority, B.A. and Odenyo, A.A. (2003) Influence of diet on the rumen protozoal fauna of indigenous African wild ruminants. *Journal of Eukaryotic Microbiology* 50, 220–223.

Dehority, B.A. and Varga, G.A. (1991) Bacterial and fungal numbers in ruminal and cecal contents of the blue duiker (*Cephalophus monticola*). *Applied Environmental Microbiology* 57, 469–472.

Demment, M.W. and Van Soest, P.J. (1985) A nutritional explanation for body-size patterns of ruminant and non-ruminant herbivores. *American Naturalist* 125, 641–672.

Ditchkoff, S.S. (2000) A decade since 'diversification of ruminants': has our knowledge improved? *Oecologia* 125, 82–84.

Dominguez-Bello, M.G., Lovera, M., Suarez, P. and Michelangeli, F. (1993a) Microbial digestive symbionts of the crop of the hoatzin (*Opisthocomus hoazin*): an avian foregut fermenter. *Physiological Zoology* 66, 374–383.

Dominguez-Bello, M.G., Ruiz, M.C. and Michelangeli, F. (1993b) Evolutionary significance of foregut fermentation in the hoatzin (*Opisthocomus hoazin*; Aves: Opisthocomidae). *Journal of Comparative Physiology* B163, 594–601.

Dominguez-Bello, M.G., Garcia Amado, M.A. and Michelangeli, F. (1999) Loss of haemolytic activity of Quillaja saponins in anaerobic bacterial cultures from the crop of the hoatzin (*Opisthocomus hoazin*). The Fifth International Symposium on the Nutrition of Herbivores. Nutritional Ecology of Herbivores: an Integration. San Antonio, Texas, 11–16 April.

Duncan, P., Foose, T.J., Gordon, I.J., Gakahu, C.G. and Lloyd, M. (1990) Comparative nutrient extraction from forages by grazing bovids and equids: a test of the nutritional model of equid/bovid competition and coexistence. *Oecologia* 84, 411–418.

Ensley, P.K., Rost, T.L., Anderson, M., Benirschke, K., Brockman, D. and Ullrey, D.E. (1982) Intestinal obstruction and perforation caused by undigested *Acacia* sp. leaves in languor monkeys. *Journal of the American Veterinary Medical Association* 181, 1351–1354.

Farlow, J.O. (1987) Speculations about the diet and digestive physiology of herbivorous dinosaurs. *Paleobiology* 13, 60–72.

Foley, W.J., McLean, S. and Cork, S.J. (1995) Consequences of biotransformation of plant secondary metabolites on acid-base metabolism in mammals – a final common pathway? *Journal of Chemical Ecology* 21, 721–743.

Froetschel, M.A., Streeter, M.N., Amos, H.E., Croom, W.J., Jr and Hagler, W.M., Jr (1995) Effects of abomasal slaframine infusion on ruminal digesta passage and digestion in steers. *Canadian Journal of Animal Science* 75, 157–163.

Gordon, G.L.R. and Phillips, M.W. (1998) The role of anaerobic gut fungi in ruminants. *Nutrition Research Reviews* 11, 133–168.

Gordon, I.J. and Illius, A.W. (1994) The functional significance of the browser-grazer dichotomy in African ruminants. *Oecologia* 98, 167–175.

Gordon, I.J. and Illius, A.W. (1996) The nutritional ecology of African ruminants: a reinterpretation. *Journal of Animal Ecology* 65, 18–28.

Grajal, A., Strahl, S.D., Parra, R., Dominguez, M.G. and Neher, A. (1989) Foregut fermentation in the hoatzin, a neotropical leaf-eating bird. *Science* 245, 1236–1238.

Harb, O.S., Gao, L.Y. and Abukwaik, Y. (2000) From protozoa to mammalian cells: a new paradigm in the life cycle of intracellular bacterial pathogens. *Environmental Microbiology* 2, 251–265.

Hofmann, R.R. (1973) *The Ruminant Stomach*. East African Literature Bureau, Nairobi, Kenya.

Hofmann, R.R. (1984) Comparative anatomical studies imply adaptive variations of ruminant digestive physiology. *Canadian Journal of Animal Science* 64, 203–205.

Hofmann, R.R. (1989) Evolutionary steps of ecophysiological adaptation and diversification of ruminants: a comparative view of their digestive system. *Oecologia* 78, 443–457.

Hofmann, R.R., Streich, W.J., Fickel, J., Hummel, J. and Clauss, M. (2008) Convergent evolution in feeding types: salivary gland mass differences in wild ruminant species. *Journal of Morphology* 269, 240–257.

Holtenius, K. and Bjornhag, G. (1985) The colonic separation mechanism in the guinea pig (*Cavia porcellus*) and the chinchilla (*Chinchilla laniger*). *Comparative Biochemistry and Physiology A* 82, 537–542.

Hume, I.D. (1999) *Marsupial Nutrition*. Cambridge University Press, Cambridge, UK.

Hume, I.D. and Warner, A.C.I. (1980) Evolution of microbial digestion in mammals. In: Ruckebusch, Y. and Thivend, P. (eds) *Digestive Physiology and Metabolism in Ruminants*. MTP Press, Lancaster, Lancashire, UK, pp. 615–634.

Illius, A.W. and Gordon, I.J. (1992) Modelling the nutritional ecology of ungulate herbivores: evolution of body size and competitive interactions. *Oecologia* 89, 428–434.

Janis, C. (1976) The evolutionary strategy of the Equidae and the origins of rumen and cecal digestion. *Evolution* 30, 757–774.

Jones, R.J. and Lowry, J.B. (1984) Australian goats detoxify the goitrogen 3-hydroxy-4(1H) pyridone (DHP) after rumen infusion from an Indonesian goat. *Experientia* 40, 1435–1436.

Jones, R.J., Garcia Amado, M.A. and Dominguez-Bello, M.G. (2000) Comparison of the digestive ability of crop fluid from the folivorous hoatzin (*Opisthocomus hoazin*) and cow rumen fluid with seven tropical forages. *Animal Feed Science and Technology* 87, 287–296.

Kay, R.N.B., Engelhardt, W.V. and White, R.G. (1980) The digestive physiology of wild ruminants. In: Ruckebusch, Y. and Thivend, P. (eds) *Digestive Physiology and Metabolism in Ruminants*. AVI Publishing Co., Westport, Connecticut, pp. 743–761.

Kearney, C.C. (2005) Effects of dietary physical form and carbohydrate profile on captive giraffe. MSc. thesis, University of Florida, Gainesville, Florida.

Knott, K.K., Barboza, P.S., Bowyer, R.T. and Blake, J.E. (2004) Nutritional development of feeding strategies in Arctic ruminants: digestive morphometry of reindeer, *Rangifer tarandus*, and muskoxen, *Ovibos moschatus*. *Zoology* 107, 315–333.

Langer, P. (1984a) Anatomical and nutritional adaptations in wild herbivores. In: Gilchrist, F.M.C. and Mackie, R.I. (eds) *Herbivore Nutrition in the Subtropics and Tropics*. The Science Press, Craighall, South Africa, pp. 185–221.

Langer, P. (1984b) Comparative anatomy of the stomach in mammalian herbivores. *Quarterly Journal of Experimental Physiology* 69, 615–625.

Langer, P. (1986) Large mammalian herbivores in tropical forests with either hindgut- or forestomach-fermentation. *Zeitschrift fur Saugetierkunde* 51, 173–187.

Ley, R.E., Hamady, M., Lozupone, C., Turnbaugh, P.J., Ramey, R.R., Bircher, J.S., Schlegel, M.L., Tucker, T.A., Schrenzel, M.D., Knight, R. and Gordon, J.I. (2008) Evolution of mammals and their gut microbes. *Science* 320, 1647–1651.

Lowry, J.B. (1989) Green-leaf fractionation by fruit bats: is this feeding behaviour a unique nutritional strategy for herbivores? *Australian Wildlife Research* 16, 203–206.

McArthur, C., Hagerman, C.T. and Robbins, C.T. (1991) Physiological strategies of mammalian herbivores against plant defences. In: Palo, R.T. and Robbins, C.T. (eds) *Plant Defenses Against Mammalian Herbivory*. CRC Press, Boca Raton, Florida, pp. 103–114.

McArthur, C., Robbins, C.T., Hagerman, A.E. and Hanley, T.A. (1993) Diet selection by a ruminant generalist browser in relation to plant chemistry. *Canadian Journal of Zoology* 71, 2236–2243.

Orpin, C.G. (1975) Studies on the rumen flagellate *Neocallimastix frontalis*. *Journal of General Microbiology* 91, 249–262.

Perez-Barberia, F.J., Elston, D.A., Gordon, I.J. and Illius, A.W. (2004) The evolution of phylogenetic differences in the efficiency of digestion in ruminants. *Proceedings of the Royal Society of London B* 271, 1081–1090.

Rasmussen, M.A., Carlson, S.A., Franklin, S.K., McCuddin, Z.P., Wu, M.T. and Sharma, V.K. (2005) Exposure to rumen protozoa leads to enhancement of pathogenicity of and invasion by multiple antibiotic-resistant *Salmonella enterica* bearing SGI1. *Infection and Immunity* 73, 4668–4675.

Robbins, C.T., Spalinger, D.E. and Van Hoven, W. (1995) Adaptations of ruminants to browse and grass diets: are anatomical-based browser-grazer interpretations valid? *Oecologia* 103, 208–213.

Rowell-Schafer, A., Lechner-Doll, M., Hofmann, R.R., Streich, W.J., Guven, B. and Meyer, H.H.D. (2001) Metabolic evidence of a 'rumen bypass' or a 'ruminal escape' of nutrients in roe deer (*Capreolus capreolus*). *Comparative Biochemistry and Physiology Part A: Molecular and Integrative Physiology* 128(2), 289–298.

Russo, S.L., Shenk, J.S., Barnes, R.F. and Moore, J.E. (1981) The weanling meadow vole as a bioassay of forage quality of temperate and tropical grasses. *Journal of Animal Science* 52, 1205–1210.

Schurg, W.A., Frei, D.L., Cheeke, P.R. and Holtan, D.W. (1977) Utilization of whole corn plant pellets by horses and rabbits. *Journal of Animal Science* 45, 1317–1321.

Shenk, J.S., Elliott, F.C. and Thomas, J.W. (1971) Meadow vole nutrition studies with alfalfa diets. *Journal of Nutrition* 101, 1367–1372.

Shipley, L.A. and Felicetti, L. (2002) Fibre digestibility and nitrogen requirements of blue duikers (*Cephalophus monticola*). *Zoo Biology* 21, 123–134.

Simpson, G.G. (1945) The principles of classification and a classification of mammals. *Bulletin of the American Museum of Natural History* 85, 1–350.

Stevens, C.E. and Hume, I.D. (1995) *Comparative Physiology of the Vertebrate Digestive System*, 2nd edn. Cambridge University Press, Cambridge.

Stevens, C.E. and Hume, I.D. (1998) Contributions of microbes in vertebrate gastrointestinal tract to production and conservation of nutrients. *Physiological Reviews* 78, 393–427.

Ullrey, D.E. (1986) Nutrition of primates in captivity. In: Benirschke, K. (ed.) *Primates. The Road to Self-Sustaining Populations.* Springer-Verlag, New York, pp. 823–835.

Van Soest, P.J. (1994) *Nutritional Ecology of the Ruminant.* Cornell University Press, Ithaca, New York.

Van Soest, P.J. (1996) Allometry and ecology of feeding behavior and digestive capacity in herbivores: a review. *Zoo Biology* 15, 455–479.

PART II
Protein, Amino Acid and Nitrogen Metabolism

This part discusses the structure, function, digestion and metabolism of proteins and their constituent amino acids.

Part Objectives

1. To describe the structure and properties of proteins and amino acids.
2. To discuss the digestion of proteins in autoenzymatic and alloenzymatic digesters.
3. To describe the metabolism of amino acids, including the formation of various metabolites.

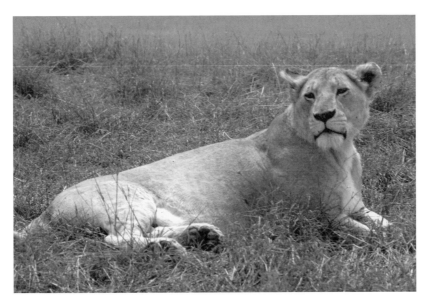

Members of the cat family have some unique aspects of protein metabolism, reflecting their carnivorous feeding behaviour.

4 Protein and Amino Acid Structures and Properties

A consideration of protein and amino acid metabolism is fundamental to the study of animal nutrition. Much of the structure of animal tissue is proteinaceous, metabolic reactions are catalysed by proteins (enzymes) and protein synthesis is intimately linked with the genetic code and the metabolism of DNA.

Proteins are macromolecules built up of building blocks (basic units) called **amino acids**. The biological properties of a protein are determined by the amino acids it contains, the sequence in which they are linked together, and the spatial relationships among amino acids within the protein molecule.

Structures and Chemical Properties of Amino Acids

There are over 300 amino acids known to exist in the plant world (perhaps as many as 900; see Chapter 1), but only about 20 of these are important constituents of animal proteins or function in animal metabolism. Some amino acids, such as ornithine and citrulline, have important roles in animal metabolism but are not used in protein synthesis. They are known as **non-protein amino acids**. In addition, some proteins contain additional amino acids that are formed by modification of an amino acid already in a peptide (e.g. cystine, hydroxyproline, hydroxylysine).

All amino acids by definition contain at least one amino group ($-NH_2$) and one carboxyl group ($-COOH$). (An exception is proline, which is an **imino acid**, lacking a free amino group.) The amino acids important in animal proteins are **alpha (α)-amino acids**, which are carboxylic acids with an amino group on the α-carbon. (The α-carbon is the first carbon attached to a functional group – in this case, the carboxylic acid group.) The general structure of an α-amino acid is shown in Fig. 4.1.

The R-group represents any other chemical group found in the structure. For example, in glycine, R is a hydrogen atom; in alanine, it is a methyl group ($-CH_3$), while in methionine it is $-CH_2-CH_2-S-CH_3$. A list of the amino acids important in animal nutrition and metabolism and their chemical structures is given in Fig. 4.2. In biological systems, the amino acids are ionized with either the amino group as $-NH_3^+$ or the carboxyl group as $-COO^-$, depending upon the pH. In some cases, both groups are ionized.

An additional amino acid used in protein synthesis, not shown in Fig. 4.2, is **selenocysteine**. It has selenium in place of the sulfur in cysteine. It is sometimes called 'the 21st amino acid'. It occurs at the active site of selenium-containing enzymes, including glutathione peroxidase and deiodinases.

Amino acids can exist in two isomeric forms, the **D- and L-isomers**. All amino acids except glycine contain an asymmetric α-carbon (four different chemical groups attached to it). Compounds with **asymmetric carbons** can exist as isomers, which rotate the plane of polarized light in opposite directions. D-isomers (dextrorotary) rotate the plane of polarized light to the right, while L-isomers (levorotary) rotate it to the left. Only the L-amino acids are used in protein synthesis. In some cases, such as methionine, animals can convert the D-isomer to the L form, whereas in other cases (e.g. lysine), they cannot. Thus DL-methionine is used as a feed additive but lysine is available only as L-lysine.

The D- and L-amino acid isomers differ in their configuration of groups around the asymmetric α-carbon. Consider D- and L-alanine (Fig. 4.3).

Imagine the carbon chain to be in the plane of the paper, while the $-NH_2$ and $-H$ groups are either sticking out towards you (to the left) or through the other side of the paper (to the right). These two isomeric forms (when considered in three-dimensional configuration, i.e. without lifting from the plane of the paper) cannot be superimposed on each other (they are mirror images), and so have distinct chemical, physical and biological properties.

The particular properties of individual amino acids reflect the nature of the R group. Where the side chain is non-ionized (e.g. in leucine) or aromatic (e.g. phenylalanine), the amino acids are non-polar,

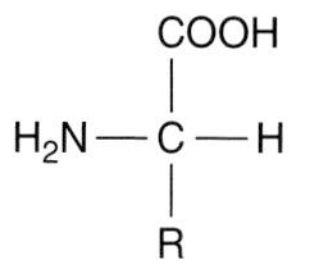

Fig. 4.1. General structure of an α-amino acid.

whereas if the side chain contains ionized groups, they will be polar (e.g. glutamic acid). The sulfhydryl group (–SH) of cysteine and the alcohol group (–OH) of serine are nucleophilic (nucleophiles are electron-rich molecules) and function at the active sites of enzymes to facilitate catalysis.

Essential amino acids

Essential amino acids are those which are **dietary essentials** for one or more species of animals. The list of essential amino acids varies somewhat according to species (chicken versus pig versus human) and age (e.g. chick versus adult hen), but as a generalization, the amino acids commonly referred to as essential are:

- arginine;
- histidine;
- isoleucine;
- leucine;
- tryptophan;
- lysine;
- methionine;
- phenylalanine;
- threonine; and
- valine.

Various memorization aids have been devised by students, such as 'Any Help In Learning Ten Little Molecules Proves Truly Valuable' (used in compiling the above list). Another memory jogger is 'Matt Hill, VP'.

The essential amino acids are essential in the diet of autoenzymatic digesters such as pigs and poultry. Ruminant animals do not generally have a dietary requirement for these amino acids because they are synthesized by rumen microorganisms. The situation in non-ruminant herbivores is variable; in some cases, as in horses, essential amino acids are required in the diet, whereas in other animals, such as rabbits, the dietary requirements are influenced by bacterially synthesized amino acids made available to the animal via coprophagy or caecotrophy. The role of microbial synthesis in obviating dietary requirements will be discussed further in Chapter 5.

Proteins and Protein Structure

Proteins consist of chains of amino acids linked together by peptide bonds. A **peptide bond** is formed by reaction of the α-amino group of one amino acid with the α-carboxyl group of another. Consider the reaction between glutamic acid and lysine to form a dipeptide (Fig. 4.4).

The peptide bond is the amide bond between the C and the N in the shaded portion. Note that it is the amino and carboxyl groups on the α-carbons, not those on the side chains, which function in peptide bond formation. By convention, peptide structures are written with the N-terminal group on the left and the carboxyl group on the right. A molecule of metabolic water is formed with each peptide bond. A **dipeptide** contains one peptide bond and two amino acids. If an additional amino acid is added, a **tripeptide** is formed. A peptide with more than ten amino acid residues is called a **polypeptide**. A protein is essentially a large polypeptide; arbitrarily a polypeptide with a molecular weight above 8000 is termed a protein. The size of large molecules can also be expressed in **daltons**. One dalton is the mass of a single hydrogen ion. A protein molecule composed only of amino acids is called a **simple protein**, while **complex proteins** contain additional constituents such as haem (e.g. haemoglobin), carbohydrate (glycoproteins) and lipid (lipoproteins).

The structure of a protein is determined first by the sequence of amino acids it contains. This is the **primary** *structure*. **Disulfide bonds** (–S–S–) are considered part of the primary structure. These are very important in keratin protein. The bonds are formed between the sulfhydryl (–SH) groups in non-adjacent cysteines, producing a new intramolecular amino acid, cystine (Fig. 4.5). In this hypothetical example, a polypeptide chain of 90 amino acids is shown. Amino acids 25 and 74 in the chain are cysteine, so they are non-adjacent (separated in the chain by 49 amino acids). In the formation of the polypeptide, the primary chain has folded so that the sulfhydryl groups of the non-adjacent cysteine molecules can react to produce a new amino acid, cystine, containing the disulfide bond. These bonds account for the tough physical properties of keratins (e.g. feathers, hair, wool, hoof, horn) and their low digestibility. The waviness or 'crimp' of wool fibres is formed by disulfide bonds of cystine. Disulfide bonds are also important in joining together two or more polypeptide chains which make up polypeptide hormones, such as insulin (Fig. 4.6).

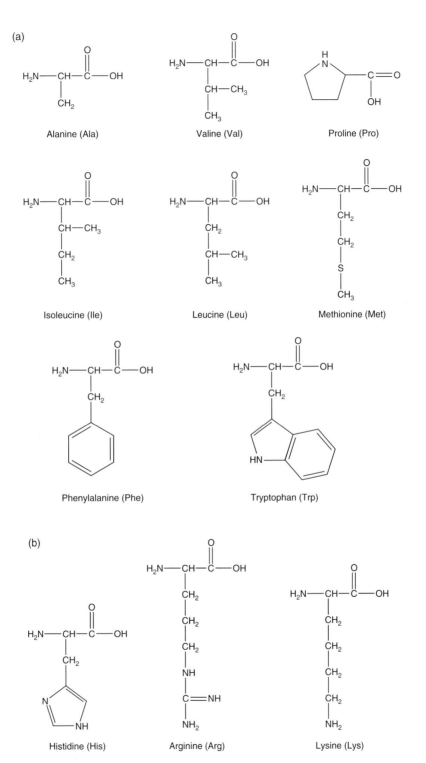

Fig. 4.2. Names and structures of essential and non-essential amino acids that participate in protein synthesis. (a) Non-polar (hydrophobic) amino acids. (b) Basic amino acids.

Continued

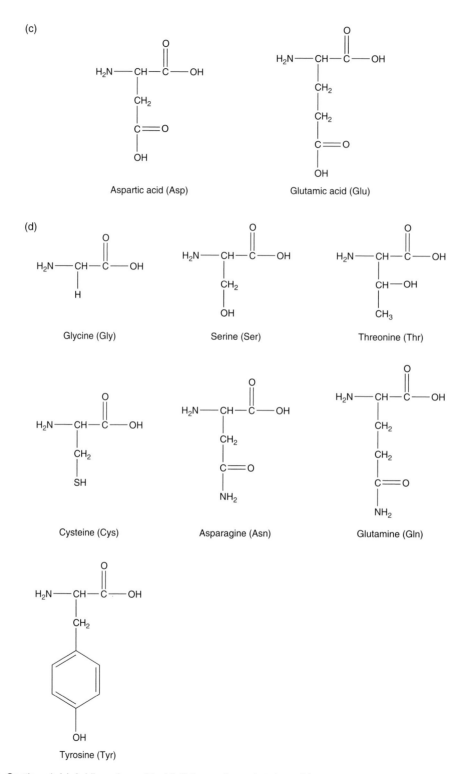

Fig. 4.2. Continued. (c) Acidic amino acids. (d) Polar, uncharged amino acids.

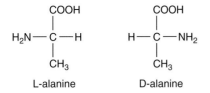

Fig. 4.3. L- and D-alanine.

The **secondary** *structure* of proteins relates to further types of interactions which give the protein molecule a particular shape. These include hydrogen bonds, electrostatic bonds and hydrophobic attraction (the side chains of non-polar amino acids tend to attract each other in an aqueous medium). Some proteins exist in a helical arrangement, such as the α-helix structure of hair and wool (keratins). The helix configuration is considered to be a secondary structural feature.

The disruption of the secondary structure is called **denaturation**. Heat treatment, acids, bases, detergents, and various other procedures may cause protein denaturation. Various toxic proteins, such as trypsin inhibitors and lectins in beans, can be denatured by heat treatment.

Chaperones are proteins that participate in the folding of proteins to create secondary bonds. Many are classified as **heat shock proteins**, so named because their expression is increased when cells are exposed to elevated temperatures or other stresses, including infection and inflammation. They bind to hydrophobic portions of unfolded and unaggregated proteins, providing a sheltered environment which allows for the formation of secondary bonds which produce folding. Chaperones prevent faulty folding and unproductive interactions of proteins. Inappropriate folding of proteins occurs in **prion diseases** (e.g. mad cow disease) and in **Alzheimer's disease**.

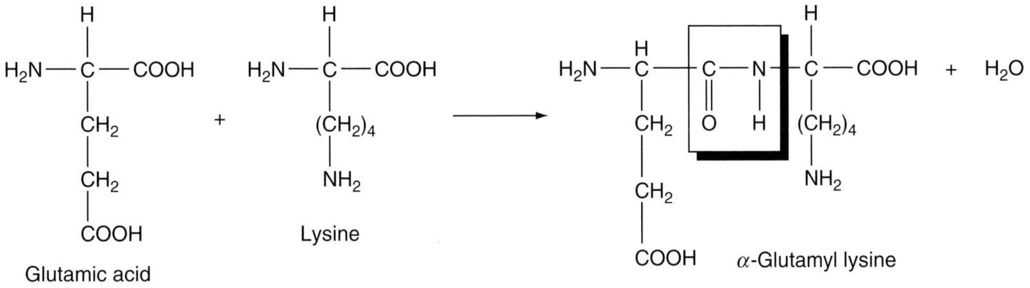

Fig. 4.4. Reaction between glutamic acid and lysine to form a dipeptide.

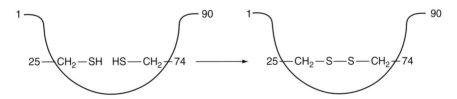

Fig. 4.5. Bonds form between sulfhydryl (–SH) groups in non-adjacent cysteines, producing a new intramolecular amino acid, cystine (see text for explanation).

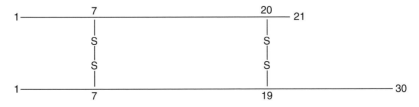

Fig. 4.6. Disulfide bonds join together two polypeptide chains which make up polypeptide hormones, such as insulin.

Classification of Proteins

Proteins have been classified in various ways, according to their solubilities, shape and function. The following list provides a classification of proteins commonly encountered in animal nutrition.

I. Globular proteins (spherical shape)
   A. Albumins
- soluble in water
- coagulated by heat
- e.g. egg albumen, serum albumin (note difference in spelling of the two types)

   B. Globulins
- sparingly soluble in water; soluble in salt solutions
- coagulated by heat
- e.g. serum globulins, glycinin in soybeans

   C. Glutelins
- insoluble in water; soluble in dilute acid or base
- e.g. glutenin in wheat

   D. Prolamines
- insoluble in water; soluble in 70–80% ethanol
- e.g. zein (maize), gliadin (wheat), hordein (barley); prolamines are storage proteins in grains
- low in lysine content

II. Fibrous proteins
   A. Collagens
- insoluble in water
- converted to **gelatin** by boiling in water or dilute acid or base
- contain a high content of hydroxyproline and some hydroxylysine, which function in cross-linking of collagen fibres; complete absence of cysteine, cystine and tryptophan
- e.g. the major protein of skeletal muscle; constitutes over 50% of total body protein

   B. Elastins
- similar to collagen but cannot be converted to gelatin
- constitute the major protein in elastic tissues
- e.g. tendons, arteries

   C. Keratins
- very insoluble and indigestible
- contain very high content of cystine
- the proteins of hair, wool, feathers, claws, nails, beak, hoofs, horns and antlers

III. Conjugated proteins
   A. Nucleoproteins
- combined with nucleic acids in cell nucleus

   B. Mucoproteins
- combined with carbohydrate (mucopolysaccharide) to form mucus

   C. Glycoproteins
- contain less than 4% carbohydrate
- e.g. egg albumen

   D. Lipoproteins
- water-soluble proteins conjugated with lipid or phospholipid
- e.g. lipoproteins of blood

   E. Chromoproteins
- simple proteins combined with a coloured prosthetic group
- e.g. haemoglobin, cytochromes, flavoproteins (FAD, FMN), visual purple, catalase

---

Questions and Study Guide

1. How many amino acids are there?
2. Is proline an amino acid?
3. What is an alpha- (α-) carbon?
4. Why does glycine not exist as D-glycine and L-glycine?
5. What causes an amino acid to be polar (e.g. glutamic acid) or non-polar (e.g. leucine)?
6. Name the ten essential amino acids.
7. What is the difference between an 'essential' and a 'non-essential' amino acid?
8. How many peptide bonds are there in a tripeptide?
9. What amino acid contains (a) a sulfhydryl group and (b) a disulfide bond?
10. Draw the structure of a tripeptide of lysine, glutamic acid and cysteine.
11. What is the difference between keratin and carotene?
12. What causes the waviness or 'crimp' of wool?
13. Heating of proteins causes them to denature. What does this mean?
14. (a) Where does albumin occur? (b) Where do you find albumen?
15. Where does gelatin come from?

5 Protein Digestion

Autoenzymatic Digestion in Simple Non-Ruminants

Digestion is the preparation of ingested material for absorption. In the case of proteins, digestion involves denaturing the protein to expose peptide bonds so they can be split through hydrolysis of the amide bonds into the component amino acids. Free amino acids are the main absorbed compounds, although there is some absorption of small peptides. Protein digesting enzymes are either endopeptidases or exopeptidases. **Endopeptidases** hydrolyse peptide bonds within the primary protein structure, and break a protein into smaller fragments, the polypeptides. **Exopeptidases** cleave amino acids off the terminal end of the protein molecule. **Carboxypeptidases** remove an amino acid from the end with a free carboxyl group, while **aminopeptidases** act on the terminal amino acid with a free amino group.

Protein digestion begins in the stomach with the secretion of **pepsinogen** from chief cells in the gastric mucosa. Pepsinogen is activated to the active enzyme, **pepsin**, by HCl secreted from parietal cells in the gastric mucosa. The activation process involves splitting off a protective polypeptide to expose active pepsin. Pepsin is an endopeptidase, specific for peptide bonds between aromatic (e.g. tyrosine, phenylalanine) or dicarboxylic (e.g. glutamic acid, aspartic acid) amino acids.

In the suckling animal, a milk-coagulating enzyme, **rennin** (chymosin, rennet) is secreted into the stomach. Rennin in the presence of calcium causes casein to coagulate or clot. Clot formation is generally considered useful in reducing the rate at which milk protein exits the stomach into the small intestine. In young calves, formation of an abomasal curd consisting of casein protein and milk fat slows the release of milk from the abomasum to the small intestine, but this process does not seem to be essential in this species, as good calf performance can be achieved with milk replacers containing non-clotting proteins (Longenbach and Heinrichs, 1998). Milk clotting is essential for numerous other species (e.g. rabbits).

The major site of protein digestion is the small intestine. Proteins and polypeptides that exit from the stomach are digested to release free amino acids and small peptides that are absorbed. A major source of the intestinal proteolytic enzymes is the pancreas. The pancreas secretes three endopeptidases secreted in a zymogen form: trypsinogen, chymotrypsinogen and proelastase, which are activated in the intestine to produce trypsin, chymotrypsin and elastase, respectively. **Trypsin** is specific for peptide bonds with basic amino acids while **chymotrypsin** is specific for bonds involving non-charged aromatic amino acids. **Elastase** is a protease with broad specificity, including the capacity to digest elastin. Elastin is the second major protein (besides collagen) in connective tissue.

Many plants contain inhibitors of pancreatic proteolytic enzymes. The best known is raw soybeans (Cheeke, 1998). Soybeans (and many other legume seeds and nuts) contain large protein molecules that combine irreversibly with trypsin and chymotrypsin. Instead of being able to break the **trypsin inhibitors** apart, the trypsin is bound to the inhibitor and excreted. This reduces protein digestibility because of the tie-up of trypsin, and creates an amino acid deficiency from the increased excretion of trypsin. The pancreas gland enlarges in an attempt to produce more trypsin to overcome its inactivation in the gut. Trypsin inhibitors are inactivated by heat treatment; all commercial soybean meal products are routinely prepared with adequate heating to inactivate trypsin inhibitors.

The secretions of some of the cells lining the intestinal villi contain digestive enzymes, including aminopeptidases and carboxypeptidases. These enzymes complete the process of protein digestion in the brush border of the villi. The free amino acids are liberated in the vicinity of the microvilli where they are readily absorbed. Amino acids are absorbed by **active transport** mechanisms. Active transport is an energy-requiring process, with the amino acid temporarily attached to a carrier protein to transport the amino acids from the intestinal cell outer membrane to the circulatory system within the villus. The active transport systems are usually coupled to a sodium-potassium pump which maintains an electrical potential difference. Although free amino acids are the primary absorbed end product of protein digestion, there is significant absorption of di-, tri- and oligopeptides. Free amino acids are absorbed by sodium-dependent active transport, with several different transport proteins specific for the nature of the amino acid side chains (large, small, neutral, acidic, basic). Dipeptides and tripeptides that enter the mucosal cells are hydrolysed to free amino acids intracellularly. Relatively large peptides that are absorbed intact may stimulate antibody formation, causing food allergies.

Nitrogen metabolism in the hindgut

Nitrogenous substances not fully digested in the small intestine enter the hindgut, where they are subjected to microbial action. Bacterial fermentation of amino acids produces odiferous compounds responsible for the characteristic odour of faeces. Many amino acids undergo decarboxylation by intestinal bacteria to produce toxic amines (**ptomaines**) (Fig. 5.1). Examples include cadaverine, putrescine, tyramine and histamine (Fig. 5.2).

Several of these amines have powerful pharmacological effects, including vasopressor activity (vascular constriction causing increased blood pressure or hypertension). For example, absorbed histamine is implicated in causing **laminitis** in horses and cattle, by affecting the blood vessels in the hoof (see Chapter 19). **Polyamines** such as putrescine, cadaverine and spermidine are promoters of cell division, protein synthesis and tissue growth. Dietary polyamines can partially alleviate the toxic effects of raw soybeans, probably by reversing the

adverse effects of lectins on the intestinal cells (Mogridge *et al.*, 1996). Putrescine also has beneficial effects on prevention of and recovery from coccidiosis in poultry (Girdhar *et al.*, 2006). This response is due to the favourable effects of polyamines on the growth of the intestinal epithelium, facilitating recovery from coccidian-induced intestinal lesions.

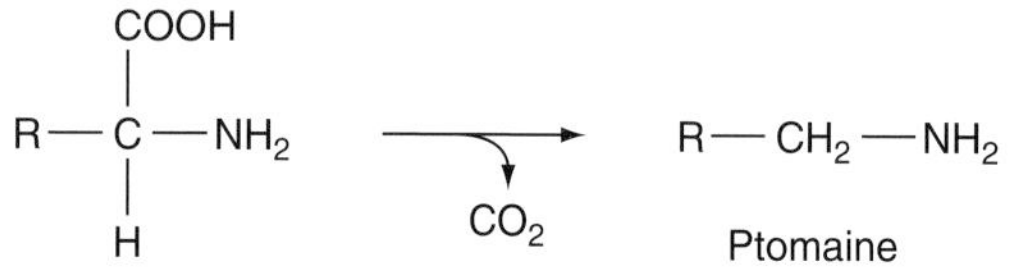

There is microbial metabolism of various other amino acids in the hindgut, producing foul-smelling compounds that contribute to the **faecal odour**. For example, the indole group of tryptophan is converted to **skatole** (3-methyl indole) (Fig. 5.3). Absorbed skatole is implicated in off-flavours of pork from intact male pigs (boar taint) (see Chapter 6).

Faecal odour is characteristic of animal species, for example pig, sheep, human and dog faeces – each have their own characteristic odour. Probably this is related to the characteristic hindgut microflora of each species, as well as the nature of the diet. Faeces of carnivores are more odiferous than those of herbivores, as amusingly related in the following poem:

> Protein Foundation
>
> How inoffensive are the feces
> Of all the graminivorous species
> That grind on grain and graze on grasses,
> Like sheep and horses, mules and asses,
> Or, practiced in regurgitation,
> Spend idle hours in rumination.
> Such are the cows, the goats, the camels
> And other ungulated mammals.
> But ah, how offal they excrete
> Who pry their protein needs from meat
> From chops and steaks and, yes, from cheeses
> And pork and everything that pleases
> From sulfurous eggs and oily fishes
> And all the highly seasoned dishes;
> Such is the orduous part of man
> Devoted to his frying pan.
>
> (van Soest, 1994)

The sulfur-containing amino acid cysteine undergoes microbial transformations to form **mercaptans**[1] (ethyl mercaptan, methyl mercaptan) and hydrogen sulfide (H_2S) (Fig. 5.4). **Phenols** are produced from the aromatic amino acids tyrosine and phenylalanine.

A large amount of **ammonia** is also produced by microbial metabolism in the hindgut. Ammonia is readily absorbed, and detoxified in the liver by conversion to urea.

Fig. 5.1. Many amino acids undergo decarboxylation by intestinal bacteria to produce ptomaines.

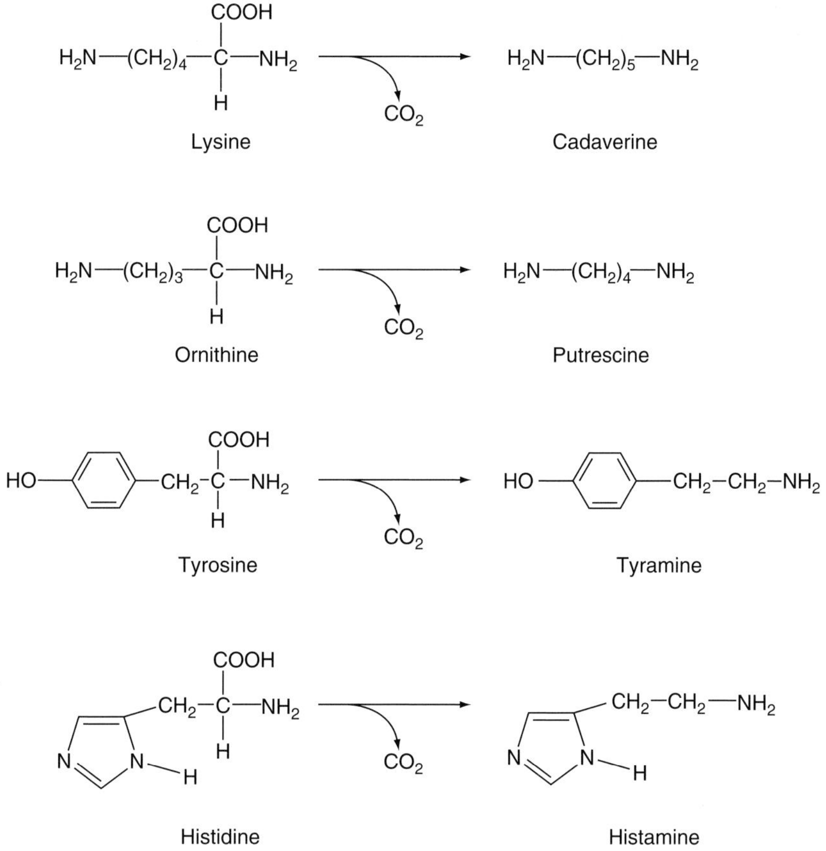

Fig. 5.2. The most common ptomaines are cadaverine, putrescine, tyramine and histamine.

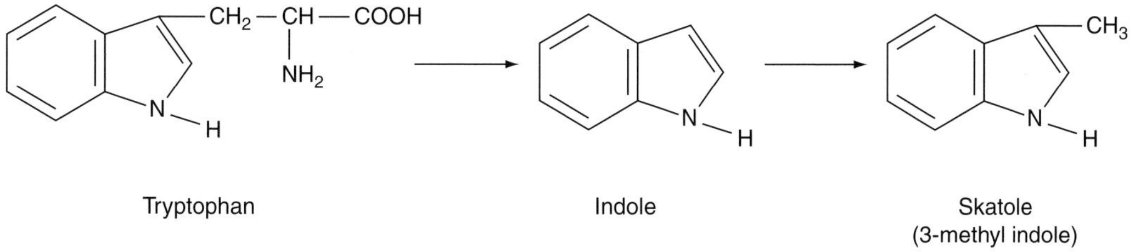

Fig. 5.3. The indole group of tryptophan is converted to skatole (3-methyl indole).

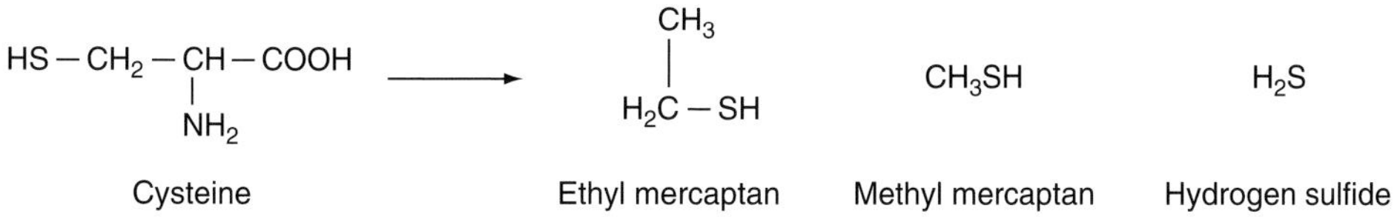

Fig. 5.4. Cysteine undergoes microbial transformations to form ethyl mercaptan, methyl mercaptan and hydrogen sulfide.

The formation of odiferous compounds by microbial metabolism of amino acids has important implications in animal production. The development of large confinement pig production facilities in the USA is very controversial, in large part because of the offensive nature of pig faecal odour. Balancing diets to provide highly digestible protein sources, minimizing entry of protein and amino acids to the hindgut, is one means of reducing faecal odour. Diet formulation to minimize odours is facilitated by using **ileal digestibility** values. These are obtained in digestibility trials in which the excreta is collected from the terminus of the ileum (using surgically-cannulated animals) rather than the traditional means of collecting faeces (total tract digestibility).

Protein Digestion in Ruminants

Protein digestion in ruminants can be subdivided into two phases: (i) alloenzymatic digestion in the stomach (reticulorumen); and (ii) autoenzymatic digestion in the abomasum and small intestine. A third, minor phase is alloenzymatic digestion in the hindgut. More so than in the simple monogastrics, protein digestion in ruminants is more or less synonymous with nitrogen metabolism, because of the ability of rumen microbes to utilize inorganic nitrogen (e.g. ammonia). Generally, in studies of protein metabolism, the fate of dietary protein is assessed by analysis of nitrogen (N intake, faecal N, urinary N, retained N, etc.). In other words, the metabolic fate of protein can be followed by tracking the fate of nitrogen.

Nitrogen metabolism in the rumen

Proteins and other nitrogenous compounds can be digested (degraded) in the rumen by **rumen microorganisms (RMO)**, with the conversion of dietary protein to microbial protein. The rumen microbes (mainly bacteria) synthesize proteins which are ultimately used by the host animal when the microbes are digested. It is important to bear in mind that the synthetic activities of the RMO are for their own benefit; there is not a higher calling that they are doing anything to benefit the host. The RMO have fortuitously found themselves in an environment that is warm, moist and anaerobic, with a continual influx of food and a continual removal of their waste products. Fortunately for the ruminant, it benefits from these 'parasites' by being able to digest them and utilize them as a source of protein.

Dietary protein can either be fermented in the rumen, or can bypass rumen fermentation and be digested in the small intestine. Several factors influence the rumen **degradability** of proteins, such as their solubility, and nature of their physical structure. Protein denaturation, such as by heat treatment, decreases degradability. Rumen bacteria produce proteases and peptidases that digest proteins. These enzymes are normally elaborated on to feed particles after the bacteria have attached to them, rather than being secreted into the rumen fluid. Amino acids and peptides are taken up by the bacterial cells at the point of their liberation from the protein, at the site of microbial attachment.

The majority of amino acids taken up by RMO are not used directly for protein synthesis, but are deaminated and used as energy sources, giving rise to ammonia, branched-chain VFAs, carbon dioxide and methane.

Rumen ammonia occupies a central role in nitrogen metabolism in the rumen. Ammonia is the nitrogenous end product of bacterial fermentation of dietary protein. It is also the starting point for microbial synthesis of bacterial amino acids and proteins. Most rumen bacteria synthesize their amino acids 'from scratch', with ammonia as the source of the amino group. Thus rumen bacteria can synthesize protein from any substrate which will yield ammonia in the rumen. **Non-protein nitrogen (NPN)** sources such as urea, biuret and uric acid (from poultry excreta) may be converted by RMO into bacterial protein.

Dietary **urea** is converted to ammonia by bacterial urease (Fig. 5.5).

There is abundant urease in the rumen, so conversion of urea to ammonia occurs very quickly.

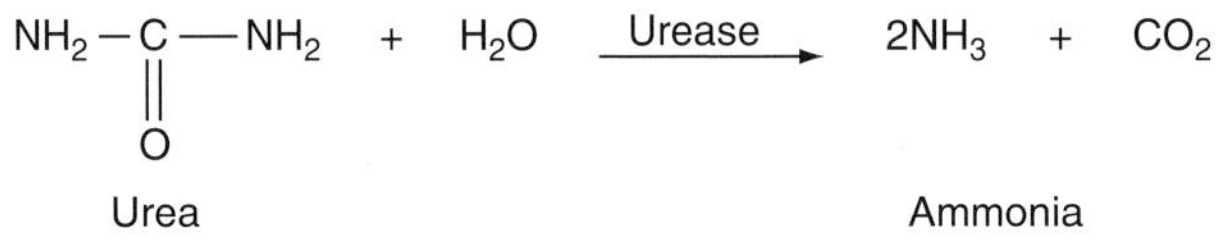

$$NH_2 - \underset{\underset{O}{\|}}{C} - NH_2 \ + \ H_2O \ \xrightarrow{\text{Urease}} \ 2NH_3 \ + \ CO_2$$

Urea   Ammonia

Fig. 5.5. Dietary urea is converted to ammonia by bacterial urease.

For urea to be effectively utilized, it must be converted to microbial protein. Ammonia in excess of what the bacteria can utilize for amino acid synthesis accumulates in the rumen (the ammonia pool), and may be absorbed. Absorption of ammonia is undesirable for several reasons. The nitrogen is of value to the host animal only if converted to microbial protein. Absorbed ammonia must be metabolized in the liver, by being converted to urea by the urea cycle enzymes. This is an energy-requiring process. If the amount of absorbed ammonia exceeds the liver's capacity to detoxify it by converting it to urea, ammonia can enter the general circulation. It is very toxic to the tissues and causes ammonia poisoning.

Urea poisoning occurs when the intake of dietary urea produces so much ammonia that the ability of the liver to detoxify absorbed ammonia is exceeded. Thus urea toxicity is really **ammonia poisoning**. Ammonia is toxic to the central nervous system; signs of poisoning in ruminants include bloat, frothing at the mouth (excessive salivation), staggering and convulsions, coma and death. Ammonia in the brain reacts with glutamic acid to produce glutamine; the drain on the α-ketoglutaric acid needed to form glutamic acid (Fig. 5.6) may affect oxidative metabolism and ATP production, causing the symptoms listed above. The depletion of α-ketoglutarate, an intermediate of the citric acid cycle, reduces ATP formation, leading to deficiency of energy for normal brain metabolism.

Urea poisoning in ruminants can be avoided by limiting dietary urea to one-third or less of the crude protein content of the diet (1 urea = 2.92 crude protein). The ability to efficiently utilize urea depends upon the carbohydrate portion of the diet. **Readily available carbohydrates** (e.g. starch from cereal grains) support rapid growth of rumen bacteria, thus utilizing much of the rumen ammonia. High energy diets supporting rapid fermentation also result in a more acid rumen pH, from the high VFA production rate. Ammonia is absorbed most rapidly in the non-ionized state, as NH_3. Under acidic conditions, it exists primarily as ammonium ion (NH_4^+) which is absorbed more slowly (Fig. 5.7).

Absorbed ammonia is converted to urea in the liver by urea cycle enzymes. The urea is secreted into the blood, and commonly measured and expressed as **blood urea nitrogen** (**BUN**). Blood urea can be recycled to the rumen; thus absorbed ammonia is not necessarily lost from the protein pool. Urea can be filtered from the blood in the salivary glands, and recycled to the rumen via the saliva. It can also diffuse into the rumen across the rumen wall. These processes are referred to as **urea recycling**. In both cattle and sheep, as much as 40–80% of the urea produced by the liver can be recycled to the digestive tract (Lapierre and Lobley, 2001). Urea is

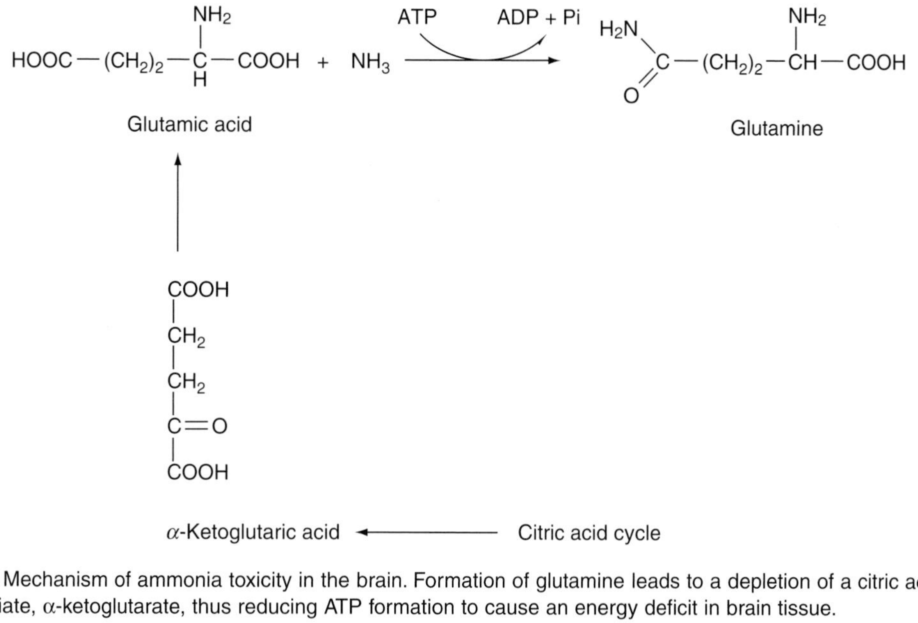

Fig. 5.6. Mechanism of ammonia toxicity in the brain. Formation of glutamine leads to a depletion of a citric acid cycle intermediate, α-ketoglutarate, thus reducing ATP formation to cause an energy deficit in brain tissue.

$$NH_3 \quad + \quad H^+ \rightleftharpoons \quad NH_4^+$$

Ammonia   Ammonium ion

Fig. 5.7. Under acidic conditions ammonia exists primarily as ammonium ion.

transported into the gastrointestinal tract by urea transporters (Simmons *et al.*, 2009), which are transport proteins. Bacteria attached to the rumen wall produce urease, which immediately hydrolyses urea diffusing across the rumen wall. This process maintains a continual concentration gradient favouring diffusion of urea from the blood to the rumen. The BUN not recycled to the rumen is excreted in the urine.

Urea is the major form of excretory nitrogen in mammals. The concentration of BUN in ruminants reflects the efficiency of utilization of dietary crude protein. Urea rapidly equilibrates throughout body fluids, including the milk. Thus, **milk urea nitrogen (MUN)** also may serve as an index of efficiency of protein utilization, particularly in the lactating dairy cow (Broderick and Clayton, 1997). For field-testing purposes, milk samples are easily obtained. Elevated concentrations of BUN are associated with decreased conception rates of dairy cattle. BUN or MUN concentrations exceeding 200 mg/L are indicative of potentially reduced reproductive rates in dairy cattle (Butler *et al.*, 1996).

Biuret is another NPN source, produced by heating urea to a high temperature, which causes two urea molecules to condense to form biuret and ammonia (Fig. 5.8). Biuret is a slow-release form of NPN which is degraded more slowly than urea to ammonia. The RMO produce biuretase, which breaks down biuret to release ammonia. An adaptation period of several weeks may be necessary to induce biuretase production by rumen microbes. Biuret theoretically may be more effective than urea as a nitrogen supplement in roughage-based diets because of its slower degradation rate. This maintains rumen ammonia concentrations for a longer period, supporting microbial growth during the prolonged interval required for fibre digestion.

However, the data do not always support this contention (Oltjen *et al.*, 1969). Biuret is not commonly used at present, probably because of a lack of commercial sources.

Another NPN source is **dried poultry waste (DPW)**, which is poultry excreta. DPW is rich in uric acid, the main nitrogenous excretory product of birds. The RMO can degrade uric acid to release ammonia. The structure of uric acid is shown in Fig. 5.9.

About 50% of the soluble protein in plant leaves is a single protein involved in photosynthesis, called ribulose-1,5-biphosphate carboxyl/oxygenase (**Rubisco**). It was formerly called Fraction 1 protein, and is considered the most abundant protein in nature. Rubisco catalyses the photosynthetic reaction by which carbon dioxide is taken up by leaves to form two molecules of phosphoglyceric acid (a constituent of the glycolysis pathway) which can be converted to glucose. Because Rubisco is identical in all green plants, and is the major protein in plants, it follows that the protein quality of all forages is quite similar. Because of the high quality (balance of essential amino acids) of Rubisco, it increases the performance (growth, wool production, lactation) of ruminants if the Rubisco bypasses rumen fermentation. Condensed tannins in some temperate forages (e.g. trefoils) reduce Rubisco fermentation by reversible binding; the protein is bound in the rumen but is released in the small intestine (Min *et al.*, 2000, 2003).

Post-ruminal protein digestion

Protein reaching the small intestine is either dietary protein that has escaped or bypassed rumen fermentation, or the microbial protein associated with rumen bacteria and protozoa. The amino acid requirements of the host animal are provided by the amino acids liberated from escape (non-degradable) protein and microbial protein.

Microbial protein

The **microbial nitrogen** is a mixture of true protein (about 60–70% of total N) and non-protein

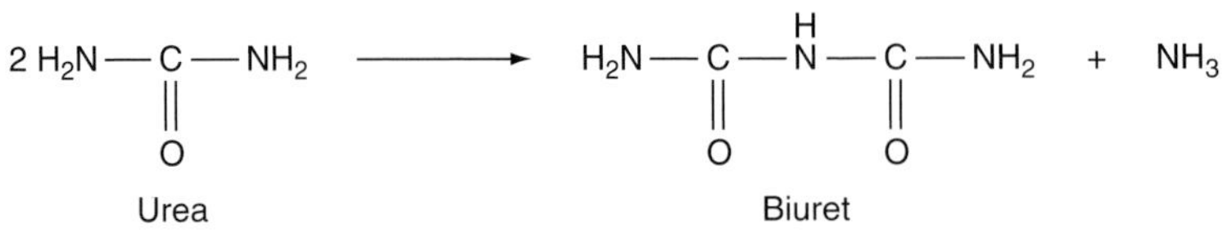

Fig. 5.8. At high temperatures two urea molecules condense to form biuret and ammonia.

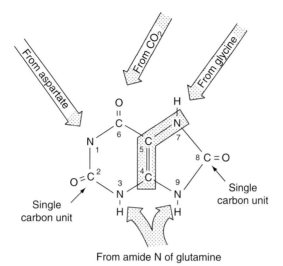

Fig. 5.9. Structure of uric acid and the metabolic origin of each atom (courtesy of University Books, Guelph, Canada.)

nitrogen such as that in bacterial amino acids and indigestible cell wall components (peptidoglycans). As microbial protein outflows from the rumen, the microbes are killed in the highly acidic abomasum. There is some acid hydrolysis and breakdown of the microbes. Microbial cell walls are composed of substituted glucosamine (muramic acid) polymers with attached peptides (Van Soest, 1994). Bacterial cell walls contain a unique amino acid, **diaminopimelic acid**. **Aminoethyl-phosphoric acid** is an amino acid unique to protozoa. These amino acids can be measured to estimate quantities of microbial protein. Microbes have a high content of nucleic acid, because of their high reproductive rate. Ruminants secrete **pancreatic ribonuclease**, which liberates purine and pyrimidine nucleotides in the intestine.

Microbial protein contains sufficient essential amino acids for maintenance and survival of ruminants. However, for the high rates of growth and lactation demanded in modern ruminant production systems, microbial protein is deficient in several amino acids including methionine and lysine. **Rumen-protected amino acids** are commercially available, encapsulated in pH-sensitive polymers that remain intact in the rumen but which dissolve in the highly acidic abomasum.

In ruminants, much of the absorbed amino acid fraction is actually absorbed in the form of di- and tripeptides (Webb *et al.*, 1992), which are converted to free amino acids after absorption. The nutritional significance of peptide absorption is unclear.

Bypass, escape, non-degradable proteins and amino acids

Microbial protein has a less favourable amino acid balance than many dietary proteins. Thus, in many cases, protein would be used more efficiently if it 'bypassed' rumen fermentation and went directly to the small intestine for digestion by the animal itself. The terms **bypass**, **escape** and **non-degradable** protein are used synonymously. There has been much interest in attempting to determine the bypass potential of protein supplements, however, total success has not been achieved to date. There is a great deal of variability in experimental values both within and among feedstuffs. Among grains, maize has the greatest bypass protein potential (Table 5.1). However, the quality (amino acid profile) of the maize protein is low. Maize protein is deficient in two of the amino acids, lysine and methionine, that are most important in a bypass protein. High-lysine maize is a good source of bypass lysine and also methionine; feedlot cattle fed high-lysine maize show improved performance over those fed normal maize (Ladely *et al.*, 1995). This result was attributed to improved energy utilization and not to the additional lysine. Some of the animal protein sources have the greatest bypass potential; blood meal, meat meal, and fish meal are among the highest in non-degradable protein content as well as

Table 5.1. Estimates of bypass protein content of common feedstuffs (adapted from National Research Council, 1985).

Feedstuff	Non-degradability (%)[a]	Feedstuff	Non-degradability (%)[a]
Grains		*By-product feeds*	
Barley	21	Blood meal	82
Maize	65	Brewers' dried grains	53
Sorghum	52	Maize gluten meal	55
Lupin	35	Distillers' dried grains	62
Oil meals		Fish meal	80
Cottonseed (solvent)	41	Meat meal	76
Soybean	28	Meat and bone meal	60
Linseed	44	*Forages*	
Groundnut (peanut)	30	Lucerne hay	28
Rapeseed	23	Dehydrated lucerne	62
Sunflower	24	Bromegrass hay	32
		Maize silage	27
		Timothy hay	42
		Subterranean clover (immature)	27

[a]Percentage of total crude protein that escapes rumen fermentation.

being of high protein quality. Drying of forages (e.g. dehydrated lucerne) increases their bypass potential because of the denaturation of soluble cytoplasmic leaf proteins. Methods of estimating rumen-undegraded protein have been described by the National Research Council (1985).

Treatment of proteins with **formaldehyde** or **tannins** renders them partially resistant to digestion in the rumen without impairing intestinal digestion. **Heat treatment** of protein sources increases their bypass potential. Soybean meal (Coenen and Trenkle, 1989) and cottonseed meal (Goetsch and Owens, 1985) prepared by the mechanical expeller or screw-press process, in which considerable heat is generated, have greater bypass activity than those prepared by solvent extraction. Controlled **non-enzymatic browning**, by reacting soybean meal with xylose in the presence of heat, increased the flow of undegraded protein to the small intestine (Cleale *et al.*, 1987) and may offer potential as a processing method to improve bypass activity of proteins.

Mir *et al.* (1984b) compared several methods of treating soybean and canola proteins to decrease their degradation in the rumen. Treatment with formaldehyde can cause overprotection of the protein, reducing its digestibility in the small intestine. (Because of potential carcinogenic effects, formaldehyde treatment of proteins in many countries, including the USA, is not permitted.) Sodium

hydroxide (2 g/100 g dry matter) was effective in reducing ruminal degradation of protein. Sodium hydroxide treatment of proteins may result in crosslinkages between amino acids in proteins, thus protecting them from microbial attack (Mir *et al.*, 1984b). These workers also found that treatment of proteins with whole blood protected them from rumen degradation, possibly by coating the protein sources and providing a physical barrier to microbial action (blood protein is not easily degraded in the rumen). A similar but lesser effect was achieved by using fish hydrolysate, which also has a high resistance to rumen degradation. Feeding trials with dairy cattle confirmed that treatment of dietary proteins with sodium hydroxide and fresh blood improved protein utilization and increased milk production (Mir *et al.*, 1984a). Another means of protecting proteins from rumen digestion is to coat them with calcium soaps of long-chain fatty acids (rumen inert fats); this procedure supplies both bypass protein and energy (Sklan, 1989).

Lysine and methionine are the two major amino acids that are often limiting in the amino acids absorbed from the intestine. Besides supplementing high-performing ruminants with bypass proteins having a high concentration of lysine and methionine, it is also possible to use rumen bypass sources of these amino acids. If lysine and methionine are added directly to the diet, they will be fermented and degraded in the rumen. **Rumen protected amino** acids (RPAA) are commercially available. Polymers that are pH sensitive have been used to encapsulate methionine and lysine (Merchen and Titgemeyer, 1992; Rulquin and Delaby, 1997). The polymers are stable in the rumen but break down in the highly acidic conditions of the abomasum. Commercial sources of RPAA include Smartamine M® (70% methionine) and Smartamine ML® (15% methionine, 50% lysine), marketed by Rhone-Poulenc; and Mepron M85®, marketed by Degussa Corporation. **Methionine hydroxy analogue (MHA)**, which has a hydroxyl group in place of the amino group, is a source of RPAA because, compared to methionine, it has a very slow rate of degradation in the rumen. MHA is converted to methionine in the liver. Organic **metal chelates** of amino acids, such as zinc methionine, are sources of RPAA, but at the concentrations at which they are used as sources of minerals, their RPAA contribution is minimal.

The suckling stimulus causes closure of the oesophageal groove and the passage of milk directly from the oesophagus to the omasum. Milk, therefore, is an excellent source of bypass protein. Suckling calves and lambs on pasture benefit from this effect. Similarly, in tropical countries or other areas where ruminants are fed low quality roughages, the bypass potential of milk protein and the ability of the dam to lactate on a poor quality diet are significant in improving the utilization efficiency of low quality feeds.

Protein Digestion in Non-Ruminant Herbivores

In hindgut-digester non-ruminant herbivores, like horses and rabbits, high quality proteins are digested in the small intestine, as in the simple non-ruminants. Less digestible dietary proteins, such as those associated with the cell walls of forages, may resist digestion in the small intestine, and pass through to the hindgut where they are subjected to microbial digestion. The processes are similar to those in the rumen, but less efficient. Microbial growth is limited by a shortage of soluble nutrients (which are absorbed in the small intestine). Unless coprophagy or caecotrophy is employed, the digestibility of microbial protein in the hindgut is low, and the microbial protein will be excreted in the faeces. In caecal fermenters, like rabbits, the consumption of caecal contents (caecotrophy, see Chapter 3) will result in digestion of most of the microbial protein in the small intestine.

Non-protein nitrogen utilization by non-ruminant herbivores

Microbes in the caecum and colon of non-ruminant herbivores can utilize NPN as a nitrogen source. This process is less efficient as a means of using NPN in place of dietary protein than it is in ruminants, primarily because the site of fermentation is at the end rather than at the beginning of the digestive tract. This presents difficulties in getting the NPN source to the hindgut, and in the animal's utilization of microbial protein. Dietary urea is used inefficiently by horses and rabbits because it is hydrolysed to ammonia by bacterial urease in the small intestine. The ammonia is absorbed and reconverted to urea in the liver. Some urea does reach the hindgut, but by secretion from the blood into the caecum rather than by transit through the small intestine. Much of the absorbed ammonia is excreted in the urine and wasted.

Non-ruminant herbivores are less susceptible to urea toxicity than cattle, presumably because some of the urea is absorbed directly and excreted in the urine, rather than all of it being converted to ammonia. **Ammonia toxicity** in horses causes neurological symptoms, such as head pressing, with the head pressed against a solid object. Biochemically, the condition is caused by the metabolism of ammonia in the brain. α-Ketoglutaric acid is converted to glutamic acid which reacts with ammonia to produce glutamine; the depletion of α-ketoglutaric acid, an intermediate of the citric acid cycle, impairs ATP production by brain tissue, leading to coma and death (Fig. 5.6). Similar signs occur with liver dysfunction, impairing the liver's ability to convert ammonia to urea. This occurs with poisoning of horses by toxic plants containing hepatotoxic alkaloids, such as *Senecio* species.

Biuret is more suitable than urea as an NPN source for horses and rabbits because it is not hydrolysed in the small intestine and so can reach the hindgut intact. In rabbits, microbial protein synthesized in the caecum can be made available to the animal via caecotrophy, the process by which caecal contents are consumed. It is less certain how horses can derive benefit from NPN sources because the microbial protein synthesized in the hindgut is excreted in the faeces. Horses fed low protein diets do practise coprophagy, which may be a mechanism to conserve nitrogen when poor quality diets are consumed.

Note

[1] A mercaptan is an alcohol with the –OH replaced by –SH.

References

Broderick, G.A. and Clayton, M.K. (1997) A statistical evaluation of animal and nutritional factors influencing concentrations of milk urea nitrogen. *Journal of Dairy Science* 80, 2964–2971.

Butler, W.R., Calaman, J.J. and Beam, S.W. (1996) Plasma and milk urea nitrogen in relation to pregnancy rate in lactating dairy cattle. *Journal of Animal Science* 74, 858–865.

Cheeke, P.R. (1998) *Natural Toxicants in Feeds, Forages, and Poisonous Plants*. Prentice Hall, Upper Saddle River, New Jersey.

Cleale, R.M., Britton, R.A., Klopfenstein, T.J., Bauer, M.L., Harmon, D.L. and Satterlee, L.D. (1987) Induced non-enzymatic browning of soybean meal. II. Ruminal escape and net portal absorption of soybean protein treated with xylose. *Journal of Animal Science* 65, 1319–1326.

Coenen, D.J. and Trenkle, A. (1989) Comparisons of expeller-processed and solvent-extracted soybean meals as protein supplements for cattle. *Journal of Animal Science* 67, 565–573.

Girdhar, S.R., Barta, J.R., Santoyo, F.A. and Smith, T.K. (2006) Dietary putrescine (1,4-diaminobutane) influences recovery of turkey poults challenged with a mixed coccidial infection. *Journal of Nutrition* 136, 2319–2324.

Goetsch, A.L. and Owens, F.N. (1985) The effects of commercial processing method of cottonseed meal on site and extent of digestion in cattle. *Journal of Animal Science* 60, 803–813.

Ladely, S.R., Stock, R.A., Klopfenstein, T.J. and Sindt, M.H. (1995) High-lysine corn as a source of protein and energy for finishing calves. *Journal of Animal Science* 73, 228–235.

Lapierre, H. and Lobley, G.E. (2001) Nitrogen recycling in the ruminant: a review. *Journal of Dairy Science* 84 (E Suppl.), E223–E236.

Longenbach, J.I. and Heinrichs, A.J. (1998) A review of the importance and physiological role of curd formation in the abomasum of young calves. *Animal Feed Science and Technology* 73, 85–97.

Merchen, N.R. and Titgemeyer, E.C. (1992) Manipulation of amino acid supply to the growing ruminant. *Journal of Animal Science* 70, 3238–3247.

Min, B.R., McNabb, W.C., Barry, T.N. and Peters, J.S. (2000) Solubilization and degradation of ribulose-1,5-bisphosphate carboxylase/oxygenase (EC 4.1.1.39; Rubisco) protein from white clover (*Trifolium repens*) and *Lotus corniculatus* by rumen micro-organisms and the effect of condensed tannins on these processes. *Journal of Agricultural Science* 134, 305–317.

Min, B.R., Barry, T.N., Attwood, G.T. and McNabb, W.C. (2003) The effect of condensed tannins on the nutrition and health of ruminants fed fresh temperate forages: a review. *Animal Feed Science and Technology* 106, 3–19.

Mir, Z., MacLeod, G.K., Buchanan-Smith, J.G., Grieve, D.G. and Grovum, W.L. (1984a) Effect of feeding soybean meal protected with sodium hydroxide, fresh blood, or fish hydrolysate to growing calves and lactating dairy cows. *Canadian Journal of Animal Science* 64, 845–852.

Mir, Z., MacLeod, G.K., Buchanan-Smith, J.G., Grieve, D.G. and Grovum, W.L. (1984b) Methods for protecting soybean and canola proteins from degradation in the rumen. *Canadian Journal of Animal Science* 64, 853–865.

Mogridge, J.L., Smith, T.K. and Sousadias, M.G. (1996) Effect of feeding raw soybeans on polyamine metabolism in chicks and the therapeutic effect of exogenous putrescine. *Journal of Animal Science* 74, 1897–1904.

National Research Council (1985) *Ruminant Nitrogen Usage.* National Academy Press, Washington, DC.

Oltjen, R.R., Williams, E.E., Jr, Slyter, L.L. and Richardson, G.V. (1969) Urea versus biuret in a roughage diet for steers. *Journal of Animal Science* 29, 816–822.

Rulquin, H. and Delaby, L. (1997) Effects of the energy balance of dairy cows on lactational responses to rumen-protected methionine. *Journal of Dairy Science* 80, 2513–2522.

Simmons, N.L., Chaudhry, A.S., Graham, C., Scriven, E.S., Thistlethwaite, A., Smith, C.P. and Stewart, G.S. (2009) Dietary regulation of ruminal bovine UT-B urea transporter expression and localization. *Journal of Animal Science* 87, 3288–3299.

Sklan, D. (1989) *In vitro* and *in vivo* rumen protection of proteins coated with calcium soaps of long-chain fatty acids. *Journal of Agricultural Science* 112, 79–83.

Van Soest, P.J. (1994) *Nutritional Ecology of the Ruminant.* Cornell University Press, Ithaca, New York.

Webb, K.E., Jr, Matthews, J.C. and DiRienzo, D.B. (1992) Peptide absorption: a review of current concepts and future perspectives. *Journal of Animal Science* 70, 3248–3257.

6 Protein and Amino Acid Metabolism and Function

Protein Structure and Synthesis

Proteins are composed of basic units, the amino acids. The relative proportions of different amino acids, and the sequence in which they are joined together, determine the physical and physiological properties of proteins. The fundamental structure of proteins is a string or chain of amino acids linked together by peptide bonds.

The control of protein synthesis lies ultimately with the genetic code. The **genetic code** is formed by the arrangement of nucleotides in DNA in the cell nucleus. Purine and pyrimidine bases (adenine, A; guanine, G; cytosine, C; uracil, U; and thymine, T) exist in animal tissue either as **nucleosides** consisting of the base covalently bonded to either D-ribose or 2-deoxy-D-ribose, or as **nucleotides** which are phosphorylated nucleosides. Nucleotides have diverse functions, such as protein and nucleic acid synthesis, and in energy metabolism (e.g. ATP).

Nucleic acids, such as DNA and RNA, consist of nucleotides arranged in a strand in which the purine and pyrimidine bases are linked together by a backbone of phosphorylated sugars (either ribose or deoxyribose). DNA, arranged in two strands around a central axis in the form of a double helix, contains the genetic code. The nucleotides A, G, T and C are organized into three-letter codes (**codons**). A linear array of nucleotides specifies the synthesis of specific RNA molecules, which in turn control the amino acid sequence during protein synthesis. The genetic information within DNA (the codons specifying specific amino acids) is transferred to RNA by the use of one strand of DNA as a template. The sequence of nucleotides in RNA is complementary to the nucleotide sequence of the DNA template.

Two types of RNA, **transfer RNA** (**t-RNA**) and **messenger RNA** (**m-RNA**) are produced from the DNA template. The t-RNA has an anticodon of three nucleotides which codes for a specific amino acid. The t-RNA picks up a specific amino acid in the cytoplasm, and transports it to the site of protein synthesis, the ribosomes. **Ribosomes** are linked together by a strand of m-RNA, which has a three-base codon that codes for amino acids. The t-RNA recognizes a specific site on the m-RNA. Thus each amino acid is placed in the correct site for the particular protein being synthesized. When the intracellular supply of a specific amino acid is exhausted, protein synthesis stops. As the peptide chain is being formed, a 'blank space' cannot be left for a missing amino acid. Thus all of the dietary essential amino acids must be present in the diet at all times.

Mechanisms of protein synthesis are described in any biochemistry text and courses in biochemistry. It is a complicated process, but one to which any student in the biological sciences should have exposure.

Amino Acid Metabolism

Synthesis of the 'non-essential' amino acids

The so-called non-essential amino acids are those that are not dietary requirements, because they can be synthesized by animals. A major process for synthesis of non-essential amino acids is **transamination**, in which an amino group from one amino acid is transferred to an organic acid to form a new amino acid (Fig. 6.1). For example, the reaction shown in Fig. 6.2 illustrates the synthesis of alanine from glutamic acid and pyruvic acid.

Enzymes called **transaminases** catalyse these reactions. The keto acids are those formed in carbohydrate and amino acid metabolism, such as pyruvic, oxaloacetic and α-ketoglutaric acids (Fig. 6.3). The liver is a major site of amino acid metabolism, and is rich in transaminase activity. Various

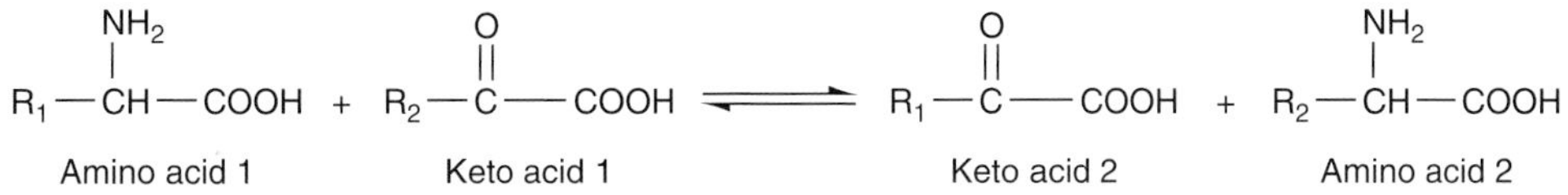

$$\underset{\text{Amino acid 1}}{R_1-\underset{\underset{NH_2}{|}}{CH}-COOH} \;+\; \underset{\text{Keto acid 1}}{R_2-\underset{\overset{O}{\|}}{C}-COOH} \;\rightleftharpoons\; \underset{\text{Keto acid 2}}{R_1-\underset{\overset{O}{\|}}{C}-COOH} \;+\; \underset{\text{Amino acid 2}}{R_2-\underset{\underset{NH_2}{|}}{CH}-COOH}$$

Fig. 6.1. Transamination, in which an amino group from one amino acid (amino acid 1) is transferred to an organic acid (keto acid 2) to form a new amino acid (amino acid 2).

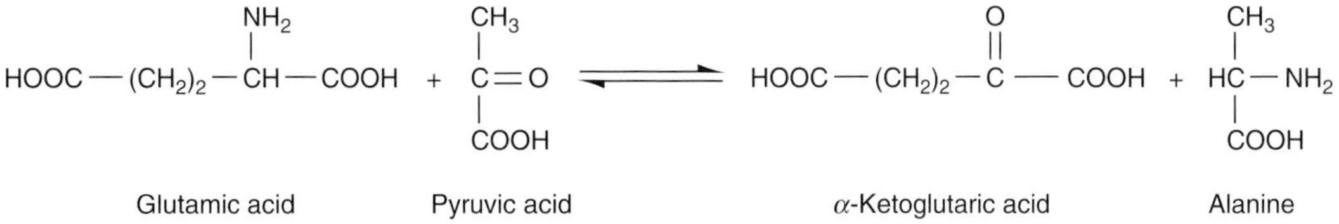

Fig. 6.2. Synthesis of alanine by transamination from glutamic acid and pyruvic acid.

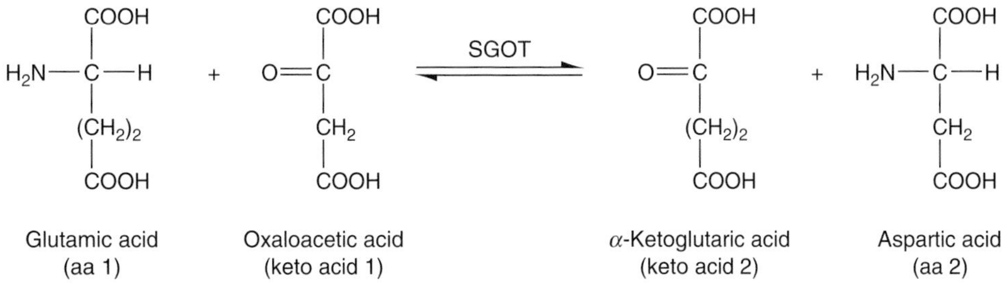

Glutamic acid + Pyruvic acid ⇌ α-Ketoglutaric acid + Alanine

Fig. 6.3. Transamination of glutamic acid to aspartic acid is catalysed by serum glutamic-oxaloacetic transaminase (SGOT).

Glutamic acid (aa 1) + Oxaloacetic acid (keto acid 1) ⇌ (SGOT) α-Ketoglutaric acid (keto acid 2) + Aspartic acid (aa 2)

transaminases, such as **serum glutamic-oxaloacetic transaminase (SGOT)** can be measured in blood as an indicator of liver damage. During liver damage, these enzymes are released into the blood by the damaged tissue, causing elevated blood transaminase activity.

Vitamin B_6 (pyridoxine) functions in transamination reactions (Fig. 6.4a). The phosphorylated form of pyridoxine, pyridoxal phosphate, forms a **Schiff base** (Fig. 6.4b) in which the aldehyde group of pyridoxal phosphate reacts with an amino group of an amino acid, to transfer it to a keto acid, forming a new amino acid.

Glutamic acid has a particularly important role in transaminations, in part because it can be formed by **ammonia fixation** (Fig. 6.5).

Glutamic acid is readily synthesized in the liver by the above ammonia fixation reaction, and can then participate in transaminations to produce other amino acids. Ammonia fixation is a means by which non-ruminant animals can utilize small amounts of dietary non-protein nitrogen sources.

Transamination reactions provide a linkage between protein and carbohydrate metabolism. All amino acids, except leucine, are gluconeogenic – in other words, their carbon skeletons can be used for glucose synthesis.

The amine formed from glutamic acid, glutamine, is considered a major fuel for the metabolism of enterocytes in the gut (Watford, 1999). Glutamine helps maintain gut mucosal glutathione concentrations; glutathione is a critical antioxidant found in high concentrations in the gut mucosa. Inhibition of glutathione synthesis leads to degeneration of the mucosa, diarrhoea and growth failure (Duggan *et al.*, 2002).

Use of amino acids for protein synthesis

The term **protein quality** refers to how well the amino acid composition of dietary protein matches the amino acid requirements of the animal. High quality proteins are those whose amino acid composition closely matches animal requirements.

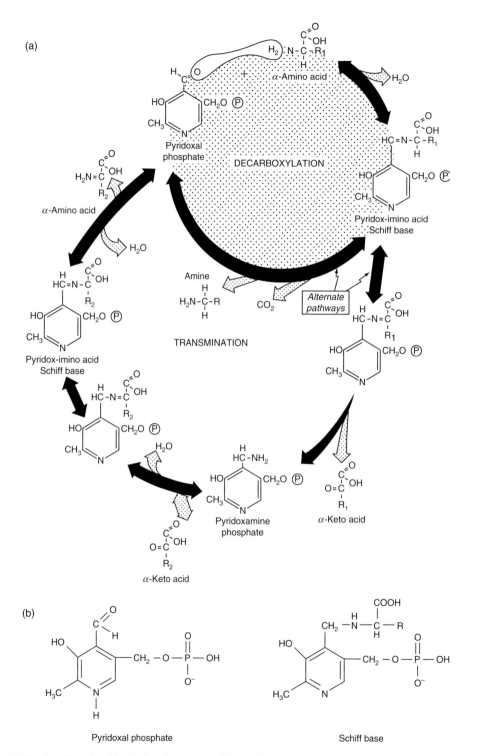

Fig. 6.4. (a) The function of pyridoxal phosphate and pyridoxamine phosphate in decarboxylation and transamination of amino acids (courtesy of University Books, Guelph, Canada). (b) Pyridoxal phosphate and Schiff base.

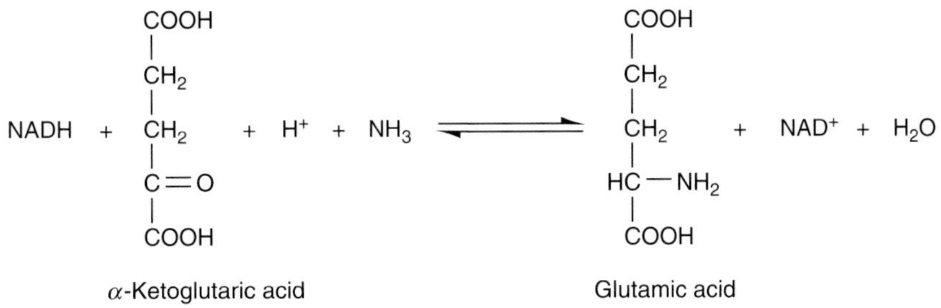

Chapter 6

Fig. 6.5. Glutamic acid can be formed by ammonia fixation.

The requirements vary with age, animal species and productive function (e.g. growth, lactation, wool growth). Amino acid requirements are high for young, rapidly growing animals and decline with age. Thus, it has been traditional to use starter, grower and finisher diets for various species, with protein and essential amino acid contents reduced in concentration as growth proceeds.

Traditionally, animal protein sources have been viewed as being of high quality. Milk and eggs are sources of high quality protein, which is not surprising because they support the growth of young animals when their requirements are highest. It is increasingly recognized that judicious selection of plant protein sources can meet most animal and human amino acid requirements. Pigs and poultry, for example, are efficiently produced on maize-soybean meal diets supplemented with synthetic amino acids (e.g. L-lysine, DL-methionine). These amino acids, produced by biotechnological techniques using 'genetically engineered' microbes, are widely used in animal nutrition. Thus the quality of dietary protein sources is of less concern than it once was, because deficiencies are readily overcome by supplementation with amino acids. The concept of an ideal protein is increasingly used. An **ideal protein** is one that meets amino acid requirements precisely, and thus optimizes nitrogen utilization and growth (Chung and Baker, 1992). Chung and Baker (1992) proposed that expression of amino acids in an ideal pattern should involve expressing them as a ratio of the lysine requirement. Lysine is usually the most limiting amino acid; it is required in the greatest quantitative amount of all amino acids, and protein synthesis is the only need for dietary lysine. Thus amino acid requirements can be expressed as a percentage of the lysine requirement, in the ideal protein concept.

In the case of humans, it has long been dogma among animal scientists that we require animal protein sources in our diets as sources of essential amino acids. This concept, discussed by Shorland (1988), is a long-held fallacy based on early work with young rats, which failed to grow with wheat as the sole source of protein unless supplemented with meat, milk or egg protein. Thus a distinction developed, with animal proteins considered first class and plant proteins second class. However, it is now recognized that the relative growth rate of humans is much slower than that of weanling rats (or chicks or pigs), and that an appropriate mixture of plant proteins can meet the human's need for essential amino acids. Although perhaps not good news for the animal science community, vegetarian and vegan diets can be and generally are nutritionally adequate for humans (Key et al., 2006). (A vegan diet is one that contains no ingredients of animal origin; some vegetarian diets may include milk or eggs.) Another great ape (besides humans), the gorilla, consumes a vegetarian diet of fruit and foliage. Captive gorillas fed diets containing meat and eggs can develop high serum cholesterol levels, premature cardiovascular disease and ulcerative colitis (Popovich et al., 1997).

Disposal of excess amino acids

Amino acids in excess of the immediate needs for protein synthesis are degraded in the liver. If the profile of absorbed amino acids does not exactly match the requirements for protein synthesis (which it virtually never does), excess amino acids are catabolized in the liver by removal of the amino group, and the carbon skeletons enter into pathways of energy metabolism. Besides absorbed amino acids, another source of amino acids that are degraded is those liberated by the intracellular digestion of proteins. Enzymes and other proteins that are 'worn out' are disposed of by either of two major pathways of *protein* **degradation**: (i) non-ATP-dependent lysosomal proteases; and (ii) an ATP-dependent ubiquitin system. **Intracellular proteases** include cathepsins and the calcium-activated calpains and calpastatins. These enzymes are located in subcellular organelles called **lysosomes. Ubiquitin** is a small protein that plays a key role in degradation of proteins in proteasomes. It is particularly involved with disposal of misfolded proteins and regulatory enzymes that have short half-lives. When a molecule of ubiquitin is attached to a protein, a number of others attach, resulting in a polyubiquinated protein. These enter subcellular organelles called **proteasomes**, located in the cytosol, for proteolysis of the 'tagged' protein. Liberated ubiquitin molecules are recycled.

The first step in amino acid degradation is **deamination**, or removal of the amino group, by transaminases which occur in the liver. Deamination is accomplished by transamination reactions involving reaction with α-ketoglutaric acid to form glutamic acid:

α-ketoglutaric acid + amino acid ® glutamic acid + α-keto acid

Glutamic acid + NAD$^+$ + H$_2$O ® α-ketoglutaric acid + NADH + H$^+$ + NH$_3$

Sum: amino acid + NAD$^+$ + H$_2$O ® α-keto acid + NADH + H$^+$ + NH$_3$

The ammonia liberated by deamination is toxic to the central nervous system. Thus it is essential that ammonia be either excreted or detoxified as soon as it is produced. In aquatic species, such as fish, the ammonia is excreted from the gills as ammonia. The elasmobranch fish (e.g. sharks, rays) produce urea, which accumulates in their flesh and causes unpleasant odours and flavours during storage and cooking. In terrestrial animals, nitrogen is excreted as urea or uric acid. Most mammals excrete urea in the urine, while birds excrete uric acid in their semi-solid excreta. **Dalmatians** are unique among dog breeds in excreting relatively large amounts of uric acid in their urine. However, the origin of the uric acid is not from protein metabolism, but from the metabolism of purines.

The Dalmatian is homozygous for a defective recessive gene regulating purine metabolism. Dalmatians are thus very susceptible to urate urolithiasis (Brown *et al.*, 2003). Their high blood uric acid concentrations are apparently a result of a defect in their hepatic uric acid transport system.

In mammals, urea is synthesized in the liver by the urea cycle enzymes. The **urea cycle** (Fig. 6.6) involves two non-protein amino acids, citrulline and ornithine. **Ornithine** reacts with carbomylphosphate, which is derived from ammonia, to produce **citrulline**, which reacts with aspartate ultimately to produce **arginine**. This is the normal pathway for arginine biosynthesis. Liver arginase splits urea off from the guanidine group of the side chain of arginine, producing ornithine, to start the cycle again.

Urea synthesis is an energy-requiring reaction. Energy (as ATP) is required for the formation of **carbamoyl phosphate**, which is the form in which the ammonia nitrogen is added to ornithine (Fig. 6.7).

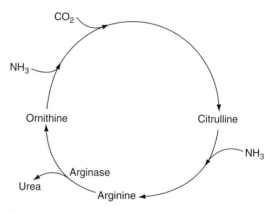

Fig. 6.6. Reactions of the urea cycle.

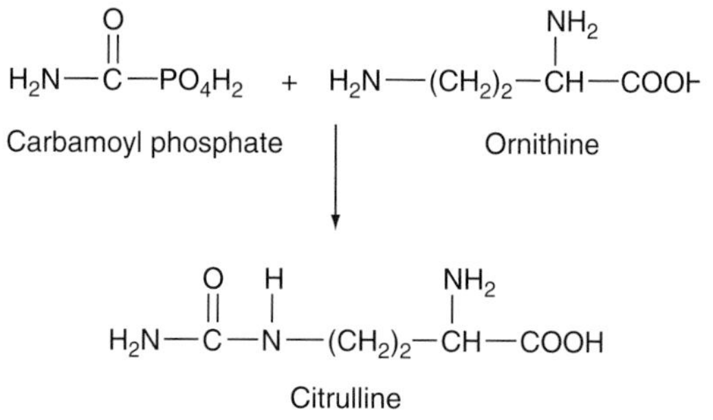

Fig. 6.7. Carbamoyl phosphate is the form in which the ammonia nitrogen is added to ornithine.

Carbamoyl phosphate is formed by the condensation of carbon dioxide, ammonia and ATP (Fig. 6.8). The formation of carbamoyl phosphate requires two molecules of ATP. Another molecule of ATP is required for the formation of argininosuccinic acid, an intermediate in the formation of arginine from citrulline (Fig. 6.9).

Poultry and other birds do not have carbamoyl phosphate synthetase, so they cannot synthesize urea or arginine. Amino nitrogen from deamination is converted to glutamic acid, which is used in the synthesis of **uric acid**. Glycine is also used in uric acid synthesis, and methyl groups derived from methionine are required (see Fig. 5.9 in Chapter 5). Thus poultry have higher dietary requirements for arginine, glycine and methionine than do mammals. Furthermore, the requirements for these amino acids increase with increasing dietary protein, because they are required for the excretion of the excess nitrogen.

Birds excrete uric acid as a supersaturated colloidal suspension, which is the white substance visible in bird excreta. They also excrete some free ammonia; this is especially true of freshwater ducks. A small amount of urea is excreted, arising from the catabolism of excess dietary arginine.

The formation of urea and uric acid requires energy as ATP. Thus the feeding of excess dietary protein or poor quality protein is undesirable, because it increases energy requirements. In addition, the excess urea or uric acid in the excreta leads to environmental problems, including elevated air ammonia in confinement buildings, and groundwater pollution with nitrates. Ammonia also leads to formation of acid rain. Although ammonia has an alkaline reaction, it can react with atmospheric sulfuric acid to form ammonium sulfate. Ammonium sulfate can react with oxygen in soils to produce nitric and sulfuric acids:

$$(NH_4)_2SO_4 + 4O_2 \circledR 2HNO_3 + H_2SO_4 + 2H_2O$$

A major part of the caloric needs of many fish species is met by the catabolism of protein and amino acids. As a result, there is a large amount of nitrogen to be excreted. The major nitrogenous excretory product in **teleost fishes** is ammonia, with lesser amounts of urea (Mommsen and Walsh, 1992). **Ammonia** is largely excreted via the gills, although ammonia excretion through the skin is important in some marine species. Ammonia exists in the toxic un-ionized form (NH_3) and as less-toxic ammonium ion (NH_4^+). The equilibrium between these two forms is influenced by water characteristics such as pH and temperature. At high water pH, the un-ionized

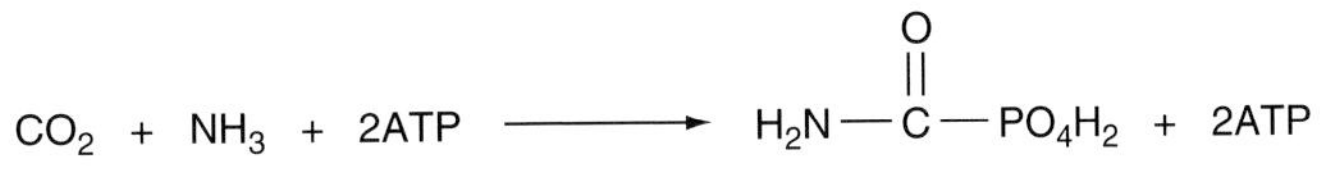

Fig. 6.8. Carbamoyl phosphate is formed by the condensation of carbon dioxide, ammonia and ATP.

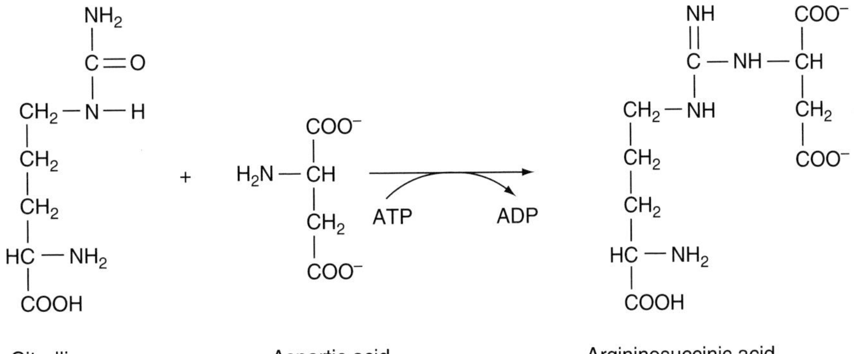

Fig. 6.9. Argininosuccinic acid is an intermediate in the formation of arginine from citrulline.

ammonia predominates, and diffusion of ammonia from the gills is impaired.

Animals can be categorized by their type of nitrogen excretion as ureotelic (urea excretion), uricotelic (uric acid excretion) and ammonotelic (ammonia excretion) (telic is from the Greek *telikos* meaning belonging to the completion or end).

Other aspects of protein and amino acid metabolism

Sulfur amino acid metabolism

The three main sulfur-containing amino acids are methionine, cystine and cysteine (Fig. 6.10). Methionine is a dietary essential, while the others can be synthesized from methionine.

Cysteine contains sulfur as a **sulfhydryl group** (–SH) while cystine has a **disulfide bond** (–S–S–), formed by the reaction of two cysteine molecules. The presence of cysteine in the diet is said to have a 'sparing effect' on methionine, because less diversion of methionine to synthesize cysteine and cystine occurs. Cysteine can also be provided in the diet as N-acetyl-L-cysteine (Dilger and Baker, 2007). The α-amino nitrogen is protected by an acetyl group, which can be removed after absorption to yield cysteine.

Methionine is known as a methyl donor because it is a source of labile methyl groups (Fig. 6.11). **Methyl groups** (–CH$_3$) are needed for the synthesis of various metabolites such as choline, betaine and creatine. The methyl group is attached to tetrahydrofolic acid for transfer reactions.

Folic acid is one of the B vitamins, as is choline.[1] Creatine occurs in muscle as phosphocreatine, and functions as an energy reserve for muscle contraction. Choline functions in lipid metabolism; a choline deficiency results in the accumulation of triacylglycerol in the liver (**fatty liver syndrome**). Betaine can substitute for choline in this role. Choline may be involved in the synthesis of lipoprotein phospholipids which transport triacylglycerols from the liver. **Choline** is a constituent of lecithin, or phosphatidylcholine, a major component of membranes and surfaces of plasma lipoproteins. Choline, methionine and other methyl donors are referred to as **lipotropes**, which aid in mobilizing lipids from liver, preventing fatty liver syndrome.

Betaine (Fig. 6.11) is an additional source of labile methyl groups. Experimentally, betaine can react with homocysteine to produce methionine. This is not usually of practical significance, because most feedstuffs are low in homocysteine content. Dietary betaine can have a sparing effect on methionine, a methyl donor, by recycling homocysteine (Kidd *et al.*, 1997). Betaine has **osmoregulatory properties** (i.e. it aids in maintaining normal osmotic pressure of cells). Osmoregulation is particularly important in marine animals, in their adaptation to salt water. Seawater tolerance of young salmon and rainbow trout is improved by dietary betaine (Kidd *et al.*, 1997). In a review of betaine nutrition of poultry, Kidd *et al.* (1997) concluded that supplemental betaine might be advantageous during certain physiologically challenging conditions,

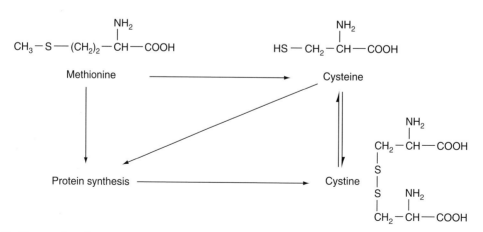

Fig. 6.10. Three main sulfur-containing amino acids: methionine, cystine and cysteine.

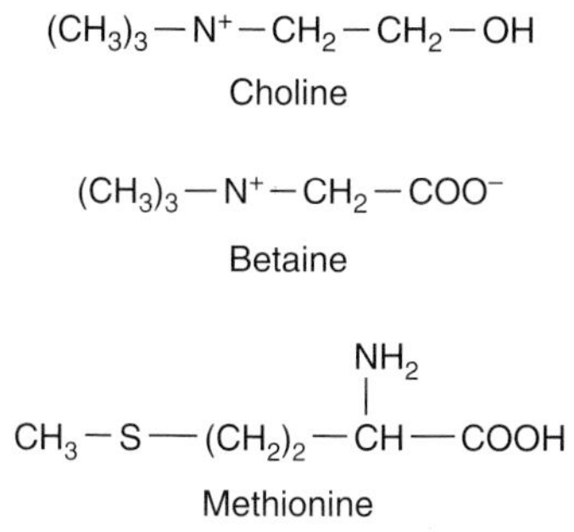

$$(CH_3)_3-N^+-CH_2-CH_2-OH$$

Choline

$$(CH_3)_3-N^+-CH_2-COO^-$$

Betaine

$$CH_3-S-(CH_2)_2-\overset{\overset{\displaystyle NH_2}{|}}{CH}-COOH$$

Methionine

Fig. 6.11. Sources of labile methyl groups.

including the high metabolic demand of rapid growth and response to disease challenge. Betaine supplementation of feed or drinking water may be useful in the control of dysfunctional osmoregulatory conditions such as diarrhoea, diuresis and ascites (Kidd *et al.*, 1997).

Ascites is the accumulation of fluid in body cavities such as the abdominal cavity. It is a consequence of impaired liver function. The serum proteins such as serum albumin and globulin are synthesized by the liver. With impaired liver function, hepatic protein synthesis is reduced and serum protein concentrations decline. Serum proteins, especially albumin, play an important role in maintaining fluid balance and fluid interchange between the blood and tissues. A decline in solutes in the blood, by osmotic action, causes a movement of water from the more dilute solution (blood) into the tissue spaces. Dietary protein deficiency also causes ascites for the same reason. This disorder in humans is called **kwashiorkor** (an African word meaning 'what happens to the first child when the next one is born'). Ascites is characterized by a swollen, fluid-containing abdomen. Another deficiency disorder of humans in Africa is **marasmus**. Marasmus is a severe deficiency of both protein and calories, causing emaciation and wasting. Basically it is starvation. Kwashiorkor affects only children; marasmus can occur in both adults and children. The distinguishing feature of kwashiorkor is ascites, whereas extreme emaciation with loss of body fat and extensive muscle wasting is characteristic of marasmus. **Starvation** results in a reduced synthesis of proteins and impaired immune response, increasing risk of disease and infection. Impairment of cell proliferation in the intestinal mucosa occurs, resulting in a reduction of surface area and impaired nutrient

absorption. Animals that have suffered from starvation may not recover even when given food and water; these substances may pass through the damaged gastrointestinal tract without being absorbed.

Homocysteine is produced when methionine serves as a methyl donor. Blood homocysteine concentrations are elevated in patients with arterial occlusive diseases (coronary, cerebral and peripheral artery occlusion or blockage) and may be a risk factor for these diseases. A review of nutritional effects of homocysteine is provided by Weir and Scott (1998).

Hair and feathers have a high content of cystine. Cystine is formed within the protein molecule by the formation of disulfide bonds between non-adjacent cysteines. This type of protein, high in cystine, is called **keratin**. Hair meal and feather meal must be steam-hydrolysed to break the disulfide bonds for use as feedstuffs; the raw products have a very low digestibility.

Creatine phosphate (Fig. 6.12) is synthesized in liver tissue from glycine, arginine and methionine. Creatine phosphate is a high-energy phosphate that is a major source of ATP in muscle tissue. **Creatinine** (Fig. 6.12) is a metabolite of creatine that is excreted in the urine. Urinary and blood creatinine concentrations are good indicators of kidney function. Creatinine is excreted primarily by kidney filtration, with little tubular resorption. If filtering by the kidney is impaired, blood creatinine concentrations increase.

Taurine is an amino sulfonic acid derivative of sulfur amino acids (Fig. 6.13). It is a dietary essential for cats, and is commonly added to pet foods. **Taurine deficiency** causes retinal degeneration and loss of vision in cats. Other deficiency signs in cats include heart failure, poor reproduction and impaired growth. Taurine is also required in the cat for the formation of bile acids in which cholic acid and other bile acids conjugate with taurine.

Taurine deficiency has also been observed in dogs. Dilated cardiomyopathy (DCM) occurs in large-breed dogs such as Newfoundlands (Backus *et al.*, 2006). Common findings in affected dogs are large body size, very low blood taurine concentrations, and maintenance feeding with a lamb and rice diet. The disorder is probably due to inadequate hepatic synthesis of taurine, as a result of the higher sulfur-amino acid requirements of large dogs. Retinal degeneration does not occur with a

Protein and Amino Acid Metabolism and Function

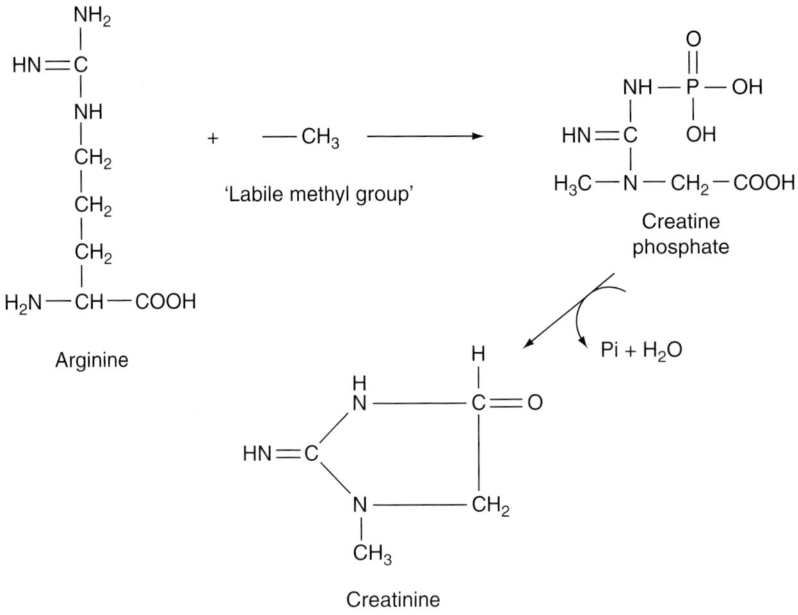

Fig. 6.12. Structures of creatine phosphate and creatinine.

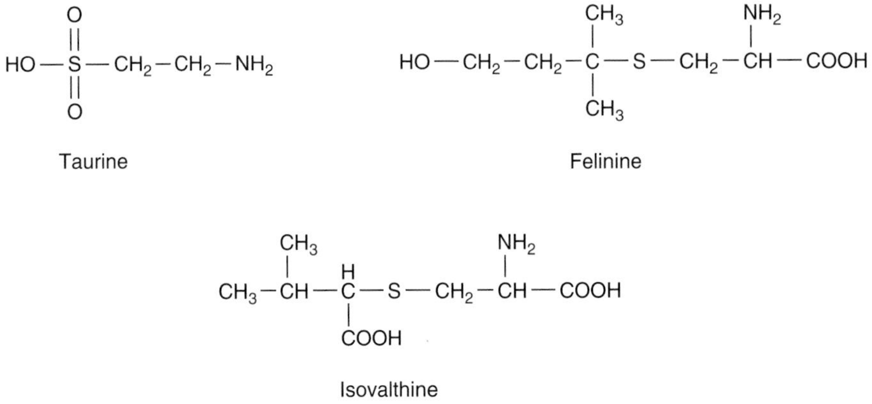

Fig. 6.13. Sulfur amino acids (felinine and isovalthine) in feline urine, and structure of taurine, a derivative of sulfur amino acids and essential nutrient for felines.

taurine deficiency in dogs, which is in contrast to that in cats. American cocker spaniels are also subject to DCM (Backus *et al.*, 2006).

Cats metabolize sulfur amino acids somewhat differently from other animals. They excrete unique sulfur-containing compounds in their urine (Fig. 6.13), accounting for its strong odour. These include isovalthine and felinine, which are both derivatives of cysteine. These compounds

function in territorial marking. **Felinine** is the source of the characteristic tomcat urine odour (Hendriks *et al.*, 1995). Felinine is synthesized from cysteine and/or methionine (Hendriks *et al.*, 2001) as part of a tripeptide via the glutathione conjugation pathway, and is excreted by the same mechanisms as used for glutathione conjugates to form mercaptic acids (Rutherfurd-Markwick *et al.*, 2006). Felinine is transported to the kidney as part of the tripeptide γ-glutamylfelinylglycine (Hendriks *et al.*, 2004).

Metabolites of tryptophan

Tryptophan contains an **indole group**. There are numerous indole-containing compounds derived from tryptophan, including niacin, serotonin, melatonin, melanin, indole alkaloids (e.g. ergot) in plants, and indolic metabolites in faeces (e.g. skatole). Niacin (a B vitamin) is derived from tryptophan but does not contain a complete indole group (Fig. 6.14). **Niacin** is the generic name for nicotinic acid and nicotinamide, which function as essential cofactors in metabolism (e.g. NAD^+, $NADP^+$). Niacin is synthesized from tryptophan, with numerous intermediates (Fig. 6.14). There are species differences in activities of enzymes involved in niacin biosynthesis, for example in the cat **picolinic acid** is formed rather than niacin. Thus the cat has a dietary requirement for niacin. In most species, dietary tryptophan has a sparing effect on the niacin requirement.

Serotonin (Fig. 6.15) is a potent vasoconstrictor and stimulator of smooth muscle contraction. It functions in the brain as a neurotransmitter. It is an indolic compound synthesized from tryptophan. Dietary tryptophan can influence brain serotonin concentrations. Serotonin has a sedative or calming effect; for this reason tryptophan is used as a neurotransmitter to control aggressive behaviour, suppress hysteria in poultry, and inhibit the response to stress (Koopmans *et al.*, 2006; Li *et al.*, 2006). In the pineal gland, serotonin is converted to **melatonin**, a hormone which functions in various physiological responses to photoperiod. These include reproduction, hair growth, hibernation and migration. The pasture grass reed canary grass contains indole (tryptamine) alkaloids that cause neurological disturbances in grazing animals, because of the structural relationship of the **tryptamine alkaloids** to neurotransmitters such as serotonin (Cheeke, 1998).

In ruminants, metabolism of tryptophan by rumen microbes produces **3-methyl indole (3-MI)**, which is a lung toxin (Cheeke, 1998). Under certain dietary conditions which favour 3-MI production, ruminants develop respiratory distress (summer pneumonia, acute bovine pulmonary emphysema). The 3-MI, also known as **skatole**, is produced by hindgut microbes as well, and is a major component of faecal odour (Jensen *et al.*, 1995). Absorbed skatole in pigs causes an unpleasant odour (**boar taint**) of meat. The association with boars is that they have high blood concentrations of the steroid hormone androstenone, which affects liver cytochrome P_{450} activity, reducing the degradation of skatole by the liver (Deslandes *et al.*, 2001). Pigs with high skatole concentrations tend to have low hepatic cytochrome $P_{450}IIE1$ concentrations (Squires and Lunstrom, 1997). Skatole is catabolized by liver enzymes to produce two major metabolites, 6-sulfatoxyskatole and 3-hydroxy-3-methyloxindole, that are excreted in the urine. Thus low cytochrome P_{450} activity results in less production of metabolites and higher blood and tissue skatole concentrations. An increase in plasma skatole in young boars at weaning is associated with changes in the intestinal microflora (Lanthier *et al.*, 2006).

Meat from grass-fattened ruminants has an undesirable taste to many consumers, sometimes referred to as pastoral flavour (Schreurs *et al.*, 2008). **Pastoral flavour** is in part caused by absorbed indole and skatole, produced in rumen fermentation. Fresh forage diets consumed by ruminants tend to be high in fibre and low in readily fermentable carbohydrate, so that the dietary protein is more rapidly solubilized and degraded in the rumen than the protein in high concentrate diets. Thus pasture and forage diets have a high protein to readily fermentable carbohydrate ratio. Pastoral flavours tend to be highest in animals consuming legume pastures, such as white clover, because of the rapid solubilization and degradation of their protein in the rumen. Production of skatole is lower in forages that contain **condensed tannins**, such as trefoil (Schreurs *et al.*, 2008). Condensed tannins bind to soluble protein in the rumen, reducing its degradation rate, and also tannins inhibit the activities of proteolytic and skatole-forming rumen microbes.

Off-flavour of grass-fed beef is also associated with phospholipids in the structural fat and with flavour constituents produced by rumen fermentation of forage lipids (Melton, 1990). A high concentration of polyunsaturated fatty acids in the phospholipids contributes to the undesirable flavour of grass-fed beef (Larick and Turner, 1989), and may lead to oxidative rancidity and off-flavours.

Metabolites of tyrosine and phenylalanine

The amino acid tyrosine is a precursor of several hormones and metabolites (Fig. 6.16). It is synthesized

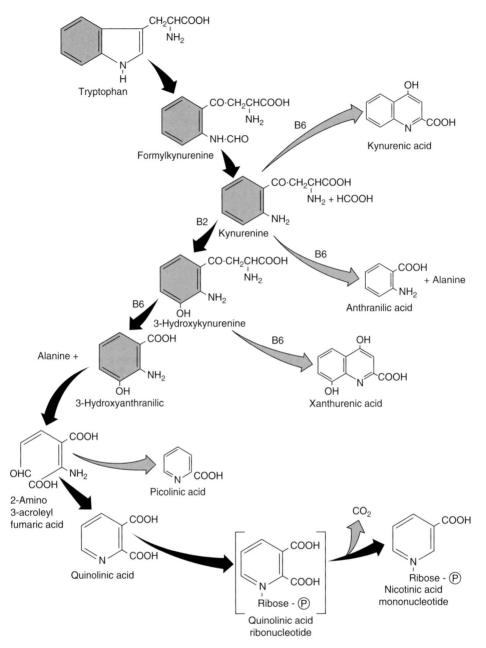

Fig. 6.14. Conversion of the amino acid tryptophan to the vitamin niacin (nicotinic acid). Numerous enzymatic steps are involved. Members of the cat family lack the terminal enzymes with the result that picolinic acid is formed. Cats have a very high activity of the enzyme picolinic acid carboxylase which diverts tryptophan metabolism away from niacin synthesis (courtesy of University Books, Guelph, Canada).

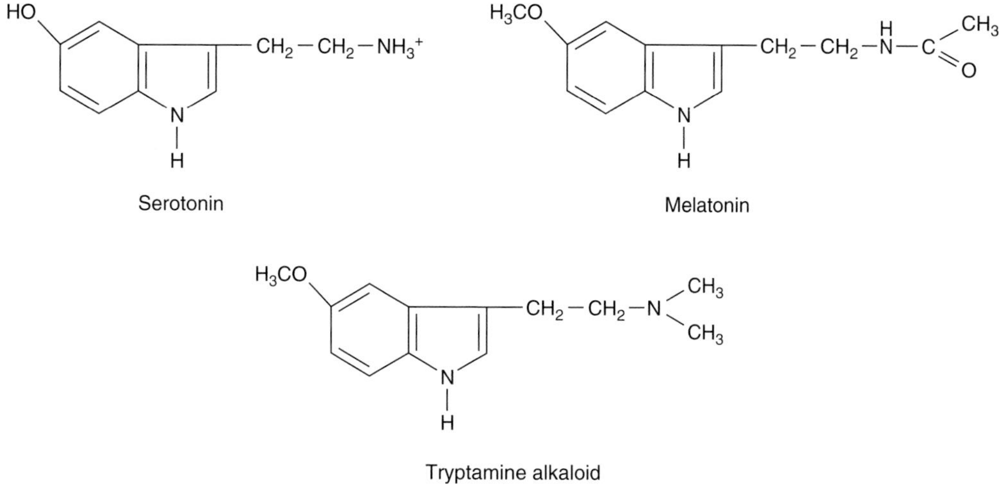

Serotonin

Melatonin

Tryptamine alkaloid

Fig. 6.15. Neurotransmitters containing an indole group derived from the amino acid tryptophan.

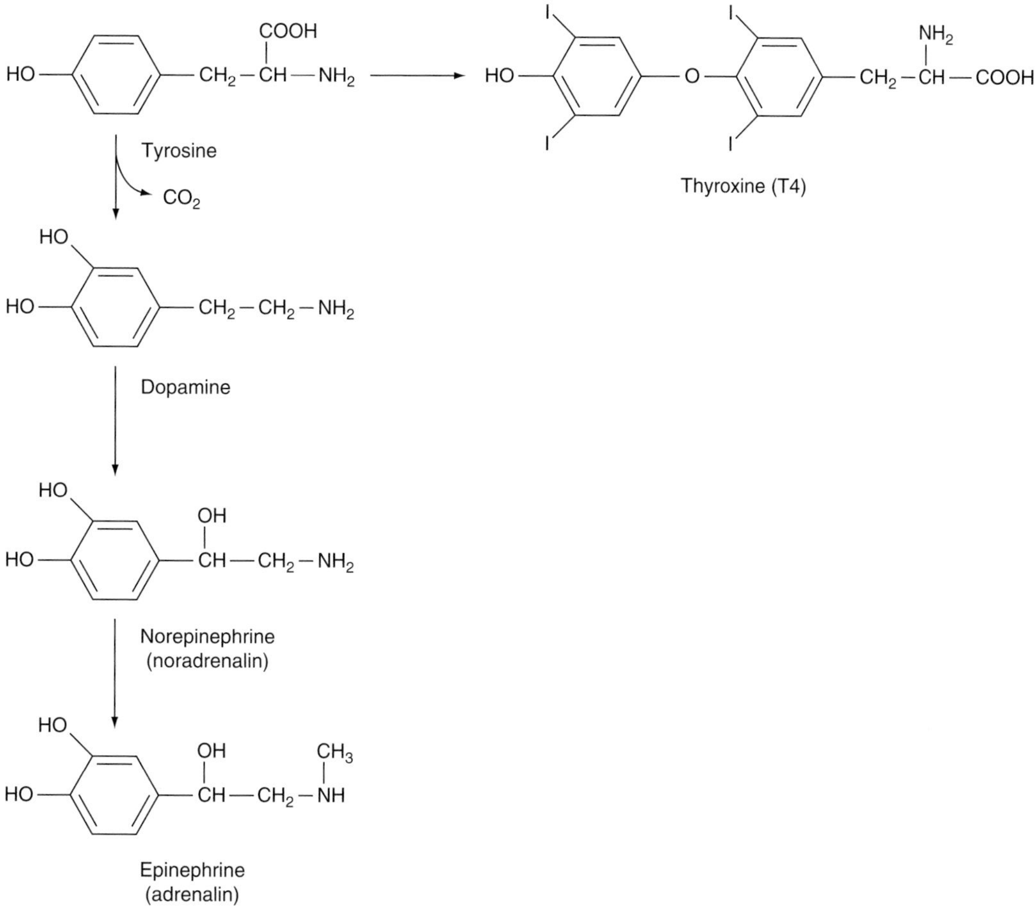

Tyrosine

CO_2

Thyroxine (T4)

Dopamine

Norepinephrine
(noradrenalin)

Epinephrine
(adrenalin)

Fig. 6.16. Hormones synthesized from tyrosine.

from phenylalanine by the addition of an hydroxyl group. Tyrosine is converted to epinephrine (adrenalin), norepinephrine (noradrenalin), and the thyroid hormone, thyroxine. **Dopamine,** an intermediate in the synthesis of epinephrine and norepinephrine, is a neurotransmitter. Dopamine deficiency is a factor in Parkinson's disease, an important disease of humans characterized by tremor and other neurologic signs. Tyrosine is also a precursor of the **melanin pigments** in hair and skin (see Chapter 19). Melanin pigments are brown and black, while pheomelanins are red and yellow. The aromatic amino acids phenylalanine and tyrosine in wool can be degraded by ultraviolet (UV) light, producing photoproducts that cause an undesirable yellowing of the wool fibres.

Black cats have a high requirement for phenylalanine-tyrosine. Morris *et al.* (2002) observed that black cats fed a diet low in phenylalanine developed reddish-brown hair. Cats have a higher dietary requirement for phenylalanine or tyrosine for melanin deposition in hair than for maximal growth (Anderson *et al.*, 2002), which is an unusual situation of a secondary nutrient requirement being greater than the requirement for growth.

Metabolism of branched chain amino acids

The branched chain amino acids are leucine, isoleucine and valine. They are metabolized in a manner similar to fatty acid metabolism, and ultimately are degraded to acetyl CoA and ketone bodies such as acetoacetate. They are also important nitrogen donors for the synthesis of the excitatory neurotransmitter glutamate and the inhibitory neurotransmitter γ-amino butyric acid (see section 'Excitatory and inhibitory amino acids', this chapter). Metabolism of branched chain amino acids is reviewed by Hutson *et al.* (2005).

Amino acids in conjugation reactions

Toxic substances are often excreted by the body in the form of conjugates, meaning that they are conjugated with another substance (see Chapter 13). The amino acid glycine is an important conjugating agent, with many toxins and drugs as well as bile acids excreted in the bile or urine as **glycine conjugates.** Phenolic acids which are absorbed in large quantity in herbivores are conjugated with glycine. For example, benzoic acid forms the glycine conjugate **hippuric acid,** excreted in the urine of ruminants and horses (Fig. 6.17).

Glutathione (Fig. 6.18) is a tripeptide containing glutamic acid, cysteine and glycine. The sulfhydryl group is important in the conjugation of numerous toxic compounds with glutathione. The glutathione conjugates are metabolized with the removal of the glutamic acid and glycine, with an acetyl group (CH_3COO-) added. The resulting compound is called a **mercaptic acid,** a conjugate of acetylcysteine, and is excreted in the urine. **Grouse** and **ptarmigan** are herbivorous northern and Arctic birds that feed on highly fibrous plant parts such as buds of shrubs (e.g. willow, heather). These plant materials contain phenolics. Grouse conjugate the smaller absorbed phenolic molecules with the amino acid ornithine, and excrete ornithuric acid (Moss, 1997). This represents a significant loss of nitrogen, particularly on winter feeds. Some nitrogen recycling is accomplished through the movement of urinary nitrogen by reverse peristalsis into the caeca (Moss, 1997).

Formation of nitric oxide

The gas **nitric oxide (NO)** has a variety of physiological roles. It is a vasodilator important in the

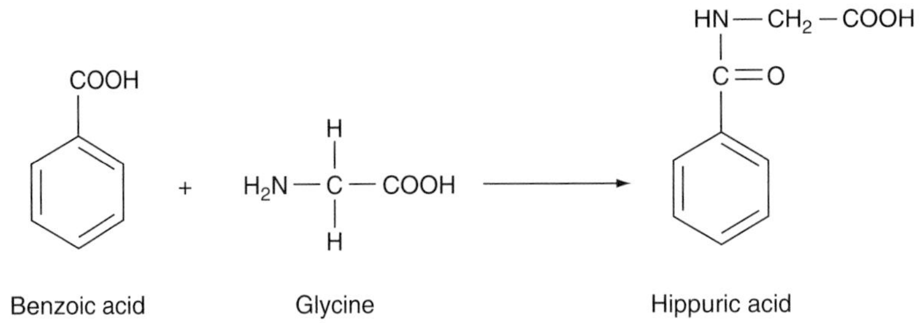

Fig. 6.17. Conjugation of benzoic acid with glycine to produce hippuric acid.

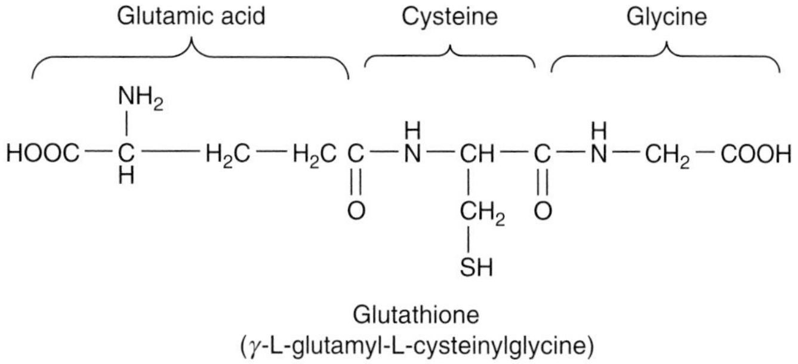

Fig. 6.18. Structure of the tripeptide glutathione.

regulation of blood pressure. NO is formed in the tissues by action of the enzyme NO synthase (NOS) on the amino acid arginine:

$$\text{Arginine} \xrightarrow{\text{NOS}} \text{Citrulline} + \text{NO}$$

The reaction is more complicated than it looks in the general equation, and involves a variety of cofactors. Drugs whose activity involves NO include the coronary artery dilator nitroglycerin, and the erectile dysfunction drug Viagra. NO can be generated in tissues by a constitutive NOS, or by an inducible enzyme (iNOS) in macrophages, neutrophils and other cells of the immune system. During the **inflammatory process**, iNOS and NO production are enhanced. Anti-inflammatory drugs can reduce NO production by inhibiting nuclear transcription factors (e.g. nuclear factor kappa-B, NFκB) which induce increased iNOS activity.

Excitatory and inhibitory amino acids

Glutamate and aspartate are **excitatory amino acids** in the brain. Glutamate is responsible for about 75% of the excitatory neurotransmission in the brain. **Excitotoxins** are chemicals that inhibit normal excitatory activity by causing the death of neurons from the release of excessive glutamate. Brain tissue contains glutamate receptors. Chronic stimulation of glutamate receptors causes an influx of calcium ions, leading to cell death. Excess intracellular calcium is very toxic to cells; calcium has an important role as a second messenger in many intracellular functions. Plants of the sweet pea family (*Lathyrus* genus) and cycad family contain amino acid derivatives called **lathyrogens**, which cause neurological problems (lathyrism) when

Lathyrus and cycad seeds are consumed. Certain plants in the locoweed group (*Astragalus* spp.) contain 3-nitropropionic acid (3-NPA), which causes neurological problems in livestock. Mouldy sugarcane toxicosis of humans in China is caused by 3-NPA produced by fungi growing on sugarcane. Sugarcane is a common confectionary consumed in China. These conditions, which involve excitotoxins, are discussed in more detail by Cheeke (1998).

γ-Amino butyric acid (GABA) arises from decarboxylation of glutamic acid by a highly active enzyme in brain (Fig. 6.19). GABA can also be synthesized from the polyamine putrescine. GABA is an **inhibitory neurotransmitter**.

Numerous diseases in humans, including Huntington's disease and stroke, have an involvement of excitatory amino acids. Ischaemia (blood vessel constriction) causes depolarization of neuronal membranes, releasing glutamate. This glutamate release overexcites glutamate receptors on adjacent neurons, leading to abnormally large influxes of calcium ions causing cell injury or death.

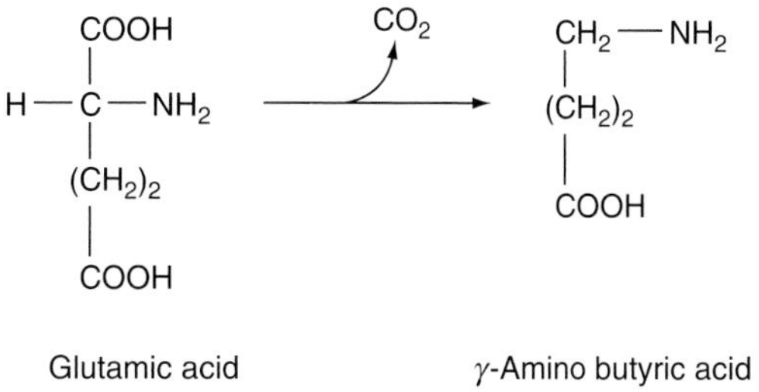

Fig. 6.19. γ-Amino butyric acid (GABA) is produced by decarboxylation of glutamic acid.

Browning reactions of amino acids (lysine tie-up)

Proteins may undergo chemical reactions in which brown, indigestible polymers are produced. There are two general types: (i) enzymatic; and (ii) non-enzymatic browning. **Enzymatic browning** is promoted by the enzyme polyphenol oxidase in plant tissue. **Polyphenol oxidase** catalyses the conversion of phenolic acids such as caffeic acid and chlorogenic acid to quinones (Fig. 6.20). The quinones react non-enzymatically to polymerize or form covalent bonds with amino, thiol and methylene groups. The epsilon amino of lysine and the thioether group of methionine can covalently bond with quinones to render these amino acids nutritionally unavailable (Fig. 6.20). Enzymatic browning occurs in fruit, causing it to turn brown when mechanically damaged and exposed to oxygen (e.g. browning of apples when peeled or cut). Various food-processing methods are used to prevent this type of browning, including heating to inactivate polyphenol oxidase, and addition of sulfites to foods (now being discontinued

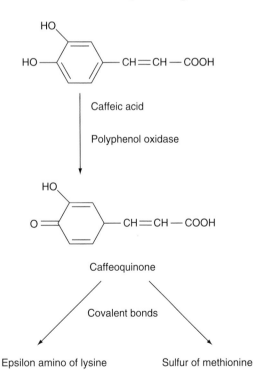

Caffeic acid

Polyphenol oxidase

Caffeoquinone

Covalent bonds

Epsilon amino of lysine   Sulfur of methionine

Fig. 6.20. Polyphenol oxidases in plants convert phenolics to quinones, which can react with amino acids such as lysine and methionine to render them nutritionally unavailable.

because of potential for asthmatic crisis in susceptible individuals).

Red clover (*Trifolium pratense*), a common and productive forage crop, quickly turns brown when harvested. Jones *et al.* (1995) demonstrated that red clover has polyphenol oxidase and soluble phenols. No other common legume forage has polyphenol oxidase activity. The browning of red clover is accompanied by a loss of proteolysis activity, probably because of the binding of oxidized phenols (quinones) to proteolytic enzymes.

Non-enzymatic browning (**Maillard reaction**) is more important in animal feeds. In the Maillard reaction, reducing sugars (those with a potential carbonyl group) react with functional groups of amino acids, and particularly the epsilon amino of lysine. Further reactions producing brown, indigestible polymers occur, resulting in a 'tie-up' of lysine in an unavailable form (Fig. 6.21), thus reducing the protein quality. The Maillard reaction is stimulated by heat and moisture. Whenever proteins are heated, such as when soybean meal is heated to inactivate trypsin inhibitors, browning and **lysine tie-up** will occur. Thus it is important that heat processing be carefully controlled to ensure detoxification but minimize amino acid tie-up. Methionine and tryptophan can also be rendered unavailable by Maillard reactions. Plant protein sources such as soybean meal and cottonseed meal that contain oligosaccharides, such as stachyose and raffinose, or with free glucose, are most susceptible to browning. Besides the reduction in protein quality, some of the products may be toxic, causing growth inhibition and possible mutagenic effects (Friedman, 1994, 1996).

Non-enzymatic browning may also have useful implications in animal production. Cleale *et al.* (1987) used controlled browning of soybean meal with xylose (as a reducing sugar) to increase the bypass protein value of soybean meal in ruminants. Nakamura *et al.* (1992) evaluated xylose-browned soybean meal as a protein source for lactating dairy cattle, and found that the protein from the non-enzymatically browned soybean meal supported the same rate of milk production at half the amount of supplemental soybean meal.

Another type of non-enzymatic browning is the **caramelization** of sugars. Caramel formation occurs when sugars are heated to a high temperature.

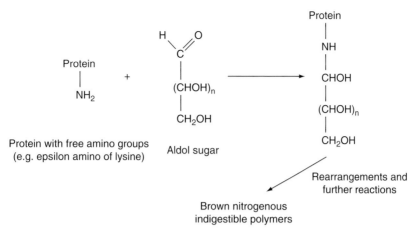

Fig. 6.21. The browning or Maillard reaction results in the 'tie-up' of lysine in an unavailable form.

It involves the removal of water from a sugar followed by isomerization and polymerization, to produce a variety of end products with unique tastes and flavours. The chemistry of caramelization is not well understood.

Foods and feeds are sometimes treated with alkali. Potatoes and fruits may be industrially peeled using strong alkali solutions, and the by-products containing the alkali are often used in animal feeds. **Alkali treatment** of proteins can result in the formation of crosslinked amino acids. For example, **lysinoalanine (LAL)** is formed by the reaction of the epsilon amino of lysine with cysteine or serine. LAL formation results in a reduction in available lysine, and a decrease in digestibility of the modified protein in the intestine (Friedman, 1992) and in the rumen (Nishino *et al.*, 1995). There is evidence that LAL is toxic, causing kidney damage in rats. Friedman (1992) suggests that this effect involves the binding of copper by LAL, within the epithelial cells of the proximal tubules of the kidney. According to Friedman (1994): 'These observations raise concern about the nutritional quality and safety of alkali-treated proteins.'

Nucleotides as Essential Nutrients

Although they are not proteins, nucleotides are discussed in this chapter because they are closely linked to protein metabolism, and nucleic acids do exist as nucleoproteins. **Nucleosides** are derivatives of purine and pyrimidine bases that have a sugar linked to a nitrogen in a ring.

Nucleotides are nucleosides with a phosphate group attached to the sugar. **Nucleotides** are the building blocks of nucleic acids (DNA and RNA). They also form a part of numerous coenzymes and serve as donors of phosphate groups (e.g. ATP). Regulatory nucleotides include cyclic AMP (cAMP).

Pyrimidines (longer name) are single rings while **purines** (short name) are larger (two rings). Examples of pyrimidines are cytosine, uracil and thymine. Purines include adenine and guanine.

The structure of ATP illustrates the structures of nucleosides and nucleotides (Fig. 6.22).

Nucleic acids associated with nucleotides are found in feeds rich in protein, such as organ meats, poultry meat and seafood, and in rapidly dividing cells rich in nucleic acids, for example single-cell proteins such as yeasts and bacteria. Nucleotides may be dietary essentials under some circumstances (Kulkarni *et al.*, 1994). Specifically, they may be required during periods of rapid growth and stress, and in immuno-compromised animals.

Dietary nucleoproteins (nucleic acids conjugated to proteins), nucleic acids (chains of nucleotides) and nucleotides are enzymatically digested prior to absorption. Only the pyrimidine and purine bases and nucleosides are absorbed. Major digestive enzymes include endonucleases, phosphodiesterases and nucleoside phosphorylase, all secreted from the intestinal mucosa (brush border). Dietary nucleotides may be required for optimal growth and disease resistance of newly weaned baby pigs (Mateo *et al.*, 2004). Dietary nucleotides may stimulate growth and maturation of intestinal epithelial cells (Carver, 1994) and have a role in maintaining intestinal health.

In humans, dietary purines may have negative effects. Humans convert adenosine and guanosine to poorly soluble uric acid (Fig. 5.9 in Chapter 5 and Fig. 6.23). In mammals other than higher primates (except the Dalmatian dog), uricase converts uric acid to a more water-soluble product called **allantoin**. Because humans lack uricase, the end product of purine catabolism is uric acid. When serum uric acid is elevated, it may crystallize in soft tissues and joints, causing the painful condition called **gout**. The primary metabolic defect in gout is an over-production of uric acid. In hereditary gout, genetic defects in enzymes involved in purine metabolism result in over-production of uric acid.

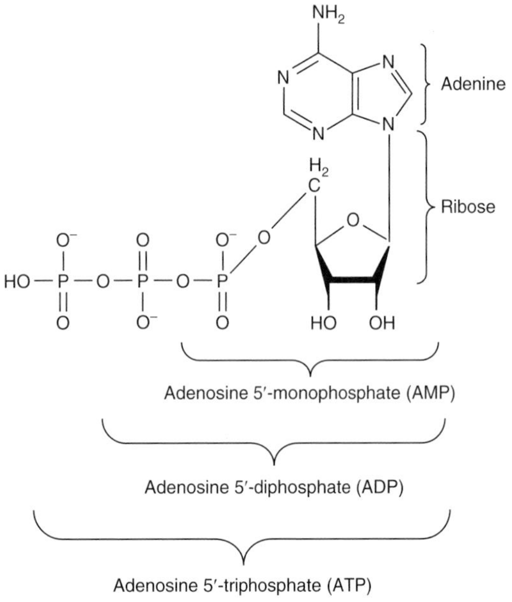

Fig. 6.22. Structures of ATP, and its di- and monophosphates.

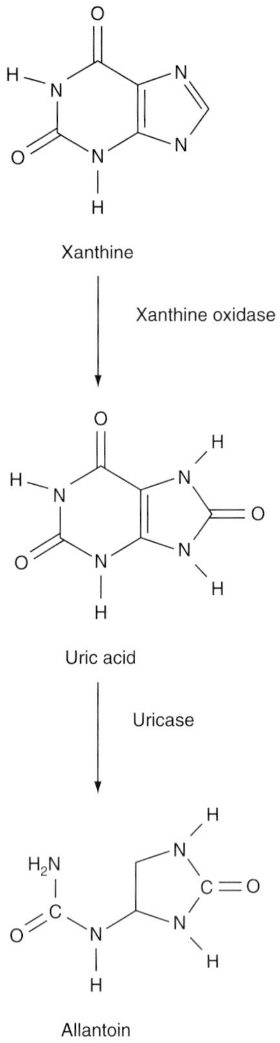

Fig. 6.23. In most animals, uric acid derived from purine metabolism is converted to allantoin. Humans lack uricase, which in some individuals leads to elevated serum uric acid, and development of gout.

Questions and Study Guide

1. Draw the structures of the reactants and products of the transamination reaction catalysed by SGOT.
2. How does a Schiff base function?
3. What is an ideal protein?

4. Are animal proteins (e.g. meat, milk, eggs) essential in the human diet or can a vegetarian diet meet our protein needs?
5. What is the function of (a) lysosomes and (b) ubiquitin?

Continued

---

6. What is unique about the urinary nitrogen of the Dalmatian dog?
7. What are the functions of ornithine and citrulline?
8. Why do chickens have higher dietary requirements for arginine, glycine and methionine than do mammals like pigs?
9. Bird excreta is white in appearance. What is the white substance in it?
10. Ammonia is an alkaline substance, but it can contribute to acid rain. Explain.
11. How do fish excrete nitrogen?
12. Give an example of a 'sparing effect'.
13. Why is choline considered a lipotrope?
14. What is the difference between creatine and creatinine?
15. What are kwashiorkor and marasmus? How do they differ?
16. Is taurine an amino acid? What animals have a dietary requirement for taurine?
17. Male cats have odiferous urine. Why?
18. What is an indole? Which amino acid has an indole group? Name a neurotransmitter, a lung toxin and a pasture grass toxin which are indolic compounds.
19. What causes boar taint?
20. Why do cats have a high dietary requirement for niacin?
21. What hormones are synthesized from tyrosine? What is the role of tyrosine in determining hair colour?
22. What is glutathione? What are some metabolic roles of glutathione? How does it function in preventing red blood cell haemolysis?
23. What animal or bird excretes ornithuric acid?
24. Name two drugs whose activity is related to the production of nitric oxide (NO).
25. Heating proteins causes them to turn brown in colour. Why?
26. Why does red clover hay often turn brown or black in colour?
27. What amino acid is most affected by the Maillard reaction?
28. Are nucleotides essential nutrients?
29. What causes gout in humans? Why don't pigs get gout?

Note

[1] Choline is often considered one of the B vitamins, although it does not strictly meet the definition of a vitamin. It can be synthesized in the liver, is required in the body in greater quantities than other vitamins, and functions in a structural role rather than as a coenzyme.

References

Anderson, J.B., Rogers, Q.R. and Morris, J.G. (2002) Cats require more dietary phenylalanine or tyrosine for melanin deposition in hair than for maximal growth. *Journal of Nutrition* 132, 2037–2042.

Backus, R.C., Ko, K.S., Fascetti, A.J., Kittleson, M.D., MacDonald, K.A., Maggs, D.J., Berg, J.R. and Rogers, Q.R. (2006) Low plasma taurine concentration in Newfoundland dogs is associated with low plasma methionine and cyst(e)ine concentrations and low taurine synthesis. *Journal of Nutrition* 136, 2525–2533.

Brown, W.Y., Vanselow, B.A. and Walkden-Brown, S.W. (2003) One dog's meat is another dog's poison – nutrition in the Dalmation dog. *Recent Advances in Animal Nutrition Australia* 14, 123–131.

Carver, J.D. (1994) Dietary nucleotides: cellular immune, intestinal and hepatic system effects. *Journal of Nutrition* 124, 144–148.

Cheeke, P.R. (1998) *Natural Toxicants in Feeds, Forages, and Poisonous Plants*. Prentice Hall, Upper Saddle River, New Jersey.

Chung, T.K. and Baker, D.H. (1992) Ideal amino acid pattern for 10-kilogram pigs. *Journal of Animal Science* 70, 3102–3111.

Cleale, R.M., Britton, R.A., Klopfenstein, T.J., Bauer, M.L., Harmon, D.L. and Satterlee, L.D. (1987) Induced non-enzymatic browning of soybean meal. II. Ruminal escape and net portal absorption of soybean protein treated with xylose. *Journal of Animal Science* 65, 1319–1326.

Deslandes, B., Garlepy, C. and Houde, A. (2001) Review of microbiological and biochemical effects of skatole on animal production. *Livestock Production Science* 71, 193–200.

Dilger, R.N. and Baker, D.H. (2007) Oral *N*-acetyl-L-cysteine is a safe and effective precursor of cysteine. *Journal of Animal Science* 85, 1712–1718.

Duggan, C., Gannon, J. and Walker, W.A. (2002) Protective nutrients and functional foods for the gastrointestinal tract. *American Journal of Clinical Nutrition* 75, 789–808.

Friedman, M. (1992) Dietary impact of food processing. *Annual Review of Nutrition* 12, 119–137.

Friedman, M. (1994) Improvement in the safety of foods by SH-containing amino acids and peptides. A review. *Journal of Agricultural and Food Chemistry* 42, 3–20.

Friedman, M. (1996) Food browning and its prevention: an overview. *Journal of Agricultural and Food Chemistry* 44, 631–653.

Hendriks, W.H., Moughan, P.J., Tarttelin, M.F. and Woolhouse, A.D. (1995) Felinine: a urinary amino acid of Felidae. *Comparative Biochemistry and Physiology B* 112, 581–588.

Hendriks, W.H., Rutherfurd, S.M. and Rutherfurd, K.J. (2001) Importance of sulfate, cysteine and methionine as precursors to felinine synthesis by domestic cats (*Felis catus*). *Comparative Biochemistry and Physiology C* 129, 211–216.

Hendriks, W.H., Harding, D.R.K. and Rutherfurd-Markwick, K.J. (2004) Isolation and characterization of renal metabolites of γ-glutamylfelinylglycine in the urine of the domestic cat (*Felis catus*). *Comparative Biochemistry and Physiology B* 139, 245–251.

Hutson, S.M., Sweatt, A.J. and LaNoue, K.F. (2005) Branched-chain amino acid metabolism: implications for establishing safe intakes. *Journal of Nutrition* 135, 1557S–1564S.

Jensen, M.T., Cox, R.P. and Jensen, B.B. (1995) Microbial production of skatole in the hind gut of pigs given different diets and its relation to skatole deposition in backfat. *Journal of Animal Science* 61, 293–304.

Jones, B.A., Hatfield, R.D. and Muck, R.E. (1995) Screening legume forages for soluble phenols, polyphenol oxidase and extract browning. *Journal of the Science of Food and Agriculture* 67, 109–112.

Key, T.J., Appleby, P.N. and Rosell, M.S. (2006) Health effects of vegetarian and vegan diets. *Proceedings of the Nutrition Society* 65, 35–41.

Kidd, M.T., Ferket, P.R. and Garlich, J.D. (1997) Nutritional and osmoregulatory functions of betaine. *World's Poultry Science Journal* 53, 125–139.

Koopmans, S.J., Guzik, A.C., van der Meulen, J., Dekker, R., Kogut, J., Kerr, B.J. and Southern, L.L. (2006) Effects of supplemental L-tryptophan on serotonin, cortisol, intestinal integrity, and behavior in weanling piglets. *Journal of Animal Science* 84, 963–971.

Kulkarni, A.D., Rudolph, F.B. and Van Buren, C.T. (1994) The role of dietary sources of nucleotides in immune function: a review. *Journal of Nutrition* 124, 1442–1446.

Lanthier, F., Lou, Y., Terner, M.A. and Squires, E.J. (2006) Characterizing developmental changes in plasma and tissue skatole concentrations in the prepubescent intact male pig. *Journal of Animal Science* 84, 1699–1708.

Larick, D.K. and Turner, B.E. (1989) Influence of finishing diet on the phospholipid composition and fatty acid profile of individual phospholipids in lean muscle of beef cattle. *Journal of Animal Science* 67, 2282–2293.

Li, Y.Z., Kerr, B.J., Kidd, M.T. and Gonyou, H.W. (2006) Use of supplementary tryptophan to modify the behavior of pigs. *Journal of Animal Science* 84, 212–220.

Mateo, C.D., Peters, D.N. and Stein, H.H. (2004) Nucleotides in sow colostrum and milk at different stages of lactation. *Journal of Animal Science* 82, 1339–1342.

Melton, S.L. (1990) Effects of feeds on flavor of red meat: a review. *Journal of Animal Science* 68, 4421–4435.

Mommsen, T.P. and Walsh, P.J. (1992) Biochemical and environmental perspectives on nitrogen metabolism in fishes. *Experientia* 48, 583–593.

Morris, J.G., Yu, S. and Rogers, Q.R. (2002) Red hair in black cats is reversed by addition of tyrosine to the diet. *Journal of Nutrition* 132, 1646S–1648S.

Moss, R. (1997) Grouse and ptarmigan nutrition in the wild and in captivity. *Proceedings of the Nutrition Society* 56, 1137–1145.

Nakamura, T., Klopfenstein, T.J., Owen, F.G., Britton, R.A., Grant, R.J. and Winowiski, T.S. (1992) Nonenzymatically browned soybean meal for lactating dairy cows. *Journal of Dairy Science* 75, 3519–3523.

Nishino, N., Uchida, S. and Ohshima, M. (1995) Formation of lysinoalanine following alkaline processing of soya bean meal in relation to the degradability of protein in the rumen. *Journal of the Science of Food and Agriculture* 68, 59–64.

Popovich, D.G., Jenkins, D.J.A., Kendall, C.W.C., Dierenfeld, E.S., Carroll, R.W., Tariq, N. and Vidgen, E. (1997) The western lowland gorilla diet has implications for the health of humans and other hominoids. *Journal of Nutrition* 127, 2000–2005.

Rutherfurd-Markwick, K.J., McGrath, M.C., Weidgraaf, K. and Hendriks, W.H. (2006) γ-Glutamylfelinylglycine metabolite excretion in the urine of the domestic cat (*Felis catus*). *Journal of Nutrition* 136, 2075S–2077S.

Schreurs, N.M., Lane, G.A., Tavendale, M.H., Barry, T.N. and McNabb, W.C. (2008) Pastoral flavour in meat products from ruminants fed fresh forages and its amelioration by forage condensed tannins. *Animal Feed Science and Technology* 146, 193–221.

Shorland, F.B. (1988) Is our knowledge of human nutrition soundly based? *World Review of Nutrition and Dietetics* 57, 126–213.

Squires, J.E. and Lundstrom, K. (1997) Relationship between cytochrome P450IIE1 in liver and levels of skatole and its metabolites in intact male pigs. *Journal of Animal Science* 75, 2506–2511.

Watford, M. (1999) Is there a requirement for glutamine catabolism in the small intestine? *British Journal of Nutrition* 81, 261–262.

Weir, D.G. and Scott, J.M. (1998) Homocysteine as a risk factor for cardiovascular and related disease: nutritional implications. *Nutrition Research Reviews* 11, 311–338.

PART III
Carbohydrates

This part is intended to describe carbohydrates, particularly with reference to their relationship with the structure of glucose, and to discuss the pathways of catabolism of carbohydrates in animals.

Part Objectives

1. To describe the chemical structure of monosaccharides and more complex carbohydrates (disaccharides, oligosaccharides, polysaccharides).
2. To discuss the digestion of carbohydrates in auto- and alloenzymatic animals.
3. To discuss the metabolism of carbohydrates in animal tissues.

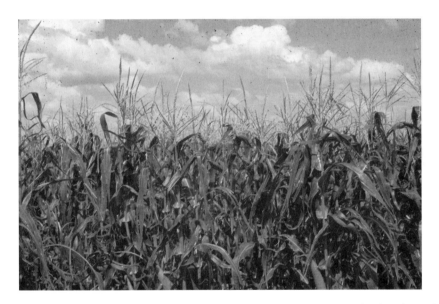

Forages and grains are major carbohydrate sources for animal feeding. Shown here is maize (corn), a major grain source that has the C4 photosynthetic pathway.

Carbohydrates were originally named because they generally contain carbon, hydrogen and oxygen, with the hydrogen and oxygen in the same proportion as in water: $C_n(H_2O)_n$; hence, **hydrates of carbon**. Carbohydrates are synthesized in plants from carbon dioxide, water and solar energy. Carbohydrate catabolism in animals is the reverse of this process, with carbohydrates oxidized to carbon dioxide and water, and release of chemical energy in the form of ATP. Carbohydrate metabolism will be described in more detail in Chapter 9.

Classification of Carbohydrates

The basic units of carbohydrate structure are the simple sugars or **monosaccharides**, that cannot be hydrolysed into simpler carbohydrates. The monosaccharides may be subdivided into groups based upon the number of carbon atoms: for example trioses (three carbons), tetroses (four carbons), pentoses (five carbons) and hexoses (six carbons). Most monosaccharides encountered in animal nutrition are pentoses (e.g. ribose) and hexoses (e.g. glucose). The simple sugars are also subdivided into aldoses and ketoses: **aldoses** have an aldehyde structure and **ketoses** are ketones. Thus glucose and fructose have the same molecular formula ($C_6H_{12}O_6$); they are both hexoses, with glucose an aldose and fructose a ketose (Fig. 7.1). This difference in orientation causes glucose and fructose to have different physical, chemical and biological properties.

Common monosaccharides important in animal nutrition include glucose, fructose (also known as levulose), galactose, mannose and ribose. Because glucose occupies a central position in carbohydrate structure and metabolism, its properties will be discussed in more detail. The chemical structure of glucose can be represented in both a straight-chain form and a cyclic form. In biological systems, glucose exists primarily in the cyclic form (Fig. 7.2).

Glucose (formerly known as grape sugar) has four **asymmetric carbons** (four different chemical groups attached to a carbon atom) which allows the formation of isomers. The number of possible isomers depends on the number of asymmetric carbons (n) and is equal to 2^n. Thus hexoses can exist in 16 isomeric forms. D- and L-glucose differ in their orientation of the hydroxyl groups on carbon 5 (Fig. 7.3). The orientation of the hydrogen and hydroxyl groups around the carbon atom adjacent to the terminal carbon (carbon 5 in glucose) determines whether a simple sugar is in the D or L series. Most of the monosaccharides metabolized by animals are of the D configuration. Isomers differing in configuration of the hydroxyls on carbons 2, 3 and 4 of glucose are known as **epimers**. The most important epimers of glucose are those with epimerization at C2 (mannose) and C4 (galactose) (Fig. 7.4). Thus there are numerous monosaccharides with the same molecular formula as glucose ($C_6H_{12}O_6$), but with completely different chemical and biological properties.

Sugars such as glucose can also exist as alpha (α) and beta (β) **anomers**, which are isomers differing in their orientation about the bond formed by reaction of the aldehyde and hydroxyl groups. Glucose exists as α and β isomers (Fig. 7.5). This apparently simple difference (to a non-chemist) in bond orientation has immense nutritional implications. **Starch** is a soft polymer consisting of α-D-glucose units, while cellulose is a rigid polymer of β-D-glucoses (Fig. 7.6). **Cellulose** is the most abundant organic compound in the world, but cannot be digested by autoenzymatic digesters such as pigs, poultry and humans because they do not produce the enzyme, cellulase, which splits the bonds joining the β-D-glucoses. Starch, on the other hand, is a pliable substance that is readily digested.

A common source of fructose in the human diet is **high fructose corn syrup (HFCS)**.[1] It is prepared by processing maize starch to yield maize syrup

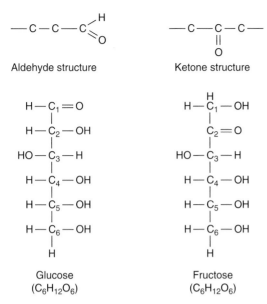

Aldehyde structure

Ketone structure

Glucose
($C_6H_{12}O_6$)

Fructose
($C_6H_{12}O_6$)

Fig. 7.1. Straight-chain structures of glucose (aldehyde on C1) and fructose (ketone on C2). Note that while these are different sugars they have the same molecular formula of $C_6H_{12}O_6$.

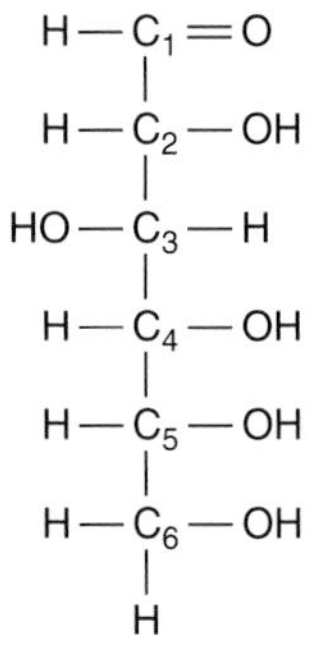

D-glucose
(straight chain)

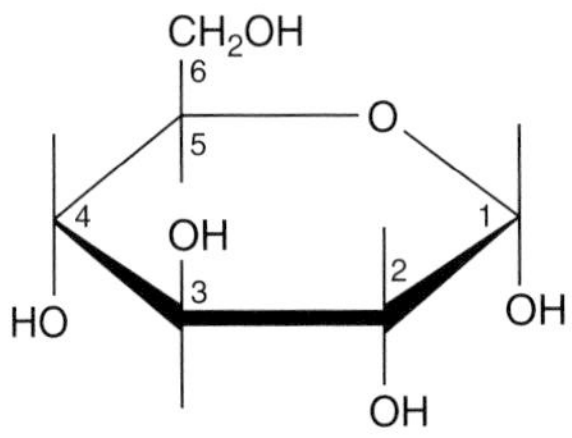

D-glucose
(cyclic or ring form)

Fig. 7.2. Monosaccharides such as glucose may occur in a straight-chain or cyclic form.

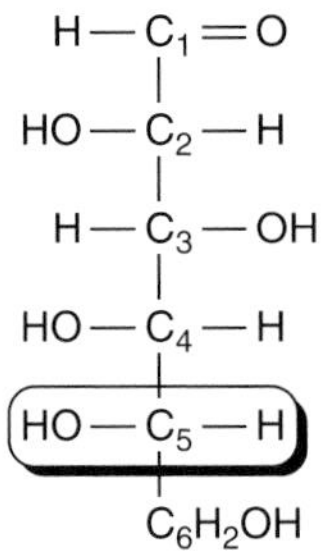

L-glucose

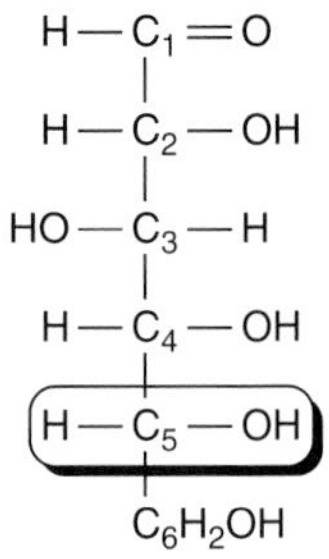

D-glucose

Fig. 7.3. L- and D-isomerism of glucose.

Disaccharides are composed of two monosaccharides linked together by a glycosidic (ether) bond. Important disaccharides in animal nutrition (Fig. 7.7) include sucrose (glucose + fructose), maltose (glucose + glucose), lactose (glucose + galactose) and cellobiose (glucose + glucose).

Sucrose (table sugar, cane sugar, beet sugar) can be hydrolysed by an enzyme (**invertase**), acid or heat to produce a mixture of glucose and fructose called **invert sugar**. The hydrolysis of sucrose causes an inversion of the rotation of polarized light. Invert sugar is sweeter than sucrose, and is widely used in food processing in the preparation of sweets, chocolates and other products. The making of jam produces invert sugar because of the acidity of the fruit and extended heating.

Reducing sugars reduce (provide hydrogen) Fehling's solution or Benedict's solution. These reagents contain alkaline cupric tartrate (Benedict's) or citrate (Fehling's). Reducing sugars reduce the cupric (Cu^{++}) ions to cuprous (Cu^+), which oxidizes to produce a brick red precipitate, cupric oxide. Reducing sugars have a free aldehyde group that can donate hydrogen. All monosaccharides and most disaccharides are reducing sugars. An exception is sucrose, which is a non-reducing sugar because it does not have a free aldehyde group. Monosaccharides that are in ring form are nonreducing, but are in equilibrium with the open chain form, so are instantaneously converted entirely to reducing sugar in the simple test for reducing sugars. Fructose is a reducing sugar, even though it does not have an aldehyde group, because under alkaline conditions the keto group isomerizes to an aldehyde group.

It is important in food and feed processing to know if reducing sugars are present. For example, they react with the amino acid lysine to reduce its

that is almost entirely glucose, and then enzymatically converting the glucose into fructose. This is done because fructose is sweeter than glucose. The widespread use of HFCS as a sweetener in the USA is largely due to import quotas and tariffs on sugar, which elevates the US price of sugar to a level much higher than the international price, along with subsidies on maize which cause the price of maize to be artificially low.

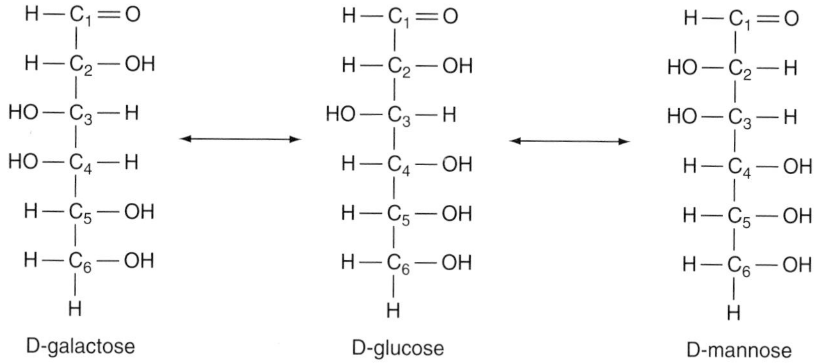

Fig. 7.4. Epimerization of glucose. Epimers differ in the orientation of the hydroxyl groups on C2, C3 and C4 of glucose.

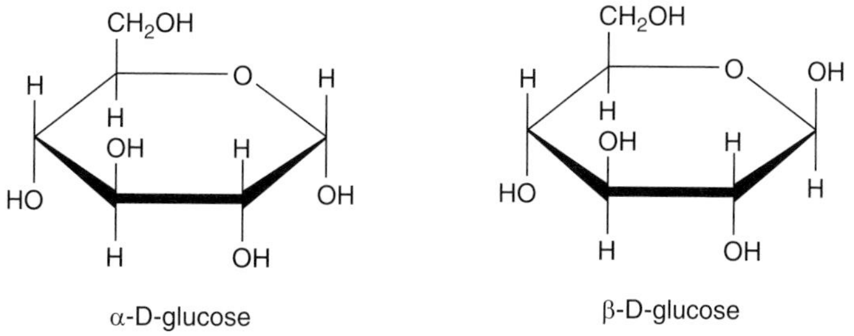

Fig. 7.5. The α and β configurations of glucose, depending on the orientation of the hydroxyl on C1.

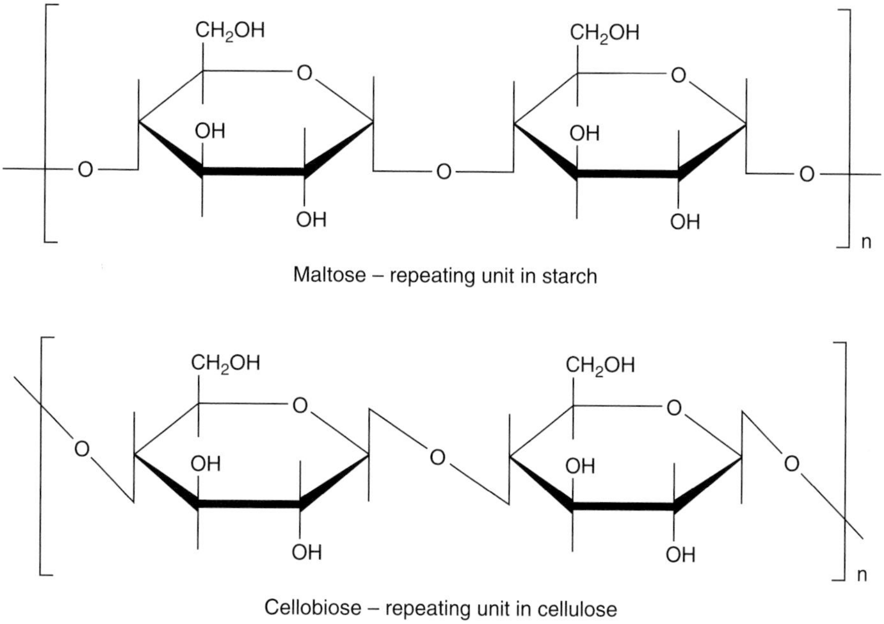

Fig. 7.6. Maltose and cellobiose, the repeating units of starch and cellulose, respectively.

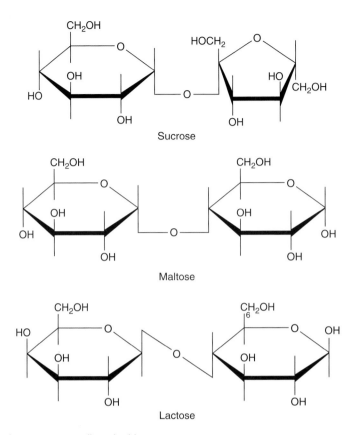

Fig. 7.7. Examples of some common disaccharides.

availability to an animal (lysine tie-up, **Maillard reaction**; see Chapter 6). Reducing sugars also react with ammonia to produce toxic **imidazoles**. Imidazoles cause bovine hyperexcitability (bovine hysteria, bovine bonkers, crazy cow syndrome, **ammoniated hay toxicosis**), as reviewed by Cheeke (1998). Ammoniation of hay containing reducing sugars, or the ammoniation of molasses, can lead to imidazole formation.

Oligosaccharides contain three or more monosaccharides linked by glycosidic bonds. **Raffinose** (glucose, fructose, galactose) is a trisaccharide, and occurs in beans and other legume seeds, as well as in rapeseed and cottonseed. **Stachyose**, a tetrasaccharide (two galactoses, glucose, fructose), occurs in legume seeds and rapeseed. These short-chain oligosaccharides are nutritionally significant because mammals do not secrete enzymes to digest them. They reduce the potential digestible energy in feeds for non-ruminants such as pigs and poultry. In these animals, they are fermented by microbes in the hindgut, causing gas production and flatulence (oligosaccharides are the flatulence-factors of beans). A number of oligosaccharides, such as mannan oligosaccharide (**MOS**), fructooligosaccharides (**FOS**) and galactooligosaccharides (**GOS**) are used as feed additives for the modification of gut microflora and stimulation of the intestinal immune system. The intestinal mucosa contains carbohydrate residues that serve as binding sites for bacterial cell walls. Dietary oligosaccharides may bind to these receptor sites on bacteria, thus preventing them from binding to the intestinal mucosa, and causing the bacteria to be flushed out of the digestive tract. Pathogenic bacteria must bind to and colonize the gut lining to cause enteric disease. The binding sites on bacteria are called **lectins**. Raw beans also contain lectins, which damage the intestinal mucosa by binding to the carbohydrate components of the microvilli. Oligosaccharides are also known as **prebiotics**, which are substances that stimulate the growth of beneficial gut microbes.

FOS, MOS and GOS are prebiotics used as feed additives for this purpose.

Polysaccharides are large polymers[2] composed of simple sugars linked together. The most important carbohydrates in feeds are polysaccharides: starch and cellulose. **Starch** is composed of α-D-glucose linked together by α-1,4-bonds (Fig. 7.8). The repeating unit in starch is the disaccharide maltose (Fig. 7.6). Starch is of two types: (i) amylose; and (ii) amylopectin. **Amylose** has a straight chain, non-branching structure, with α-D-glucoses linked by α-1,4-bonds, with the molecule curled in a helical structure. **Amylopectin** has a branched structure, with glucoses linked by α-1,4-bonds, with branches with α-1,6-bonds (Fig. 7.8). Most starch in cereal grains and tubers (e.g. potatoes) is a mixture of 15–20% amylose and 80–85% amylopectin.

Cellulose consists of a straight chain of glucose molecules, with the glucoses joined by β-1,4-bonds (Fig. 7.6). The repeating disaccharide unit in

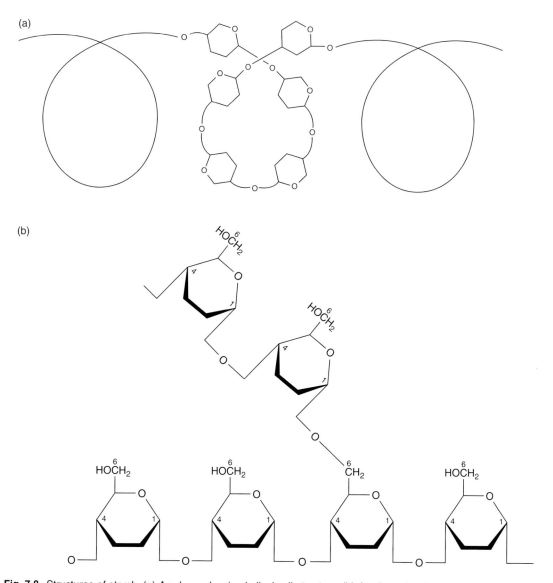

Fig. 7.8. Structures of starch. (a) Amylose, showing helical coil structure. (b) Amylopectin, showing the α1 → 6 branch point.

cellulose is **cellobiose**. Cellulose is the major component of plant cell walls and plant fibre. It is remarkable that starch and cellulose, so different in physical structure and function, are both composed solely of glucose, differing only in the orientation of the bond linking the glucoses together. The nature of the bond influences the molecular shape of the molecule, and its ability to pack into a solid structure.

Lactulose is a synthetic sugar used in the treatment of constipation in humans. It is a disaccharide of fructose and galactose. It is indigestible in the small intestine, but is fermented in the colon, producing short-chain fatty acids that have a cathartic effect through osmotic action.

Sucralose (Splenda®) is an artificial disaccharide sweetener manufactured from sucrose. Three of the hydroxyl groups (two on fructose and one on glucose) of sucrose are substituted with chlorine atoms. It is up to 1000 times sweeter than sucrose. Sucralose has no recognized toxicity, but is frowned upon by some critics because it is not 'natural'.

There are various **non-starch polysaccharides** (NSP) in feeds. For example, barley and oats contain β-**glucans**, which are branched structures containing β-1,3- and β-1,4-linkages. They are partially soluble in water, forming viscous, gummy solutions. There are a variety of other NSP, containing various monosaccharides. They are found in plant gums, seeds and in the cell walls of forages. Examples include xylans, mannans, pentosans and arabinoxylans. They are collectively referred to as **hemicellulose**.

Polymers of fructose are called **fructans**. As with glucose polymers, they exist both as storage and as structural polysaccharides in plants. **Inulin**, with β-2,1-linkages between fructoses, is a fructose polymer occurring as a storage carbohydrate in Jerusalem artichoke tubers and chicory. Jerusalem artichokes are grown to a minor extent as substitutes for potatoes in the human diet, while chicory is a perennial broadleaved plant grown as a forage crop, especially in New Zealand. **Jerusalem artichokes** (neither from Jerusalem nor a real artichoke!) resemble sunflowers in above-ground appearance. Below ground, they produce knobby, misshapen tubers rich in inulin. Inulin is a polymer of about 35 fructose units (Rumessen *et al.*, 1990). Animals do not produce an inulin-degrading enzyme, so consumption of inulin by humans does not result in absorbable monosaccharides. For this reason, Jerusalem artichokes are sometimes recommended in diets for

diabetics (Rumessen *et al.*, 1990). Grasses contain structural fructans, with β-2,6-linkages. The fructan content of temperate grasses may be as much as 30% of the dry matter. Fermentation of fructans in the hindgut of the horse may play a role in laminitis (see Chapter 19).

Pectins are NSP rich in galacturonic acid that occur in plant cell walls, where they function as the 'glue' cementing plant cells together. Pectins have a galacturonic acid central chain with arabinan and galactan side chains. The acid groups on the side chains may occur as methyl esters, or with complexed calcium ions. Weak acids in combination with sucrose precipitate pectins in the form of a gel, which is important in food processing in the preparation of jams and jellies.

Carbohydrates occur primarily in plants. In animal tissue, the main carbohydrate is **glycogen**, a polysaccharide similar in structure to amylopectin (hence it is also known as animal starch). Glycogen is stored in liver and muscle. Liver glycogen is used to maintain the blood glucose level, while muscle glycogen is an energy reserve for muscular work. The other carbohydrate of animal origin is **lactose** (milk sugar), a disaccharide of glucose and galactose.

Miscellaneous Carbohydrates

Although quantitatively carbohydrate is not a major constituent of animal tissues, some carbohydrates do have important roles in tissue structure. Most of these are combinations of carbohydrate with protein (glycoproteins) or lipid (glycolipids). **Mucopolysaccharides** (**mucins**) are glycoproteins which constitute mucus secretions. They are also known as **glycosaminoglycans**. Mucins help lubricate and form a protective physical barrier on epithelial surfaces in the digestive, respiratory and reproductive tracts. These glycoproteins contain amino sugars and uronic acids. **Amino sugars**, such as glucosamine, contain an amino group that may participate in forming bonds with other substances. **Uronic acids**, such as glucuronic acid, have a carboxyl group in place of an hydroxyl group on a sugar molecule. Examples of mucopolysaccharides include hyaluronic acid, chondroitin sulfate and heparin. Their functions will be discussed in Chapter 18.

Chitin is a structural polysaccharide in invertebrates. It is a major component of the exoskeleton of crustaceans and insects. Some feedstuffs (e.g. crab meal, shrimp meal) contain chitin. It is composed of

N-acetyl-D-glucosamine units joined by β-1,4-linkages.

Sialic acids are derivatives of a nine-carbon sugar, neuramininc acid. Sialic acids are constituents of glycoproteins and glycolipids, such as gangliosides. Glycolipids are important components of nerve tissue.

Carbohydrate Analysis of Forages

The time-honoured system of feed analysis is the **proximate analysis scheme** or Weende system (named after the Weende Experiment Station at Gottingen, Germany, where it was developed). Components of the proximate analysis scheme are crude protein, ether extract, ash, crude fibre and nitrogen-free extract (NFE). Feed carbohydrates are the crude fibre and NFE fractions.

The **crude fibre** content of feeds and forages is measured by boiling an ether-extracted feed sample in dilute acid, then in dilute alkali, drying, and burning in a muffle furnace. The difference in weight before and after burning is the crude-fibre fraction. In the modified crude-fibre determination, the correction for ash content is not done. This procedure was developed in the early days of nutrition research in an attempt to estimate the indigestible portion of food in the human digestive tract by simulating the acid condition of the stomach and alkaline condition of the intestine. In spite of well-recognized inadequacies, crude-fibre values are still widely used (mainly because crude fibre analyses are legally required on feed tags).

New procedures to estimate the fibre content of forages have been developed. These methods, such as acid detergent fibre and neutral detergent fibre, are described in more detail below.

Nitrogen-free extract (NFE) is derived by subtracting the sum of the other proximate components from 100:

Percentage NFE = 100 – Percentage of
[Water (%) + Crude protein (%) + Ether
extract (%) + Ash (%) + Crude fibre (%)]

The NFE theoretically represents mainly starch, sugars and other readily available carbohydrates. In practice, the inaccuracies associated with crude fibre are such that neither crude fibre nor NFE are nutritionally very meaningful. The proximate analysis system is inaccurate when applied to roughages because it does not accurately separate the carbohydrate fraction into the true fibrous fractions and the non-fibre components. Van Soest (1994) of Cornell University has developed a better system based on the use of neutral and acid detergents. Refluxing (boiling) a forage sample in a detergent solution solubilizes proteins, sugars, minerals, starch and pectins. These compounds, known as the **cell contents**, are highly digestible in the rumen. The detergent-insoluble fraction corresponds to the fibrous cell wall material, referred to as the **cell wall constituents** (CWC).

In the Van Soest procedure, a dried, ground forage sample is refluxed first in a neutral-detergent solution of sodium lauryl sulfate and ethylenediaminetetraacetate (EDTA) at pH 7.0. The detergent solubilizes the proteins and dissolves minerals, sugars, starch and pectins. The dissolved material is called 'cell contents' and is completely digestible in ruminants. The insoluble residue is called **neutral detergent fibre (NDF)**. The NDF (or a new sample of the forage) is then boiled in an acid detergent solution (cetyl trimethylammonium bromide in 1 N H_2SO_4). In addition to solubilizing the cell contents, the acid detergent dissolves hemicellulose. The residue is called **acid detergent fibre (ADF)**. Thus hemicellulose = NDF – ADF. The ADF fraction consists largely of cellulose, lignin, silica and **cutin** (cutin is the waxy material on the surface of leaves). The ADF fraction can be further categorized by boiling in concentrated (72%) H_2SO_4. This dissolves cellulose and leaves a residue of lignin, silica and cutin. This can be treated with a permanganate solution that oxidizes and destroys lignin. The **silica** content can be measured by ashing a sample of ADF; the residue is silica. Thus, by these methods, the plant cell wall material can be completely classified. Dairy nutritionists also use effective NDF (eNDF), which is described in Chapter 17.

The cell contents fraction, consisting of those components soluble in neutral detergent, is also known as the **neutral detergent-soluble carbohydrates (NDSC)** fraction (Hall *et al.*, 1999; Hall, 2003). The NDSC can be partitioned into four fractions that reflect ruminal and mammalian digestion properties (Hall *et al.*, 1999): (i) organic acids; (ii) mono-, di- and oligosaccharides; (iii) starch; and (iv) **neutral detergent-soluble fibre (NDSF)** (fructans, pectins and glucans).

Differential solubilities of carbohydrates in aqueous ethanol and in neutral detergent with heat-stable α-amylase can be used to estimate the NDSC fractions. Aqueous ethanol (80:20 V/V ethanol/water)

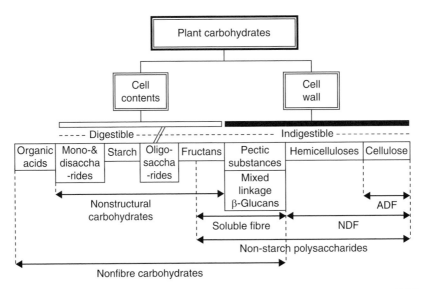

Fig. 7.9. Carbohydrate fractions of plants. ADF, acid detergent fibre; NDF, neutral detergent fibre; NDSF, neutral detergent-soluble fibre; NFC, non-NDF carbohydrates (courtesy of M.B. Hall, USDA, Madison, Wisconsin, USA).

solubilizes low molecular-weight carbohydrates (organic acids, mono- and oligosaccharides), leaving starch and NDSF as an ethanol-insoluble residue. The starch content of the ethanol/water insoluble residue is measured using amylase to convert the starch to glucose, which is measured colorimetrically. Detailed descriptions of the methodology of NDSC components is provided by Hall (2003). The relationship of plant carbohydrates to the typical forage cell structure is shown in Fig. 7.9.

Structural Carbohydrate Characteristics of Forages

The predominant chemical characteristic of forages is their high content of cell wall material. The structure of plant cells is shown in Fig. 7.10. They consist of a fibrous cell wall, with the cell contents inside. The cell wall is composed of metabolically inert, highly fibrous material, whereas the cell contents contain the metabolically active components. Dominant **cell contents** components include the chloroplasts, in which photosynthesis occurs, and the mitochondria and cellular protoplasm containing the enzymes involved in carbohydrate and protein synthesis. The major components of the **cell wall** include cellulose, lignin, hemicellulose and silica. Cellulose and lignin provide structural strength to the cell wall. The polysaccharides

(complex carbohydrates) of the cell wall occur either in crystalline (microfibrils) or non-crystalline (matrix) form.

The microfibrils consist of cellulose molecules ordered together in rod-like chains to form bundles of fibres. They form a three-dimensional crystal lattice. The matrix is made up of hemicelluloses and pectins. **Hemicelluloses** are complex carbohydrates containing mixtures of monosaccharides; the main types are xylans, mannans and galactans, containing the simple sugars xylose, mannose and galactose, respectively. The **cell wall** can be compared to reinforced concrete: the matrix polysaccharides are the cement and the cellulose fibres are the reinforcing rods. The matrix contains a considerable amount of water, forming a viscous gel. As the growth of the cell ceases, the space occupied by water becomes progressively filled with lignin so that the matrix becomes permeated with this compound. This process is called **lignification**, and it occurs after the deposition of the polysaccharide components. Lignin is a highly indigestible phenolic substance. In some plants, especially some grasses and *Equisetum* (horsetail) species, the matrix may contain considerable quantities of silica. The space between cells (intercellular space) is called the middle lamella. This is composed largely of pectin. In woody tissues, the pectin is permeated with lignin.

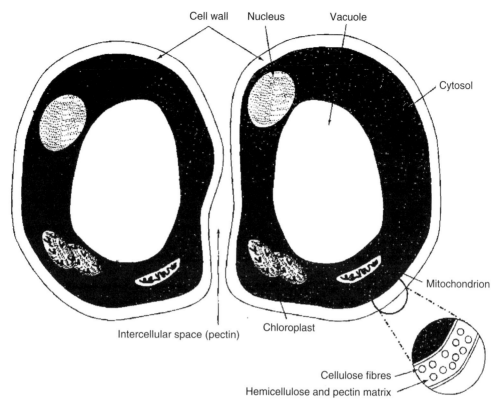

Fig. 7.10. Simplified diagram of cells of forage plant tissue. The highly digestible cell contents are encased in the less digestible cell wall. The nutritive value of a forage depends in part on the accessibility of the cell contents to microbial enzymes, which in turn depends on the structure of the cell wall.

The **cell contents** are the metabolically active part of the plant cell and consist of the cytosol and vacuole(s) (Fig. 7.10). The cytosol contains the nucleus, mitochondria and chloroplasts and is the part of the cell where the photosynthetic work is taking place. The interior vacuole, which may be one large vacuole or numerous small ones, is an aqueous phase that helps keep the cell in turgid condition. It is also a storage area for cell wastes, food reserves and toxic substances, such as alkaloids, tannins and glycosides. It has lysosomal activity for intracellular digestion. Thus, the vacuoles are a water solution of free sugars, organic acids, minerals and secondary compounds (secondary compounds are alkaloids, glycosides and tannins, which are chemical defences from the plant perspective and toxins from the animal perspective).

The nutritional value of forages depends largely on the relative proportions of cell contents and cell wall constituents, and on the degree of lignification of the cell walls. The carbohydrate content of forages shows **diurnal variation**. Sugars (photosynthate) are synthesized by photosynthesis during daylight hours, and accumulate in the cell contents. A point that is often overlooked by animal scientists is that plants catabolize carbohydrate by glycolysis and the citric acid cycle, just as animals do. This metabolism continues at night, using up sugars that were photosynthesized during the day. Thus the soluble carbohydrate content of forages tends to be lowest in the early morning, and highest at midday and the afternoon. For this reason, hay cut in the afternoon has a higher digestible energy content than hay cut in the morning. Because of the higher sugar content, afternoon-cut hay tends to be more palatable and nutritious for ruminants than hay cut in early morning (Fisher *et al.*, 1999). For horses, the higher sugar content of afternoon forages may play a role in the etiology of laminitis and equine metabolic disorder (see Chapter 16). Therefore, early morning grazing for horses may be preferable over late morning or afternoon grazing.

Notes

[1] In North America, *Zea mays* is known as corn. In most of the rest of the world, it is referred to as maize.

[2] A polymer is a large molecule composed of multiples of a specific repeating unit.

References

Cheeke, P.R. (1998) *Natural Toxicants in Feeds, Forages, and Poisonous Plants*. Prentice Hall, Upper Saddle River, New Jersey.

Fisher, D.S., Mayland, H.F. and Burns, J.C. (1999) Variation in ruminant's preference for tall fescue hays cut at sundown or sunup. *Journal of Animal Science* 77, 762–768.

Hall, M.B. (2003) Challenges with nonfiber carbohydrate methods. *Journal of Animal Science* 81, 3226–3232.

Hall, M.B., Hoover, W.H., Jennings, J.P. and Webster, T.K.M. (1999) A method for partitioning neutral detergent-soluble carbohydrates. *Journal of the Science of Food and Agriculture* 79, 2079–2086.

Rumessen, J.J., Bode, S., Hamberg, O. and Gudmand-Hoyer, E. (1990) Fructans of Jerusalem artichokes: intestinal transport, absorption, fermentation, and influence on blood glucose, insulin, and C-peptide responses in healthy subjects. *American Journal of Clinical Nutrition* 52, 675–681.

Van Soest, P.J. (1994) *Nutritional Ecology of the Ruminant*. Cornell University Press, Ithaca, New York.

8 Carbohydrate Digestion and Absorption

Carbohydrate Digestion and Absorption in Monogastric Animals

In autoenzymatic digester monogastrics, carbohydrate digestion involves the enzymatic hydrolysis of complex carbohydrates with the release of free sugars (monosaccharides) which are absorbed. The primary site of carbohydrate digestion is the small intestine. Because most dietary carbohydrate (e.g. starch) contains glucose, the primary product of carbohydrate digestion is glucose.

Starch occurs in plants in the form of **starch granules**, which vary in size and shape depending upon the plant source. The membrane of the starch granule is resistant to water entry and enzyme attack. Heat treatment of grains causes starch **gelatinization**, in which the hydrogen bonds holding the starch molecules together are denatured. This allows the granules to absorb water and swell. During grain processing, such as with steam rolling, the swollen starch granules are torn apart by the rolling or flaking, increasing the area of starch exposed to digestive enzymes.

Carbohydrate digestion in many animals (not in ruminants) begins in the mouth, with the secretion of **salivary amylase**. This activity is not usually physiologically significant; almost all starch digestion occurs in the small intestine. The major enzyme involved in starch digestion is **pancreatic amylase**. There are two amylases: one that cleaves α-1,4-bonds in random fashion while the other successively removes disaccharide units (maltose) from the polysaccharide chain. Neither enzyme splits the α-1,6-bonds that form the branch points in the structure of amylopectin. The action of amylases gives rise to a mixture of glucose, maltose and **limit dextrins**, which are the residues containing α-1,6-branch points. Dextrins are digested by α-1,6-glucosidase. Pancreatic amylase acts on starch granules in the lumen of the intestine (Fig. 8.1). The products of starch digestion diffuse into the **brush border** (unstirred water layer) where the final

digestive processes occur. Various **disaccharidases** such as maltase complete the degradation of starch fragments to free glucose, which is then absorbed into the enterocytes. The advantage of having free glucose released in the brush border is that it is not swept away by the luminal contents, but is trapped in the unstirred water layer, facilitating its absorption at active transport sites (Moran, 1985). The disaccharidases are anchored to the enterocyte membrane. Nectar-feeding birds such as hummingbirds have very high intestinal sucrase activity (Schondube and Martinez del Rio, 2004). Hummingbirds are unique in their capacity to rapidly hydrolyse sucrose, a result of their sucrose-based diet and high metabolic activity.

There is evidence that modern humans have adapted biochemically to high starch diets. Following domestication of cereal grains and tubers, starch has become an increasingly important component of the human diet in agricultural societies and hunter-gatherers in arid environments. In contrast, rainforest and circum-Arctic hunter-gatherers consume much less starch. Perry *et al.* (2007) studied the human salivary amylase gene in diverse human populations, including European Americans, Japanese, Hadza hunter-gatherers who rely extensively on starch-rich roots and tubers, and low starch-intake populations including rainforest hunter-gatherers, Datog pastoralists and Arctic (Yakut) pastoralists with a fish-based diet. As predicted, populations with a traditional high starch diet had higher salivary amylase gene expression levels (which correlates with levels of salivary amylase), which probably improves the digestion of starchy foods and may buffer against intestinal disease. This situation represents recent biochemical evolution in response to diet.

In the chicken, the chick at hatching has full development of its carbohydrate digestive enzyme activity (Moran, 1985), whereas this is not the case for species that consume crop milk (e.g. pigeons). In contrast to the chicken, these crop-milk species

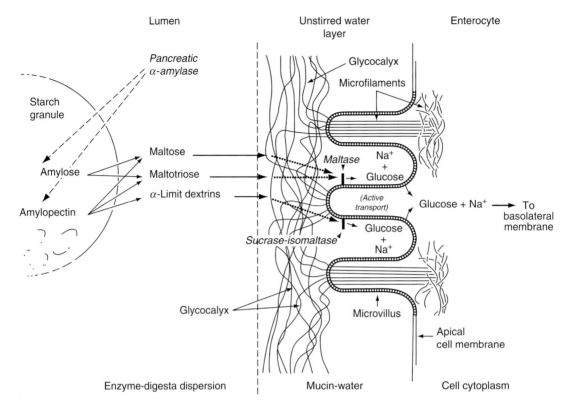

Fig. 8.1. Postulated sequence of events in the digestion of starch by fowl. Starch is normally in granular form and pancreatic α-amylase progressively hydrolyses constituent amylose and amylopectin to maltose, maltotriose and α-limit dextrins. Enterocytes lining the small intestine project microvilli and a fibrous glycocalyx into the lumen. An aqueous dispersion of mucin from nearby goblet cells is immobilized in these structures to form the 'unstirred water layer'. Dissolved products from starch digestion must diffuse through this barrier to reach carbohydrases anchored on the surface in order to finalize digestion; however, glucose accrues near active transport sites, and its rate of absorption is improved (courtesy of E.T. Moran, Jr, Auburn University, Auburn, Alabama, USA).

develop digestive enzyme activity and diet shifts over the first few weeks of life. Similarly, in the pig and other mammals, the neonate initially consumes only milk, so at birth has a low activity of amylase, sucrase and other carbohydrases involved in digestion of plant-origin carbohydrates. Only lactase is needed by the newborn mammal. Development of digestive enzyme activity is stimulated by the consumption of solid feed by the young animal.

Monosaccharides are absorbed both by simple diffusion and by **active transport** against a concentration gradient. A sodium-dependent glucose transport protein binds both glucose and Na$^+$ at separate sites and transports them through the enterocyte plasma membrane, releasing them into the cytosol. Active transport is an energy (ATP)-requiring process.

Mammals do not secrete enzymes that can digest cellulose, chitin, the non-starch polysaccharides (NSP) such as β-glucans, and short-chain oligosaccharides such as raffinose and stachyose. **Cellulose**, a major component of plant fibre, is not nutritionally useful to pigs and poultry except as a source of bulk and as a diet diluent (e.g. gestating sows). The pig has substantial hindgut microbial activity, with some apparent fibre digestion, but the end products of microbial action (volatile fatty acids, VFAs) do not make a significant contribution to the pig's energy needs. The NSP such as β-glucans in barley and oats are not digestible in the small intestine of pigs and poultry. Glucans and other viscous, poorly water-soluble plant gums tend to 'clog up' the brush border because of their high viscosity, and interfere with the digestion and absorption of other substances, especially lipids. The NSP in grains cause a specific **fat malabsorption syndrome** in poultry, due to the increased viscosity of the gut contents. The adverse nutritional effects of NSP are primarily explained by their influence on viscosity of intestinal contents (Annison and Choct, 1991). The hydroscopic nature of NSP causes increased water retention in the gut, as well as increased endogenous secretion of water via the saliva and intestinal tract (Low, 1989). This causes significant management problems in poultry, because of the increased excretion of water, causing wet, soupy litter.

Wheat contains NSP that are **pentosans**, which are polymers of pentoses such as xylose and arabinose (arabinoxylans). The presence of these substances reduces the apparent metabolizable energy (AME) of wheat for poultry (Annison, 1991; Annison and Choct, 1991). The digestive problems caused by NSP in barley, oats, wheat and rye in poultry can be minimized by inclusion of **feed enzymes** such as β-glucanases and pentosanases. Commercial products of fungal origin are available to the feed industry (Campbell and Bedford, 1992). The best responses are seen in poultry; the NSP have less adverse effects in pigs because of the high water content of the digesta, diluting the viscosity effect. The response to enzyme supplements is due to reduced viscosity, rather than to release of free sugars and their metabolism as energy sources (Campbell and Bedford, 1992).

Lactose is synthesized in the mammary gland of all mammals, except the sea lion (Montgomery *et al.*, 1991). The lactose content of milk is inversely related to the fat and protein contents. Primate milk has the highest lactose content (about 7%) of all species, whereas marine species (e.g. seals, sea lions) have very low milk lactose concentrations (Robbins, 1993). **Lactose intolerance** is caused by the inability to digest lactose (milk sugar), a disaccharide in milk. **Lactase** is the enzyme that splits lactose into glucose and galactose. The chemical and molecular properties of lactase have been described in detail by Montgomery *et al.* (1991). Lactase activity in the intestine is high in young animals, and declines with age. Normally, weaned animals would not require lactase, because milk would not be part of the normal diet. In humans, lactase activity is retained into adulthood, particularly in those whose ethnic background involved a dairy product tradition. People of ethnic groups without an evolutionary history of milk consumption may have low lactase secretion, and are intolerant of dietary lactose. This is one of only a few recent biochemical adaptations to diet in humans. Human populations have adapted to milk drinking in 5000 years or less (Wrangham and Conklin-Brittain, 2003). Lactose intolerance results in symptoms of digestive upset such as diarrhoea, gas production and flatulence. Because of the lack of lactase, undigested lactose transits the small intestine, and is fermented by microbes in the hindgut. Digestive disturbance is related to microbial fermentation (gas, organic acid irritation of mucosa) and **osmotic diarrhoea** caused by a high concentration of solute (lactose) in the hindgut (Fig. 8.2).

Young mammals secrete low concentrations of carbohydrate-digesting enzymes except lactase, and

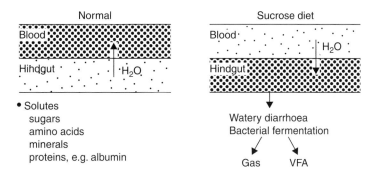

Fig. 8.2. The physiological events accounting for osmotic diarrhoea. In the normal situation, the concentration of solutes is greater in the blood than in the hindgut, because most solutes have been absorbed in the small intestine. By osmosis, water moves from the more dilute solution (hindgut) to the more concentrated solution (blood). In osmotic diarrhoea, such as with sucrose in the diet of a baby pig, the dissolved but non-absorbed sucrose in the hindgut draws water into the hindgut by osmosis.

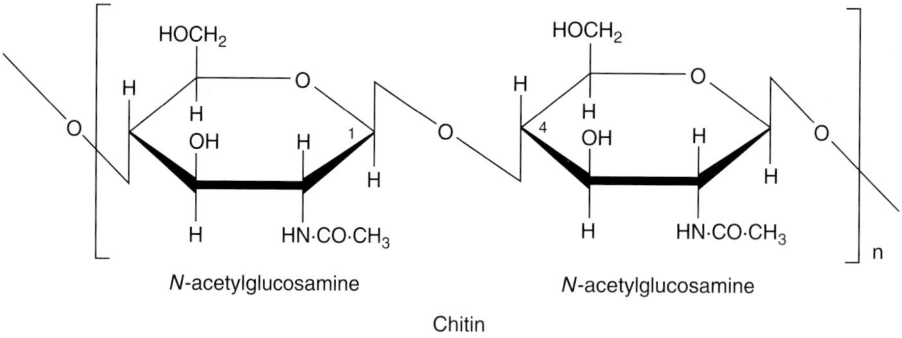

Fig. 8.3. Structure of chitin, a polymer of chitobiose.

are intolerant of carbohydrates they cannot digest. Neonatal animals are sucrose intolerant. Feeding a baby lamb with milk containing added **sucrose** (table sugar) may cause symptoms of diarrhoea and dehydration and can be fatal (the three Ds: diarrhoea, dehydration and death). The undigested sucrose causes osmotic diarrhoea, and dehydration (Fig. 8.2). Molasses is a common source of sucrose in livestock diets. Fructose (e.g. HFCS) is acceptable as a sweetener in milk replacers because it is absorbed directly, without requiring digestion.

Chitin (Fig. 8.3) is a structural carbohydrate of animals, and is present in bacterial and fungal cell walls and the exoskeleton of insects and many marine invertebrates (Stevens and Hume, 1995). Chitin is hydrolysed by chitinase to chitobiose (β-1,4-linked N-acetylglucosamine) which can be hydrolysed by chitobiase. Many species, particularly those which feed on insects or marine invertebrates like crabs, have gastric chitinase activity. Stevens and Hume (1995) provide an extensive list of chitinase activity in mammals, birds, reptiles and amphibians.

Carbohydrate Digestion in Ruminants

Carbohydrate digestion in ruminants is largely the result of microbial fermentation in the rumen. Fermentation is anaerobic respiration. Dietary carbohydrates are fermented, mainly by rumen bacteria, and the absorbed energy sources for the animal are the bacterial waste products, the **VFAs**. The VFAs were originally termed steam-volatile fatty acids, because they are volatilized from solution by the action of passing steam through the solution. Steam distillation of volatile compounds was a common technique in the early days of biochemistry.

They are also known as **short-chain fatty acids (SCFA)**. The three major VFAs are: (i) acetic (C2); (ii) propionic (C3); and (iii) butyric (C4) acids. Others include lactic acid, valeric acid and branched-chain VFAs such as isobutyric and isovaleric acids (Fig. 8.4). As a generalization, ruminants meet their protein needs by digesting rumen microbes, while they meet their energy needs by absorbing the waste products (VFAs) of rumen bacterial fermentation.

Rumen fermentation of carbohydrates

Bacteria, protozoa and fungi are the three types of **rumen microorganisms (RMO)**. They all have roles in carbohydrate digestion, although bacteria are the most important. Bacteria secrete enzymes that split the bonds linking sugars together in oligosaccharides and polysaccharides, resulting in the release of free sugars. These are taken up immediately by the bacteria, and metabolized as energy sources. Because the rumen is primarily anaerobic, the bacteria cannot oxidize sugars completely to carbon dioxide and water (luckily for the ruminant!) They excrete carbon fragments in the form of VFAs, carbon dioxide and methane (CH_4). Small amounts of oxygen may enter the rumen, as air swallowed during feeding. Although oxygen is toxic to obligate anaerobic bacteria, it is quickly utilized by facultative anaerobes.

Cellulose fermentation

Bacteria that produce cellulase are called **cellulolytic bacteria**. They attach to fibre particles and the cell walls of fibrous plant material consumed by the animal. There is little or no free cellulase in the rumen

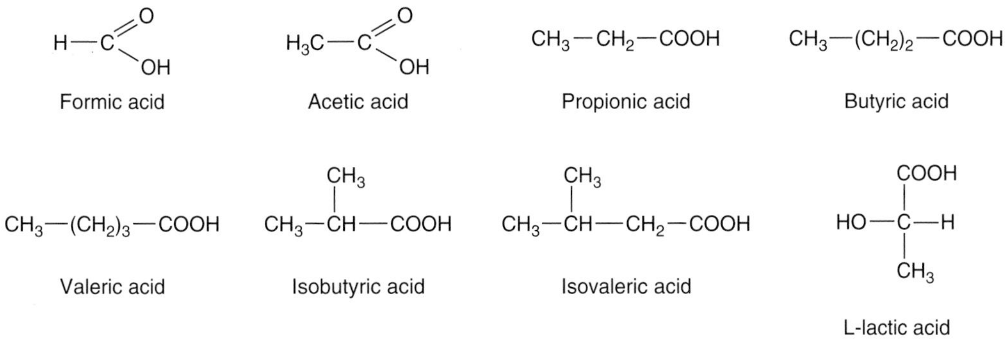

Fig. 8.4. Structures of the rumen VFAs.

contents. Cellulolytic bacteria invade the plant cells, and tend to digest them from the inside, which protects them from predatory protozoa. Rumen bacteria tend to form **consortia** with a common feeding strategy, so that the end products of one organism are often the substrate for another. Some of the common cellulolytic bacteria are *Bacteroides succinogenes*, *Ruminococcus albus* and *Ruminococcus flavefaciens*. The major VFA produced by cellulolytic bacteria is **acetic acid (C2)**. Thus high roughage diets result in a high molar proportion of acetic acid as a percentage of total VFA.

Cellulolytic bacteria digest cellulose, hemicellulose and pectins. **Rumen fungi** have a role in fibre digestion. They invade highly lignified mature plant fibre (e.g. straw) and aid in its penetration by cellulolytic bacteria. At least four genera of rumen fungi have been identified: *Neocallimastix*, *Caecomyces*, *Pyromyces* and *Orpinomyces* (Van Soest, 1994). The latter genus is named in honour of Colin Orpin, who first identified rumen fungi (Orpin, 1975). Previously, the flagellated swimming body (zoospore) was mistakenly believed to be a flagellated protozoan. Rumen fungi produce a fruiting body (sporangium) that produces free-swimming **zoospores** (see Fig. 3.9 in Chapter 3). These attach to fibre particles, and develop filaments (hyphae) which penetrate the plant cell walls. They secrete cellulase, and the penetration of the cell walls by the hyphae may pave the way for bacterial invasion. While the fungi do not directly digest lignin, they facilitate the breakdown of lignified plant material such as straw (see Fig. 3.8 in Chapter 3). Rumen fungi produce spore-like cysts that are shed from the animal, and can be a means of transmission to other animals. There is evidence that inoculating the rumen with fungi can improve fibre digestion, feed intake and growth in young ruminants (Van Soest, 1994). Propionic acid and its salts are well-known mould (fungi) inhibitors. The effect of this VFA on rumen fungi is unknown, but it could be speculated that with high concentrate diets, the high rumen propionate might suppress rumen fungi.

The role of **rumen protozoa** in fibre digestion is uncertain. Protozoa are single-celled animals visible without using microscopy. They are difficult to study because they cannot be cultured in the absence of rumen bacteria. Protozoa feed on bacteria, and engulf starch granules and small feed particles. Cellulolytic activity of protozoa may actually be attributed to cellulolytic bacteria engulfed by the protozoa. Van Soest (1994) speculates that protozoa may be 'miniruminants', harbouring a population of metabolically active bacteria. Elimination of protozoa from the rumen is called **defaunation**, and can be accomplished using various chemicals such as copper sulfate and detergents. There are two general groups of rumen protozoa: the **holotrichs** and **entodiniomorphs**. The holotrichs are ciliated over the entire body surface, while in entodiniomorphs the cilia are restricted to a ciliary band encircling the mouth (Hungate, 1968). Hungate (1968) provides a comprehensive discussion of rumen protozoa. The majority of rumen protozoa are ciliated, while some are flagellates. Ciliates include the genera *Entodinium*, *Diplodinium*, *Epidinium* and *Ophryoscolex*. They actively feed on rumen bacteria; proteolysis of bacteria by protozoa is a major source of rumen ammonia. Theoretically, defaunation should increase outflow of bacterial protein from the rumen. Low protein diets usually achieve best results of defaunation. However, the procedure is not practical because of the ease in which animals become re-populated with protozoa.

Lignin[1] is not well defined chemically, and its composition varies according to the method of isolation. Lignin is indigestible under anaerobic conditions, and has survived for thousands of years in anaerobic sites such as peat bogs. Lignin is a highly polymerized substance containing phenolic constituents such as cinnamic acid and an abundance of aromatic (benzene ring) groups. There is extensive crosslinking through the phenolic groups and structural carbohydrates, contributing to a rigid cell wall structure. The digestibility of highly lignified plant material such as straw and wood can be increased by chemical treatments which dissolve lignin. Alkaline conditions are necessary. Sodium hydroxide (lye), anhydrous ammonia and alkaline hydrogen peroxide are some of the treatments used to increase fibre digestibility. **Ammoniation**, performed by covering a straw stack with black plastic and introducing anhydrous ammonia gas, is a practical and effective means of increasing the nutritive value of straw for ruminants.

White-rot fungi secrete lignolytic enzymes such as laccases that cause depolymerization and solubilization of lignin. These are wood-decaying fungi that cause the eventual decomposition of rotting logs. Inoculation of wheat straw and other fibrous low-quality roughages with white-rot fungi increases their ruminal degradation (Rodrigues *et al.*, 2008). Extracts of these fungi may have potential as feed additives for ruminants.

Starch fermentation

Starch is a major dietary constituent of concentrate-fed ruminants, such as dairy and feedlot cattle. Starch-digesting or **amylolytic rumen bacteria** include *Bacteroides amylophilus*, *Streptococcus bovis*, *Succinimonas amylolytica* and *Succinivibrio dextrinosolvens*. The rate of degradation of starch depends upon its source and feed processing method. Most grains are processed in some manner for ruminant feeding with such techniques as dry or steam rolling, extrusion, popping and grinding. Amylolytic bacteria attach to feed particles and starch granules. They secrete amylase at the point of attachment, degrading starch to maltose and free glucose units. Glucose and other sugars are taken up by **saccharolytic** (sugar digesting) **bacteria**, such as *Bacteroides ruminicola*, *Butyrivibrio fibrisolvens* and *Selenomonas ruminantium*. Fermentation of

the sugars occurs by the Embden-Meyerhof pathway (glycolysis) with production of ATP for bacterial metabolism. The end product of glycolysis, pyruvate, is converted to VFAs, carbon dioxide and methane. The major end product of starch fermentation is propionic acid. Most propionate is synthesized by the dicarboxylic acid pathway: pyruvate → oxaloacetate → malate → fumarate → succinate → methylmalonyl CoA → propionate (Fig. 8.5). Another pathway for propionate formation is the **acrylate pathway**: pyruvate → lactate → acrylate → propionate (Fig. 8.6). The main organism using the acrylate pathway is *Megasphaera elsdenii*.

End products of rumen fermentation

The main end products of rumen fermentation are microbial cell mass, gases, heat (the heat of fermentation) and the VFAs. Microbial cell mass (bacterial or microbial protein) has been discussed in Chapter 5. The main gases produced during rumen fermentation are carbon dioxide, methane and small amounts of hydrogen and hydrogen sulfide. Rumen gas is typically about 65% carbon dioxide and 25% methane. Methane in the rumen is a hydrogen sink. The rumen is a reducing environment, with excess hydrogen. One means of hydrogen disposal is the formation of methane. Rumen methane production has several adverse consequences. Because methane is eliminated from the rumen by eructation, it represents a loss of energy (about 10% of gross energy intake). Methane is a '**greenhouse gas**', which accumulates in the upper atmosphere, contributing to the 'greenhouse effect' and **global warming**. Ruminant methane makes a small but significant contribution to the global methane pool. Methane production can be minimized in several ways. Feeding **ionophores** such as Rumensin® and lasalocid inhibits hydrogen producers such as *Ruminococcus* and *Butyrivibrio*, favouring propionate production. Production of propionate uses more hydrogen than acetate production, so an increase in molar proportion of propionate reduces methane production. Metabolism of propionate by the animal liberates more energy than from acetate metabolism, because there are more hydrogens and carbons to be oxidized (see Chapter 9). Experimentally, certain halogenated compounds (e.g. dibromomethane) function as **methane inhibitors**, by suppressing methane-generating bacteria.

The proportions of the three major VFAs, acetate (C2), propionate (C3) and butyrate (C4), produced

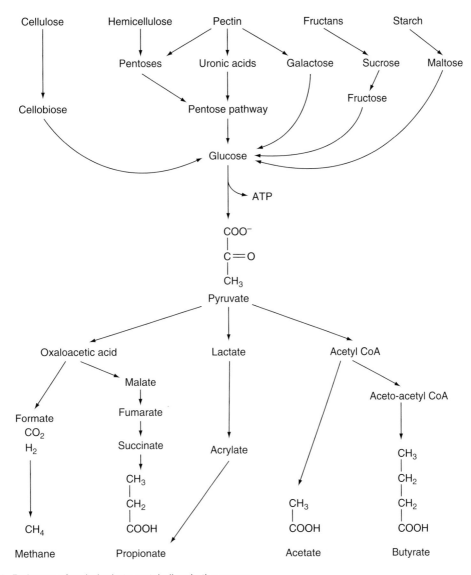

Fig. 8.5. Pathways of carbohydrate metabolism in the rumen.

in the rumen are influenced by diet. Cellulolytic bacteria tend to produce more C2, so acetate makes up 75% or more of total VFAs with a roughage-based diet. With high concentrate diets, propionate is the major VFA. Typically, the molar ratios (moles of acetate:propionate:butyrate) are 65:25:10 with roughage diets and 50:40:10 with concentrate diets. Ruminal VFA concentrations represent the balance between VFA production and absorption rates. Under conditions of lactic acidosis, lactic acid is a major rumen VFA.

Disorders of Carbohydrate Digestion in Herbivores

Ruminants fed diets high in grain are subject to a number of digestive or metabolic problems, including lactic acidosis, rumenitis, laminitis, displaced abomasum, liver abscesses, polioencephalomalacia and enterotoxaemia. Many of these conditions are secondary to acute acidosis. Some may also occur in non-ruminant herbivores such as horses, and are often significant health issues in zoo hoofstock.

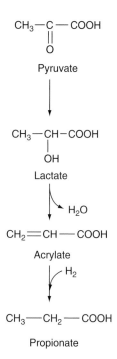

CH₃—C—COOH
‖
O

Pyruvate

↓

CH₃—CH—COOH
|
OH

Lactate

↘ H₂O

CH₂=CH—COOH

Acrylate

↙ H₂

CH₃—CH₂—COOH

Propionate

Fig. 8.6. The acrylate pathway for the synthesis of propionate in the rumen.

Acute lactic acidosis can occur in ruminants when there is an abrupt increase in the intake of readily fermentable carbohydrates. For example, when range- or pasture-fed cattle are brought into a feedlot and fed high grain diets, it is desirable to make the change from roughage to concentrate slowly. If the amount of grain fed exceeds the ability of the rumen microbes to switch from a primarily cellulolytic microflora to a starch-digesting (amylolytic) microflora, a change in normal rumen microbial ecology can occur. When ruminants with a cellulolytic microflora are switched abruptly to a high starch diet, there may be an initial shortage of amylolytic bacteria. This void is quickly occupied by fast-growing opportunistic amylolytic bacteria, particularly *S. bovis*, which has a generation interval of just a few minutes. *S. bovis* proliferates and becomes the dominant organism. It produces lactic acid as a fermentation end product, and particularly D-lactate, which is poorly absorbed. Lactate-producing *Lactobacillus* spp. also proliferate. The accumulation of D-lactic acid in the rumen causes the pH to drop, inhibiting the growth of other rumen microbes. A downward spiral of ever-increasing lactate and lower rumen pH occurs. Lactic acid is a stronger acid than the other VFAs (pKa of 3.0 for lactic versus 4.8 for acetic acid) and causes a severe drop in rumen pH to as low as 4.0. This strong acid has a corrosive effect on the rumen wall, causing the papillae to slough off (**parakeratosis**). Absorption is impaired, and bacteria may invade the rumen wall and enter the blood, infecting the liver to cause liver abscesses. Chronic **liver abscesses** are associated with acidosis in feedlot cattle, and reduced growth rate, feed efficiency and carcass value. The incidence of liver abscess in American feedlot cattle is typically 12–32% (Nagaraja and Chengappa, 1998).

As lactic acid concentrations build up in the rumen, the growth of all organisms, including *S. bovis*, is inhibited. The increased osmolality of the rumen contents draws water from the blood, causing dehydration and haemoconcentration. Absorbed acid may cause metabolic acidosis, with lowered blood pH, electrolyte imbalance and kidney failure. Haemoconcentration may cause arterioles in the extremities to rupture, leading to laminitis or founder. Laminitis is characterized by sore, tender feet, unnatural stance and abnormal overgrowth of hoof tissue. Lactic acidosis may be either acute or chronic. **Chronic acidosis** reduces feed intake and animal performance in feedlot and dairy cattle. Acidosis in concentrate-fed cattle is prevented by making a gradual conversion from a roughage-based to a high concentrate diet by gradually increasing the proportion of grain in the diet. **Acute acidosis** can rapidly lead to death, because of the extensive damage to the rumen (parakeratosis). Lactic acid is also a factor in development of laminitis in horses (Chapter 19).

Questions and Study Guide

1. What are two biochemical differences among human populations that have developed in response to the development of agriculture? (Hint: think grains and dairy products.)

2. Feeding barley to poultry can cause some nutritional and management problems. Explain.
3. Describe how the use of feed enzymes can improve the utilization of cereal grains by poultry.

Continued

Questions and Study Guide Continued.

4. Some people are lactose intolerant. What effect would eating pizza or cheese have on this condition? Why?

5. What are the major VFAs produced in rumen fermentation?

6. Why is the addition of table sugar to the milk given to a bottle-fed baby goat undesirable?

7. What is the significance of rumen fungi to ruminant animals?

8. What is the difference between holotrichs and entodiniomorphs?

9. How can ruminants be defaunated?

10. What is the acrylate pathway?

11. What is the effect of ionophores on methane production by ruminants?

12. Why does feeding ionophores to ruminants improve feed conversion efficiency?

13. Why is *Streptococcus bovis* of concern in feedlot cattle?

14. What is parakeratosis in cattle? What are the signs of parakeratosis in pigs? (See Chapter 19.)

15. Sodium and calcium propionate are mould inhibitors used in feeds and foods, for example bread. A biologist has analysed blood of wild bighorn sheep in a remote part of North America, and discovered sodium and calcium propionate in their blood. Where did it come from?

Note

[1] Note that in addition to lignin, plants contain phenolic compounds termed lignans. The similarity in their names could cause confusion. Lignans have mild oestrogenic activity and may have beneficial effects on human health.

References

Annison, G. (1991) Relationship between the levels of soluble nonstarch polysaccharides and the apparent metabolizable energy of wheats assayed in broiler chickens. *Journal of Agricultural and Food Chemistry* 39, 1252.

Annison, G. and Choct, M. (1991) Anti-nutritive activities of cereal non-starch polysaccharides in broiler diets and strategies minimizing their effects. *World's Poultry Science Journal* 47, 232–242.

Campbell, G.L. and Bedford, M.R. (1992) Enzyme applications for monogastric feeds: a review. *Canadian Journal of Animal Science* 72, 449–466.

Hungate, R.E. (1968) *The Rumen and Its Microbes*. Academic Press, New York.

Low, A.G. (1989) Secretory response of the pig gut to non-starch polysaccharides. *Animal Feed Science and Technology* 23, 55–65.

Montgomery, R.K., Buller, H.A., Rings, E.H.H.M. and Grand, R.J. (1991) Lactose intolerance and the genetic regulation of intestinal lactase-phlorizin hydrolase. *FASEB Journal* 5, 2824–2832.

Moran, E.T., Jr (1985) Digestion and absorption of carbohydrates in fowl and events through perinatal development. *Journal of Nutrition* 115, 665–674.

Nagaraja, T.G. and Chengappa, M.M. (1998) Liver abscesses in feedlot cattle: a review. *Journal of Animal Science* 76, 287–298.

Orpin, C.G. (1975) Studies on the rumen flagellate, *Neocallimastix frontalis*. *Journal of General Microbiology* 91, 249–262.

Perry, G.H., Dominy, N.J., Claw, K.G., Lee, A.S., Fiegler, H., Redon, R., Werner, J., Villanea, F.A., Mountain, J.L., Misra, R., Carter, N.P., Lee, C. and Stone, A.C. (2007) Diet and the evolution of human amylase gene copy number variation. *Nature Genetics* 39, 1256–1260.

Robbins, C.T. (1993) *Wildlife Feeding and Nutrition*. Academic Press, San Diego, California.

Rodrigues, M.A.M., Pinto, P., Bezerra, R.M.F., Dias, A.A., Guedes, C.V.M., Cardoso, V.M.G., Cone, J.W., Ferreira, L.M.M., Colaco, J. and Sequeira, C.A. (2008) Effect of enzyme extracts isolated from white-rot fungi on chemical composition and *in vitro* digestibility of wheat straw. *Animal Feed Science and Technology* 141, 326–338.

Schondube, J.E. and Martinez del Rio, C. (2004) Sugar and protein digestion in flowerpiercers and hummingbirds: a comparative test of adaptive convergence. *Journal of Comparative Physiology* 174, 263–273.

Stevens, C.E. and Hume, I.D. (1995) *Comparative Physiology of the Vertebrate Digestive System*. Cambridge University Press, Cambridge, UK.

Van Soest, P.J. (1994) *Nutritional Ecology of the Ruminant*. Cornell University Press, Ithaca, New York.

Wrangham, R. and Conklin-Brittain, N. (2003) Review, 'Cooking as a biological trait'. *Comparative Biochemistry and Physiology A* 136, 35–46.

9 Cellular Metabolism of Carbohydrates

Cellular metabolism is based on the catabolism of glucose, which involves the sequential degradation of the molecule through a series of enzymatic reactions. The end result is the conversion of glucose to carbon dioxide and water, with the release of energy as ATP and heat. The total energy released is equivalent to the solar energy required to synthesize glucose from carbon dioxide and water via photosynthesis. There are two major pathways of glucose catabolism: (i) glycolysis; and (ii) the citric acid cycle (Krebs cycle, tricarboxylic acid cycle or TCA cycle).

Hydrogen plays a prominent role in energy metabolism. In photosynthesis, solar energy splits water into hydrogen and oxygen. The light energy is transferred to hydrogen, which then binds with carbon to produce hydrocarbons (e.g. carbohydrates). During the catabolism of glucose by animals, hydrogen is transferred from glucose to hydrogen receptors, such as NAD^+, $NADP^+$ and FMN. These hydrogen acceptors are reduced (**biological reduction** is gain of hydrogen) when they accept hydrogen (e.g. NADH). The reduced hydrogen acceptors are oxidized in the reactions of the respiratory chain:

$$H_2 + \tfrac{1}{2}O_2 \circledR H_2O + Energy$$

In a hydrogen-powered automobile, the energy from this reaction is in the form of electricity (produced in a fuel cell that combines hydrogen with oxygen – the proton from hydrogen combines with oxygen to produce water, while the electron is released as electricity). In biological systems, the oxidation of hydrogen is coupled with synthesis of ATP from ADP (coupling of oxidative phosphorylation with hydrogen metabolism). Certain substances (e.g. carbon tetrachloride, 2,4-dinitrophenol) are toxic because they cause 'uncoupling of oxidative phosphorylation', so that energy is wasted as heat instead of being used to synthesize high-energy bonds of ATP.

Fats yield more energy (9 kcal/g) than do carbohydrates (4 kcal/g) because they are less oxidized. In comparing the fatty acid palmitic acid with glucose, for example, palmitic acid contains 16 carbons and two oxygens, while glucose has six carbons and six oxygens. Thus per atom of carbon, palmitic acid is much less oxidized, so there is more carbon to be oxidized (to yield energy) in animal catabolism (see Chapter 12).

Carbohydrate Metabolism

The catabolism of glucose to carbon dioxide and water occurs in a series of steps, known as the two metabolic pathways of glycolysis and the citric acid cycle. **Glycolysis** enzymes are located in the cytosol of the cell. Gycolysis can function either aerobically or anaerobically. The glycolysis pathway involves the breakdown of glucose (six carbons) to two molecules of a three-carbon end product (pyruvic acid in aerobic metabolism, lactic acid in anaerobic metabolism) (Fig. 9.1). In this process, ATP is generated. In the initial step of glycolysis, glucose is phosphorylated to form glucose-6-phosphate and then fructose-1,6-bisphosphate (diphosphate in older literature). The phosphorylations are energy (ATP)-requiring, but subsequently ATP is generated. Glycolysis is also the pathway by which other sugars such as fructose and galactose are catabolized. For example, **fructose** is phosphorylated by fructokinase to form fructose-1-phosphate, which is cleaved to dihydroxyacetone-phosphate and glyceraldehyde. This catabolic process bypasses phosphofructokinase, the enzyme that converts fructose-6-phosphate to fructose 1, 6-biphosphate. This reaction is an important regulatory step in glycolysis. Thus fructose undergoes more rapid glycolysis than glucose. This difference between glucose and fructose catabolism may be significant in human health. Diets high in sucrose or HFCS syrup used in manufactured foods and beverages

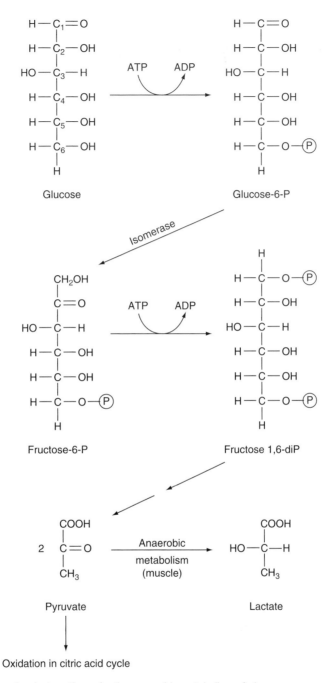

Fig. 9.1. Reactions of the glycolysis pathway for the anaerobic metabolism of glucose.

may cause enhanced fatty acid synthesis and increased serum cholesterol due to the lack of regulatory control of fructose metabolism. Other monosaccharides can enter the glycolysis pathway.

Dietary **galactose** (e.g. as lactose in dairy products) is converted to galactose-1-phosphate by galactokinase. Galactose-1-phosphate is converted to glucose first, then to glycogen, from which glucose can

---

be liberated. Thus galactose, like fructose, is ultimately catabolized in the glycolysis pathway.

Under aerobic conditions, pyruvic acid enters the mitochondria, and after conversion to acetyl CoA, is oxidized to carbon dioxide by the reactions of the citric acid cycle. Red blood cells (rbc) have no mitochondria, so are totally dependent on glycolysis for their metabolic fuel. A genetic deficiency of glucose-6-phosphate dehydrogenase (G6PD), the enzyme that catalyses the oxidation of glucose-6-phosphate, causes a susceptibility to rbc haemolysis and haemolytic anaemia. The metabolic basis of this problem will be described in the discussion of the pentose phosphate pathway.

The end product of glycolysis, pyruvate, is produced in the cytosol. It is transported into the mitochondria, where it is decarboxylated into **acetyl CoA** by the pyruvate dehydrogenase complex. Three B vitamins, thiamin, niacin and pantothenic acid, are involved in this step. Niacin functions as a component of NAD. **Thiamin** (vitamin B_1) is a coenzyme for decarboxylation reactions, while **pantothenic** acid is a component of CoA. In thiamin deficiency, glucose metabolism is impaired at this step, and pyruvate accumulates. Acetyl CoA, a two-carbon compound, enters the reactions of the citric acid cycle (Krebs cycle or TCA cycle) by combining with oxaloacetic acid (OAA), a four-carbon compound, to form citric acid, a six-carbon compound (Fig. 9.2). Citric acid undergoes a series of enzymatic reactions, leading to the loss of two molecules of carbon dioxide, and the end product of OAA, which can combine with another acetyl CoA to start the cycle anew. In the process, reduced cofactors ($FADH_2$ and NADH) are formed. Oxidation of these cofactors in the respiratory chain (also referred to as the electron transport system), involves coupling of the oxidation with phosphorylation (**oxidative phosphorylation**) to generate ATP from ADP. In one 'turn' of the citric acid cycle, three NADH and one $FADH_2$ are produced, which results in production of nine ATP when oxidized.

Four B vitamins have key roles in the citric acid cycle: (i) **thiamin** functions as the coenzyme for decarboxylation reactions in the formation of acetyl CoA from pyruvate and the conversion of α-ketoglutaric acid to succinic acid (as succinyl CoA); (ii) **niacin**, as a constituent of NAD, is a coenzyme for dehydrogenases (isocitrate, α-ketoglutarate and malate dehydrogenases); (iii) **riboflavin** has a similar coenzyme role as a constituent of FAD; and (iv) **pantothenic acid** is a constituent of CoA, attached to carboxylic acids (acetyl CoA, succinyl CoA). Deficiencies of these vitamins result in impaired energy metabolism, and deficiency symptoms which may reflect this impairment. For instance, **thiamin deficiency** blocks energy metabolism at the decarboxylation reactions involved in formation of acetyl CoA and succinyl CoA, causing symptoms of energy deficiency, including **polyneuritis** (ataxia, opisthotonus or star gazing, convulsions), anorexia and hypothermia (lowered body temperature) (Fig. 9.3). Clinically, there is elevated blood pyruvate, which inhibits the appetite centre to cause anorexia. Recovery from thiamin deficiency is extremely rapid. As soon as the vitamin is provided, the decarboxylation reactions resume normal activity.

A significant cause of thiamin deficiency is the presence of dietary factors which destroy or inactivate the vitamin. **Thiaminases** are enzymes which split thiamin into its two constituent rings (Fig. 9.4), inactivating it. A co-substrate, usually an amine or a sulfhydryl-containing compound such as proline or cysteine, is required. The pyrimidine analogue produced when thiamin is cleaved can also be a thiamin antagonist, depending upon the structure of the co-substrate, which increases the severity of thiamin deficiency. Examples of sources of thiaminases include bracken fern (Cheeke, 1998), certain fish such as carp (Wistbacka *et al.*, 2002), and certain rumen bacteria such as *Clostridium sporogenes* (Haven *et al.*, 1983). Thiamin deficiency in mink and foxes fed raw carp is known as **Chastek's paralysis**, named after the Minnesota fox farmer who first noted the problem. Thiamin deficiency has occurred in dogs fed raw carp (Houston and Hulland, 1988). Atlantic salmon in the Baltic Sea sometimes develop thiamin deficiency, as a result of consuming Baltic herring which have the thiaminase activity (Wistbacka *et al.*, 2002). A similar condition occurs in the Great Lakes in lake trout consuming thiaminase-rich alewife and smelt (Fitzsimons *et al.*, 1999). The source of the thiaminases in certain fish may be thiaminase-producing bacteria in their diets; the enzyme content is enhanced by blue-green algae and environmental toxins such as DDT (dichlorodiphenyltrichloroethane) (Wistbacka *et al.*, 2002).

Polioencephalomalacia (PEM), also known as cerebral cortical necrosis, is a disorder of feedlot cattle fed high concentrate diets. It is associated

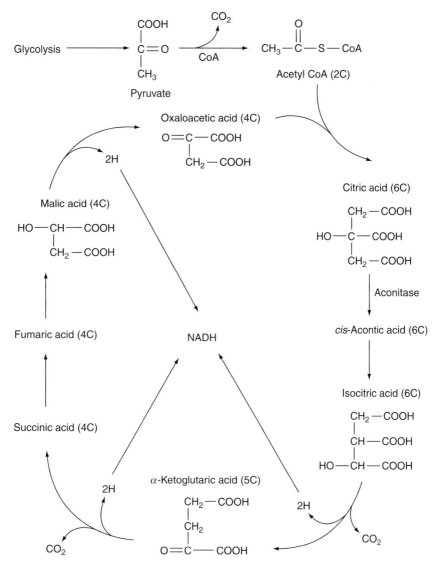

Fig. 9.2. The citric acid cycle. Energy is released when NADH is oxidized in the respiratory chain, resulting in phosphorylation of ADP to produce ATP.

with high rumenal concentrations of thiaminase in affected animals. Several thiaminase-producing bacteria, such as *C. sporogenes* and certain *Bacillus* spp., have been implicated (Haven *et al.*, 1983). Other causes of PEM include high sulfate content of drinking water (Gould, 1998) and consumption of the desert range plant *Kochia scoparia*.

The reduced cofactors (NADH and $FADH_2$) produced in the TCA cycle reactions are oxidized via the **respiratory chain** (the electron transport system,

cytochrome system). In the final stage of the respiratory chain hydrogen ions react with oxygen to form water. The respiratory chain consists of flavoproteins linked to iron-containing enzymes called **cytochromes**. Hydrogen and electrons flow through the system to the terminal cytochrome (cytochrome oxidase) where hydrogen ions react with oxygen to produce water. The respiratory chain is the site of a large proportion of total ATP production in cellular metabolism, by the process of **oxidative**

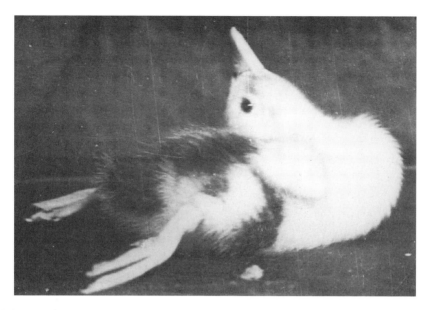

Fig. 9.3. Opisthotonus (star gazing posture) caused by thiamin deficiency.

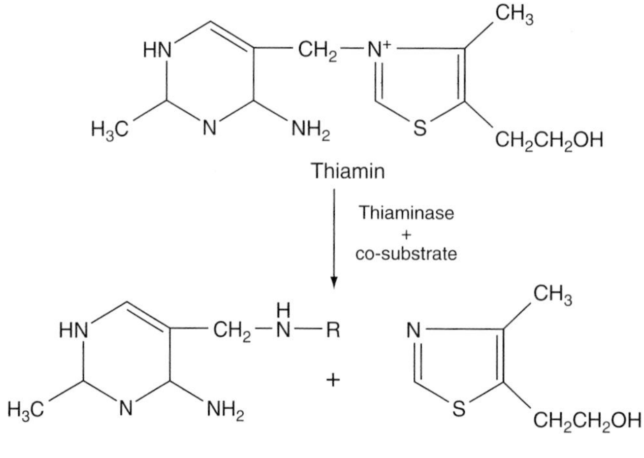

Thiamin

Thiaminase
+
co-substrate

+

Fig. 9.4. Destruction of thiamin by the enzyme thiaminase.

phosphorylation. As the flow of electrons through the respiratory chain proceeds, energy is transferred from the respiratory chain to the synthesis of high-energy phosphate bonds in ATP.

One of the components of the respiratory chain is **coenzyme Q**, also known as **ubiquinone**. Coenzyme Q is a quinone with an isoprenoid side chain of ten isoprene units, somewhat similar in structure to vitamins E and K (Fig. 9.5). Coenzyme Q (CoQ, CoQ_{10}) shares a common biosynthetic pathway with cholesterol. The synthesis of mevalonate, one of its intermediary precursors, is inhibited by statin drugs. Supplementation with coenzyme Q may be warranted in humans whose normal synthesis of coenzyme Q might be impaired, such as those on statin therapy.

Cytochrome oxidase, the terminal enzyme in the respiratory chain, contains iron as a component of haem. The iron atoms oscillate between Fe^{3+} and Fe^{2+} during oxidation and reduction. Cytochrome oxidase also contains two copper atoms, each associated with a haem unit. The enzyme has a high

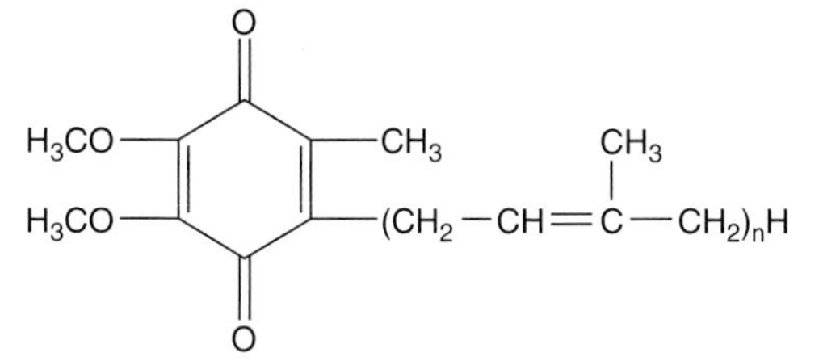

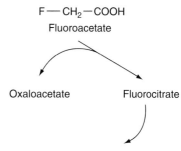

Fig. 9.6. Fluoroacetate enters the citric acid cycle by combining with oxaloacetic acid (OAA). The resulting fluorocitrate inhibits aconitase, the enzyme that converts citric acid to *cis*-aconitic acid.

Inhibits formation of *cis*-aconitic acid; citrate accumulates

---

Ubiquinone (coenzyme Q)

Fig. 9.5. Structure of the respiratory pigment ubiquinone.

affinity for oxygen, but an even higher affinity for cyanide. **Cyanide poisoning** of livestock, associated with forage sorghums and poisonous plants such as chokecherries (Cheeke, 1998), is a result of total inhibition of cytochrome oxidase and lack of ATP production.

In the initial reactions of the citric acid cycle, citrate is converted to *cis*-aconitic acid and then isocitrate by aconitase (aconitate hydratase). This enzyme is inhibited by **fluoroacetate** (compound **1080**). Fluoroacetate was formerly used in poisonous baits for coyotes and other 'pests'. Its use was banned in the USA because of 'collateral damage'; the carcasses of animals killed by 1080 were poisonous to scavengers (e.g. eagles). Interestingly, a number of plants in Australia, South America and Africa contain fluoroacetate, and are deadly poisonous to many animals. In Australia, 1080-containing plants occur primarily in Western Australia (WA). Many native herbivores in WA have evolved resistance to 1080, and can safely consume fluoroacetate-containing plants. For example, the LD_{50} (lethal dose for 50% of individuals) for 1080 in the brush-tailed possum in WA is about 100 mg/kg, whereas for the same species in eastern Australia the LD_{50} is 0.68 mg/kg, a 150-fold difference (Mead *et al.*, 1979). In Australia, numerous species of small marsupials are threatened with extinction from predation by introduced predators such as cats and foxes. In many cases, these alien predators can be controlled with 1080-containing baits to which the native animals are resistant. Twigg and King (1991) provide a good review of coevolution of Australian animals and 1080-containing plants. The toxic mode of action of fluoroacetate involves the substitution of this compound for acetyl CoA. The resulting fluorocitrate (Fig. 9.6) competitively inhibits aconitase, blocking the TCA cycle at the citrate stage. This results in accumulation of citrate, ATP deprivation and death.

Another pathway of carbohydrate metabolism is the **pentose phosphate pathway** (hexose monophosphate shunt, pentose shunt). It does not generate ATP, but has two major functions: the formation of NADPH, and the synthesis of ribose for nucleic acid formation. Glucose enters the pentose shunt as glucose-6-P. Glucose-6-P is oxidized with formation of 6-phosphogluconic acid. This reaction is coupled with the reduction of $NADP^+$ with H^+ from glucose, producing NADPH. NADPH is required for the reduction of oxidized glutathione (G-S-S-G) to regenerate reduced glutathione (GSH) by glutathione reductase, and for a variety of other reductive reactions, especially in fatty acid and cholesterol synthesis. GSH is used to reduce (add hydrogen) oxidants such as hydrogen peroxide, in a reaction catalysed by a selenium-containing enzyme, **glutathione peroxidase** (see Chapter 13).

In rbc, the pentose phosphate pathway is necessary for the generation of GSH to protect the rbc membrane from oxidants. In humans, some individuals have a genetic deficiency of glucose-6-phosphate dehydrogenase, with consequent impairment of NADPH and GSH production. This deficiency is manifested by erythrocyte haemolysis when susceptible individuals are subjected to oxidants. One type of oxidant is glycosides in fava beans (*Vicia faba*). Susceptible people, mainly of Mediterranean and African origin, can develop severe haemolytic anaemia following consumption of fava beans, a condition known as **favism**. In livestock, haemolytic anaemia is characteristic of onion toxicity, brassica anaemia and red maple poisoning. These conditions are caused by oxidants

---

that deplete the rbc of GSH. These have been reviewed by Cheeke (1998).

A second function of the pentose phosphate pathway besides generation of NADPH is the production of pentoses. The action of glucose-6-P dehydrogenase produces 6-phosphogluconic acid as an end product. This six-carbon compound is oxidatively decarboxylated to produce pentoses such as ribose and xylose, and NADPH. Three molecules of glucose-6-P gives rise to three molecules of carbon dioxide and three five-carbon sugars.

Volatile Fatty Acid (VFA) Metabolism in Ruminants

In contrast to simple non-ruminants, ruminants absorb very little glucose. Their major absorbed energy sources are the VFAs, the end products of microbial fermentation in the rumen. Absorbed acetate and butyrate are incorporated directly into the citric acid cycle reactions by being converted to acetyl CoA. Butyrate is split into two acetyl CoAs. Propionate also enters the citric acid cycle, by being converted to succinyl CoA (Fig. 9.7). Absorbed propionate reacts with CoA, with input of energy from ATP. Propionyl CoA is converted to

D-methylmalonyl CoA by a biotin-containing carboxylase, with the addition of carbon dioxide. L-methylmalonyl CoA undergoes rearrangement by a vitamin B_{12}-containing isomerase, to produce succinyl CoA. Thus three B-complex vitamins (pantothenic acid, biotin, vitamin B_{12}) are involved in propionate entry into the citric acid cycle. Propionate metabolism is consequently impaired with vitamin B_{12} deficiency. Vitamin B_{12} is a complex molecule containing chelated cobalt (Fig. 9.8). The only known metabolic function of cobalt is its role as a constituent of vitamin B_{12}.

Cattle and sheep on cobalt-deficient pastures become extremely emaciated. Lack of dietary **cobalt** reduces ruminal synthesis of vitamin B_{12} by the rumen bacteria. Ruminants have a relatively high cobalt requirement, and may develop wasting disease on pastures that support grazing horses with no sign of deficiency. Two factors that contribute to the high cobalt requirement of ruminants are an inefficiency in ruminal vitamin B_{12} synthesis, and a low ability to absorb vitamin B_{12}. Only a small portion of ruminal cobalt is used for vitamin B_{12} synthesis; other cobalt-containing compounds without vitamin activity are synthesized. Cobalt (and thus vitamin B_{12})-deficient ruminants are unable to

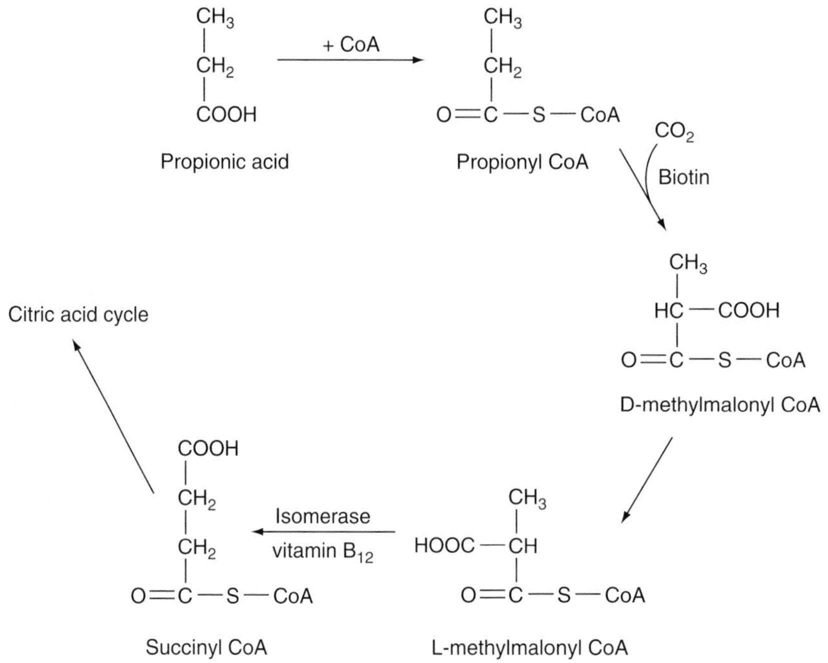

Fig. 9.7. Metabolism of propionate.

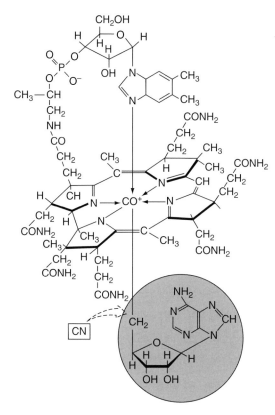

Fig. 9.8. Cobamide coenzyme, the structure of the coenzyme form of vitamin B_{12}. The usual form in which vitamin B_{12} is isolated has the cyanide group replacing the 5′ deoxyadenosine shown in the shaded area (courtesy of University Books, Guelph, Canada).

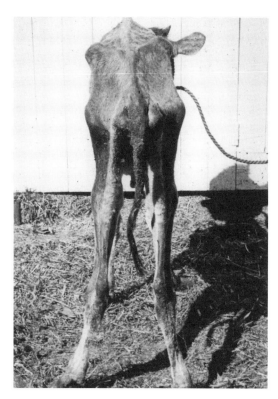

Fig. 9.9. Cobalt-deficient cow. Cobalt-deficient ruminants are unable to metabolize VFA (propionate) because of vitamin B_{12} deficiency and become extremely emaciated as a result.

metabolize propionate, so they suffer from a lack of cellular ATP and glucose. A build-up of propionate in the blood impairs appetite. As a result of these factors, the animals become extremely emaciated (Fig. 9.9). They are also anaemic, because vitamin B_{12} functions in haemoglobin formation. The anaemia is actually a folic acid deficiency; vitamin B_{12} deficiency blocks the metabolism of folic acid, leading to folate deficiency. Because propionate metabolism yields a net increase in OAA, propionate is glucogenic whereas acetate and butyrate are not. The normal blood glucose concentration of ruminants (around 50 mg/100 ml serum) is about half the normal level of non-ruminants. Inadequate ruminal production of propionate leads to hypoglycaemia and ketosis (Chapter 16).

Vitamin B_{12} was the last vitamin to be discovered, in 1948. It has a complex structure, containing chelated cobalt (Fig. 9.8). Its discovery was a result of several seemingly unrelated observations. A fatal anaemia in humans (pernicious anaemia) was related both to a deficiency of a factor in the stomach (the intrinsic factor) and to a dietary deficiency which could be overcome by treatment with liver extracts. It was discovered that the liver factor was also essential for the growth of the bacterium *Lactobacillus lactis*. This organism was used to test substances for their ability to treat pernicious anaemia, and ultimately to isolate vitamin B_{12}. It was also well known that pigs, poultry and rats would grow poorly on diets lacking animal proteins. Adding animal protein (meat, milk, liver) to the diet overcame the deficiency. Cow manure also had activity. These substances were called the animal protein factor and the cow manure factor. Several research groups isolated vitamin B_{12} as the active principle of these various factors, at approximately the same time.

Shortly after the discovery of vitamin B_{12}, it was found to be effective in treating cobalt deficiency in ruminants.

Vitamin B_{12} is not synthesized by plants; it is produced only by certain species of bacteria. The vitamin B_{12} requirements of herbivores are met by microbial synthesis in the gut, while autoenzymatic digesters such as pigs, poultry and humans must receive a dietary source (animal products or synthetic vitamin B_{12}).

Methane production by ruminants is nutritionally significant. Methane, also known as natural gas, represents a major loss of energy in rumen metabolism. From 4 to 10% of the gross energy intake is lost to the animal as a result of rumen methane production (McAllister *et al.*, 1996). Development of ways to reduce ruminal methane would increase the efficiency of ruminant production. The amount of methane produced in ruminants is determined in large part by diet. There are two major types of rumen fermentation: (i) amylolytic; and (ii) cellulolytic. **Amylolytic (starch-digesting) bacteria** produce propionic acid as the major VFA end product, while **cellulolytic bacteria** produce mainly acetic acid as their end product of fermentation. The stoichiometry of propionate and acetate production is indicated by the following equations:

Eqn 9.1 (amylolytic bacteria):

$$C_6H_{12}O_6 \rightarrow 2CH_3CH_2COOH$$
glucose   propionic acid

Eqn 9.2 (cellulolytic bacteria):

$$C_6H_{12}O_6 \rightarrow CH_3COOH + CO_2 + CH_4$$
glucose   acetic acid carbon   methane
                        dioxide

Thus more methane is produced with fibre than with starch digestion. When propionate is produced, all of the carbon and hydrogen present in the glucose are still present in the VFA (see Eqn 9.1 and add up the C and H). In contrast, when acetate is produced, both carbon and hydrogen are lost as CO_2 and CH_4 (see Eqn 9.2). The rumen contains a vast array of microbes, so the actual overall reactions are more involved than these shown above. However, with high fibre diets, more acetate and methane are produced; with high grain diets, more propionate and less acetate and methane are produced. For example, suppose a high grain diet is fed, giving an acetate:propionate molar ratio of 1:1:

Eqn 9.3:

3 Glucose ® 2 Acetate + 2 Propionate
    + Butyrate + $3CO_2$ + CH_4 + $2H_2O$

In contrast, a high forage diet might give an acetate:propionate ratio of 3:1:

Eqn 9.4:

5 Glucose ® 6 Acetate + 2 Propionate
    + Butyrate + $5CO_2$ + $3CH_4$ + $6H_2O$

Thus per mole of glucose, Eqn 9.3 (high grain diet) would yield one-third of a mole of methane, whereas with Eqn 9.4 (high fibre diet), the methane yield would be three-fifths of a mole of methane per mole of glucose. For each mole of glucose, the high forage diet yielded almost twice as much methane as the high concentrate diet (Eqns 9.3 and 9.4 are from Fahey and Berger, 1988).

The **ionophore feed additives** such as Rumensin® improve the efficiency of rumen fermentation by stimulating propionate production and decreasing the production of methane. Thus the use of ionophores can help to decrease methane emissions from cattle and have a small beneficial effect in alleviating global warming. Intensive cattle production, using high concentrate diets and ionophore feed additives, can reduce the contribution of cattle to global warming by the following means:

1. Methane production per unit of feed is reduced on high concentrate diets.
2. Ionophores lower methane production in the rumen by altering rumen fermentation.
3. Ionophores decrease the amount of feed required to produce a given amount of weight gain, further reducing methane production.
4. Both high concentrate diets and ionophores (and other feed additives and implants) increase growth rate, reducing the age at slaughter. Thus with a shorter lifespan, the animal has a lower lifetime methane production.

The energy yield to the animal is higher when propionate rather than acetate is produced by rumen fermentation. As shown in Eqns 9.1 and 9.2 (above), when glucose is fermented to propionate, all of the carbon and hydrogen are still present, and can be oxidized by the animal, yielding ATP. In contrast, with acetate production (Eqn 9.2), some of the carbon and hydrogen are lost as carbon dioxide and methane, reducing the potential ATP yield in the animal's cellular metabolism.

Questions and Study Guide

1. Name the two major pathways of carbohydrate catabolism.
2. What is the significance of hydrogen in energy metabolism?
3. How does thiamin function in energy metabolism?
4. Four vitamins function in the citric acid cycle. Name them, and indicate how they function.
5. What causes Chastek's paralysis?
6. How is glucose catabolism involved in preventing red blood cell haemolysis?
7. Describe how the major absorbed VFAs are catabolized by ruminants.
8. What is the relationship between dietary cobalt concentrations and emaciation and anaemia in cattle?
9. Why does the acetate:propionate ratio affect methane production and metabolic efficiency of ruminants?

References

Cheeke, P.R. (1998) *Toxicants in Feeds, Forages, and Poisonous Plants.* Prentice Hall, Upper Saddle River, New Jersey.

Fahey, G.C., Jr and Berger, L.L. (1988) Carbohydrate nutrition of ruminants. In: Church, D.C. (ed.) *The Ruminant Animal. Digestive Physiology and Nutrition.* Prentice Hall, Upper Saddle River, New Jersey, pp. 269–297.

Fitzsimmons, J.D., Brown, S.B., Honeyfield, D.C. and Hnath, J.G. (1999) A review of early mortality syndrome (EMS) in Great Lakes salmonids: relationship with thiamine deficiency. *Ambio* 1, 9–15.

Gould, D.H. (1998) Polioencephalomalacia. *Journal of Animal Science* 76, 309–314.

Haven, T.R., Caldwell, D.R. and Jensen, R. (1983) Role of predominant rumen bacteria in the cause of polioencephalomalcia (cerebrocortical necrosis) in cattle. *American Journal of Veterinary Research* 44, 1451–1455.

Houston, D.M. and Hulland, T.J. (1988) Thiamine deficiency in a team of sled dogs. *Canadian Veterinary Journal* 29, 383–385.

McAllister, T.A., Okine, E.K., Mathison, G.W. and Cheng, K.-J. (1996) Dietary, environmental and microbiological aspects of methane production in ruminants. *Canadian Journal of Animal Science* 76, 231–243.

Mead, R.J., Oliver, A.J. and King, D.R. (1979) Metabolism and defluorination of fluoroacetate in the brush-tailed possum (*Trichosurus vulpecula*). *Australian Journal of Biological Sciences* 32, 15–26.

Twigg, L.E. and King, D.R. (1991) The impact of fluoroacetate-bearing vegetation on native Australian fauna: a review. *Oikos* 61, 412–430.

Wistbacka, S., Heinonen, A. and Bylund, G. (2002) Thiaminase activity of gastrointestinal contents of salmon and herring from the Baltic Sea. *Journal of Fish Biology* 60, 1031–1042.

PART IV
Lipids

This part provides a discussion of lipids that are important in animal nutrition and their metabolic roles.

Part Objectives

1. To present the chemical structures of lipids that are important in animal nutrition.
2. To discuss digestion and metabolism of lipids.
3. To discuss lipid-related issues relevant to animal production, including human health concerns (hypercholesterolaemia, conjugated linoleic acid (CLA) and *trans*-fatty acids).
4. To discuss the roles of antioxidant nutrients such as vitamin E, vitamin C and selenium on lipid metabolism.

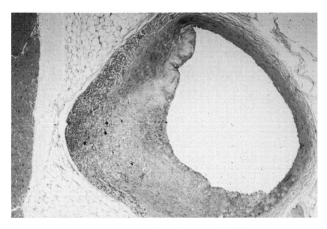

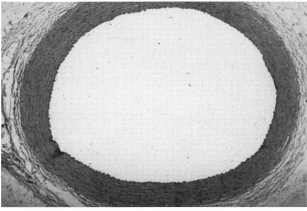

Atherosclerosis (hardening of the arteries) involves deposition of lipids, including cholesterol, in artery walls. Cross-sections of arteries (above) are from subjects with and without lipid deposition, or plaque.

10 Lipid Structure

Lipids are components of plant and animal tissue that are relatively insoluble in water and soluble in organic solvents such as ether, benzene and hexane. In nutritional terms, they are mainly fats and oils. Plant pigments (e.g. chlorophyll, carotenoids) and waxes are lipids as are fat-soluble vitamins. Lipids are important in animal nutrition as sources of energy. They also function as components of cell membranes and as the 'insulation' of nerves. The lipid component of animal products (body fat, cholesterol) is important in human nutrition, and is implicated in various human health pathologies such as obesity, cancer, atherosclerosis and coronary heart disease.

Chemical Structures of Lipids

The following is a simplified scheme of the chemical structure of lipids important in animal nutrition.

Fatty acids

Somewhat analogous to amino acids as basic units of protein structure and simple sugars as basic units of carbohydrates, the basic units of more complex lipids are fatty acids. **Fatty acids** consist of simple carboxylic acids of various hydrocarbon chain lengths and degrees of unsaturation. The carbon chain may be either saturated or unsaturated. **Saturated fatty acids** contain all the hydrogen that they are chemically capable of containing (they are saturated with hydrogen). Some of the most common saturated fatty acids are listed in Table 10.1. **Unsaturated fatty acids** contain one or more double bonds between adjacent carbon atoms (Fig. 10.1) in the hydrocarbon chain (all fatty acids contain one double-bonded oxygen in the carboxyl group). Fatty acids are normally synthesized from acetic acid (C2) residues, so they generally contain an even number of carbon atoms. Fatty acids in complex lipids tend to have at least ten or 12 carbon atoms – they

are **long-chain fatty acids (LCFA)**. The **short-chain fatty acids (SCFA)**, such as acetic, propionic and butyric acids, are the VFA of rumen fermentation and are not generally viewed as lipids as they are water soluble. Most fatty acids in fats and oils contain 16, 18 or 20 carbon atoms.

Unsaturated fatty acids may be either **monounsaturated fatty acids (MUFA)** or **polyunsaturated fatty acids (PUFA)**. MUFA have one double bond, while PUFA have two or more double bonds. The position of double bonds is generally indicated by nutritionists by using the **omega (ω)** carbon designation. The ω carbon is the first carbon with a double bond, counted from the terminal methyl end of the carbon chain. Double bonds are generally **methylene interrupted**, with a $-CH_2-$ between each double bond, so when the location of the first double bond is known, the others can be deduced. Common PUFA are of either the ω-3 or ω-6 series (Fig. 10.2). Dietary omega-3 fatty acids occur in fish oils and some vegetable oils (e.g. flaxseed oil), while most vegetable oils are of the omega-6 type. The location of double bonds can also be indicated by the Greek letter Δ (delta), which denotes the position of the double bond from the carboxyl terminus (see Table 10.2). The Δ system is the one preferred by organic chemists.

While most unsaturated fatty acids have double bonds of the methylene-interrupted type, there is considerable interest in **conjugated linoleic acid (CLA)** in milk, which seems to have healthful properties such as anticarcinogenic activity (Parodi, 1997). In CLA, the two double bonds have a conjugated arrangement (i.e. lacking a methylene group separating the double bonds) (Fig. 10.3).

Unsaturated fatty acids can be geometric isomers, with either the *cis* or *trans* configuration of groups around a double bond. Most natural fatty acids of animal and plant origin are of the *cis* configuration, whereas those of bacterial origin contain both *cis* and *trans* configurations. *Trans*-fatty

Table 10.1. Common saturated fatty acids of nutritional significance.

Common name	Number of carbons	Occurrence
Acetic	2	Rumen VFA
Propionic	3	Rumen VFA
Butyric	4	Rumen VFA
Valeric	5	Rumen VFA
Caproic	6	Rumen VFA
Lauric	12	Tropical (palm) oils
Myristic	14	Tropical (palm) oils
Palmitic	16	Plant and animal fats
Stearic	18	Plant and animal fats

acids (e.g. elaidic acid) are formed in the chemical hydrogenation of vegetable oils to produce margarine, as well as biohydrogenation in the rumen. As just implied, **hydrogenation** is the addition of hydrogen to double bonds to convert unsaturated fatty acids to a more saturated form. Naturally occurring unsaturated LCFA are usually of the *cis* configuration, with the fatty acid being bent at 120° at the double bond. Thus oleic acid, which is 18:1 *cis*-9, is bent, whereas elaidic acid (18:1 *trans*-9) remains as a straight chain (Fig. 10.4). More *cis* double bonds in an unsaturated fatty acid produce a variety of spatial configurations, such as in arachidonic acid (20:4 *cis*) which has a U shape. Derivatives of arachidonic acid, such as prostaglandins, also have a U shape.

Characteristics of common saturated and unsaturated fatty acids are listed in Tables 10.1 and 10.2.

Lipids containing glycerol

Neutral lipids

The major neutral (uncharged) lipids in animal nutrition are the triglycerides, also known as triacylglycerols. Triglycerides are the fats and oils. The term **triacylglycerol (TAG)** is now the preferred term, and will generally be used here in place of triglyceride.

TAGs are the esters of three fatty acids with glycerol (Fig. 10.5). In most cases, the fatty acids are not the same. When there is a preponderance of saturated fatty acids, the lipid tends to be a solid at room temperature and is called a **fat**. **Oils** have mainly unsaturated fatty acids. The major properties of fatty acids which affect the physical nature of the TAGs are the length of the carbon chain and the degree of unsaturation. The shorter the carbon chain and the more unsaturated the fatty acids, the greater the tendency to be a liquid at room temperature (i.e. the lower the melting point). This phenomenon is because the carboxyl group is water soluble and the hydrocarbon chain is lipophilic. Thus the greater the contribution of the carbon chain (longer chain) to the size of the molecule, the less water soluble it will be. Tropical oils (palm oil, coconut oil) are almost completely saturated, but are liquids at room temperature because they have SCFA (C_{12}). A simple test for assessing the degree of unsaturation of fats and oils is the **iodine number**. Iodine reacts with the double bonds of unsaturated fatty acids. The iodine number is the

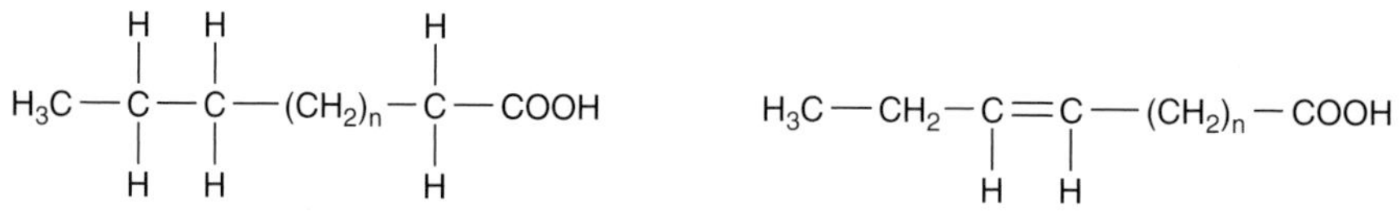

Saturated fatty acid · Unsaturated fatty acid

Fig. 10.1. General structures of saturated and unsaturated fatty acids.

ω-3 Fatty acid

ω-6 Fatty acid

Fig. 10.2. The omega (ω) designation indicates the location of the first double bond from the terminal methyl group.

Table 10.2. Common unsaturated fatty acids of nutritional significance.

Number of carbons and position of double bonds[a]	Family	Common name	Isomers	Occurrence
18:1; Δ9	ω-9	Oleic	*Cis*	Most vegetable oils and fats
18:1; Δ9	ω-9	Elaidic	*Trans*	'*Trans*-fats', hydrogenated vegetable oils
18:2; Δ9,12	ω-6	Linoleic	All *cis*	Most plant oils
18:3; Δ6,9,12	ω-6	γ-Linolenic	All *cis*	Evening primrose, borage oils
18:3; Δ9,12,15	ω-3	α-Linolenic	All *cis*	Linseed (flax) oil
20:4; Δ5,8,11,14	ω-6	Arachidonic	All *cis*	Groundnut (peanut) oil

[a]Δ indicates the location of the double bond(s) beginning from the carboxyl end, in contrast to ω which indicates the location of the double bond(s) beginning at the methyl end of the fatty acid (e.g. 18:3ω6 is the same as 18:3Δ6,9,12). 18:3ω9 means that the fatty acid has 18 carbons and three double bonds, with the first one in the ω-9 position.

$$-CH=CH-CH_2-CH=CH---COOH \qquad -CH=CH-CH=CH---COOH$$

Methylene-interrupted double bonds   Conjugated double bonds

Fig. 10.3. Double bonds in fatty acids may be either methylene interrupted or conjugated.

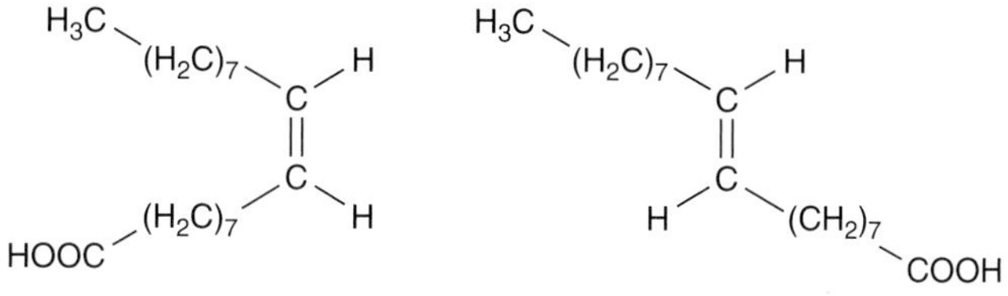

Oleic acid
cis form (bent)

Elaidic acid
trans form (straight)

Fig. 10.4. The *cis* (oleic) and *trans* (elaidic) isomers of ω-3 18:1. Note that the *trans* configuration tends to give a linear structure while the *cis* isomer is bent.

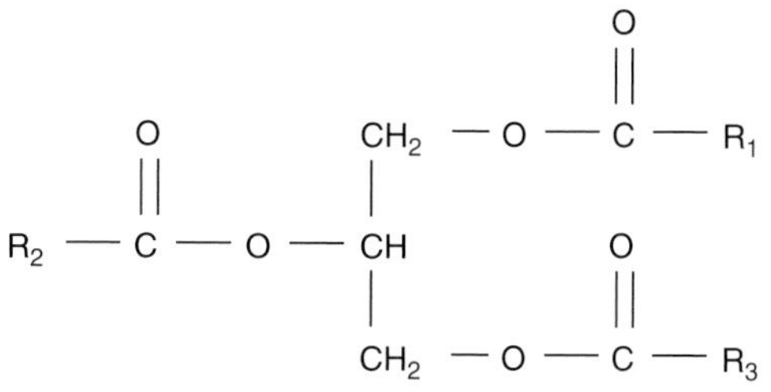

Triacylglycerol

Fig. 10.5. Structure of a triacylglycerol (TAG), also known as a triglyceride (fats and oils). R_1, R_2 and R_3 are fatty acids.

number of grams of iodine reacting with 100 g of lipid. The iodine number of saturated fatty acids is 0 (zero); of oleic acid, 90; of linoleic acid, 181; and of linolenic acid, 274. Physical and chemical properties of common vegetable oils are shown in Table 10.3. Oils of marine fish (e.g. cod liver oil) contain long chain (20 carbons or more), highly unsaturated fatty acids, which is important in cold-water fish species to maintain the body lipids in a non-solid state to maintain mobility. During digestion, carboxylesters of fatty acids are hydrolysed from the glycerol moiety, producing diacylglycerols, monoacylglycerols and free glycerol.

Table 10.3. Physical and chemical properties of common vegetable oils.

Fat or oil	Iodine number	Melting point (°C)	Fatty acids (% of total)[a]					
			16:0	18:0	18:1	18:2	18:3	20:4
Canola	114	–	4.3	1.7	**59.1**	22.8	8.2	0.5
Coconut[b]	8–10	20–35	8.0	2.8	5.6	1.6	–	–
Maize	115–127	–10	12.0	2.7	30.1	**54.7**	1.4	0.2
Cottonseed	97–115	10–16	20.9	1.9	16.0	**59.6**	0.1	–
Linseed	–	–	6.4	3.3	17.0	15.6	**57.7**	–
Olive	79–90	0	14.0	2.6	**74.0**	8.1	1.0	0.4
Palm	48–56	27–50	**42.0**	5.4	39.1	10.6	–	0.2
Groundnut	84–100	–2	11.1	3.0	**52.1**	27.8	0.5	0.7
Rapeseed[c]	81	–9	1.7	0.1	**14.3**	13.4	8.9	0.9
Safflower	145	–17	12.3	1.8	11.2	**74.3**	–	0.5
Soybean	130–138	–21	11.5	4.3	27.3	**49.7**	6.9	0.2
Sunflower	125–136	–17	6.8	3.9	15.7	**73.5**	–	–

[a]The major fatty acids in each oil are set in bold.
[b]The major fatty acids in coconut oil have fewer than 16 carbons.
[c]The major fatty acid in rapeseed oil is erucic acid (22:1), which is 40% or more of total fatty acids.

Phospholipids

Phospholipids contain one or more phosphate groups. Phospholipids are important constituents of cell membranes and nerve tissue. An example is lecithin. **Lecithin** (Fig. 10.6) contains a phosphate group linked to a diacylglycerol and choline, a trimethyl compound. Lecithin is a surfactant, with the phosphatidylcholine side chain providing polarity. Other phosphoacylglycerols found in cell membranes include phosphatidylethanolamine and phosphatidylserine, with ethanolamine and serine replacing choline.

Lipids not containing glycerol

Waxes

The surfaces of plants are often covered in a protective layer of wax or cutin. **Waxes** are lipids with fatty acids esterified to an alcohol other than glycerol. For example, jojoba oil from the desert plant jojoba (*Simmondsia californica*) is actually a wax, with a fatty acid esterified with a long-chain alcohol. **Cutin** is a type of wax. It is a complex polymer of hydroxy fatty acids linked by ester bonds to give a three-dimensional network. Waxes occur as components of forages, but are of low digestibility.

Sphingolipids

Sphingolipids contain a long-chain alcohol, sphingosine (Fig. 10.7). Sphingomyelins are phospholipids containing **ceramide**, the fatty-acid derivative of sphingosine (Fig. 10.7).

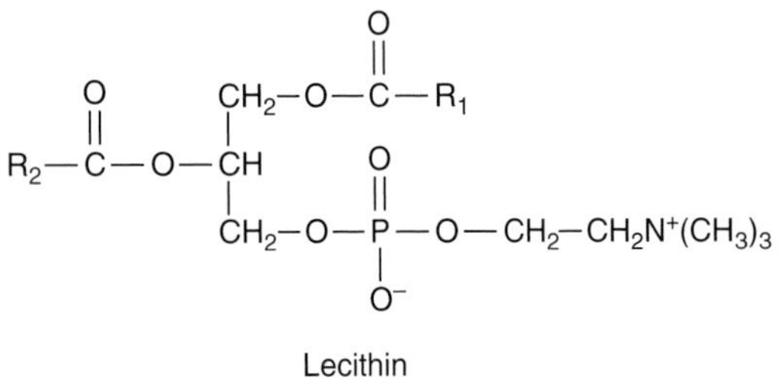

Fig. 10.6. Lecithin is a methylated compound with amphoteric properties, giving it surfactant activity. R_1 and R_2 are fatty acids.

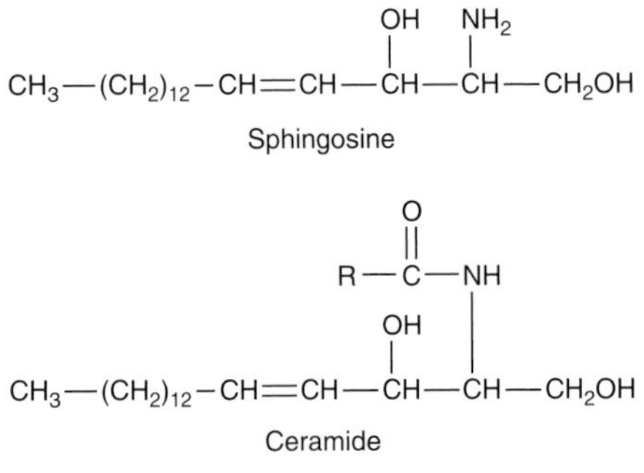

Fig. 10.7. Sphingosine is a long-chain alcohol that is a constituent of sphingolipids. Ceramide is the fatty-acid derivative of sphingosine. R is a fatty acid.

Sphingolipids are major constituents of nerve tissue (cerebrosides and gangliosides) and they occur in cell membranes in general. Some are involved in intercellular communication and as blood-group substances. The myelin sheath of nerves is particularly rich in sphingolipids.

A common mycotoxin in maize, **fumonisin**, is structurally similar to sphingosine (Fig. 10.8). Fumonisins inhibit sphingosine biosynthesis, causing impaired brain synthesis of sphingolipids. Fumonisins cause a neurological disease of horses (**equine leucoencephalomalacia**) characterized by necrosis of the white matter of the cerebrum (Thiel *et al.*, 1991). This disorder can be explained by the impaired sphinoglipid biosynthesis. In humans, various neurological diseases such as multiple sclerosis result from defects in sphingolipid metabolism. Fumonisin-contaminated maize (corn) used in tortillas has been linked to disrupted sphingolipid metabolism, neural tube and craniofacial defects and impaired folate metabolism in Central American populations (Marasas *et al.*, 2004).

Plants contain glycolipids, which have a diacylglycerol structure with galactose instead of a fatty acid on C1. They are important components of membranes (e.g. the chloroplast membrane in leaf tissue). Some leaf galactolipids are sulfated and are referred to as **sulfolipids**. Because galactolipids are the major lipids in leaves, they are a predominant lipid source of forage-fed animals. Seeds, in contrast to leaves, contain lipid mainly as TAGs.

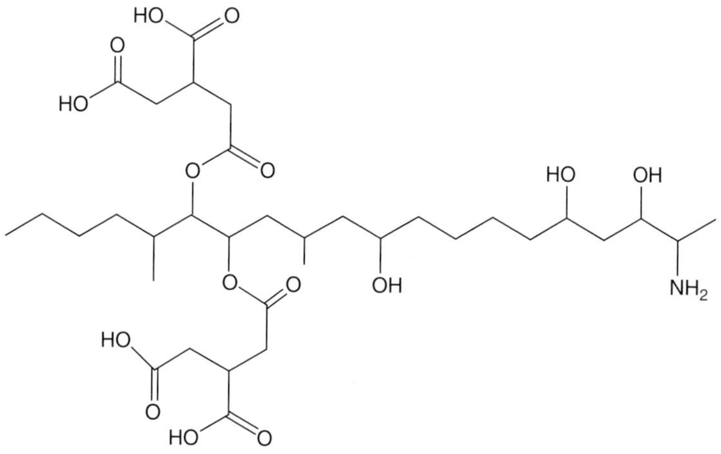

Fumonisin B1

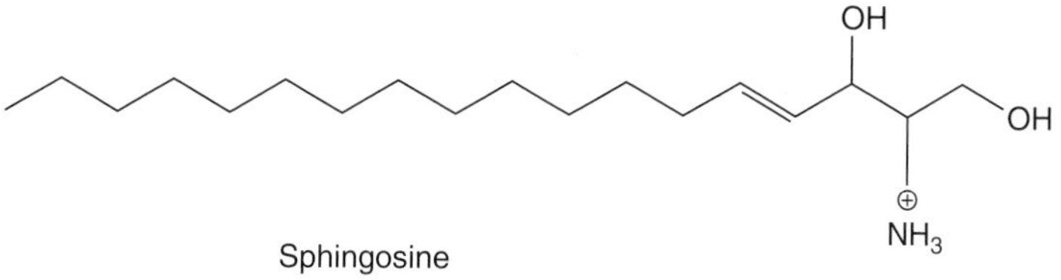

Sphingosine

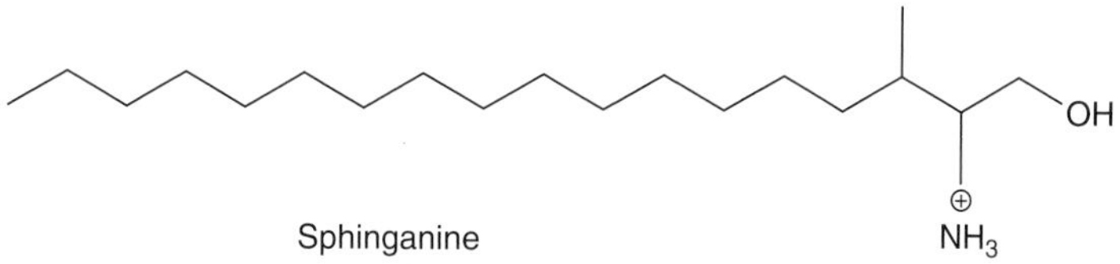

Sphinganine

Fig. 10.8. Fumonisins are mycotoxins that are structurally similar to sphingosine and sphinganine, thus disrupting normal sphingolipid synthesis and causing neurological problems.

Other lipids

Steroids

Steroids are fat-soluble substances that contain the steroid nucleus. Cholesterol is the best-known steroid, and is the ultimate precursor of many others, including vitamin D, bile acids, sex hormones (testosterone, oestrogen, progesterone), corticosteroid hormones (cortisol, corticosterone, aldosterone), anabolic steroids, etc. **Sterols** have the steroid nucleus with one or more hydroxyl groups. **Cholesterol** is a sterol, containing the steroid nucleus with an hydroxyl group (Fig. 10.9). Examples of steroid hormones synthesized from cholesterol are shown in Fig. 10.10.

Cholesterol is an important component of animal tissue, not only as a precursor of other steroids but also as a major component of cell membranes. It is especially important in nerve tissue. Although commonly but erroneously believed to be a major constituent of animal fat, cholesterol is actually higher in muscle tissue because cell membranes are more abundant in muscle than in adipose tissue. Adipose tissue cells are large, so the membrane is a smaller part of the cell mass than is the case with smaller cells.

Steroids, such as cholesterol, vitamin D, bile acids, sex hormones (androgens, oestrogens, progesterones), corticosteroid hormones (e.g. cortisol) and mineralocorticoids (e.g. aldosterone) are essential metabolites. The word 'steroids' has acquired a bad reputation because **anabolic steroids** derived from androgens are used as illegal drugs to enhance anabolism (build-up of body tissue, especially protein). This usage is, for many people, their only awareness of steroids, so the word has acquired a bad name with the general public.

Cholesterol is synthesized by plants, but it has a fleeting existence as an intermediate in the synthesis of other steroids. Unlike the cell membranes of animals, plant cell walls do not contain cholesterol, but instead contain other sterols (plant- or phytosterols).

Eicosanoids

Eicosanoids are compounds derived from 20-carbon and 22-carbon fatty acids, and include prostaglandins, prostacyclins, thromboxanes and leukotrienes. These substances have hormone or hormone-like roles in vasoconstriction and blood

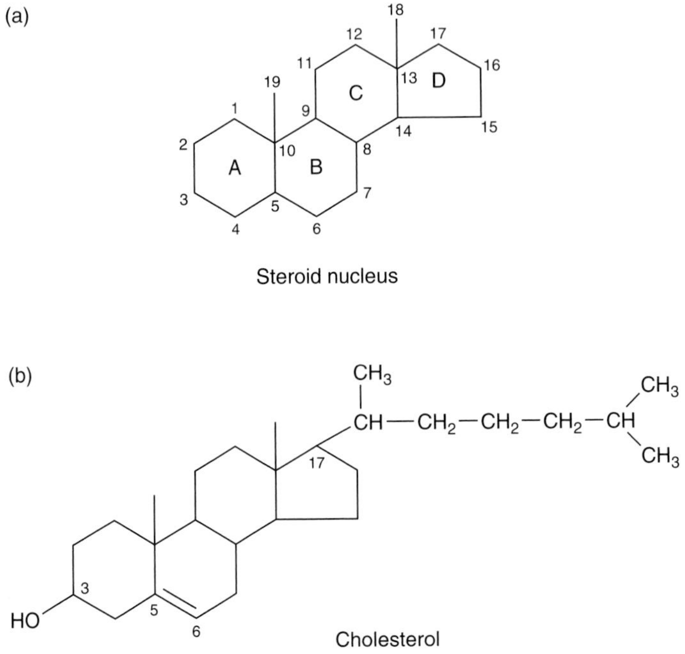

Fig. 10.9. The steroid nucleus (a) and cholesterol, an example of a steroid (b).

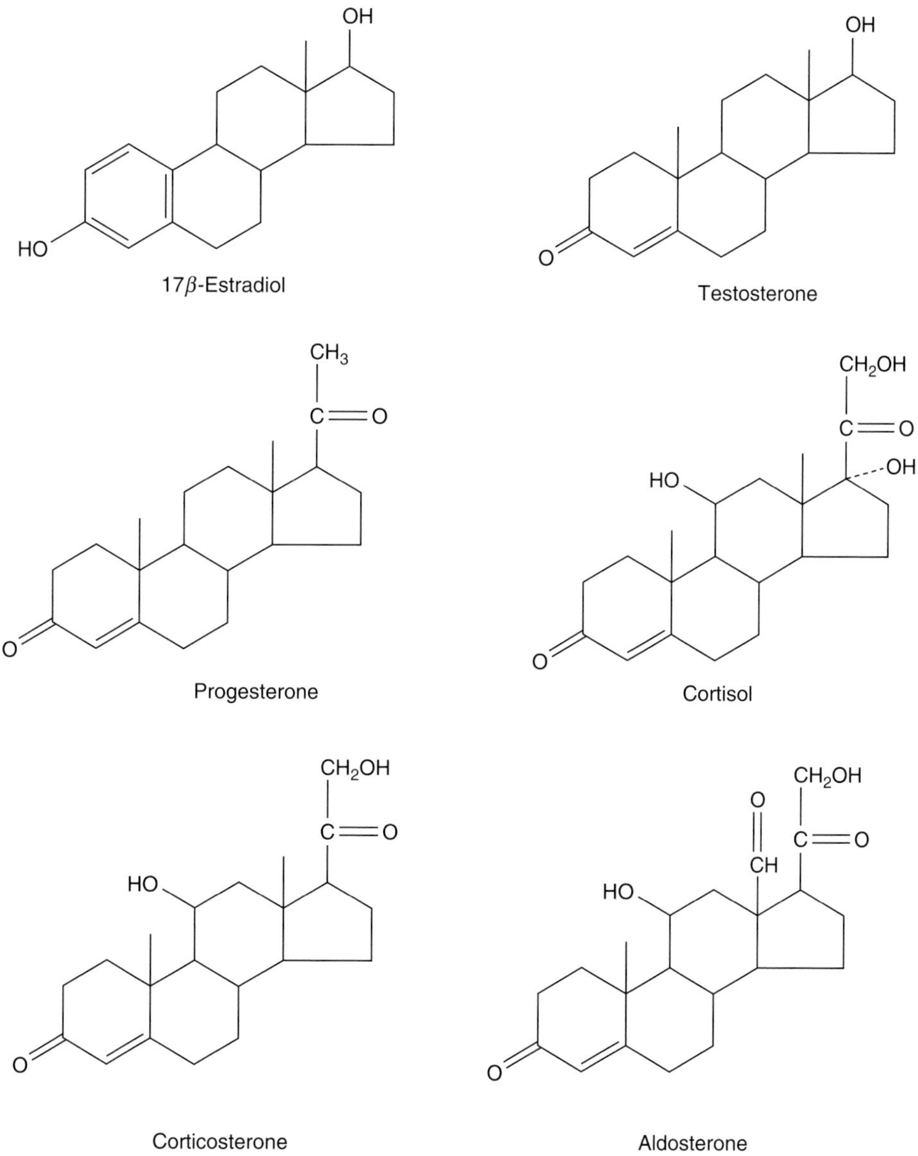

Fig. 10.10. Examples of steroid hormones derived from cholesterol.

platelet aggregation. Prostaglandins and other eicosanoids are synthesized mainly from arachidonic acid.

Two other fatty acids from which eicosanoids are synthesized are **docosahexaenoic acid (DHA; 22:6ω3)**, which is present in fish oils, and **eicosapentaenoic acid (EPA; 20:5ω3)**. Changing prostaglandin profiles through elevated intakes of DHA and EPA from fish

and fish oils can decrease clotting capacity and platelet aggregation.

Some of the major ω-3 essential fatty acids are:

- C18:3ω3 – linolenic acid (LNA);
- C20:5ω3 – eicosapentaenoic acid (EPA);
- C22:5ω3 – docosapentaenoic acid (DPA); and
- C22:6ω3 – docosahexaenoic acid (DHA).

Some of the major ω-6 are:

- C18:2ω6 – linoleic acid (LA); and
- C20:4ω6 – arachidonic acid (AA).

Some of these fatty acids are referred to as **essential fatty acids**, because for most animals, they are required metabolically for the synthesis of essential metabolites. Those that are dietary essentials for many species of animals, including humans, are LA and α-LNA. In most animals, AA can be formed from LA. Double bonds can be introduced at the Δ4, Δ5, Δ6 and Δ9 positions in most animals, but never beyond Δ9. Plants, in contrast, can introduce double bonds at the Δ12 or Δ15 positions.

The lipid content of the retina and grey matter in the mammalian brain is high in both AA and DHA. These long-chain PUFA are derived from their respective dietary essential fatty-acid precursors, LA and LNA, through desaturation and chain elongation. The conversion of LNA to long-chain ω-3 fatty acids is not efficient. The AA and DHA accumulate rapidly in the human brain during the third trimester of pregnancy and in the early postnatal period (Wainwright, 2000), when the rate of brain growth is maximal. Broadhurst *et al.* (1998) and Cunnane and Crawford (2003) proposed that the evolution of the enlarged brain of *Homo sapiens*, in the East African Rift Valley widely considered the cradle of human origins, was due to the consumption of fish, which provided the fatty-acid nutrients necessary for brain growth. They claim that the uniquely complex human neurological system could not have evolved in the absence of consumption of animal-based foods. The lipid profile of tropical freshwater fish has a DHA:AA ratio that is closer to human brain phospholipids than any other food source known (Broadhurst *et al.*, 1998). Fish are also an excellent source of zinc, copper, iodine and other trace elements necessary for PUFA metabolism and for normal brain development and function. According to Broadhurst *et al.* (1998, p.18):

> There is good evidence today that lack of abundant, balanced DHA and AA *in utero* and infancy leads to lower intelligence quotient and visual acuity, and in the longer term contributes to clinical depression and attention-deficit hyperactivity disorder. We are not so far removed from our Paleolithic ancestors that we can expect our present agricultural, processed-food-based diet to provide indefinitely for our continued intellectual development.

Aliphatic alcohols

Aliphatic alcohols occur in some lipid sources, such as sperm whale oil and beeswax. For example, sperm whale oil (head oil) contains cetyl alcohol esterified with palmitic acid, producing cetyl palmitate (spermaceti). Cetyl alcohol is palmitic acid with an hydroxyl (alcohol group) in place of the carboxyl group.

Terpenes

Terpenes contain multiples of a five-carbon structure called isoprene (Fig. 10.11). This class of compounds includes essential oils and the carotenoids (carotenes, lycopene, xanthophylls). Vitamin E and vitamin K contain terpenoid side chains.

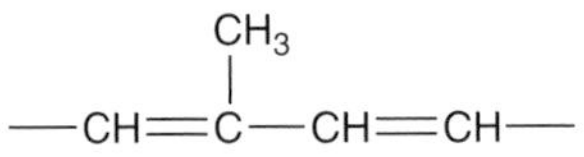

Isoprene unit

Fig. 10.11. The five-carbon isoprene unit.

Questions and Study Guide

1. What is the difference between saturated and unsaturated fatty acids?
2. Draw the structures of 18:3ω6 and 18:3Δ6,9,12.
3. What is the difference between oleic acid (18:1) and elaidic acid (18:1)?
4. What is the difference between methylene-interrupted double bonds and conjugated double bonds?
5. How do fats and oils differ chemically?
6. Many people regard steroids as harmful substances. Why? Are they harmful?
7. What is an eicosanoid? What are DHA and EPA?
8. What are the fatty acids that are dietary essentials for most species?

References

Broadhurst, C.L., Cunnane, S.C. and Crawford, M.A. (1998) Rift Valley lake fish and shellfish provided brain-specific nutrition for early Homo. *British Journal of Nutrition* 79, 3–21.

Cunnane, S.C. and Crawford, M.A. (2003) Survival of the fattest: fat babies were the key to evolution of the large human brain. *Comparative Biochemistry and Physiology A* 136, 17–26.

Marasas, W.F.O., Riley, R.T., Hendricks, K.A., Stevens, V.L., Sadler, T.W., Waes, J.G., Missmer, S.A., Cabrera, J., Torres, O., Gelderblom, W.C.A., Allegood, J., Martinez, C., Maddox, J., Miller, J.D., Starr, L., Sullards, M.C., Roman, A.V., Voss, K.A., Wang, E. and Merrill, A.H., Jr (2004) Fumonisins disrupt sphingolipid metabolism, folate transport, and neural tube development in embryo culture and *in vivo*: a potential risk factor for human neural tube defects among populations consuming fumonisin-contaminated maize. *Journal of Nutrition* 134, 711–716.

Parodi, P.W. (1997) Cows' milk fat components as potential anticarcinogenic agents. *Journal of Nutrition* 127, 1055–1060.

Thiel, P.G., Shephard, G.S., Sydenham, E.W., Marasas, W.F.O., Nelson, P.E. and Wilson, T.M. (1991) Levels of fumonisins B_1 and B_2 in feeds associated with confirmed cases of equine leukoencephalomalacia. *Journal of Agricultural and Food Chemistry* 39, 109–111.

Wainwright, P. (2000) Invited commentary. Nutrition and behaviour: The role of ω-3 fatty acids in cognitive function. *British Journal of Nutrition* 83, 337–339

11 Lipid Digestion

Non-Ruminants

Lipids are hydrophobic, meaning that they are not soluble in water. Therefore, a fundamental aspect of lipid digestion is to 'dissolve' fat in water, that is, in the aqueous medium of the digestive tract. This is accomplished by **emulsification**, or the dispersal of lipid in water in the form of very small droplets. In practical terms, most dietary lipid in typical pig and poultry diets consists of fats and/or oils, or **triacylglycerols** (**TAGs**). The TAGs are emulsified in the small intestine by the emulsifying activity of bile salts (also known as bile acids) and phospholipids (e.g. lecithin). Emulsification actually begins in the stomach, caused by the churning action of muscular contractions accompanied by some activity of gastric lipase. As the stomach contents are propelled into the duodenum, emulsification is completed by the action of bile salts and phospholipids excreted in the bile. **Bile salts** are derivatives of cholesterol and have **amphipathic properties**, meaning that they are both water soluble and fat soluble because of variations in polarity within the molecule. **Emulsified lipid droplets** are formed, consisting of a droplet of lipid surrounded by a layer of bile salts and phospholipids. The water-soluble 'head' of the bile salt is at the surface of the droplet, causing the droplet to essentially be in solution. Thus lipids are dispersed in water by forming very small, emulsified droplets.

Primary bile acids are synthesized in the liver from cholesterol. The first steps are hydroxylation of cholesterol on carbon 7 and 12, followed by binding to coenzyme A (CoA) to form cholyl-CoA (Fig. 11.1). Cholyl-CoA may conjugate with taurine to form **taurocholic** acid or with glycine to form **glycocholic** acid (Fig. 11.1). Detergents are toxic to intestinal mucosal cells; the conjugated bile acids are less toxic than the free bile acids. In birds, bile acids are conjugated only with taurine, while in mammals there may be a mixture of taurine and glycine conjugates. The bile acids of herbivores tend to have glycine conjugates, except for those of ruminants that have primarily taurine conjugates. Under the acidic conditions of the upper small intestine in ruminants, taurine-conjugated bile acids remain in a partially ionized condition, and are more effective at solubilizing fatty acids than glycine-conjugated bile acids. Glycine-conjugates are much less soluble under acidic conditions than taurine-conjugated bile acids. Carnivore bile acids are conjugated with taurine (e.g. cats). Omnivores tend to have a mixture of the two types (Moran, 1982). **Secondary bile acids** are formed by microbial metabolism of primary bile acids in the hindgut. In human nutrition, secondary bile acids are of concern because they are carcinogens, and may be involved in development of colon cancer (Govers *et al.*, 1996). Through a surfactant effect, secondary bile acids and soluble fatty acids damage the colonic epithelium and stimulate the proliferation of colonic crypt cells, which increases the risk of colon cancer (Govers *et al.*, 1996). Most of the bile acid secreted in the bile is reabsorbed from the lower small intestine and removed from the blood by the liver. This is known as **entero-hepatic recycling** of bile. This recycling contributes to maintaining a constant metabolic pool of cholesterol. Serum cholesterol can be decreased by dietary agents that bind bile acids and cause them to be excreted. These include cholesterol-lowering drugs (e.g. cholestyramine) and natural substances (e.g. saponins).

Bile pigments are the metabolic end products of haem metabolism and account for the characteristic colour of bile. Red blood cells are degraded in the liver, releasing the porphyrin haem from haemoglobin. Haem is metabolized by liver enzymes to the bile pigments **biliverdin** (green) and **bilirubin** (reddish orange). Bilirubin is conjugated with glucuronic acid to form bilirubin glucuronide before excretion from the liver. In the intestine, conjugated

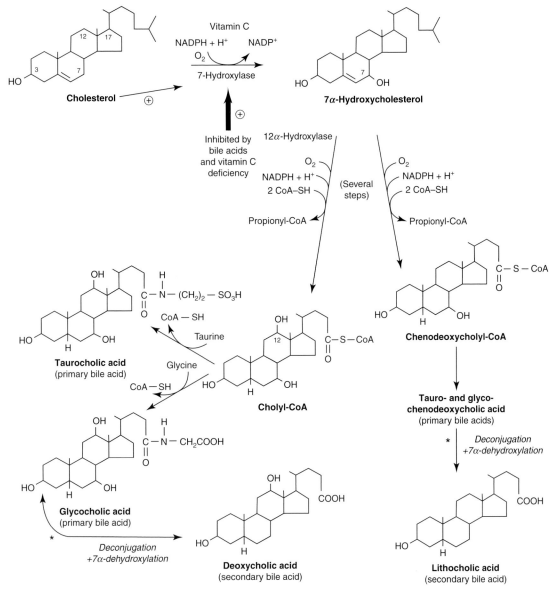

Fig. 11.1. Biosynthesis and degradation of bile acids. A second pathway in mitochondria involves hydroxylation of cholesterol by sterol 27-hydroxylase. *, Catalysed by microbial enzymes (courtesy of E.T. Moran, Jr, Auburn University, Auburn, Alabama, USA).

bilirubin is reduced to **urobilinogens** by intestinal microbes. Urobilinogens are colourless, but are oxidized to brown pigments in the faeces upon exposure to air. Birds and reptiles excrete only biliverdin in the bile, while mammals excrete mainly bilirubin. Liver damage may impede the normal excretion of bile pigments, leading to accumulation of bilirubin in the blood (jaundice or icterus).

Digestion of **TAGs** involves hydrolysis of ester bonds by which fatty acids are esterified with glycerol. **Pancreatic lipase** acts at the lipid–water interface of the emulsified oil droplet (Fig. 11.2). The polar ends of the fatty acids on the C-1 and C-3 positions of glycerol 'stick out' into the aqueous phase at the interface. The water-soluble lipase enzyme then splits off fatty acids from the C-1 and C-3 positions, liberating free fatty acids (**FFAs**), diacylglycerols (**DAGs**) and monoacylglycerols (**MAGs**). Pancreatic lipase is specific for fatty acids esterified at the C-1 and C-3 positions of glycerol. There is an isomerization enzyme to move fatty acids from the C-2 position to C-1 or C-3, so that complete degradation to three FFAs and glycerol is possible. There may be some absorption of 2-MAGs in addition to the FFAs released by lipase at the C-1 and C-3 positions. **Colipase** is a protein factor required for optimal lipase activity. It is secreted by the pancreas in an inactive form, and is activated in

the intestinal lumen by trypsin. Its function is to prevent the inhibitory effects of bile salts on hydrolysis of long-chain fatty acids (LCFAs) from TAGs.

The next step in the fat digestion process is that the products of lipase activity (DAGs, MAGs, FFAs) form water-soluble **micelles**, which are temporary associations of lipids with amphipathic bile salts. The micelle consists of an aggregation of hydrophobic portions of these molecules, surrounded by a layer of bile salts with the water-soluble portion (head) of the bile salt at the lipid–water interface (Fig. 11.3)

The micelles are thus dispersable in water, and transport the fat-soluble substances to the intestinal surface for absorption. During absorption, the micelle breaks down and bile salts return to the intestinal lumen to be re-used in making micelles.

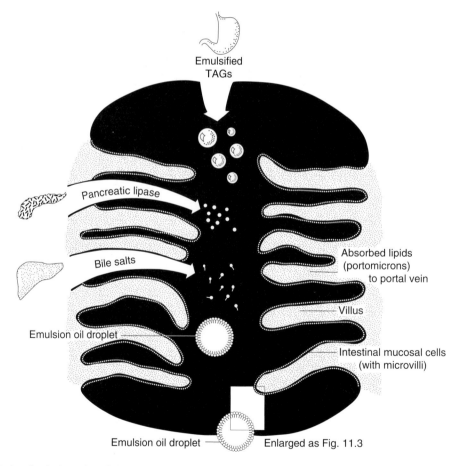

Fig. 11.2. Intraluminal section of the duodenum showing the initial stages of fat digestion (courtesy of University Books, Guelph, Canada).

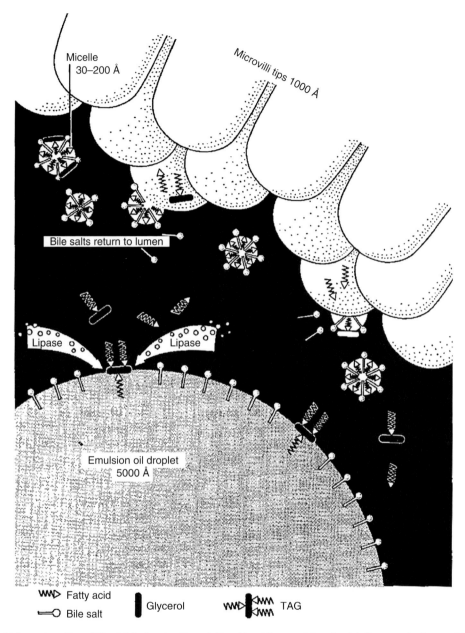

Fatty acid	Glycerol		TAG
Bile salt			

Fig. 11.3. Enlarged section of Fig. 11.2 showing the relationship of the emulsion droplet, lipase, micelles, and the tips of the microvillus during fat digestion and absorption (courtesy of University Books, Guelph, Canada).

Mixed micelles can contain a variety of lipid digestion end products, and other lipid-soluble substances such as the fat-soluble vitamins and cholesterol.

Several factors influence the absorbability of fats and fatty acids. The ability to form micelles is an important consideration. Saturated fatty acids, either as free fatty acids or as components of TAGs (at the 1 and 3 positions) do not form micelles well unless some unsaturated fatty acids are present. Thus the utilization of saturated fatty acids and animal fats is improved when a source of unsaturated lipid is included in the diet.

Ruminants

The natural diets of ruminants tend to have a low concentration of lipids. Leaf lipids are mainly galactolipids and phospholipids, and miscellaneous substances such as waxes, plant pigments (chlorophyll, carotenoids) and essential oils. Seed lipids are primarily TAGs; therefore, modern feedlot and dairy diets based on grains have a preponderance of dietary lipid as TAGs.

Rumen microbes utilize lipids inefficiently. In non-ruminants, fats are eumulsified by bile before digestion in the small intestine. In the rumen, there is a lack of emulsifying agent and pancreatic lipase, so high (above 5%) amounts of dietary fat can cause reductions in fibre digestibility by a physical coating action on feed particles. Fats also have an inhibitory effect on rumen microbes; unsaturated fatty acids are toxic to rumen bacteria.

Unsaturated fatty acids are partially or completely hydrogenated in the reducing (high hydrogen) conditions of the rumen. The positions of the double bonds are altered, and generally they are converted to the more stable *trans* form (Bessa *et al.*, 2000). There is also the formation of odd-carbon and branched-chain acids. Linoleic acid, in which the double bonds are methylene interrupted, is converted to several **conjugated fatty acids**, in which the double bonds are not separated by a methylene (CH_2) group (see Fig. 10.3 in Chapter 10 and Fig. 11.4). The fatty acids are intermediates in the conversion of linoleic and linolenic acids to stearic acid (Fig. 11.5). They are of interest in human health. Studies in laboratory animals have shown that they have anticancer activity, as well as beneficial effects on immune function and atherosclerosis. It is not yet firmly established whether or not these favourable effects occur in humans.

In ruminants, lipolysis, or the release of fatty acids from TAGs, occurs mainly in the rumen.

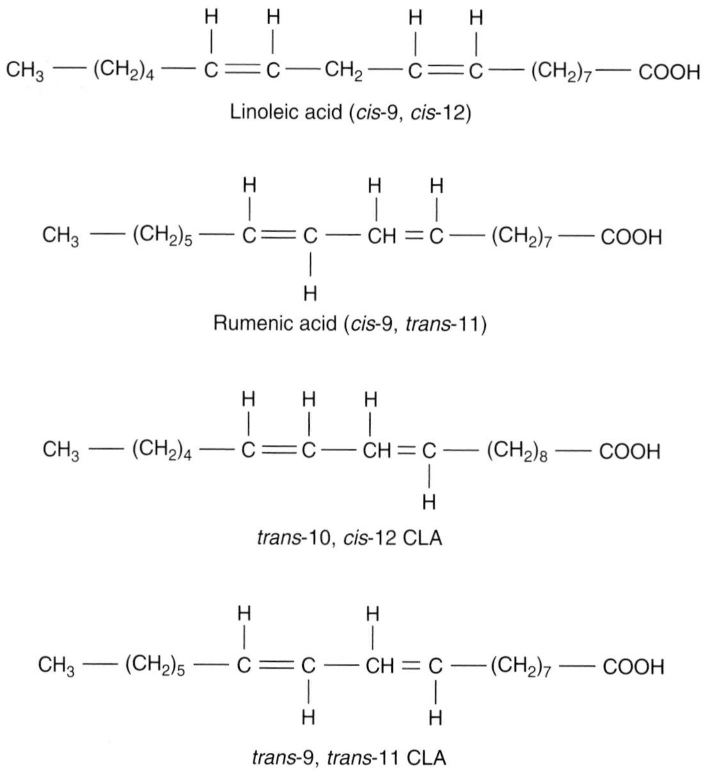

Fig. 11.4. Linoleic acid and its main conjugated isomers produced in the rumen.

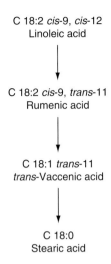

C 18:2 *cis*-9, *cis*-12
Linoleic acid

↓

C 18:2 *cis*-9, *trans*-11
Rumenic acid

↓

C 18:1 *trans*-11
trans-Vaccenic acid

↓

C 18:0
Stearic acid

Fig. 11.5. Pathway of biohydrogenation of linoleic acid in the rumen.

Fatty acids are neutralized at the rumen pH and converted to **soaps**, which are salts of fatty acids. Potassium soaps are readily absorbed in the small intestine, whereas calcium soaps have lower absorbability.

Ruminants secrete a high proportion of taurine-conjugated bile acids, which facilitates solubilization of fatty acids in the acidic duodenum of ruminants. In ruminants, the majority of lipid entering the small intestine is in the form of FFAs (80–90%) in contrast to non-ruminants, in which most lipid is in the esterified form. The duodenum of ruminants is acidic, because of the low concentration and rate of secretion of bicarbonate in ruminant pancreatic secretions. The predominant fatty acid exiting the rumen is stearic acid, which is saturated. In non-ruminants, saturated fatty acids are absorbed more poorly than the unsaturated forms, because of less effective micelle formation. In ruminants, pancreatic enzymes (phospholipases) convert biliary lecithin to **lysolecithin**, which 'desorbs' the fatty acids from feed particles and microbes. Because most of the fatty acids leaving the rumen are saturated (stearic and palmitic acids), ruminants have evolved an efficient lysolecithin system for solubilizing these fatty acids. Lipid metabolism of ruminants has been reviewed by Doreau and Ferlay (1994).

As described in Chapter 3, Hofmann proposed three categories of ruminants: (i) concentrate selectors (browsers); (ii) grazers; and (iii) intermediate feeders. Hofmann indicated that concentrate selectors have a less well-developed rumen, with a rapid rumen pass-through of liquids and soluble plant cell contents. Meyer *et al.* (1998) postulated that a large reticular groove and copious salivary secretion to facilitate passage of solubles should result in a greater bypass of unsaturated fatty acids in concentrate selectors, producing a more unsaturated body fat than is typical of grazers and intermediate feeders. They examined the body fat of a variety of ruminants (roe deer, moose, deer, giraffe, goats, sheep, cattle, bison, camel) and non-ruminants (wild boar, elephant) for fatty acid composition. As hypothesized, the concentrate-selector ruminants (roe deer, moose) had significantly higher percentages of polyunsaturated fatty acids (PUFA) in their adipose tissue than the grazer and intermediate-feeder ruminants. The non-ruminant wild boar and elephant had, as predicted, much higher concentrations of PUFA than any of the ruminant species. These results support the validity of Hofmann's physiological interpretation of concentrate-selector ruminants; because of the rapid flow-through of solubilized material, there is less opportunity for hydrogenation of unsaturated fatty acids in the rumen.

One of the microbial transformations of lipids in the rumen is the synthesis of odd- and branched-chain fatty acids, which aid in maintaining optimal fluidity of microbial cell membranes (Or-Rashid *et al.*, 2007). The main fatty acid in mixed rumen bacteria is stearic acid, whereas palmitic acid is predominant in protozoa (Or-Rashid *et al.*, 2007). Protozoa contain a greater proportion of unsaturated fatty acids and CLA than do bacteria.

The flavour and odour of lamb and mutton are offensive to many people. These odours and flavours are due to medium-length **branched-chain fatty acids** (BCFAs) (4-methyloctanoic, 4-methylnonanoic and 4-ethyl analogues) which occur as TAGs in the adipose tissue (Wong *et al.*, 1975, cited by Schreurs *et al.*, 2008). The high concentration of BCFAs in adipose tissue is unique to sheep and goats. They are formed from methylmalonate, which is produced from propionate. The concentration of BCFAs in body fat is higher in grain-fed than in pasture-raised sheep, because of the higher propionate production with high concentrate diets.

Questions and Study Guide

1. What is the difference between primary and secondary bile acids?
2. How do micelles function in lipid absorption?
3. What causes the brown coloration of faeces?
4. How do ruminants differ from non-ruminants in fat digestion and absorption?
5. The fat of sheep meat has an odour that some people find offensive. What causes this odour? It is lower in grass-fed sheep than in those fed grain in feedlots. Why?

References

Bessa, R.J.B., Santos-Silva, J., Ribeiro, J.M.R. and Portugal, A.V. (2000) Reticulo-rumen biohydrogenation and the enrichment of ruminant edible products with linoleic acid conjugated isomers. *Livestock Production Science* 63, 201–211.

Doreau, M. and Ferlay, A. (1994) Digestion and utilisation of fatty acids by ruminants. *Animal Feed Science and Technology* 45, 379–396.

Govers, M.J.A.P., Termont, D.S.M.L., Lapre, J.A., Kleibeuker, J.H., Vonk, R.J. and Van der Meer, R. (1996) Calcium in milk products precipitates intestinal fatty acids and secondary bile acids and thus inhibits colonic cytotoxicity in humans. *Cancer Research* 56, 3270–3275.

Meyer, H.H.D., Rowell, A., Streich, W.J., Stoffel, B. and Hofmann, R.R. (1998) Accumulation of polyunsaturated fatty acids by concentrate selecting ruminants. *Comparative Biochemistry and Physiology Part A* 120, 263–268.

Moran, E.T., Jr (1982) *Comparative Nutrition of Fowl and Swine. The Gastrointestinal Systems*. University of Guelph, Guelph, Canada.

Or-Rashid, M.M., Odongo, N.E. and McBride, B.W. (2007) Fatty acid composition of ruminal bacteria and protozoa, with emphasis on conjugated linoleic acid, vaccenic acid, and odd-chain and branched-chain fatty acids. *Journal of Animal Science* 85, 1228–1234.

Schreurs, N.M., Lane, G.A., Tavendale, M.H., Barry, T.N. and McNabb, W.C. (2008) Pastoral flavour in meat products from ruminants fed fresh forages and its amelioration by forage condensed tannins. *Animal Feed Science and Technology* 146, 193–221.

12 Fat and Fatty Acid Metabolism

Dietary fats are subject to partial digestion in the gut, with release of fatty acids and monoacylglycerols (MAGs). These are resynthesized into triacylglycerols (TAGs) in the intestinal mucosa. TAGs are incorporated into **chylomicrons** in the lymphatic system draining the intestine. Chylomicrons are basically droplets of lipid with a protein and phospholipid surface layer; they are the lowest density (because of high lipid content) of the serum lipoproteins. Shortly after the ingestion of a fatty meal, the blood serum is opaque because of the high chylomicron content. The chylomicrons are rapidly degraded by an enzyme, **lipoprotein lipase**, located in the capillary walls in many tissues, liberating glycerol and free fatty acids (FFAs; non-esterified fatty acids). As a consequence, the serum opaqueness clears rapidly. Some of the FFAs remain in the blood attached to albumin, while the remainder are taken up by the tissues.

Because lipids are insoluble in water, they are transported in blood in association with serum proteins, forming **lipoproteins**. The main lipoproteins (as determined by centrifugation) are:

- chylomicrons;
- very low density lipoprotein (VLDL);
- low density lipoprotein (LDL); and
- high density lipoprotein (HDL).

Characteristics of lipoproteins are shown in Table 12.1. Because lipid is less dense than water, the density of lipoproteins decreases as the proportion of lipid to protein increases. Lipoproteins consist of an inner core of very hydrophobic lipid, surrounded by a single surface layer of phospholipid and cholesterol, with their polar groups oriented outwards to the aqueous medium. The outer protein is called an **apolipoprotein** (or apoprotein); some of these are firmly attached (integral apoprotein) while others (perpipheral apoproteins) are free to transfer to other lipoproteins. The main apoprotein of HDL is designated A, while the main

apoprotein in LDL is B. Apoproteins C and D are small polypeptides transferable between lipoproteins. Apoprotein E functions in the uptake of chylomicron remnants by the liver.

The liver has a central role in lipid transport and metabolism, with the following major functions:

1. It facilitates the digestion and absorption of lipids by secretion of bile.
2. It synthesizes and oxidizes fatty acids.
3. It converts fatty acids to ketone bodies.
4. It is involved in the synthesis and catabolism of lipoproteins.

The **VLDL** are involved in the transport of TAGs from the liver to the extrahepatic tissues. FFAs are released from VLDL by the action of lipoprotein lipase. The **HDL** is synthesized and secreted from both the liver and the intestine. A major function of HDL is to act as a repository for the apoproteins required in the metabolism of chylomicrons and VLDL.

Cholesterol Metabolism

Lipoproteins have major roles in **cholesterol metabolism**. Cholesterol is present either as free cholesterol or combined with a long-chain fatty acid (LCFA) as cholesterol ester. In plasma, both forms are transported with lipoproteins. Cholesterol is amphipathic, meaning that it has both polar and non-polar properties, and thus is soluble in both water and lipid. Because of this property, it is a constituent of cell membranes and the outer layer of lipoproteins. All carbon atoms in cholesterol are derived from acetyl CoA. It is synthesized in many tissues, particularly the liver, and is the precursor of all other steroids in the body (vitamin D, bile acids, androgens, oestrogens, corticosteroids). Cholesterol is transported to the tissues with **LDL** ('**bad cholesterol**') and removed from the tissues by HDL ('**good cholesterol**'). (The good and bad

Table 12.1. Composition of serum lipoproteins.

Lipoprotein	Source	Density	Protein (%)	Lipid (%)	Main lipid components	Apolipoproteins
Chylomicrons	Intestine	<0.95	1–2	98–99	TAGs	A, B, C, E
VLDL	Liver (intestine)	0.95–1.006	7–10	90–93	TAGs	B, C
LDL	VLDL	1.019–1.063	21	79	Cholesterol	B
HDL	Liver, intestine, VLDL, chylomicrons	1.019–1.210	32–57	43–68	Phospholipids, cholesterol	A, C, D, E
Albumin	Adipose tissue	>1.281	99	1	FFAs	

designations are for the nature of transport; the cholesterol molecule is the same in each case.) It is transported to the liver by HDL (**reverse cholesterol transport**).

Cholesterol in the body is derived from both dietary sources and *de novo* synthesis in the liver and other tissues. The biosynthesis of cholesterol (Fig. 12.1) can be divided into several steps:

1. Mevalonate is synthesized from acetyl CoA by the same reaction involved in synthesis of ketone bodies but in an extramitochondrial compartment (see Fig. 12.2). An intermediate, 3-hydroxy-3-methylglutaryl-CoA (HMG-CoA), is produced in these reactions.
2. Mevalonate is phosphorylated to an active isoprenoid unit, isopentenyl diphosphate.
3. Six isoprenoid units condense to form squalene.
4. Squalene cyclizes to produce the parent sterol, lanosterol.
5. Cholesterol is synthesized from lanosterol.

Regulation of cholesterol biosynthesis (the rate-limiting step) is near the beginning of the pathway, at the HMG-CoA reductase step. This reaction is inhibited by **statins** (Fig. 12.2), drugs which are used to lower serum cholesterol in humans (e.g. Lipitor®, Pravachol®, Lovastatin®). LDL receptors occur on cell surfaces. LDL apoprotein binds to the receptors and then LDL is taken up intact by the cells. The LDL cholesterol is hydrolysed to free cholesterol, which is used within the cell for cell membranes and steroid hormone synthesis. The number of LDL receptors is regulated by the cellular requirement for cholesterol. Increased cellular cholesterol down-regulates synthesis of the LDL receptors.

Reverse cholesterol transport involves association of cholesterol ester with HDL and transport to the liver. The HDL cholesterol is taken up by the liver and excess cholesterol in the liver is either excreted as such in the bile or converted to bile acids. Most of the cholesterol and bile acids excreted in the bile are reabsorbed via the portal circulation (**enterohepatic circulation**). Dietary additives (e.g. cholestyramine, plant sterols, saponins) bind cholesterol and bile acids in the gut, reducing cholesterol reabsorption and lowering serum cholesterol. Thus two major mechanisms for lowering serum cholesterol are: (i) the use of statins to reduce cholesterol biosynthesis; and (ii) the use of dietary additives to bind cholesterol in the gut, causing it to be excreted in the faeces rather than being reabsorbed.

The dietary fat has an influence on **serum cholesterol** concentrations. In general, serum cholesterol is elevated (hypercholesterolaemic effect) when the dietary fat is high in saturated fatty acids, and lowered when the dietary lipid is mainly unsaturated. Lauric (C12) and myristic (C14) acids, found mainly in butterfat and tropical oils, are the two major hypercholesterolaemic fatty acids. Stearic acid (18:0), one of the main saturated fatty acids in beef fat, is not hypercholesterolaemic. Saturated fatty acids increase LDL-cholesterol by inhibiting the LDL receptors in the liver for removing LDL-cholesterol from the blood. On the other hand, the association of unsaturated fatty acids with HDL may facilitate removal of cholesterol from the serum lipoproteins by the liver and its excretion in the bile.

Fatty Acid Metabolism

Pathways of fatty acid metabolism involve fatty acid biosynthesis, oxidation (β-oxidation, ketogenesis) and metabolism of essential fatty acids. These processes, especially fatty acid biosynthesis and degradation, are intertwined with pathways of carbohydrate metabolism because of the central roles of acetyl CoA in both fat and carbohydrate metabolism.

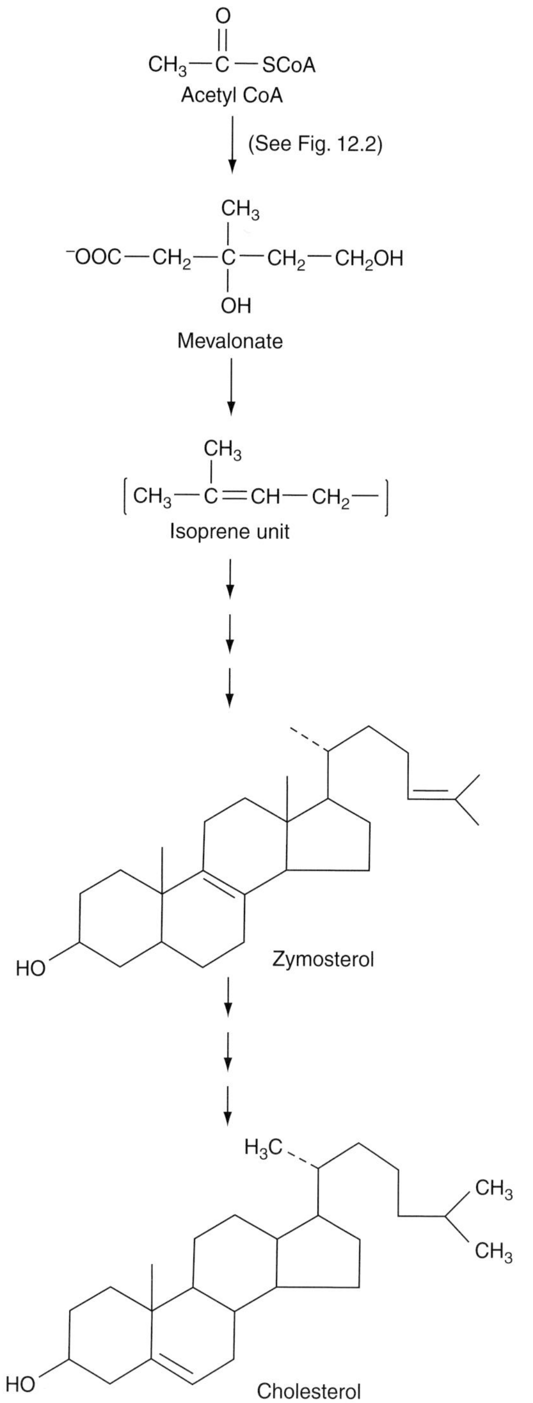

Fig. 12.1. Biosynthesis of cholesterol from acetyl CoA.

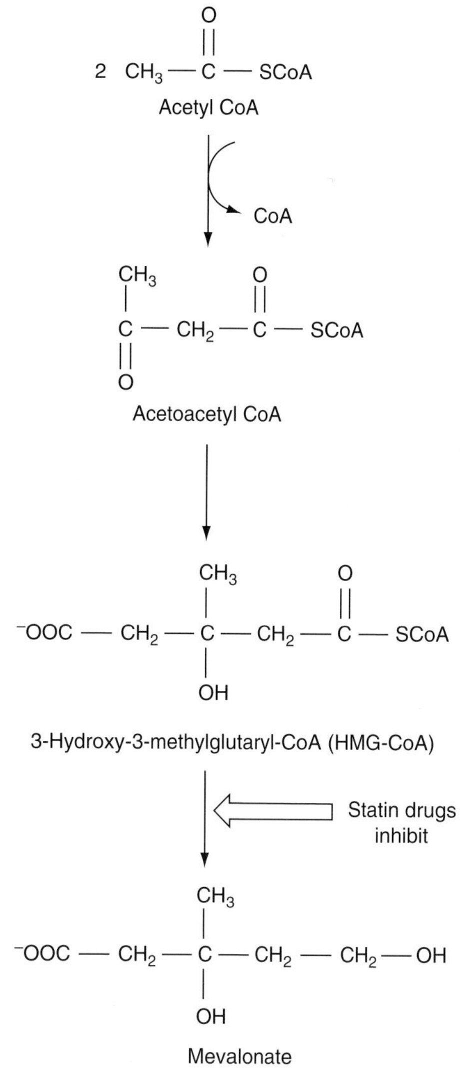

Fig. 12.2. Biosynthesis of mevalonate. HMG-CoA reductase is inhibited by statin drugs (e.g. Pravachol®, Lipitor®).

Fatty acid oxidation

Fatty acids are oxidized in the mitochondria by being converted to acetyl CoA, which is then catabolized in the citric acid (or TCA) cycle reactions. Fatty acids react with coenzyme A (CoA) intracellularly to produce **activated fatty acids (acyl CoA)** (Fig. 12.3). This step requires ATP. The activated fatty acids are transported across the mitochondrial

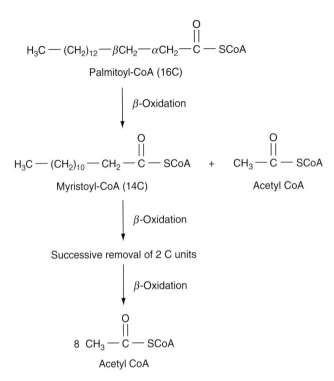

Fig. 12.3. Overview of β-oxidation of fatty acids.

membrane in association with **carnitine**, a trimethylated derivative of butyrate (Fig. 12.4). In β-oxidation, two carbons at a time are cleaved from the fatty acid-CoA, starting at the carboxyl end. The bond between the α- and β-carbons is broken (in this nomenclature system, the α-carbon is the first carbon from the carboxyl end); hence the β-carbon is oxidized to produce a new terminal carboxyl group, leaving a fatty acid shorter by two carbons (Fig. 12.3).

During β-oxidation, hydrogens are removed from the fatty acid and taken up by hydrogen acceptors such as FAD and NAD⁺. The oxidation of FADH$_2$ and NADH + H⁺ in the respiratory chain produces a high yield of ATP. Thus oxidation of fats gives high yields of cellular energy (9 kcal/g of dietary fat versus 4 kcal/g for carbohydrate).

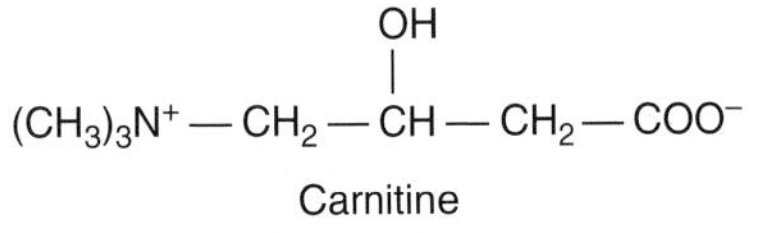

$$OH$$
$$(CH_3)_3N^+ - CH_2 - CH - CH_2 - COO^-$$

Carnitine

Fig. 12.4. Structure of carnitine.

Fatty acids have a higher energy content than carbohydrates because they are less oxidized, as shown by Table 12.2.

β-Oxidation functions in the metabolism of the usual dietary fatty acids, with 16 and 18 carbons. Very long chain fatty acids (C20, C22) are metabolized in subcellular organelles called **peroxisomes**. Peroxisomes are rich in oxidative enzymes, which produce hydrogen peroxide and other peroxides as by-products of the oxidation of LCFAs. The peroxisomes also contain enzymes such as catalase and peroxidases, which convert hydrogen peroxide to water and oxygen. Peroxisomal enzymes also shorten the side chain of cholesterol in bile acid formation.

β-oxidation of unsaturated fatty acids occurs until the first double bond is reached. The double bonds are isomerized from *cis* to *trans*, and then hydrated, by isomerases, ultimately yielding acetyl CoA.

With a high rate of fatty acid mobilization, the rate of acetyl CoA production may exceed the rate at which it enters the citric acid cycle, resulting in hepatic synthesis of **ketone bodies** (ketogenesis).

Table 12.2. Proportion of carbon, hydrogen and oxygen in glucose and palmitic acid.

	Carbon	Hydrogen	Oxygen	Hydrogen:carbon	Oxygen:carbon
Glucose	6	12	6	2	1
Palmitic acid	16	32	2	2	0.125

The ketone bodies are acetoacetic acid, β-hydroxybutyric acid and acetone (Fig. 12.5). (Technically, the term 'ketone bodies' is incorrect in this usage; hydroxybutyrate is not a ketone.) **Ketosis** is a metabolic disorder in which excessive quantities of ketone bodies are produced. Ketosis can occur in starvation or a negative energy balance, and is a common condition in ruminants (twin lamb disease or pregnancy paralysis in sheep, ketosis in lactating dairy cattle). These syndromes result from an insufficiency of carbohydrate metabolism and a high rate of catabolism of fatty acids (or absorbed acetate in ruminants). Ketosis is described in Chapter 16.

Fatty acid synthesis

Fatty acid synthesis, like β-oxidation, involves metabolism of two carbons at a time, in the form of acetyl CoA. However, fatty acid synthesis is not simply the reversal of β-oxidation, but involves different enzymes located at a different intracellular site. This separation allows each process to be individually regulated and integrated according to metabolic needs. β-Oxidation occurs in the mitochondria, whereas fatty acid biosynthesis occurs in the cytosol. Two carbons at a time, derived from acetyl CoA, are combined, yielding palmitic acid (16:0) as the end product. Other LCFAs are synthesized from palmitate by elongation and desaturation reactions.

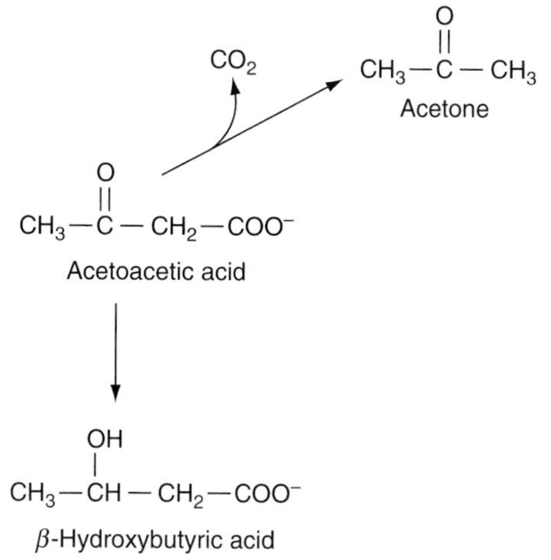

Fatty acid synthesis begins with the addition of carbon dioxide (as bicarbonate) to acetyl CoA to form malonyl CoA. The enzyme acetyl CoA carboxylase requires the B vitamin **biotin** (biotin typically is required for carboxylation reactions). Malonyl CoA reacts with acetyl CoA, elongating the molecule with two carbons to produce a five-carbon compound. This compound is decarboxylated, producing a four-carbon butyryl group that reacts with another malonyl CoA in the next reaction sequence. This reaction is repeated until a palmitoyl group is produced, which is hydrolysed, releasing palmitate. Thus in each step in fatty acid synthesis, a three-carbon group (malonyl CoA) is added to a short-chain fatty acid (SCFA), with the loss of a carbon dioxide, so the net effect is the sequential addition of two carbons at a time. A fatty-acid synthase enzyme complex, containing **pantothenic acid**, carries out these reactions. NADPH is required as a source of hydrogens. The reactions of the pentose phosphate cycle are the major source of the NADPH needed. The main source of the acetyl CoA is carbohydrate, as an end product of glycolysis. Acetyl CoA is produced in the mitochondria. It reacts with oxaloacetic acid (OAA) to produce citrate. Citrate is transported across the mitochondrial membrane; it is then cleaved by citrate lyase to yield acetyl CoA and OAA. The acetyl CoA is then available in the cytosol for fatty acid synthesis. Palmitic acid can be elongated to become a longer chain fatty acid by an enzyme system called **fatty acid elongase**. Unsaturated fatty acids are synthesized from saturated fatty acids by the introduction of double bonds by **desaturases**. The first double bond is nearly always introduced on the Δ9 carbon (Δ9 means carbon 9 starting from the carboxy end). Additional double bonds can be formed in the **oleic family (18:1Δ9)** of fatty acids by a

Fig. 12.5. The 'ketone bodies'. Note that β-hydroxybutyrate is not actually a ketone.

combination of chain elongation and desaturation. Most mammals have Δ4, Δ5, Δ6 and Δ9 desaturases, but cannot insert double bonds beyond the Δ9 position. Linoleic (18:2Δ9,12) and linolenic (18:3Δ9,12,15) acids must be supplied in the diet to produce the linoleic and linolenic series of fatty acids. Thus these two are referred to as **essential fatty acids**. Arachidonic acid (20:4Δ5,8,11,14) can be synthesized from linolenic acid. Cats are unable to convert linoleic acid to arachidonic acid, due to a lack of Δ6 desaturase, and therefore must have a dietary source of arachidonic acid. This is true for wild felines such as the lion and cheetah, as well as for domestic cats (Bauer, 1997). Felines are obligate carnivores. Because of their evolutionary history as carnivores, they have lost the enzymatic capacity to synthesize linoleic acid, linolenic acid, arachidonic acid, eicosapentaenoic acid (EPA) and docosahexaenoic acid (DHA). They rely on their prey as sources of these fatty acids (Bauer, 1997).

Fatty acid synthesis: ruminants versus non-ruminants

Ruminants and non-ruminants differ in some aspects of fatty acid and TAG synthesis. In non-ruminants, LCFAs are synthesized from acetyl CoA. Acetyl CoA is produced in the mitochondria, while fatty acid synthesis occurs in the cytosol. The mitochondrial membrane is impermeable to acetyl CoA. To obtain acetyl CoA extramitochondrially, citrate from the citric acid cycle is transported across the mitochondrial membrane and cleaved by the **citrate cleavage enzyme** (ATP-citrate lyase) into acetyl CoA and OAA:

Citrate + ATP + CoA ® Acetyl CoA + OAA
+ ADP + Pi

The OAA is converted to malate (a citric-acid-cycle constituent) by the **malic enzyme** (malate dehydrogenase) and then to pyruvate. The NADPH generated provides reducing equivalents for fatty acid synthesis (Fig. 12.6).

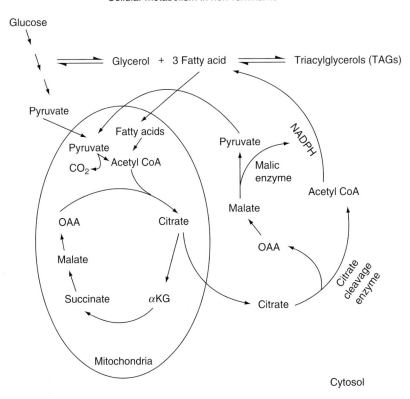

Cellular metabolism in non-ruminants

Fig. 12.6. Integration of fat and carbohydrate metabolism in non-ruminants.

Chapter 12

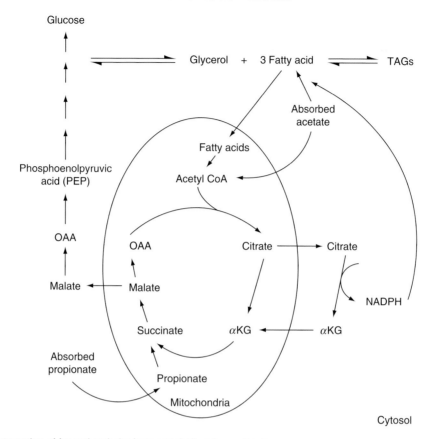

Fig. 12.7. Integration of fat and carbohydrate metabolism in ruminants.

Ruminants lack significant amounts of the citrate cleavage enzyme and the malic enzyme. They derive acetyl CoA directly from absorbed acetate rather than from absorbed glucose. Citrate is transported across the mitochondrial membrane and is converted to α-ketoglutaric acid (αKG), with the production of cytosolic NADPH. The αKG re-enters the mitochondria, while the NADPH is used in fatty acid synthesis from acetate (Fig. 12.7). The result of these reactions in ruminants is to prevent the conversion of glucose or glucogenic precursors to acetyl CoA for fatty acid synthesis. It is a means for ruminants to conserve glucose and glucogenic precursors.

Synthesis and Functions of Eicosanoids

Eicosanoids are substances derived from the eicosa- (20-carbon) polyunsaturated fatty acids.

Eicosanoids include the **prostanoids** (prostaglandins (PG), prostacyclins (PG1), thromboxanes (TX), leukotrienes (LT) and lipoxins (LX)). Prostaglandins act as hormones in mammalian tissues. They are formed by the cyclization of the centre of the carbon chain (Fig. 12.8). The thromboxanes are similar but have an oxygen in the cyclopentane ring (Fig. 12.8). The leukotrienes and lipoxins have three or four conjugated double bonds, respectively (Fig. 12.8). The prostanoids (PG, PG1, TX) are synthesized by the **cyclooxygenase enzyme system** (COX1 and COX2). Leukotrienes are synthesized in leucocytes, platelets and macrophages by the lipoxygenase pathway. Lipoxygenases insert oxygen into arachidonic acid.

Prostaglandins function as inflammatory agents, which may be a desirable response of the immune system when there is a disease challenge.

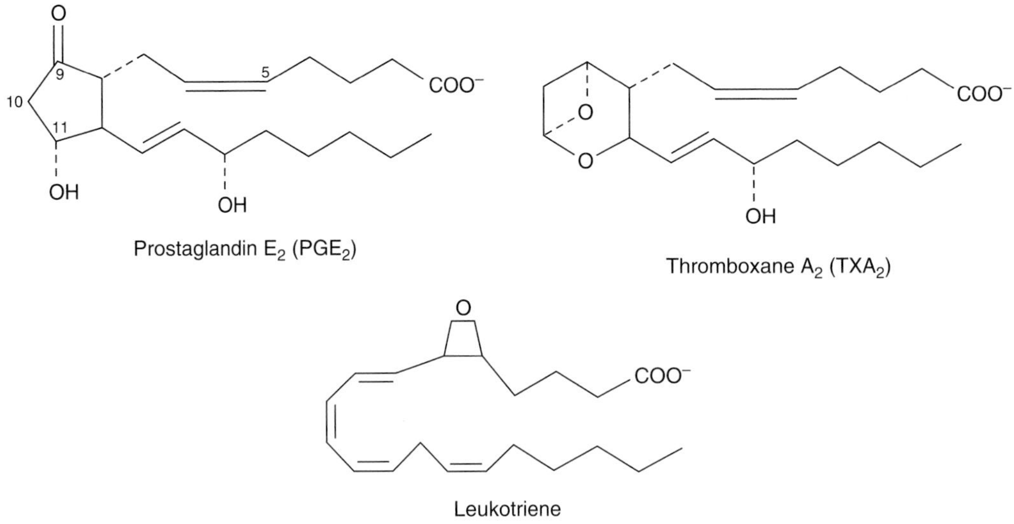

Prostaglandin E₂ (PGE₂)

Thromboxane A₂ (TXA₂)

Leukotriene

Fig. 12.8. Eicosanoids are derived from the eicosa- (20-carbon) polyunsaturated fatty acids.

Anti-inflammatory agents such as aspirin act by inhibiting prostaglandin synthesis. **Thromboxanes** are synthesized in platelets and cause vasoconstriction and platelet aggregation. **Prostacyclins** are produced by blood vessel walls and are inhibitors of platelet aggregation. Thus thromboxanes and prostacyclins are antagonistic. **Leukotrienes** and **lipoxins** have roles in vascular and immunoregulatory functions. Leukotrienes cause bronchoconstriction and may have a role in asthma. They are also potent pro-inflammatory agents. Besides their roles in eicosanoids, essential fatty acids function as constituents of cell membranes and in phospholipid synthesis.

Essential Fatty Acids

The dietary essential fatty acids for most species are linoleic (18:2ω6) and α-linolenic (18:3ω3) acids. Longer chain and/or more unsaturated fatty acids are synthesized from these two by action of chain elongation enzymes and desaturases. The first double bond introduced into a saturated fatty acid (e.g. stearic acid) is the Δ9 double bond. Additional double bonds are always separated by a methylene group (methylene interrupted) in animals, but not necessarily so in bacteria (thus the formation of conjugated linoleic acid (CLA) derivatives in the rumen). Essential fatty acids are required for the synthe-

sis of eicosanoids (prostaglandins, thromboxanes, leukotrienes and lipoxins). They also are constituents of cell membranes, including the mitochondrial membrane. Signs of essential fatty acid deficiency include poor growth, dermatitis, increased water loss through the skin (caused by deranged membrane structure) and increased water consumption (**polydipsia**) and infertility. In chickens, linoleic acid deficiency results in depressed egg production, small egg size, reduction in fertility and early embryonic mortality.

Trans-fatty acids

Unsaturated fatty acids may have either the *cis* or *trans* configuration. Nearly all naturally occurring unsaturated LCFAs produced by animals and plants are of the *cis* configuration, with a 120° bend at the double bonds(s). Naturally occurring *trans*-fatty acids arise from bacterial synthesis. The two geometric isomers of 18:lω9 are oleic acid (*cis*) and elaidic acid (*trans*). Oleic acid has an L shape, whereas elaidic acid is a straight chain (see Fig. 10.4 in Chapter 10). These differences in shape, caused by the *cis–trans* isomerism, have important implications in the formation of membranes, lipoproteins and prostanoids. The bacterial and artificial hydrogenation of unsaturated vegetable oils, such as in the conversion of maize oil into margarine, results in the formation of *trans*-isomers (*trans*-fatty acids). These partially hydrogenated vegetable oils, found in margarines and baked goods, have the same hypercholesterolaemic properties as saturated fatty acids (Zock and Katan, 1992). Thus they are implicated in various disorders such as atherosclerosis and increased risk of coronary heart disease (Nestel *et al.*, 1992). Beginning in 2006, the contents of *trans*-fatty acids must be listed on food labels in the USA. As compared with the consumption of an equal number of calories from saturated or *cis*-unsaturated fatty acids, the consumption of *trans*-fatty acids raises levels of LDL cholesterol, reduces HDL cholesterol, promotes inflammation that can cause endothelial dysfunction, and increases plasma TAGs (Mozaffarian *et al.*, 2006). *Trans*-fats promote the inflammatory response with increased activity of the tumour necrosis factor system, interleukins, C-reactive protein and endothelial cell dysfunction (Harvey *et al.*, 2008). They also bind to and modulate nuclear receptors that regulate gene transcription (Mozaffarian *et al.*, 2006), such as nuclear factor kappaB (NFκB).

Another source of *trans*-fatty acids in the human diet in addition to industrially hydrogenated vegetable oils is the carcass and milk fat of ruminants. Linoleic acid is partially biohydrogenated in the rumen to produce a number of unsaturated fatty acids collectively referred to as **conjugated linoleic acid (CLA)**. These are a group of geometric and positional isomers of linoleic acid (18:2ω6). They have double bonds separated by a single carbon-carbon bond instead of the usual methylene-interrupted double-bond system. The CLA isomers include *cis–cis*, *cis–trans* and *trans–trans* geometry with double bonds at 9 and 11, 10 and 12, or 11 and 13 positions (Bessa *et al.*, 2000). The main one is *cis*-9, *trans*-11 octadecadienoic acid, with the common name **rumenic acid**. The end product of linoleic acid biohydrogenation is stearic acid. An intermediate in this process is *trans*-11 18:1, also called *trans*-vaccenic acid (see Fig. 11.5 in Chapter 11). (Note that it is not a CLA; there is only one double bond so no conjugated double bonds.) *Trans*-vaccenic acid is the major *trans*-fatty acid in ruminant tissues. Milk contains over 20 isomers of CLA but the predominant one is cis-9, *trans*-11 (Lock and Bauman, 2004).

There is a great deal of interest in CLA in ruminant products such as meat and milk, following the discovery of anticarcinogenic properties of fried beef extracts (Bessa *et al.*, 2000). A variety of beneficial effects of CLA have been reported, including anticancer activity, enhancement of immune function and reduction in atherosclerosis (Lock and Bauman, 2004). The main dietary sources of CLA are ruminant meat and dairy products. *Trans*-vaccenic acid is probably detrimental, so enhancement of rumen production of CLA should be done without increasing vaccenic acid. Thus rumen biohydrogenation should be manipulated to increase CLA with a low *trans*-18:1. High forage diets supplemented with a linoleic-rich fat source may be a way of accomplishing this goal of a low *trans*-18:1 to CLA ratio (Bessa *et al.*, 2000).

Trans-fatty acids in the human diet can be categorized as industrial (e.g. margarine production) or ruminant-derived. The adverse effects on human health are associated to a greater extent with industrial rather than ruminant-derived *trans*-fatty acids (Chardigny *et al.*, 2008; Motard-Belanger *et al.*, 2008). *Trans*-fats have been extensively used in the food industry because of their extended half-life and flavour stability, and have displaced natural solid fats and liquid oils in many areas of food processing. According to Willett and Mozaffarian (2008), 'Current TFA [*trans*-fatty acid] consumption accounts for many thousands of premature deaths each year, and continued efforts to eliminate the consumption of partially-hydrogenated vegetable oils are strongly warranted.'

Intermediates and products from the biohydrogenation of linoleic acid in the rumen may be incorporated into microbial biomass (Or-Rashid *et al.*, 2007). The main fatty acids in both rumen bacteria and protozoa are palmitic (16:0) and stearic (18:0) acids. Or-Rashid *et al.* (2007) found that protozoa had much more palmitic acid than bacteria, while bacteria had greater amounts of stearic acid than protozoa. The total odd-chain plus branched-chain fatty acids were 16.5% of bacterial fatty acids and 11.0% of protozoal fatty acids. The protozoa had higher concentrations of vaccenic acid (18:*trans*-11) and *cis*-9, *trans*-11 CLA than the bacterial fraction. Or-Rashid *et al.* (2007) suggested that the rumen protozoa might increase the supply of CLA and other unsaturated fatty acids for intestinal absorption by ruminants.

Branched-chain fatty acids in rumen microbes are formed by elongation of propionate or valerate. Odd- or branched-chain fatty acids with an *iso-* or *anteiso-*structure are advantageous to rumen microbes because they provide optimal fluidity of microbial cell membranes (Or-Rashid *et al.*, 2007). Protozoa contain more than twice the *anteiso-*17:0 fraction than bacteria, making the *anteiso-*17:0 a possible biomarker of protozoal biomass (Or-Rashid *et al.*, 2007). *Iso-*fatty acids have a methyl group at the penultimate (*iso*) position (penultimate = last but one), while *anteiso-*fatty acids have a methyl at the antepenultimate (*anteiso)* position (antepenultimate = last but two).

Milk Fat Depression (Low Milk Fat)

Although low-fat milk is preferred by consumers, low milk fat is a problem in the dairy industry. Generally, milk prices paid to producers are based in part on milk fat content. Of course, for milk used in cheese manufacturing, milk fat is very important.

Van Soest (1994) and Bauman and Griinari (2001, 2003) reviewed various historical explanations that account for low milk fat. Milk fat depression is associated with concentrate diets deficient in coarse roughage. This dietary state results in the alteration of rumen fermentation towards high propionate:low acetate. Originally it was proposed that low levels of absorbed acetate limits milk fat synthesis, but most mammary gland lipogenesis involves preformed fatty acids. Suppression of fatty acid mobilization from adipose tissue, associated with increased insulin secretion stimulated by elevated propionate, has been suggested as a causative factor.

Bauman and Griinari (2001) divided theories of milk fat depression into two broad categories: (i) those that suggest substrate supply for milk fat synthesis is limiting; and (ii) those suggesting that direct inhibition of milk fat synthesis in the mammary gland is involved. Substrate limitation theories include acetate insufficiency, β-hydroxybutyrate insufficiency, and the glucogenic-insulin theory. This theory proposes that high propionate absorption leads to high rates of glucogenesis in the liver, and subsequently increased circulating insulin. Increased serum insulin was proposed to divert substrates to non-mammary gland sites of lipogenesis such as adipose and muscle tissue.

The 'biohydrogenation theory', discussed below, suggests that intermediates of ruminal biohydrogenation of linoleic acid are involved in milk fat depression.

The 'biohydrogenation theory' (Lock and Bauman, 2004, 2007) provides a unifying concept to explain diet-induced milk fat depression. The basis of this explanation is that intermediates of fatty acid biohydrogenation escape the rumen, are absorbed, and cause a decreased expression of lipogenic enzymes and a reduction in milk fat synthesis in the mammary gland (Bauman *et al.*, 2008). Increased absorption of *trans-*10, *cis*-12 CLA reduces milk fat (deVeth *et al.*, 2004), with as little as 2.0 g/day being sufficient to cause a 20% reduction in milk fat production. Two other intermediates of ruminal biohydrogenation that regulate milk fat synthesis are *trans-*9, *cis*-11 CLA (Perfield II *et al.*, 2007) and *cis*-10, *trans*-12 CLA (Saebo *et al.*, 2005). Several dietary factors influence the '*trans-*10 shift' in biohydrogenation (Fig. 12.9). The three main ways in which dietary components impact milk fat depression are: (i) increased dietary supply of C18 unsaturated fatty acids; (ii) alterations in rumen environment such as low rumen pH; and (iii) changes in the rate of biohydrogenation by feed additives (e.g. Rumensin®) or dietary fat. Linoleic and linolenic acids are the major dietary fatty acids in diets based on maize, maize silage and oil seeds. Intakes of linoleic acid can be as high as 400–500 g/day (Lock and Bauman, 2007), providing ample substrate for the '*trans-*10 shift' in biohydrogenation. Relatively small depressions in rumen pH can lead to changes in ruminal biohydrogenation. High concentrate diets and insufficient physically effective neutral detergent fibre (peNDF) can result in lower rumen pH. Reduced size of silage particles is associated with reduced rumination, lower secretion of salivary buffers and a lower rumen pH. Cows with high dry matter intakes (i.e. high producing cows) are at higher risk of milk fat depression due to a greater 'flushing' of biohydrogenation intermediates out of the rumen (Lock and Bauman, 2007). Rumensin® alters rumen microbes by inhibiting Gram-positive bacteria. It is these bacteria that carry out the conversion of *trans-*10, 18:1 to stearic acid (18:0). Thus their suppression leads to a build-up of biohydrogenation intermediates (Fig. 12.9).

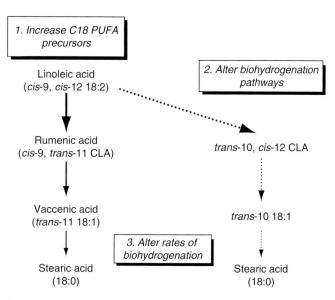

Fig. 12.9. Generalized scheme of ruminal biohydrogenation of linoleic acid under normal conditions (left) and during diet-induced milk fat depression (right) (adapted from Lock and Bauman, 2007).

Questions and Study Guide

1. What is meant by the common terminology of 'good cholesterol' and 'bad cholesterol'?
2. What characteristic causes a blood lipoprotein to have either a high density or low density?
3. Do chylomicrons have high density or low density? Why?
4. Why is the liver important in fat metabolism?
5. Many people take statin drugs (e.g. Lipitor®) to reduce their blood cholesterol concentration. How do statins work?
6. What is enterohepatic circulation?
7. Why do most plant and animal fats and oils have an even number of carbon atoms (e.g. C16, C18, C20)?
8. Carbohydrates such as glucose can be converted by the body into fat, but fat cannot be converted to glucose (no net synthesis). Explain.
9. What are eicosanoids?
10. Why are so-called 'trans-fats' considered undesirable in the human diet? What are the major dietary sources (for humans) of trans-fatty acids? What are trans-fatty acids?
11. Why does beef fat contain odd-chain and branched-chain fatty acids, while poultry fat usually does not?
12. Many people today buy low-fat or skimmed milk. Why, then, is milk fat depression (low milk fat) generally considered undesirable by the dairy industry?
13. Explain the 'biohydrogenation theory' of milk fat depression.
14. Cats require a dietary source of arachidonic acid, whereas most other animals do not. Explain.
15. What is the function of the citrate cleavage enzyme in ruminants and non-ruminants?
16. What are rumenic and vaccenic acids? How do they differ from linoleic and stearic acids?

References

Bauer, J.E. (1997) Fatty acid metabolism in domestic cats (*Felix catus*) and cheetahs (*Acinonyx jubatas*). *Proceedings of the Nutrition Society* 56, 1013–1024.

Bauman, D.E. and Griinari, J.M. (2001) Regulation and nutritional manipulation of milk fat: low-fat milk syndrome. *Livestock Production Science* 70, 15–29.

Bauman, D.E. and Griinari, J.M. (2003) Nutritional regulation of milk fat synthesis. *Annual Review of Nutrition* 23, 203–227.

Bauman, D.E., Perfield, J.W., II, Harvatine, K.J. and Baumgard, L.H. (2008) Regulation of fat synthesis by conjugated linoleic acid: lactation and the ruminant model. *Journal of Nutrition* 138, 403–409.

Bessa, R.J.B., Santos-Silva, J., Ribeiro, J.M.R. and Portugal, A.V. (2000) Reticulo-rumen biohydrogenation and the enrichment of ruminant edible products with linoleic acid conjugated isomers. *Livestock Production Science* 63, 201–211.

Chardigny, J.-M., Destaillats, F., Malpuech-Brugere, C., Moulin, J., Bauman, D.E., Lock, A.L., Barbano, D.M., Mensink, R.P., Bezelgues, J.-B., Chaumont, P., Combe, N., Cristiani, I., Joffre, F., German, J.B., Dionisi, F., Boirie, Y. and Sebedio, J.-L. (2008) Do *trans* fatty acids from industrially produced sources and from natural sources have the same effect on cardiovascular disease risk factors in healthy subjects? Results of the *Trans* Fatty Acids Collaboration (TRANSFACT) study. *American Journal of Clinical Nutrition* 87, 558–566.

de Veth, M.J., Griinari, J.M., Pfeiffer, A.M. and Bauman, D.E. (2004) Effect of CLA on milk fat synthesis in dairy cows: comparison of inhibition by methyl esters and free fatty acids, and relationships among studies. *Lipids* 39, 365–372.

Harvey, K.A., Arnold, T., Rasool, T., Antalis, C., Miller, S.J. and Siddiqui, R.A. (2008) *Trans*-fatty acids induce pro-inflammatory responses and endothelial cell dysfunction. *British Journal of Nutrition* 99, 723–731.

Lock, A.L. and Bauman, D.E. (2004) Modifying milk fat composition of dairy cows to enhance fatty acids beneficial to human health. *Lipids* 39, 1197–1206.

Lock, A.L. and Bauman, D.E. (2007) Milk fat depression: what do we know and what can we do about it? In: *Proceedings of the Pacific North West Animal Nutrition Conference*, Portland, Oregon, 16–18 October, pp. 21–32.

Motard-Belanger, A., Charest, A., Grenier, G., Paquin, P., Chouinard, Y., Lemieux, S., Couture, P. and Lamarche, B. (2008) Study of the effect of *trans* fatty acids from ruminants on blood lipids and other risk factors for cardiovascular disease. *Amercian Journal of Clinical Nutrition* 87, 593–599.

Mozaffarian, D., Katan, M.B., Ascherio, A., Stampfer, M.J. and Willett, W.C. (2006) *Trans* fatty acids and cardiovascular disease. *New England Journal of Medicine* 354, 1601–1613.

Nestel, P., Noakes, M., Belling, B., McArthur, R., Clifton, P., Janus, E. and Abbey, M. (1992) Plasma lipoprotein lipid and Lp[a] changes with substitution of elaidic acid for oleic acid in the diet. *Journal of Lipid Research* 33, 1029–1036.

Or-Rashid, M.M., Odongo, N.E. and McBride, B.W. (2007) Fatty acid composition of ruminal bacteria and protozoa, with emphasis on conjugated linoleic acid, vaccenic acid, and odd-chain and branched-chain fatty acids. *Journal of Animal Science* 85, 1228–1234.

Perfeld II, J.W., Lock, A.L., Saebo, A., Griinari, J.M., Dwyer, D.A. and Bauman, D.E. (2007) *Trans*-9, *cis*-11 conjugated linoleic acid (CLA) reduces milk fat synthesis in lactating dairy cows. *Journal of Dairy Science* 90, 2211–2218.

Saebo, A., Saebo, P.C., Griinari, J.M. and Shingfield, K.J. (2005) Effect of abomasal infusions of geometric isomers of 10,12 conjugated linoleic acid on milk fat synthesis in dairy cows. *Lipids* 40, 823–832.

Van Soest, P.J. (1994) *Nutritional Ecology of the Ruminant*. Cornell University Press, Ithaca, New York.

Willett, W. and Mozaffarian, D. (2008) Ruminant or industrial sources of *trans* fatty acids: public health issue or food label skirmish? *American Journal of Clinical Nutrition* 87, 515–516.

Zock, P.L. and Katan, M.B. (1992) Hydrogenation alternatives: effects of *trans* fatty acids and stearic acid versus linoleic acid on serum lipids and lipoproteins in humans. *Journal of Lipid Research* 33, 399–410.

13 Lipid Peroxidation and Antioxidant Nutrients

Peroxidation (auto-oxidation) of lipids exposed to oxygen is an important factor in the deterioration (**rancidity**) of fat-containing feeds and also for damage to tissues *in vivo*, where it may be important as a cause of cancer, inflammatory diseases, atherosclerosis and ageing. The deleterious effects of lipid peroxidation are caused by free radicals produced during peroxide formation from polyunsaturated fatty acids. A chain reaction occurs, in which the peroxidation processes generate **free radicals** which initiate further peroxidation. Other sources of free radicals and lipid oxidants (**reactive oxygen species; ROS**) are the superoxide free radical anion and hydrogen peroxide. The **superoxide ion** O_2^- is a by-product of normal metabolism. Free radicals have an unpaired electron and are very electrophilic (i.e. they react to gain another electron). Superoxide is detoxified by the enzyme **superoxide dismutase**, producing hydrogen peroxide (Fig. 13.1). **Hydrogen peroxide** is also a potent oxidant, and is detoxified by the reaction with reduced glutathione (GSH) catalysed by glutathione peroxidase (Fig. 13.2) and with catalase.

Lipid peroxidation is prevented by **antioxidants**. A number of antioxidants are used as preservatives to prevent auto-oxidation of lipids in foods and feeds. These include **butylated hyroxyanisole (BHA)**, **butylated hydroxytoluene (BHT)** and **ethoxyquin**. Naturally occurring antioxidants include vitamin E and vitamin C. Selenium has antioxidant activity by way of its role in glutathione peroxidase. Polyphenols from plant sources also have antioxidant activity. The phenolic group(s) of antioxidants is the active site; most antioxidants are phenolics, including vitamin E.

Lipid peroxidation occurs in three phases: (i) initiation; (ii) propagation; and (iii) termination. Initiation begins with a fatty acid reacting with a metal (e.g. iron) or an existing free radical ($X^•$):

$$ROOH + Metal^{n+} \circledR ROO^• + Metal^{n-1} + H^+, \text{ or}$$

$$X^• + RH \circledR R^• + XH$$

The free radicals formed are $ROO^•$ (hydroperoxide), $RO^•$ and $OH^•$, with R being the hydrocarbon portion of a fatty acid. Propagation involves reaction of the free radicals with oxygen to produce more free radicals.

Antioxidants either reduce the rate of initiation or interfere with chain propagation. Those that reduce initiation include catalase and other peroxidases that react with hydroperoxides, and chelators of metal ions (e.g. ethylenediaminetetraacetic acid, EDTA). Principal chain-breaking antioxidants include superoxide dismutase, which traps superoxide free radicals, and vitamin E, which traps peroxide free radicals. The tocopheroxyl free radical product is reduced back to tocopherol by ascorbic acid (vitamin C). The ascorbate free radical is converted to ascorbate and dehydroascorbate, which are not free radicals.

Unsaturated fatty acids are susceptible to peroxidation, because they have double bonds which react with oxygen. The more double bonds (i.e. the more unsaturated), the greater the susceptibility to auto-oxidation. Unsaturated fatty acids include **monounsaturated fatty acids (MUFA)** with one double bond, and **polyunsaturated fatty acids (PUFA)** with more than one double bond. Both MUFA and PUFA have serum cholesterol-lowering properties in humans. However, the PUFA are more susceptible to auto-oxidation and the production of free radicals which damage cell membranes. Thus vegetable oils high in MUFA, such as olive and canola oils, are considered to be more healthy than other vegetable oils because they have maximal positive effects (on cholesterol) and minimal negative effects (auto-oxidation).

The Antioxidant Nutrients

Vitamin E

Vitamin E was discovered in the 1920s as a fat-soluble factor that prevented fetal resorption in

$$O_2^- + O_2^- + 2H^+ \xrightarrow{\text{Superoxide}\atop\text{dismutase}} H_2O_2 + O_2$$

Fig. 13.1. Superoxide dismutase converts (reduces) superoxide to hydrogen peroxide.

rats. This led to its reputation as the 'fertility vitamin', a reputation it still holds in the public mind. However, the only metabolic function of vitamin E is as a cellular antioxidant, responsible for stabilizing cell membranes. All symptoms of vitamin E deficiency are in fact manifestations of peroxidation of cell membranes. Cell membranes contain PUFA, which are stabilized against free radical damage by the presence of vitamin E as an integral part of membranes.

Vitamin E is a generic name for two classes of isoprenoid compounds, the **tocopherols** and **tocotrienols** (Fig. 13.3). They differ in the saturation of the 16-carbon isoprenoid side chain. In the tocopherols, the side chain is fully saturated, while the side chain of tocotrienols has three double bonds. The nomenclature of vitamin E is very complicated.

In addition to the general categorization of vitamin E as tocopherols and tocotrienols, there are isomers involving mirror image (chiral) centres in the chromane ring at C-2 and in the side chain at C-4′ and C-8′ of tocopherols. The **stereoisomers** are given the designations **R** and **S**. All of the natural isomers of the tocopherols and tocotrienols have the R configuration at C-2 of the chromane ring, indicated in Fig. 13.3 by showing the methyl group at the ring position pointing up. The tocopherols have two additional chiral centres in the side chain, that also have the R configuration in the natural isomer, with the methyl groups pointed down (bond indicated by dashes). Thus the natural vitamin E isomer of α-tocopherol is called 2R, 4′R, 8′R-α-tocopherol, or **RRR-α-tocopherol**. Because the tocopherols have three chiral centres, each of which can be R or S, there are eight possible stereoisomers of the tocopherols.

In addition to these stereoisomers, both the tocopherols and the tocotrienols occur as homologues – **alpha (α)**, **beta (β)**, **gamma (γ)** and **delta (δ)** – that differ in the number or location of methyl groups in

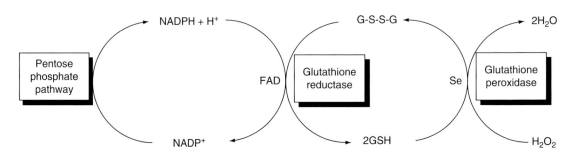

Fig. 13.2. Role of the pentose phosphate pathway in the glutathione peroxidase reaction of erythrocytes. G-S-S-G, oxidized glutathione; GSH, reduced glutathione; Se, selenium cofactor.

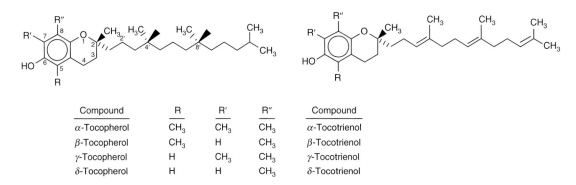

Compound	R	R′	R″	Compound
α-Tocopherol	CH₃	CH₃	CH₃	α-Tocotrienol
β-Tocopherol	CH₃	H	CH₃	β-Tocotrienol
γ-Tocopherol	H	CH₃	CH₃	γ-Tocotrienol
δ-Tocopherol	H	H	CH₃	δ-Tocotrienol

Fig. 13.3. The structures of various forms of vitamin E.

the chromane ring. For example, α-tocopherol has four methyl groups at positions 2, 5, 7 and 8, β has methyls at 2, 5 and 8, γ has methyls at 2, 7 and 8, and δ has methyls at 2 and 8. The chemistry of vitamin E is discussed in detail by Kamal-Eldin and Appelqvist (1996), Pryor (2001) and Traber (2006).

The **natural form** of vitamin E is RRR-α-tocopherol (older name d-α-tocopherol). **Synthetic vitamin E** consists of a mixture of all eight stereoisomers (RRR, RSR, RRS, RSS, SRR, SSR, SRS, SSS) and is called all-racemic-α-tocopherol or **all-rac-α-tocopherol** (older name dl-α-tocopherol). All the eight stereoisomers have equal antioxidant but different biological activities. The biopotency of the various tocopherols is shown in Table 13.1.

The name 'tocopherol' is derived from the Greek *tocos* (childbirth), *pherein* (to bear) and the alcohol designation *ol*, from its discovery as a factor preventing fetal resorption in rats. Various isomers of tocopherols and tocotrienols exist. The most active as a source of vitamin E activity is RRR-α-tocopherol. Biological activities are given as **International Units (IU)** or the newer α-**tocopherol equivalent (α-TE)**. The relationship between these units is that 1 mg RRR-α-tocopherol has an activity of 1 α-TE and is equal to 1.49 IU. One IU of vitamin E is equivalent to 1 mg of all-rac-α-tocopherol acetate; all-rac-α-tocopherol has a potency of 1.1 IU/mg. Activities of RRR-α-tocopherol acetate and RRR-α-tocopherol are 1.36 and 1.49 IU/mg, respectively. Because plants contain an array of tocopherols and tocotrienols, a statement of exact activities is imprecise, but natural-source vitamin E has approximately twice the biological activity of the all-rac synthetic form. In the feed industry, vitamin E is available commercially as all-rac-α-tocopherol acetate and RRR-α-tocopherol acetate. The acetate group is esterified on to the hydroxyl group of tocopherol, stabilizing it and rendering it resistant to oxidation. These acetate forms have antioxidant activity only after they are hydrolysed in the digestive tract, so they do not protect feeds against development of rancidity. The free hydroxyl (phenolic) group is necessary for tocopherol to function as an antioxidant.

Vitamin E associates with lipid micelles in the intestine, and is absorbed coincidently with fat absorption (Chapter 11). It is transported in the blood in association with lipoproteins and within cells is associated with tocopherol-binding proteins. In functioning as an antioxidant, the phenolic hydroxyl group on the chromanol ring of tocopherol reacts with free radicals, causing termination of the auto-oxidation chain reaction, particularly within the membranes where vitamin E resides. This action is called **free-radical scavenging**, and involves donation of the phenolic hydrogen to a fatty acid free radical. This action is also called free-radical quenching. In this process, an inactive tocopheroxyl free radical is formed, which is converted to tocopherylquinone. The quinone form is reduced back to the tocopherol form by ascorbic acid; thus vitamin E molecules are recycled and can repeatedly function as antioxidants.

Vitamin E deficiency syndromes include nutritional muscular dystrophy in most species, liver necrosis in rats and pigs, fetal resorption in rats and encephalomalacia (brain degeneration) in

Table 13.1. Biopotencies of various forms of the tocopherols.

Tocopherol	Biopotencies	
	IU/mg[a]	α-Tocopherol equivalent/mg
RRR-α-tocopherol (natural)	1.49	1.00
RRR-α-tocopherol acetate (natural)	1.36	0.91
RRR-α-tocopherol succinate (natural)	1.21	0.81
All-rac-α-tocopherol (synthetic)[b]	1.10	0.74
All-rac-α-tocopherol acetate (synthetic)	1.00	0.67
All-rac-α-tocopherol succinate (synthetic)	0.89	0.59
RRR-β-tocopherol	0.30	0.20
RRR-γ-tocopherol	0.15	0.10
RRR-δ-tocopherol	0.01	0.01

[a]IU, International Units.
[b]All-rac, All-racemic, with all eight stereoisomers present.

poultry. A classic sign of vitamin E deficiency is *in vitro* red blood cell (rbc) haemolysis (Fig. 13.4). Most vitamin E deficiency syndromes are also preventable with dietary synthetic antioxidants.

The feeding of high dietary concentrations of vitamin E to beef animals improves meat visual quality (Liu *et al.*, 1995). Animals fed high vitamin E for several weeks before slaughter store increased quantities of the vitamin in the muscle tissue. Because of its antioxidant activity, vitamin E in the muscle reduces lipid oxidation, delaying the discoloration of fresh and frozen meat, and thus extending **shelf life** (Faustman *et al.*, 1998).

Vitamin E in zoo animal nutrition

The significance of **vitamin E** in zoo animal nutrition has been reviewed by Dierenfeld (1989, 1994) and Dierenfeld and Traber (1992). Some of the characteristic signs of deficiency include cardiac and skeletal myopathy (white muscle disease) in herbivores, with steatitis (yellow fat), anaemia and poor reproduction reported more in birds and reptiles, particularly in carnivores. Plasma vitamin E concentrations in free-ranging animals have been used as a measure of normal status for captives of the same species (Dierenfeld *et al.*, 1988; Ghebremeskel and Williams, 1988; Dierenfeld, 1989; Dierenfeld and Traber, 1992), because of

concern that the vitamin E status of zoo animals may often be inadequate. According to Dierenfeld (1989) and Dierenfeld and Traber (1992), dietary vitamin E requirements of wild species may be up to ten times higher than the National Research Council requirements for domestic counterparts because of longer longevity, stresses and the general low concentrations of this nutrient in zoo diets. To standardize across hoofstock species, Dierenfeld (1989) suggests that plasma cholesterol concentrations can be used to estimate minimal plasma vitamin E concentrations expected, by dividing normal cholesterol (mg/dl) by 100. For example, a giraffe with a cholesterol value of 40 mg/dl would have an expected minimal plasma vitamin E level of 0.40 mg/ml. Domestic ruminants appear to provide a good comparative physiologic model for vitamin E nutrition of zoo ruminants.

On the contrary, **rhinoceros** and **elephants** have unique vitamin E metabolism, and normally display quite low blood concentrations of this nutrient (Dierenfeld *et al.*, 1998; Savage *et al.*, 1999; Clauss *et al.*, 2002b). The domestic horse does not appear to be a suitable comparative model for vitamin E nutrition of the pachyderms, although these species share similar gut anatomy. Plasma vitamin E concentrations of free-ranging Przewalski horses in the Ukraine were substantially higher than normal values for domestic horses (Dierenfeld, 1997).

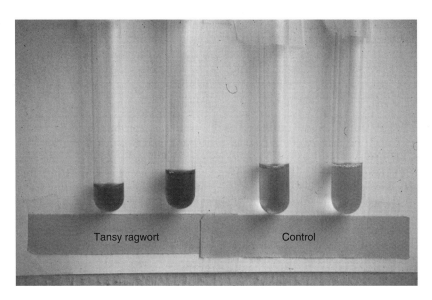

Fig. 13.4. Erythrocytes from pyrrolizidine-alkaloid-poisoned rats are susceptible to *in vitro* haemolysis, suggestive of vitamin E deficiency. Tansy ragwort contains pyrrolizidine alkaloids.

Vitamin-E-deficient elephants develop cardiac lesions similar to those seen in pigs (mulberry heart disease), whereas rhinos develop skeletal and cardiac myopathies, and rbc haemolysis. **Vitamin E** concentrations in browse plants consumed in the wild by rhinos and elephants are much higher than in grasses and pelleted diets typically fed to zoo animals (Dierenfeld, 1994).

Neither perissodactyls (horses) nor the pachyderms have a gall bladder. This might be significant in captive animals, which are usually fed meals followed by a need for large amounts of bile for **emulsification of lipids**. Ghebremeskel *et al.* (1991) suggested that the lower plasma vitamin E concentrations of captive versus wild rhinos may reflect a lack of sufficient **bile** in intermittent-fed animals to emulsify and absorb vitamin E efficiently. In contrast, wild rhinos and elephants browse continuously, requiring less bile at any one time than meal-fed animals.

Inadequate bile production in captive animals may be a limiting factor in the absorption of fat-soluble vitamin E, but similar circulating concentrations are seen in both free-ranging and supplemented zoo rhinos (Clauss *et al.*, 2002b); hence, dietary concentrations appear to underlie the previous deficiency issues reported. Also, the nature of the fatty acids in the diets of wild and captive rhinos differs (Ghebremeskel *et al.*, 1991; Wright and Brown, 1997). Ingestion of seeds and kernels favours **linoleic acid** intake, while ingestion of native browse leaves favours **linolenic acid** (Clauss *et al.*, 2008). Rapid degradation of unsaturated fatty acids occurs in stored feed, while no loss at all would occur with browsed feed in the wild (Grant *et al.*, 2002). These factors could increase the vitamin E requirements of captive rhinos.

The five rhinoceros species still surviving are in great danger of extinction. About 85% of the world's rhino population has been lost since 1970. Some species number fewer than 100 surviving animals and others are under constant armed guard to minimize poaching. **Rhino horn** is in great demand in China as a medicine (Mainka and Mills, 1995) and in Yemen for dagger handles. The International Rhinoceros Foundation has been formed to help preserve the remaining species. In 1992, an attempt was made to move a small herd of black rhinos from Africa, where they were likely to succumb to poachers in Zimbabwe, to establish a captive herd in Australia. Several animals died, probably of vitamin E deficiency, exacerbated by exposure to creosote in corral timbers (Kelly *et al.*, 1995).

Creosote is an oxidant that would increase antioxidant (vitamin E) requirements, and black rhinos have been shown to have poor oxidant enzyme activity. This example illustrates the critical need for knowledge of nutritional requirements and peculiarities of wild species, particularly endangered species, where every animal that dies is a critical loss to the gene pool. Other disease problems also occur with black rhinos that may be linked to nutritional status. Captive black rhinos, but not white rhinos, accumulate excessive **iron** as haemosiderin deposits in the liver (**haemosiderosis**). Smith *et al.* (1995) suggest that in the wild, the black rhino is a browser that has adapted to a diet of low bioavailable iron by increasing the efficiency of iron absorption. In captivity, they are usually fed a diet of grass or lucerne hay, along with concentrate pellets, which may contain a higher content of available iron than the black rhino's normal diet. Furthermore, captive diets are often low in tannins, which may serve to bind dietary iron in the wild. Black (but not white) rhinos have been shown, however, to react to feeding of dietary tannins with increased salivary tannin-binding proteins (Clauss *et al.*, 2002a, 2005), hence having differing physiologic mechanisms for dealing with a single nutrient. The role of excessive tissue iron in the suite of health syndromes affecting captive black rhinos is not known. However, iron is one of the most potent stimulators of auto-oxidation of unsaturated fatty acids, which would increase the vitamin E requirement. It appears from a recent summary (Dierenfeld *et al.*, 2005) that dietary iron concentrations are not the sole factor underlying iron status in this species, but rather interrelationships among feed type, feeding behaviour, bile secretion, stress, vitamin E, and iron may be involved in the high mortality of captive black rhinos.

Clauss (2003) reviewed the roles of tannins in the nutrition of wild animals. Many of the plants consumed by browsing animals contain tannins. Clauss (2003) proposed that because tannins reduce iron availability, the exposure on an evolutionary scale to high tannin diets could have led to selection for efficient iron absorption, leaving these animals vulnerable to the effects of low tannin, high iron diets in zoos.

Selenium

Vitamin E and the trace element selenium share the property of preventing peroxidation of unsaturated fatty acids in cell membranes. Virtually all of the disorders and deficiency signs associated with these two nutrients can be explained by their antioxidant properties (an exception is the role of selenium in the thyroid gland). Although these nutrients can be replaced by other antioxidants, vitamin E and selenium have properties that make them uniquely suited as cellular antioxidants. In most cases, either vitamin E or selenium is effective. The dietary requirement for each is influenced by the dietary concentration of the other. Thus selenium has a **sparing effect** on the vitamin E requirement (a sparing effect occurs when one nutrient or substance reduces the requirement for another nutrient, usually by replacing it in some aspect of its metabolic function).

Selenium helps protect against auto-oxidation of cell membranes by virtue of being a component of an enzyme, **glutathione peroxidase,** that reduces (by providing hydrogen) peroxides, thus converting them to innocuous products (Fig. 13.2). Glutathione peroxidase occurs mainly in the cytosol and reduces peroxides before they can attack cell membranes, whereas vitamin E acts within the membrane itself as a second line of defence. Selenium also functions as a component of a **deiodinase** that converts the thyroid hormone thyroxine (T4) into its metabolically active form (triiodothyronine) by the removal of one of the four iodines in thyroxine (Burk and Hill, 1993). In total, selenium functions as a component of three deiodinases that regulate the synthesis and degradation of triiodothyrone (T3). Also, selenoperoxidases protect the thyroid gland from hydrogen peroxide produced during the synthesis of thyroid hormones (Arthur *et al.*, 1999). Thus selenium has a nutritional interrelationship with iodine. Selenium is also a component of some **selenoproteins** in blood and muscle, for which functions have not yet been identified (Yeh *et al.*, 1997).

There are problems with both deficiency and toxicity of selenium. Selenium-deficient soils are often of volcanic origin; selenium is a volatile element and is volatilized into the atmosphere during volcanic episodes. Areas where it has re-entered the soil often have toxic selenium contents. For example, the US Pacific Coast states are selenium deficient, whereas the Great Plains states (North Dakota, South Dakota, Wyoming and Nebraska) have soils with high selenium concentrations (Fig. 13.5). Certain plants growing in these areas (e.g. *Astragalus* spp.) may accumulate very high toxic concentrations of selenium and cause livestock

poisoning. **Selenium toxicity** causes alkali disease and blind staggers, which are characterized by abnormal hoof and hair growth, abdominal distress, diarrhoea, difficult breathing, prostration and death. **Selenium deficiency** conditions include nutritional muscular dystrophy in all species (white muscle disease, stiff lamb disease), exudative diathesis in chickens (subcutaneous haemorrhages), liver necrosis in pigs and rats, unthriftiness (ill-thrift) in ruminants and reproductive disorders in many species. Some of these deficiency conditions respond to either vitamin E or selenium. For example, the form of nutritional muscular dystrophy in ruminants, **white muscle disease** (the white colour is due to the deposition of calcium salts in the degenerating muscle tissue), is responsive mainly to selenium, although high vitamin E concentrations have some protective activity (Fig. 13.6). Some species, such as rabbits and horses, seem to depend more on vitamin E than on selenium for their antioxidant protection. There is a non-selenium containing form of glutathione peroxidase, which occurs at higher concentrations in some species, making them less dependent on dietary selenium.

Subclinical selenium deficiency may increase the incidence of **retained placenta** in dairy cattle. Selenium supplementation of animals on diets of marginal selenium status enhances immune status and the ability of the immune system to respond to disease challenges (Knight and Tyznik, 1990).

For most livestock species, a dietary concentration of 0.1 ppm selenium is adequate to prevent signs of deficiency with an added margin of safety. The true metabolic requirement is closer to 0.05 ppm. Thus, selenium is required in extremely small quantities.

Vitamin E and selenium have complementary roles as antioxidants. Vitamin E is incorporated into the structure of cell membranes, and thus is a **first line of defence** against oxidant and free radical damage. It is situated so as to immediately neutralize oxidants before they can initiate chain reactions. If any oxidants escape the protective action of vitamin E, selenium (as a component of glutathione peroxidase) is a second line of defence. There is considerable variation among species and tissues in their reliance on either vitamin E or selenium as antioxidants. For example, ruminant muscle tissue is highly dependent on selenium to prevent nutritional muscular dystrophy (white muscle disease) whereas in chickens, vitamin E is more effective.

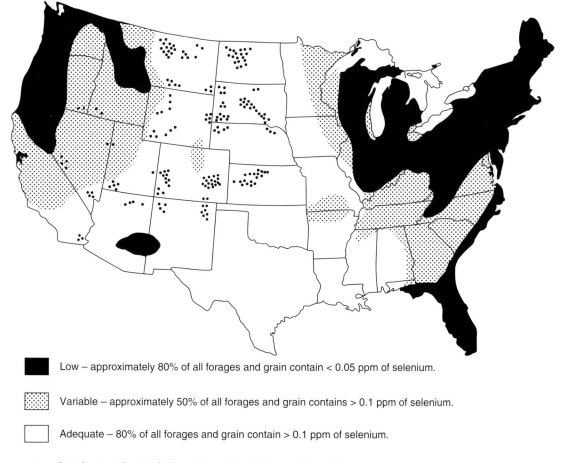

Low – approximately 80% of all forages and grain contain < 0.05 ppm of selenium.

Variable – approximately 50% of all forages and grain contains > 0.1 ppm of selenium.

Adequate – 80% of all forages and grain contain > 0.1 ppm of selenium.

● Local areas where selenium accumulator plants contain > 50 ppm.

Fig. 13.5. Selenium status of feedstuffs throughout the USA. Selenium-deficient areas include the Pacific Northwest, Great Lakes region and Northeast, and Florida. Areas with selenium toxicity occur throughout the Great Plains states (courtesy of J. Kubota, US Plant, Soil and Nutrition Laboratory, Ithaca, New York).

Some species, such as rabbits, have non-selenium dependent glutathione peroxidase and therefore are not susceptible to selenium deficiency.

Various methods of administration of selenium to livestock include its use in salt mixtures, as a direct additive to the feed, by periodic injections or oral doses, and by administration of selenium 'bullets' to ruminants. The 'bullets' may be pellets formed from iron or glass boluses, in each case containing a soluble selenium salt. In the USA, selenium concentrations in the feed permitted by the Food and Drug Administration are 0.1 μg/g in the complete feed for beef and dairy cattle, sheep, chickens, ducks and pigs (but 0.3 μg/g in starter

and prestarter diets) and 0.2 μg/g for turkeys (Levander, 1986). Selenium addition to salt is also permitted with up to 20 and 30 μg selenium/g of salt mix for beef cattle and sheep, respectively, so as not to exceed daily intakes of 0.23 and 1 mg selenium/animal/day.

The usual form of selenium addition to feeds or salt is **sodium selenite**. It has a high bioavailability. The selenium in plants is largely in the form of seleno-amino acids and has a high bioavailability. The selenium in fish meals often has a low availability, possibly because of complexing with heavy metals (e.g. mercury). The bioavailability of selenium to ruminants is greater with high concentrate diets than

(a)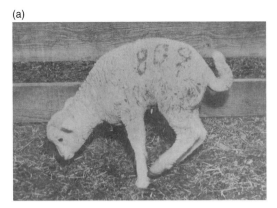

(b)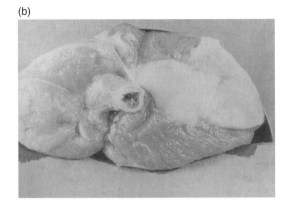

Fig. 13.6. White muscle disease in a lamb caused by selenium deficiency (a). Degeneration of skeletal muscles occurs, causing lameness. Degeneration of the heart muscle also occurs, causing heart attack and death. The muscle tissue (b) from a selenium-deficient lamb shows extensive areas of calcification, accounting for the name white muscle disease (courtesy of J.E. Oldfield, Oregon State University, Corvallis, Oregon, USA).

with high roughage diets (Koenig *et al.*, 1997). Rumen microbes convert a large proportion of dietary selenium into unavailable forms that are excreted in the faeces (Hartmann and van Ryssen, 1997). High concentrate diets may increase selenium bioavailability as a result of a lower rumen pH.

There is little information on selenium nutrition of wild animals. **Pronghorn antelope** are native to areas of western North America that tend to have high-selenium soils. They often occur on reclaimed strip-mined areas where selenium in mine spoil becomes oxidized to plant-available forms. The natural diet of pronghorns includes selenium-accumulating plant species. These observations suggest that pronghorn may be somewhat resistant to **selenium toxicity**. Raisbeck *et al.* (1996), in a feeding trial with high-selenium hay (15 ppm Se), found no evidence of clinical signs of selenium toxicity in captive

pronghorns, suggesting that they may be tolerant of selenium toxicity. (A dietary selenium level of about 2 ppm is toxic to most species.)

Vitamin C

Vitamin C, or **ascorbic acid,** functions as an antioxidant, in addition to its role in vitamin E recycling. It is a simple molecule (Fig. 13.7), derived from glucose, and can readily undergo oxidation and reduction. Its synthesis involves formation of L-gulonolactone from glucose, which is converted to ascorbic acid by the enzyme **L-gulonolactone oxidase** (Fig. 13.8). Most animals have this enzyme. A few, including humans, other primates, guinea pigs, fruit-eating bats, some fruit-eating birds and some fish lack this enzyme and so have a dietary requirement for vitamin C. Besides its role as an antioxidant, ascorbic acid is

$$
\begin{array}{ccc}
\text{Ascorbate} & \text{Monodehydroascorbate} & \text{Dehydroascorbate} \\
& \text{(semidehydroascorbate)} &
\end{array}
$$

Fig. 13.7. Ascorbic acid or vitamin C. Dehydroascorbate is the oxidized form; monodehydroascorbate has one oxygen reduced; and ascorbic acid has both oxygens reduced.

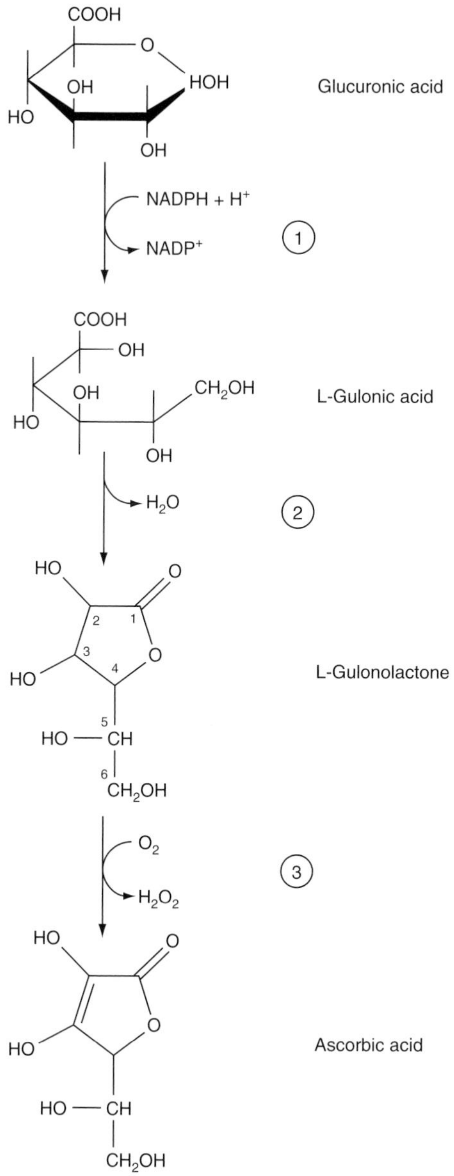

Fig. 13.8. Synthesis of vitamin C from glucose.

also required in collagen synthesis. It functions in the formation of hydroxyproline and hydroxylysine in the collagen molecule. Because of its reducing properties, vitamin C enhances iron absorption. Ascorbic acid deficiency is called **scurvy**, and is caused by faulty collagen synthesis. In humans, signs of scurvy include gum disorders (gingivitis and loosening of the teeth), anaemia, delayed healing of soft tissue injuries, and bone formation abnormalities.

The anaemia is a consequence of reduced iron absorption in the absence of ascorbic acid (see Chapter 21).

The ability to synthesize vitamin C has been lost by some species in which fruit (an excellent source of ascorbic acid) has been a major component of the diet. Benzie (2003) speculated that the ability of humans to synthesize ascorbic acid (which was present in ancestral humanoid species) was lost because it was metabolically more efficient to obtain it from the habitually consumed plant-rich diet. Ascorbic acid plays a major role as an antioxidant in plants, protecting them from ROS formed in photosynthetic reactions. Thus plants are rich in antioxidants in general (vitamin C, vitamin E, carotenoids, polyphenols). Plant parts rich in antioxidants are usually brightly coloured. Fruit-eating birds, humans and other primates have well developed colour vision which aids in selection of an antioxidant-rich diet. Carnivores, which do not rely directly on plants for antioxidants, have poor colour vision (Benzie, 2003).

Carotenoids

Carotenoids are an abundant group of plant pigments; over 600 individual carotenoids are known. They contain a long chain of conjugated double bonds, and most (e.g. β-carotene) but not all (e.g. lycopene) have a β-ionone ring (which is necessary for vitamin A activity). The chain of conjugated double bonds has antioxidant activity. In plants, carotenoids are found in the chloroplasts and function in photosynthesis. Carotenoids are discussed further in Chapter 19, as skin and feather pigments. They contribute to the antioxidant defences of animals.

Synthetic Antioxidants (Preservatives)

Synthetic antioxidants include ethoxyquin (Santoquin®), BHT and BHA. They are phenolic compounds, and are very effective at preventing oxidation (rancidity) of stored feeds and are commonly used for this purpose. (Ethoxyquin is not actually a phenolic (Fig. 13.9); it is a quinoline compound.) Synthetic antioxidants are also used as preservatives in food products such as potato chips. When included in the diet, they are absorbed and function as tissue antioxidants. Thus they have a sparing effect on vitamin E. Although they have been demonstrated to be safe, many consumers are suspicious of synthetic antioxidants (preservatives).

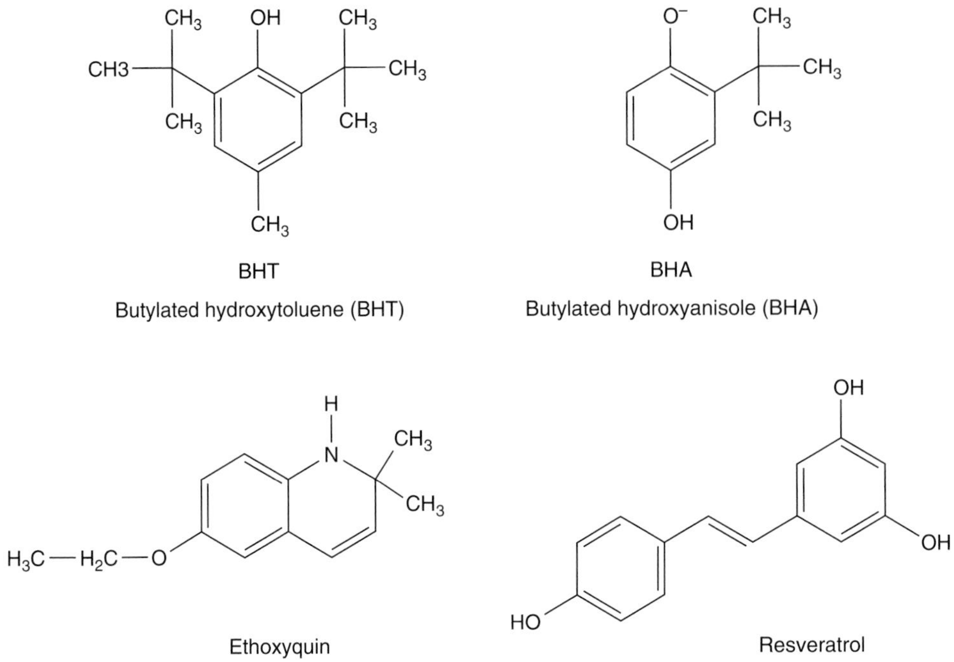

Fig. 13.9. Examples of synthetic antioxidants (BHT, BHA, ethoxyquin) and resveratrol, an antioxidant in grapes and red wine.

Polyphenolic Antioxidants

There is a great deal of interest in polyphenolics in fruits and vegetables. They are believed to have beneficial effects on human health by functioning as tissue antioxidants. Phenolic compounds contain aromatic rings with hydroxyl groups; polyphenolics have more than one hydroxyl group. These phenolic groups function as antioxidants by providing hydrogen to reduce oxidants. (Note that this is how vitamin E functions: it has a labile phenolic group on position 6 (Fig. 13.3).) An example of a phenolic antioxidant is **resveratrol** (Fig. 13.9). It occurs in grape skins and is the substance responsible for the healthful effects of red wine. Numerous phenolic compounds with antioxidant activity have been identified in a variety of plants. Phenolics may have developed in flowering plants to provide antioxidant protection against UV radiation, which was much more intense when plants first evolved than it is now. Structures of phenolic antioxidants are shown in Fig. 13.9.

There is widespread interest in the use of plant polyphenols as antioxidants in food processing, in place of synthetic antioxidants such as BHA and BHT. Many fruits and berries are good sources of antioxidants due to their flavonoid and polyphenol contents. **Plums** are a good source. The addition of plum juice concentrates to meat products aids in their preservation by reducing lipid peroxidation and off-flavour (Nunez de Gonzalez *et al.*, 2008). Native Americans and French Canadian fur trappers made use of plums and berries to prepare pemmican, a dried meat-fruit product that was stable for extensive periods.

Oxidation of Toxins: Mixed-function Oxidases

Toxicants are absorbed as lipid-soluble substances and are metabolized in the tissues to water-soluble metabolites that can be excreted in the urine. This metabolism is largely carried out in the liver by enzymes referred to collectively as the **mixed-function oxidases (MFO)**. This name is derived from the double role of the oxygen molecule in MFO-catalysed reactions, both as an oxidizing (to form water) and as an oxygenating agent. The MFO system has a remarkable degree of non-specificity, in contrast to most enzymes, so it metabolizes many diverse compounds. The MFO enzymes catalyse numerous oxidative reactions, producing more polar, water-soluble metabolites. Another attribute of MFOs in detoxification is that they respond very quickly to the presence of dietary toxicants with a marked increase in concentration or activity. This process is called **enzyme induction**, whereby the presence of a toxicant induces increased concentration of the enzymes that detoxify it. Along with the MFO system, a variety of other enzymes such as esterases, reductases and transferases are involved in detoxification.

The MFO system can metabolize a great variety of foreign lipophilic substances that are commonly encountered by animals in the course of their normal life processes. Many of these are natural toxicants in plants, since presumably the MFO system in animals and insects has evolved to allow the organisms to cope with these compounds in their food supply (Nebert *et al.*, 1989). Much of the knowledge of specific MFO reactions is concerned with man-made chemicals such as pesticides, drugs and industrial chemicals, rather than with natural toxicants.

Most MFO reactions are oxidations. The MFO enzymes are present in the endoplasmic reticulum of cells, particularly the smooth endoplasmic reticulum. When tissue is homogenized and subjected to ultracentrifugation, the endoplasmic reticulum

fragments are fractionated out as a pellet called the microsomal pellet or **microsomes**. The MFO system is often referred to as microsomal enzymes. The MFO system has several components: (i) cytochrome P_{450}; (ii) NADPH; (iii) a flavoprotein enzyme called NADPH-cytochrome P_{450} reductase; and (iv) phosphatidylcholine.

Cytochrome P_{450} is the terminal oxidase of the MFO system. It is a b-type cytochrome (a haemoprotein containing haem) that binds carbon monoxide. The reduced cytochrome–carbon monoxide complex has an absorption peak at 450 nm, hence its name. The mechanism of action of the MFO system is that the toxicant reacts with the oxidized cytochrome P_{450}, producing a complex which then is reduced by picking up hydrogen from the reduced flavoprotein, and subsequently reacts with molecular oxygen to produce water, reoxidized cytochrome P_{450} and the toxicant with a hydroxyl group attached. These reactions are shown in Fig. 13.10. The net result is that an aromatic substrate has been hydroxylated, so it can then be conjugated with polar compounds to produce a water-soluble metabolite (Parke *et al.*, 1990).

There are several isozymes of cytochrome P_{450} with different substrate specificities. Some of the animal species differences in susceptibility to toxins may be associated with differences in cytochrome

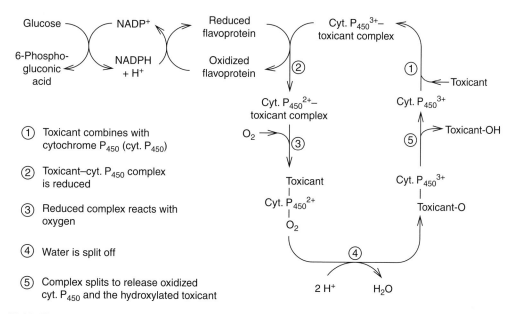

Fig. 13.10. The mixed-function oxidase (MFO) enzyme system.

P_{450} isozyme activities (Ioannides and Parke, 1990; Smith, 1991). At least eight major gene families for cytochrome P_{450} have been identified, with the types and amounts varying with species, organ, age, gender, stress and toxicant exposure (Ioannides and Parke, 1990; Sipes and Gandolfi, 1991). Thus individual isozymes are relatively substrate specific, but the full complement of P_{450} enzymes provides for a remarkably broad capacity for toxin metabolism.

Specific MFO Reactions

The MFO reactions are referred to as **biotransformation** because the substrate is transformed into metabolites. Biotransformation reactions are often referred to as **phase I reactions**. In the phase I reactions, reactive functional groups are added or exposed (e.g. –OH, –SH, –NH$_2$, –COOH). The MFO system is the primary mediator of phase I reactions. Phase II involves conjugation of the metabolites produced in the MFO-mediated phase I reactions.

Biotransformation in general is a detoxification process, converting toxic lipophilic compounds to non-toxic water-soluble metabolites, although sometimes the metabolites are more toxic than the original compounds. An example of increased toxicity is the conversion of aflatoxin to the carcinogenic epoxide.

Factors affecting MFO activity

The MFO enzyme activities are generally much higher in the liver than in other organs, so that the liver is the major site of detoxification. All other tissues do possess MFO activity. Both the liver and the lungs are important sites for detoxification enzymes, because the portal vein and the lungs are the major routes for entrance of toxicants into the internal environment. The nasal mucosa contains cytochrome P_{450} activity, which presumably aids in detoxification of toxins that are inhaled (Longo *et al.*, 1991). Nasal detoxifying enzymes could perhaps have some relevance to the ability of animals to detect poisonous plants, by producing metabolites in the nasal tissue, eliciting an olfactory response. Rumen and intestinal mucosa tissues have cytochrome P_{450} activity. Smith (1992) speculated that biotransformation of absorbed toxins in gut mucosal tissue may be more important than currently recognized.

Fetal and newborn animals have very low MFO activity, and thus lack the ability to metabolize many toxicants and drugs. Children may be more sensitive to pesticide residues on food than are adults (National Research Council, 1993), for example. There are numerous gender-related differences in MFO activity, presumably related to steroid hormone balance. Steroid hormones are metabolized by the MFO enzymes.

There are pronounced species differences in microsomal enzyme activities. Ducklings and trout are extremely sensitive to aflatoxins because of a rapid rate of metabolism to the epoxide, whereas sheep and rats metabolize aflatoxin more slowly and are much more resistant to it. Animals that are resistant to the toxic effects of pyrrolizidine alkaloids, such as sheep, guinea pigs and Japanese quail, have a much lower rate of hepatic alkaloid metabolism than susceptible species such as cattle, horses and rats (Cheeke, 1994).

Nutritional factors influence MFO activity. Low dietary protein generally results in lower MFO function. Thus the toxicity of aflatoxin is reduced on low protein diets because less of the active metabolite is produced. Vitamin and mineral deficiencies may affect MFO status.

Factors that stimulate MFO synthesis are called **inducers** or inducing agents. Most toxicants are inducers and therefore exposure to toxicants results in an increased ability of animals to detoxify them. Enzyme induction, of course, is a sound strategy for coping with environmental hazards. Certain drugs are widely used for research purposes to induce MFO activity. The most common is phenobarbital. Pretreatment of animals with barbiturates markedly increases their microsomal enzyme activities. This pretreatment increases the toxicity if the product of biotransformation is more toxic than the original toxicant.

Phase II: conjugation reactions

Metabolites produced by MFO activity are generally excreted in the urine as conjugated compounds; that is, they are conjugated with other substances such as glutathione, glycine, glucuronic acid and sulfate to increase their water solubility. These reactions are catalysed by group transferase enzymes, such as **glutathione-S-transferase**. This enzyme results in the reaction of an hydroxylated metabolite with glutathione. Glutathione is a tripeptide containing glycine, glutamic acid and cysteine. The sulfhydryl (–SH) group of cysteine reacts with the toxin metabolites. A series of enzymatic reactions converts the toxins to a mercaptic acid (a derivative of N-acetylcysteine) that is excreted in the urine. UDPglucuronosyltransferase catalyses the formation of a β-glucuronide.

Sulfotransferases result in the formation of water-soluble sulfates. There are species differ-ences in activities of conjugating enzymes. Cats lack glucuronosyltransferase and so cannot form glucuronides. Therefore they are more susceptible than other species to intoxication by benzoic acid and phenol. Guinea pigs lack the ability to synthe-size mercaptic acid metabolites from glutathione conjugation.

Questions and Study Guide

1. What is rancidity?
2. How do antioxidants work?
3. Many food products for humans are advertised as containing no preservatives. Why would 'no preservatives' be appealing to many people?
4. How does vitamin C function as a preservative?
5. What property of olive and canola oils is responsible for their reputation as being more healthy than other vegetable oils for humans?
6. What is vitamin E?
7. Which is of higher vitamin E potency: natural vitamin E or synthetic vitamin E?
8. What is a quinone?
9. Feeding a high amount of vitamin E to feedlot cattle for a few weeks prior to slaughter may extend the shelf life of the meat. Why?
10. Why do captive rhinoceros in zoos have higher vitamin E requirements than their wild counterparts?
11. What is the metabolic function of selenium?
12. Most species of animals do not require a dietary source of vitamin C. Humans and other primates do require a dietary source. Why?
13. Vitamin-C-deficient people may develop anaemia. Why?
14. What is resveratrol?
15. Feeding the insecticide DDT to rats for a few days increases their ability to metabolize it. Why?
16. What are the functions of cytochrome P_{450}?

References

Arthur, J.R., Beckett, G.J. and Mitchell, J.H. (1999) The interactions between selenium and iodine deficiencies in man and animals. *Nutrition Research Reviews* 12, 55–73.

Benzie, I.F.F. (2003) Review, Evolution of dietary antioxidants. *Comparative Biochemistry and Physiology Part A* 136, 113–126.

Burk, R.F. and Hill, K.E. (1993) Regulation of selenoproteins. *Annual Review of Nutrition* 13, 65–81.

Cheeke, P.R. (1994) A review of the functional and evolutionary roles of the liver in the detoxification of poisonous plants, with special reference to pyrrolizidine alkaloids. *Veterinary and Human Toxicology* 36, 240–247.

Clauss, M. (2003) Tannins in the nutrition of wild animals: a review. In: Fidgett, A., Clauss, M., Ganslofser, U., Hatt, J.-M. and Nijboer, J. (eds) *Zoo Animal Nutrition*, Vol. 2. Filander Verlag, Fürth, Germany, pp. 53–89.

Clauss, M., Gehrke, J., Fickel, J., Lechner-Doll, M., Flach, E.J., Dierenfeld, E.S. and Hatt, J.-M. (2002a) Induction of salivary tannin-binding proteins in captive black rhinoceros (*Diceros bicornis*) by dietary tannins. *Proceedings of the Comparative Nutrition Society* 4, 119–120.

Clauss, M., Jessup, D.A., Norkus, E.C., Holick, M.F., Streich, W.J. and Dierenfeld, E.S. (2002b) Fat soluble vitamins in blood and tissues of free-ranging and captive rhinoceros species. *Journal of Wildlife Diseases* 38(2), 402–413.

Clauss, M., Gehrke, J., Hatt, J.M., Dierenfeld, E.S., Flach, E.J., Hermes, R., Castell, J., Streich, W.J. and Fickel, J. (2005) Tannin-binding salivary proteins in three captive rhinoceros species. *Comparative Biochemistry and Physiology Part A: Molecular and Integrative Physiology* 140, 67–72.

Clauss, M., Dierenfeld, E.S., Bigley, K.E., Wang, Y., Ghebremeskel, K., Hatt, J.-M., Flach, E.J., Behlert, O., Castell, J.C., Streich, W.J. and Bauer, J.E. (2008) Fatty acid status in captive and free-ranging black rhinoceroses (*Diceros bicornis*). *Journal of Animal Physiology and Animal Nutrition* 92, 231–241.

Dierenfeld, E.S. (1989) Vitamin E deficiency in zoo reptiles, birds, and ungulates. *Journal of Zoo and Wildlife Medicine* 20, 3–11.

Dierenfeld, E.S. (1994) Vitamin E in exotics: effects, evaluation and ecology. *Journal of Nutrition* 124, 2579S–2581S.

Dierenfeld, E.S. (1997) Captive wild animal nutrition: a historical perspective. *Proceedings of the Nutrition Society* 56, 989–999.

Dierenfeld, E.S. and Traber, M.G. (1992) Vitamin E status of exotic animals compared with livestock and domestics. In: Packer, L. and Fuchs, J. (eds) *Vitamin E in Health and Disease*. Marcel Dekker Inc., New York, pp. 345–360.

Dierenfeld, E.S., du Toit, R. and Miller, R.E. (1988) Vitamin E in captive and wild black rhinoceros (*Diceros bicornis*). *Journal of Wildlife Diseases* 24, 547–550.

Dierenfeld, E.S., Karesh, W.B., Raphael, B.L., Cook, R.A., Kilbourn, A.M., Bosi, E.J. and Andau, M. (1998) Circulating α-tocopherol and retinol in free-ranging and zoo ungulates. *Proceedings of the Comparative Nutrition Society* 2, 42–46.

Dierenfeld, E.S., Atkinson, S., Craig, A.M., Walker, K.C., Streich, W.J. and Clauss, M. (2005) Mineral concentrations in serum/plasma and liver tissue of captive and free-ranging rhinoceros species. *Zoo Biology* 24, 51–72.

Faustman, C., Chan, W.K.M., Schaefer, D.M. and Havens, A. (1998) Beef color update: the role for vitamin E. *Journal of Animal Science* 76, 1019–1026.

Ghebremeskel, K. and Williams, G. (1988) Plasma retinol and alpha tocopherol levels in captive wild animals. *Comparative Biochemistry and Physiology Part A* 89, 279–283.

Ghebremeskel, K., Williams, G., Brett, R.A., Burek, R. and Harbige, L.S. (1991) Nutrient composition of plants most favoured by black rhinoceros (*Diceros bicornis*) in the wild. *Comparative Biochemistry and Physiology* 98, 529–534.

Grant, J.B., Brown, D.L. and Dierenfeld, E.S. (2002) Essential fatty acid profiles differ across diets and browse of black rhinoceros. *Journal of Wildlife Diseases* 38, 132–142.

Hartmann, F. and van Ryssen, J.B.J. (1997) Metabolism of selenium and copper in sheep with and without sodium bicarbonate supplementation. *Journal of Agricultural Science* 128, 357–364.

Ioannides, C. and Parke, D.V. (1990) The cytochrome P_{450} I gene family of microsomal hemoproteins and their role in the metabolic activation of chemicals. *Drug Metabolism Reviews* 22, 1–85.

Kamal-Eldin, A. and Appelqvist, L.A. (1996) The chemistry and antioxidant properties of tocopherols and tocotrienols. *Lipids* 7, 671–701.

Kelly, J.D., Blyde, D.J. and Denney, I.S. (1995) The importation of the black rhinoceros (*Diceros bicornis*) from Zimbabwe into Australia. *Australian Veterinary Journal* 72, 369–374.

Knight, D.A. and Tyznik, W.J. (1990) The effect of dietary selenium on humoral immunocompetence of ponies. *Journal of Animal Science* 68, 1311–1317.

Koenig, K.M., Rode, L.M., Cohen, R.D.H. and Buckley, W.T. (1997) Effects of diet and chemical form of selenium on selenium metabolism in sheep. *Journal of Animal Science* 75, 817–827.

Levander, O.A. (1986) Selenium. In: Mertz, W. (ed.) *Trace Elements in Human and Animal Nutrition*, 5th edn. Academic Press, Orlando, Florida, pp. 209–279.

Liu, Q., Lanari, M.D. and Schaefer, D.M. (1995) A review of dietary vitamin E supplementation for improvement of beef quality. *Journal of Animal Science* 73, 3131–3140.

Longo, V., Mazzaccaro, A., Naldi, F. and Gervasi, P.G. (1991) Drug-metabolizing enzymes in liver, olfactory and respiratory epithelium of cattle. *Journal of Biochemical and Molecular Toxicology* 6, 123–128.

Mainka, S.A. and Mills, J.A. (1995) Wildlife and traditional Chinese medicine – supply and demand for wildlife species. *Journal of Zoo and Wildlife Medicine* 26, 193–200.

National Research Council (1993) *Pesticides in the Diets of Infants and Children*. National Academy Press, Washington, DC.

Nebert, D.W., Nelson, D.R. and Feyereisen, R. (1989) Evolution of the cytochrome P_{450} genes. *Xenobiotica* 19, 1149–1160.

Nunez de Gonzalez, M.T., Hafley, B.S., Boleman, R.M., Miller, R.K., Rhee, K.S. and Keeton, J.T. (2008) Antioxidant properties of plum concentrates and powder in precooked roast beef to reduce lipid oxidation. *Meat Science* 80, 997–1004.

Parke, D.V., Ioannides, C. and Lewis, D.F.V. (1990) The role of the cytochromes P_{450} in the detoxication and activation of drugs and other chemicals. *Canadian Journal of Physiology and Pharmacology* 69, 537–549.

Pryor, W.A. (2001) Vitamin E. In: Brown, B.A. and Russell, R.M. (eds) *Present Knowledge in Nutrition*, 8th edn. ILSI Press, Washington, DC, pp. 156–163.

Raisbeck, M.F., O'Toole, D., Schamber, R.A., Belden, E.L. and Robinson, L.J. (1996) Toxicologic evaluation of a high-selenium hay diet in captive pronghorn antelope (*Antilocapra americana*). *Journal of Wildlife Diseases* 32, 9–16.

Savage, A., Leong, K.M., Grobler, D., Lehnhardt, J., Dierenfeld, E.S., Stevens, E.F. and Aebischer, C.P. (1999) Circulating levels of α-tocopherol and retinol in free-ranging African elephants (*Loxodonta Africana*). *Zoo Biology* 18, 319–323.

Sipes, I.G. and Gandolfi, A.J. (1991) Biotransformation of toxicants. In: Amdur, M.O., Doull, J. and Klaassen, C.D. (eds) *Casarett and Doull's Toxicology, the Basic Science of Poisons*, 4th edn. Pergamon Press, New York, pp. 88–126.

Smith, D.A. (1991) Species differences in metabolism and pharmacokinetics: are we close to an understanding? *Drug Metabolism Reviews* 23, 355–373.

Smith, G.S. (1992) Toxification and detoxification of plant compounds by ruminants: an overview. *Journal of Range Management* 45, 25–30.

Smith, J.E., Chavey, P.S. and Miller, R.E. (1995) Iron metabolism in captive black (*Diceros bicornis*) and white (*Ceratotherium simum*) rhinoceroses. *Journal of Zoo and Wildlife Medicine* 26, 525–531.

Traber, M.G. (2006) Vitamin E. In: Brown, B.A. and Russell, R.M. (eds) *Present Knowledge in Nutrition*, Vol. 1, 9th edn. ILSI Press, Washington, DC, pp. 211–219.

Wright, J.B. and Brown, D.L. (1997) Identification of 18:3 (n-3) linolenic acid, 18:3 (n-6) linolenic acid and 18:2 (n-6) linoleic acid in Zimbabwean browses preferred by wild black rhinoceroses (*Diceros bicornis*) determined by GC-MS analysis. *Animal Feed Science and Technology* 69, 195–199.

Yeh, J.-Y., Gu, Q.-P., Beilstein, M.A., Forsberg, N.E. and Whanger, P.D. (1997) Selenium influences tissue levels of selenoprotein W in sheep. *Journal of Nutrition* 127, 394–402.

PART V
Integration of Metabolism

This part is intended to 'pull together' the metabolism of the major nutrient categories. Various metabolic disorders and their causes are discussed.

Part Objectives

1. To discuss energy metabolism in terms of units of measurement (e.g. calories versus joules) and measures of whole-animal metabolism.
2. To indicate how amino acids and lipids function as metabolic fuels by entering the major metabolic pathways of carbohydrate metabolism.
3. To discuss metabolic events that occur in the hibernation process.
4. To discuss energy storage in animals, primarily as glycogen or adipose tissue.
5. To discuss current human health problems (e.g. obesity) related to evolutionary history and differences between current and ancestral diets.
6. To discuss disorders of energy metabolism, such as ketosis, diabetes, insulin resistance and metabolic syndrome.
7. To discuss the relationship between dietary energy, caloric restriction and longevity.
8. To discuss the role of the thyroid hormones as major integrators of metabolism.
9. To discuss feeding behaviour and the regulation of feed intake.

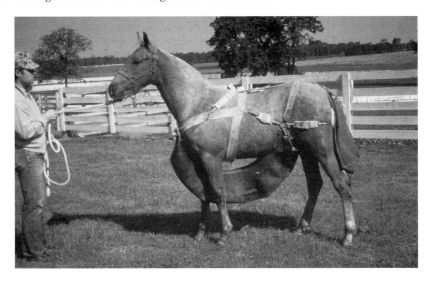

A horse equipped with a harness to facilitate collection of feces and urine. This procedure is used to collect the excreta for conducting nutrient balance and digestibility trials, such as those used to measure various energy categories such as digestible and metabolizable energy.

14 Energy Metabolism, Hibernation and Amino Acids and Lipids as Metabolic Fuels

The carbohydrate-metabolizing pathways such as glycolysis and the citric acid cycle are the basic cellular metabolic machinery. Amino acids and fats are used as energy sources by being converted to intermediate compounds ('intermediates') that enter the pathways of carbohydrate metabolism at specific locations.

Measurement of Energy Metabolism

On a practical basis, energy metabolism of animals is assessed by measuring some general aspect of metabolism. For example, in the utilization of carbohydrates, lipids and amino acids as energy sources, oxygen is consumed and carbon dioxide, water and heat are end products. All of these (except water) can be measured in animals confined in special chambers called **respirometers**. Gaseous exchange is obtained by measuring oxygen consumption and carbon dioxide output. The ratio of these gases (moles carbon dioxide produced/moles oxygen consumed), the **respiratory quotient** (**RQ**), gives an indication of the nature of the metabolic fuel being used. During metabolism of carbohydrate the RQ is 1.0. Fatty acid metabolism is associated with an RQ of 0.7. The RQ for protein is between 0.7 and 1.0. Heat production can also be measured, and used as an indicator of metabolic rate.

Examples of RQ determinations are as follows:

Carbohydrate catabolism:

$$C_6H_{12}O_6 + 6O_2 \rightarrow 6CO_2 + 6H_2O$$

$$RQ = CO_2/O_2 = 6/6 = 1.0$$

Fatty acid metabolism, e.g. stearic acid:

$$CH_3(CH_2)10COOH + 26O_2 \rightarrow 18CO_2 + 18H_2O$$

$$RQ = CO_2/O_2 = 18/26 = 0.692 \text{ (approximately 0.7)}$$

Amino acid metabolism, e.g. alanine:

$$4CH_3CH(NH_2)COOH + 12O_2 \rightarrow 10CO_2 + 10H_2O + 2CO(NH_2)_2 \text{ [urea]}$$

$$RQ = CO_2/O_2 = 10/12 = 0.83$$

Estimation of Feed Energy

In the USA, feed energy is expressed in **calories**. In most other countries, the **joule** is used as the measure of energy. Although the use of the joule in nutrition is not logical (joules are measures of electrical energy), it has been adopted because it is the unit of energy measurement used in the metric system. Feed energy is actually measured as calories, by bomb calorimetry, and then converted to joules by a conversion factor (below). Appropriate definitions and conversions are as follows:

- 1 calorie (small calorie) = the amount of heat required to raise the temperature of 1 g of water by 1°C degree centigrade, measured from 14.5 to 15.5°C;
- 1 kilocalorie (kcal) = 1000 calories = 1 Calorie (large calorie);[1]
- 1 megacalorie (Mcal) = 1000 kilocalories;
- 1 calorie = 4.184 joules (J);
- 1 kilocalorie = 4.184 kilojoules (kJ); and
- 1 kilojoule = 0.239 kcal.

The caloric content of biological materials is determined in a **bomb calorimeter** (Fig. 14.1). In brief, the sample is burned in a combustion chamber (bomb) inserted in a vessel containing a known weight of water. As the sample burns, it releases heat, which is taken up by the water. From the weight of the sample, weight of the water, and rise in temperature of the water, the number of calories of heat energy released can be calculated. When a feed sample is burned in a bomb calorimeter, its **gross energy** is determined.

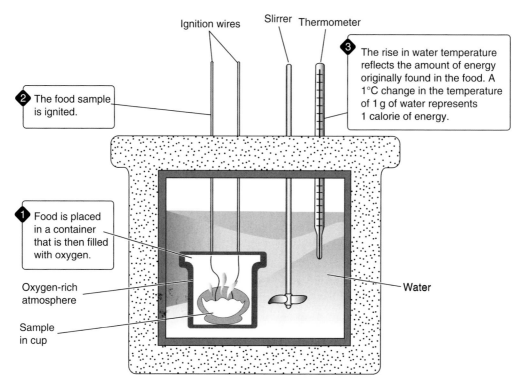

Ignition wires   Slirrer Thermometer

② The food sample is ignited.

③ The rise in water temperature reflects the amount of energy originally found in the food. A 1°C change in the temperature of 1 g of water represents 1 calorie of energy.

① Food is placed in a container that is then filled with oxygen.

Oxygen-rich atmosphere

Sample in cup

Water

Fig. 14.1. The bomb calorimeter is used to measure the gross energy content of feeds.

To determine the fraction of the gross energy that the animal can actually utilize, a metabolism trial must be conducted to account for various losses, yielding values for digestible, metabolizable and net energy:

Digestible energy (DE) = Gross energy (GE) – Faecal energy

Metabolizable energy (ME) = DE – (Urinary energy + Rumen gas losses)

Net energy (NE) = ME – Heat loss

Thus the NE represents the fraction of the GE actually utilized for productive purposes.

In the preceding determinations, faeces and urine arising from test feed are collected and their energy content determined by bomb calorimetry. Because the urinary energy is usually quite low, DE values are satisfactory for expression of energy requirements of most species. In poultry, faeces and urine are voided together, so ME values are commonly used. For determination of NE, a respiration chamber allowing measurement of heat loss is needed. Alternatively, the NE can be estimated by measuring energy retention by the animal, using a specific-gravity determination on the carcass (the comparative slaughter technique).

The **comparative slaughter technique**, also referred to as the California net energy system, is a procedure for measuring net energy of a feedstuff for growth (gain) (NE_g) and maintenance (NE_m) of beef cattle (Lofgreen and Garrett, 1968). In brief, the relationship between the specific gravity of a carcass and its energy content was determined to establish the system. The energy content of the carcass was measured by grinding up the entire carcass and measuring the caloric content of a sample by bomb calorimetry. The specific gravity of the carcass depends on the lipid content. Lipid has a low density (floats on water). The volume of water displaced by a carcass varies with its caloric content. In routine application of the procedure, a group of animals is fed the test diet. A similar group is slaughtered at the beginning of the trial. After a period of feeding the test diet, and a known intake of gross energy, the energy gain is determined as the energy content of the carcass at the end of the feeding period minus the initial energy content. The carcass energy content is estimated from the specific gravity measurement: the carcass is suspended in water and the volume of water displaced is measured. This is an application of the classic **Archimedes' principle**.

Hibernation

Hibernation is a state of hypometabolism entered into by some animals as a response to anticipated nutritional stress (Guppy and Withers, 1999). While generally viewed as a means of avoiding winter-feed scarcity and cold, hibernation is employed by some animals (e.g. California ground squirrel) to avoid hot summer months when grass seeds are unavailable (Boyer and Barnes, 1999) (also called **aestivation**). Aestivation in hot, dry conditions is common among reptiles. Hibernation is characterized by an extreme drop in body temperature (to as low as –2.9°C) and metabolic rate can be as low as 1% of normal (Carey *et al.*, 2003). This state is known as **torpor**. A typical hibernation season is characterized by several bouts of torpor, interrupted by short periods of intense metabolic activity. With the exception of bears, which become only moderately hypothermic (Tomasi *et al.*, 1998), no hibernating mammal remains deeply hypothermic for more than a few weeks. For reasons as yet unknown, they expend significant amounts of energy to periodically rewarm back to normal body temperature for less than a day before recooling (Boyer and Barnes, 1999). The molecular and cellular mechanisms of hibernation are still largely a mystery.

Hibernators are of two types: (i) fat storing; and (ii) food storing. Fat-storing hibernators do not consume food during the hibernation season and instead rely on metabolism of stored fat (**white adipose tissue; WAT**). Food-storing hibernators (e.g. chipmunks) store caches of food, which they ingest during their periodic arousals. Fat-storing hibernators, such as ground squirrels and marmots, can virtually double their body weight prior to hibernation, with 60–80% of the weight as WAT. Adipose tissue is the most efficient form of fuel storage, because body fat is energy dense and non-hydrated. Body protein is also catabolized for energy during hibernation. Hibernating bears utilize protein for energy and recycle urea back into amino acids by ammonia fixation (Barboza *et al.*, 1997). However,

black bears show no loss of skeletal muscle cell number, size or strength (Tinker *et al.*, 1998). Lipid accumulation in WAT results from cell enlargement rather from increased numbers of adipocytes. Insulin concentrations are high in late summer, promoting the synthesis and activity of lipoprotein lipase, which promotes deposition of lipid into adipose tissue. Hibernating rodents also increase their brown adipose tissue, which provides the metabolic heat needed for arousal (ATP production is uncoupled from oxidative phosphorylation – see Chapter 15).

During hibernation, several mechanisms shift metabolism from carbohydrate to lipids. During the transition to torpor, several key carbohydrate-metabolizing enzymes are phosphorylated, and thereby inactivated. These include glyceraldehyde-3-phosphate dehydrogenase and pyruvate dehydrogenase, the enzyme that converts pyruvate (end product of glycolysis) to acetyl CoA (entry to the citric acid cycle) (Storey, 1997). Pancreatic triacylglycerol lipase (PTL), normally expressed only in the pancreas, occurs in other tissues in hibernators, converting stored fat (triacylglycerols, TAGs) to free fatty acids. Reliance on fatty acid catabolism during hibernation is indicated by a respiratory quotient (RQ) of about 0.7, indicating that fatty acids are the main source of energy (RQ, see 'Measurement of Energy Metabolism' this chapter).

Black bears and grizzly bears consume considerable amounts of berries and fruits prior to hibernation (Rode and Robbins, 2000), which contributes to a positive energy balance. However, fruit and berries are poor sources of protein. The opportunity to consume sources of meat, including fish, is critical for bears in the pre-hibernation energy-storing period (Hilderbrand *et al.*, 1999a, b). Bears reduce their feed intake shortly before hibernation begins. Plasma thyroid hormone concentrations decrease at this time also (Tomasi *et al.*, 1998).

Catabolism of Amino Acids

The use of amino acids as energy sources begins with deamination (removal of the α-amino group) in the liver. The remaining carbon skeleton is then converted to intermediates of either glycolysis or citric acid cycle reactions. For example, aspartic acid is converted to oxaloacetic acid (OAA). Glycine, serine, alanine, cysteine and two carbons of threonine form pyruvate and subsequently acetyl CoA. At least 12 amino acids can form acetyl CoA (Fig. 14.2). The branched-chain amino acids (valine, leucine, isoleucine) are converted

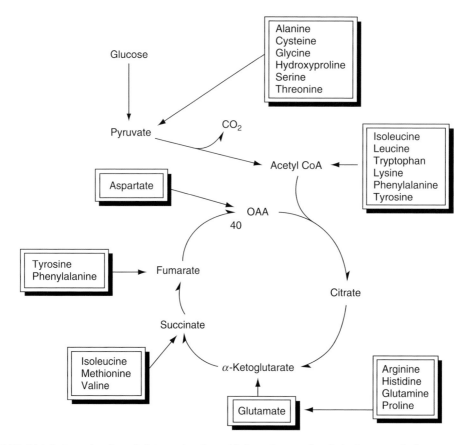

Fig. 14.2. Metabolism of carbon skeletons of amino acids in pathways of carbohydrate metabolism.

to acetyl CoA and/or succinyl CoA (Fig. 14.2). Breakdown products of lysine and tryptophan can also be converted to acetyl CoA.

Catabolism of Lipids

As discussed in Chapter 12, fatty acids are catabolized by β-oxidation to yield acetyl CoA, which enters the citric acid cycle reactions. The glycerol liberated from TAGs is converted to pyruvate, the end product of the glycolysis pathway. With odd-chain fatty acids, the final step of β-oxidation yields a three carbon short-chain fatty acid, propionate, which is converted to succinate in the citric acid cycle (see Fig. 12.7 in Chapter 12).

Questions and Study Guide

1. What is the respiratory quotient and of what use is it?
2. What is a calorie? How is the total calorie content of a food or feed measured?
3. What is the purpose of the comparative slaughter technique?
4. What are the roles of white adipose tissue and brown adipose tissue in hibernating animals?
5. How are amino acids used as energy sources?
6. There can be a net synthesis of glucose from amino acids but not from fatty acids. Explain why.

Note

[1] The kcal was formerly called a large Calorie, written with a capital letter C. This understandably caused confusion between large and small calories (written with a small c).

References

Barboza, P., Farley, S. and Robbins, C. (1997) Whole-body urea cycling and protein turnover during hyperphagia and dormancy in growing bears (*Ursus americanus* and *U. arctos*). *Canadian Journal of Zoology* 75, 2129–2136.

Boyer, B.B. and Barnes, B.M. (1999) Molecular and metabolic aspects of mammalian hibernation. *BioScience* 49, 713–724.

Carey, H.V., Andrews, M.T. and Martin, S.L. (2003) Mammalian hibernation: cellular and molecular responses to depressed metabolism and low temperature. *Physiological Reviews* 83, 1153–1181.

Guppy, M. and Withers, P. (1999) Metabolic depression in animals: physiological perspectives and biochemical generalizations. *Biology Review* 74, 1–40.

Hilderbrand, G.V., Schwartz, C.C., Robbins, C.T., Jacoby, M.E., Hanley, T.A., Arthur, S.M. and Servheen, C. (1999a) The importance of meat, particularly salmon, to body size, population productivity, and conservation of North American brown bears. *Canadian Journal of Zoology* 77, 132–138.

Hilderbrand, G.V., Jenkins, S.G., Schwartz, C.C., Hanley, T.A. and Robbins, C.T. (1999b) Effect of seasonal differences in dietary meat intake on changes in body mass and composition in wild and captive brown bears. *Canadian Journal of Zoology* 77, 1623–1630.

Lofgreen, G.P. and Garrett, W.N. (1968) A system for expressing net energy requirements and feed values for growing and finishing beef cattle. *Journal of Animal Science* 27, 793–806.

Rode, K.D. and Robbins, C.T. (2000) Why bears consume mixed diets during fruit abundance. *Canadian Journal of Zoology* 78, 1640–1645.

Storey, K.B. (1997) Metabolic regulation in mammalian hibernation: enzyme and protein adaptations. *Comparative Biochemistry and Physiology* 118, 1115–1124.

Tinker, D.B., Harlow, H.J. and Beck, T.D. (1998) Protein use and muscle-fiber changes in free-ranging, hibernating black bears. *Physiological and Biochemical Zoology* 71, 414–424.

Tomasi, T.E., Hellgren, E.C. and Tucker, T.J. (1998) Thyroid hormone concentrations in black bears (*Ursus americanus*): hibernation and pregnancy effects. *General and Comparative Endocrinology* 109, 192–199.

15 Energy Storage and the Ancestral Human Diet

Energy Storage

Energy is stored mainly as triacylglycerol (TAG, in adipose tissue) or carbohydrate (glycogen). More energy is stored in a given weight of tissue as TAG than as carbohydrate. TAGs are energy-rich (9 kcal/g) as compared to carbohydrate (4 kcal/g), so per unit of body weight, more energy can be stored as TAG. Adipose tissue is relatively free of water, whereas glycogen is highly hydrated. Thus storage of energy as TAG is a more effective use of body mass. Saturated fatty acids yield more energy than unsaturated fatty acids, because they contain more hydrogen (ATP is formed when hydrogen-containing cofactors, e.g. $FADH_2$, NADH, NADPH, are oxidized in the respiratory chain). TAG is stored in a liquid state; the lipid that is stored subcutaneously is as saturated as is compatible with being a liquid. The lipid deposits of marine mammals and fish are highly unsaturated, in order for the adipose tissue to be liquid under cold-water conditions.

Storage of glycogen

Glycogen is the major storage carbohydrate in animals. It is sometimes called animal starch, and like plant starch, it is a branched polymer of α-D-glucose. Glycogen is stored in the liver and muscle tissue. The main function of liver glycogen is to provide glucose to maintain the blood glucose concentration (glucose homeostasis), to provide a constant supply of glucose for extrahepatic cellular metabolism. Muscle glycogen is a readily available source of fuel for muscle contraction. **Glycogenolysis** is the process of glycogen breakdown. In liver, this process yields glucose, while in muscle the major end product is lactic acid. Insulin and glucagon, two hormones produced in the pancreas, have opposing activities. **Insulin** is secreted in response to hyperglycaemia, and promotes synthesis of liver glycogen. **Glucagon** secretion is stimulated by hypoglycaemia. Glucagon stimulates glycogenolysis by activating phosphorylase. It also enhances **gluconeogenesis** (reversal of glycolytic pathway to synthesize glucose, often from non-carbohydrate sources) from amino acids and lactate. The uptake of glucose from the blood by the tissue cells, especially muscle and adipose tissue, is regulated by insulin, via regulation of membrane glucose-transporters.

Glucose tolerance refers to the body's ability to regulate the blood glucose concentration after the oral administration of a test dose of glucose to a fasting subject. **Impaired glucose tolerance** (low insulin activity) is evident by a prolonged hyperglycaemia after consumption of the test dose (Fig. 15.1). In a normal subject, the blood glucose should return to the initial value within 2 h.

Glycogenolysis in muscle tissue releases primarily glucose-6-phosphate, which is catabolized anaerobically by glycolysis to pyruvic acid. Pyruvic acid is converted to lactic acid, which is released into the blood. Lactate is taken up by the liver, converted back to pyruvate, with the reformation of glucose-6-phosphate by the reversal of glycolysis and formation of glycogen (Fig. 15.2). Under aerobic muscle metabolism, carbon dioxide is the major end product.

Energy storage as body fat

Body fat is stored as TAGs in specialized fat cells (adipocytes). As with glycogen, body fat is mobilized or deposited in accordance with energy needs of the tissue cells, with these processes controlled by hormones. Some of these include insulin, epinephrine (adrenalin), norepinephrine (noradrenalin) and adrenocorticotropic hormone (ACTH). Insulin inhibits the catecholamine-stimulated release of free fatty acids (FFAs) from adipose tissue, and is a major regulator of adipose tissue metabolism. A body weight regulatory hormone, **leptin**, stimulates lipolysis and inhibits

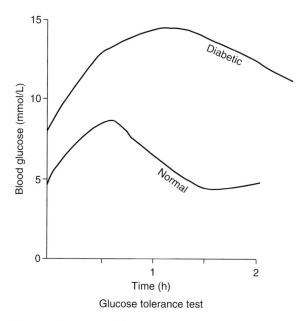

Fig. 15.1. An example of a glucose tolerance test. Blood glucose curves of a normal and a diabetic subject after oral administration of 1g glucose/kg BW. In a normal subject, the blood glucose should return to normal within 2 h.

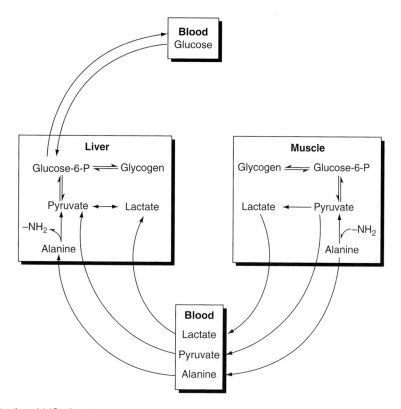

Fig. 15.2. The lactic acid (Cori) cycle.

lipogenesis by influencing the activity of enzymes involved in fatty acid synthesis and degradation. The main influence of leptin is in regulation of feed intake (Chapter 17).

TAGs in adipose tissue undergo continual breakdown and deposition, regardless of the need for energy storage or mobilization (**the dynamic state of body fat**). For this reason, and the lack of modification of dietary-derived fatty acids, the carcass fat of non-ruminant animals tends to resemble (in fatty acid composition) the dietary fat. If a pig is fed a diet with mainly saturated fatty acids, its body fat will be saturated; if it is fed unsaturated fatty acids, its body fat will be unsaturated (Fig. 15.3). In the case of ruminants, the carcass fat tends to be more saturated, regardless of the diet. Explanations for this include the biohydrogenation of unsaturated fatty acids in the rumen, and the fact that much of the body fat in ruminants is synthesized from absorbed acetate, producing palmitic acid (16:0) and stearic acid (18:0). Palmitic acid represents about 30% and stearic acid about 12% of fatty acids in subcutaneous adipose tissue of ruminants, while oleic acid represents about 50% because of Δ9 desaturase activity.

Brown adipose tissue (brown fat) is a special type of body fat especially important in newborn animals and animals that hibernate. Brown fat is characterized by a well-developed blood supply, an abundance of mitochondria and respiratory chain enzymes, and a low activity of ATP synthase. It is brown in colour because of the large numbers of mitochondria. Oxidation of fatty acids in brown fat is not efficiently coupled with phosphorylation (ATP production), increasing the amount of energy liberated as heat. (This is an example of the uncoupling of oxidative phosphorylation from electron transport.) This heat production is important in **non-shivering thermogenesis** in newborns and in animals in arousal from hibernation. Shivering thermogenesis, on the other hand, increases heat production as a result of increased muscular activity.

TAG may accumulate in the liver under certain conditions. Mobilization of body fat with increased concentrations of plasma FFAs is one cause. This condition can occur in starvation and with the feeding of high fat diets. Fatty liver is seen with diabetes and ketosis in cattle and sheep. Inadequate hepatic synthesis of lipoproteins may reduce the release of TAGs from the liver, allowing it to accumulate. **Fatty liver and kidney syndrome** in poultry affects mainly young birds. Dietary biotin is effective in preventing the syndrome. **Fatty liver haemorrhagic syndrome** is caused by excessive lipid accumulation in the livers of laying hens. High energy diets provoke the condition. **Idiopathic hepatic lipidosis (IHL)** is a common problem in cats.

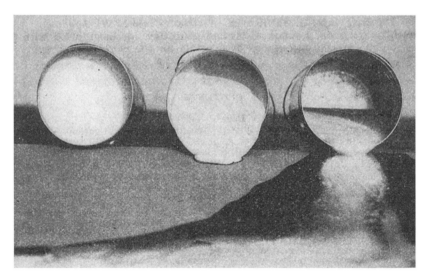

Fig. 15.3. The effect of diet fatty acid composition on carcass fat of non-ruminant animals. These are lard samples from pigs fed saturated (left), unsaturated (middle), and polyunsaturated (right) fats in the diet. The more unsaturated a fat, the greater the tendency for it to be liquid at room temperature (from Hankins *et al.*, 1928).

Dietary supplementation with carnitine helps alleviate IHL (Zoran, 2002).

Lipotropes are factors that aid in preventing fatty liver. They include choline, betaine, vitamin B_{12} and methionine. Their function is not totally clear, but may involve facilitating the production of lipoproteins.

Omega-3 (ω-3) Fatty Acids and Palaeolithic Nutrition (the Caveman Diet)

Human nutritional requirements reflect our evolutionary history extending millions of years into the past (Eaton and Konner, 1985; Eaton, 2006). Genetically, today's humans are basically the same biological organisms as our ancestors when they took up agriculture a scant 3000–10,000 years ago (Eaton *et al.*, 1996). Thus our ancestral dietary pattern has continuing relevance to the nutritional needs of contemporary humans. Small populations of hunter-gatherers still exist. These populations have a low dietary intake of fats rich in saturated fatty acids, because of the leanness of wild game. However, their cholesterol intake is high, about 480 mg/day (Eaton *et al.*, 1996). Despite this, they maintain very low serum cholesterol concentrations (about 1250 mg/l) (Eaton, 1992). Their high ratio of polyunsaturated to saturated (P:S) intakes (1.4 for hunter-gatherers, 0.4 for contemporary Americans), low saturated fatty acid intake and low total fat intake apparently offsets the high cholesterol intake (Eaton *et al.*, 1996). Hunter-gatherers do not consume cereal grains, but have a high intake of fruits and vegetables, providing a high intake of phytochemicals, vitamins and minerals. Ancestral human diets contained much more protein and fibre than do contemporary diets. Thus meat consumption is consistent with good health, which, based on archaeological evidence, hunter-gatherers apparently enjoyed. However, the fatty acid composition of contemporary intensively fattened meat animals deviates markedly, in an undesirable manner, from the lipid content and fatty acid composition of wild game animals (Crawford, 1968). The high intake of fruits and plants (vegetables) and minimal grain and dairy consumption made ancestral diets base-yielding diets, rather than today's acid-producing pattern (Frassetto *et al.*, 2001; Sebastian *et al.*, 2002; Eaton, 2006). Cereal grains and dairy foods are net acid yielding, and over prolonged periods (decades), the corrective metabolic measures necessary to offset persistent acid-yielding diets have deleterious effects, including urinary calcium loss (to balance H^+ excretion), accelerated skeletal calcium depletion (osteoporosis), calcium urolithiasis, age-related muscle wasting and progressive renal function deterioration (Frassetto, *et al.*, 2001). An excess acid load is buffered by bone minerals and in the process calcium is lost (Jajoo *et al.*, 2006). A major difference between ancestral and current diets is sodium intake. For ancestral humans, potassium intake exceeded that of sodium; now the situation is reversed (Eaton, 2006). Excessive sodium intake has been linked to numerous pathological states in humans, such as hypertension and osteoporosis (Logan, 2006).

A reasonable assumption is that the diets of the few remaining populations of hunter-gatherers reflect the diets of pre-agricultural humans. In other words, the diets of modern-day hunter-gatherers may represent a standard reference for modern human nutrition and a model for defence against diseases of affluence (Cordain *et al.*, 2000). In general, pre-industrial societies show a high dependence on animal-origin foods (O'Dea, 1991; Brand-Miller and Holt, 1998; Cordain *et al.*, 2000). Ratios of stable isotopes in bones can be used to assess the nature of the diet. Carbon-13-enriched bones of early hominids suggest that hominids consumed high-quality animal foods before the development of stone tools and the origin of the genus *Homo* (Sponheimer and Lee-Thorp, 1999). Extensive discussion on the importance of meat in the evolution of the human diet is presented in proceedings of a symposium, 'Foraging strategies and natural diet of monkeys, apes and humans', edited by Widdowson and Whiten (1991); in a book, *The Hunting Apes: Meat Eating and the Origins of Human Behavior*, reviewed by Boesch (1999); and in a book, *Meat Eating and Human Evolution*, edited by Stanford and Bunn (2001). Cordain (2002) has popularized his work on the Palaeolithic diet as 'the Paleo diet' for modern humans.

In a review of **palaeolithic nutrition** (the caveman diet), Eaton and Konner (1985) point out that, while early humans consumed a diet high in meat, the actual nutrients consumed may have been quite different from those in today's Western-type diet. The importance of meat in the caveman diet is revealed by the abundance of animal bones and hunting tools in archaeological sites, and the absence of much evidence of plant foods and tools for processing plant foods. The dawn of agriculture about 10,000 years ago marked a shift away from a meat diet to one with more plant foods (as indicated by seed-grinding tools such as mortar and pestle in archaeological sites).

There are considerable differences in the lipid composition of wild ruminants compared to modern sheep and cattle. Wild ruminants are generally much leaner, having lower quantities of depot fat and intramuscular fat (marbling). A greater proportion of the tissue lipid of wild ruminants consists of structural lipids such as phospholipids in cell membranes. Crawford and Gale (1969) and Gale et al. (1969) surveyed a number of wild African herbivores such as eland, wildebeest and buffalo and found much higher levels of long-chain PUFA such as C20:4ω3, C22:5ω3 (EPA), and C22:6ω3 (DHA). The total percentage of ω-6 PUFA of total fatty acids was about 30% in wild ruminants versus 12% in domestic cattle, while for ω-3 PUFA the averages were 9 and 4%, respectively. Thus the lipid of wild ruminants seems to contain a much higher proportion of the cholesterol-lowering ω-3 and ω-6 PUFA, reflecting the greater proportion of structural lipid in addition to diet differences. The main fatty acid in grass is C18:3ω3 (linolenic acid) whereas seeds (e.g. cereal grains) contain mainly C18:2ω6 (linoleic acid). Crawford and Gale (1969) speculated that seed capsules of herbage consumed by wild ruminants might bypass hydrogenation in the rumen, and serve as a source of higher ω-6 PUFA through desaturation and chain elongation. These differences in fatty acid composition could be of importance in meat products produced by game farming (e.g. deer, eland). However, the high PUFA in structural phospholipids of wild ruminants contributes to undesirable flavours and odours of the meat. For example, in studies by Larick and Turner (1989), meat from forage-finished American bison exhibited off-flavours including ammonia, gamey, bitter, liverish, old, rotten and sour perceptions by taste-panel participants.

While the human genetic profile has not changed much in the past 40,000 years (Simopoulos, 1998), our current Western diet has changed markedly over this time, with an increase in total fat, saturated fatty acids, trans-fatty acids and ω-6 essential fatty acids, but a decrease in ω-3 fatty acids. The ratio of ω-6 to ω-3 fatty acids is 10–20:1 today, whereas in pre-agricultural times it was about 1:1. This change arose because of our use of vegetable oils (mainly ω-6) and grain-fed meat animals, with carcass fat high in saturated and ω-6 fatty acids. Simopoulos (1998) proposes that the high incidence of 'diseases of Western civilization' such as coronary heart disease, hypertension, arthritis and diabetes, is related to a diet out of step with our evolutionary heritage. Archaeological evidence suggests that early humans cracked bones to eat bone marrow, and ate brains and other high fat tissues (Eaton et al., 1998). These tissues are excellent sources of C20 and C22ω-3 fatty acids (Cordain et al., 1998). In addition, the body fat of concentrate-selector wild ruminants such as deer has higher unsaturated fatty acid levels than that of grazers such as cattle (Meyer et al., 1998). Small, concentrate-selector ruminants probably were important food sources for pre-industrial peoples. The growing popularity of grass-fed beef may help to alter ω-3:ω-6 fatty acid intakes of contemporary humans in a beneficial manner.

A symposium entitled 'Meat or wheat for the next millennium' (Millward, 1999) was a forum for discussing the optimal human diet. An **optimal diet** is one that maximizes health and longevity, prevents nutrient deficiencies, reduces risks for chronic diseases and is composed of foods that are available, safe and palatable. An apparent irony is that human nutritionists and the general public in developed countries are emphasizing diets based largely on foods from plant sources, while in developing countries (where most humans live), plant-based diets are associated with extreme poverty and poor health. When economic conditions improve, these populations increase their consumption of meat, and display improved health (Nestle, 1999). Meat consumption in many cultures is associated with celebration and ceremony. In developing countries, there is often resentment of what is seen as a somewhat arrogant and proselytizing attitude of vegetarians from developed countries, who have purchasing power and choices enabling the selection of varied and appealing meatless diets that are clearly out of reach of people in developing countries (Millward, 1999). Millward (1999, p. 210) concludes 'For a number of highly complex social, political and economic reasons, meat occupies a pivotal position in the global food chain, which is unlikely to change much in the forseeable future.' Reduction in meat consumption in developed countries (where it is higher than optimal) will do little to improve the health of people in developing countries (through release of grain); significant dietary improvement in developing countries mainly requires economic growth, which will allow more people to add animal products to their diets (Rosegrant *et al.*, 1999).

The major dietary energy sources for modern humans are the cereal grains (cereal grains are the edible seeds of grasses). Three cereal grains, wheat, maize (corn) and rice, make up over 75% of world grain production, providing over half of the food energy consumed by humans. Cordain (1999) has called cereal grains our double-edged sword. He claims that except for the last 10,000 years, for the vast majority of human existence we rarely if ever consumed cereal grains. Humans have existed as non-cereal-eating hunter-gatherers since the emergence of *Homo erectus* 1.7 million years ago. Thus, he claims, 'We have had little time (<500 generations) to adapt to a food type which now represents humanity's major source of both calories and protein.' Archaeological evidence of when cereal grains entered the human diet is the appearance of stone processing tools (mortar and pestle) needed for grinding and cooking seeds. These artefacts are irrefutable evidence of when and where cultures began to include cereal grains in their diets. According to Cordain (1999), when cereal grains replaced the animal-based diets of hunter-gatherers, there were characteristic negative effects such as reduction in stature, increased infant mortality, reduced lifespan, increase in infectious diseases, increase in iron-deficiency anaemia, increased osteomalacia, and increased dental caries and enamel defects. Cereal grains are a 'double-edged sword' because without them, civilization as we know it, stemming from the invention of agriculture, would not have developed. On the positive side, the enormous increase in human knowledge would not have taken place without the agricultural revolution. On the other hand, agricultural development has led to societal ills including whole-scale warfare, starvation, tyranny, epidemic diseases and class divisions (Diamond, 1997). While we are no longer hunter-gatherers, our genetic make-up is still that of a palaeolithic hunter-gatherer who is optimally adapted to a diet of meat, fruits and vegetables, not to cereal grains.

Cordain (1999) discusses in considerable detail the nutritional shortcomings of cereal grains. For example, cereal grains are deficient in vitamins (vitamin A activity and several B-complex vitamins such as thiamin, niacin and vitamin B_{12}). Two of the major deficiency diseases that have plagued agricultural humans are **pellagra** and **beriberi**, exclusively associated with consumption of cereal grains. Several B vitamins in grains have a low bioavailability to humans (niacin, pyridoxine, biotin). Cereal grains are extremely deficient in calcium, and they contain phytic acid that greatly reduces bioavailability of phosphorus, zinc, iron and other trace elements. In populations where cereal grains are a major source of calories, osteomalacia, rickets, osteoporosis and iron-deficient anaemia are common. Zinc deficiency is common in some countries like Iran, where bread contributes over 50% of calories. Grains have a high ω-6:ω-3 fatty acid ratio, which may lead to essential-fatty-acid deficiencies. Grains are deficient in essential amino acids. Many people are allergic to proteins in grains. Thus, an important role of meat and other animal products in the human diet is to provide a dietary source for which we are evolutionarily adapted, to make up for problems associated with a food source (grains) for which we are not well adapted.

Shorland (1988) uses the term **nutritional distortion** to indicate the addition to the diet of a component that has been selectively removed from plant or animal tissues, such as fats and oils or sugar, or the incorporation of the residue (e.g. white flour) after removal of a component (e.g. bran). The diseases of Western civilization, including obesity, diabetes and heart disease, may be due in part to caloric concentration by **food processing and refining**. Table sugar and vegetable oils are two obvious examples. Refined flour is energy-concentrated, because the fibre (bran) has been removed. Especially in the case of vegetable oils, this processing may have other implications. Oils in plant tissues occur with natural antioxidants such as tocopherol (vitamin E) and certain phenolic compounds. Shorland (1988, p.193) expresses the concern, 'The indications are that polyunsaturated oils taken out of context of the tissues in which they reside may have adverse nutritional effects.' Perhaps the production of ruminants rich in fat (marbling) by feedlot feeding on concentrates can be viewed as nutritional distortion. The ruminant evolved as a forage eater, not as a seed eater. As discussed earlier, the wild ruminant has a much higher content of ω-3 PUFA in its body fat than the feedlot fed animal, which has been fed an unnatural diet to load its intramuscular tissue with TAGs.

References

Boesch, C. (1999) A theory that's hard to digest. A review: Stanford, C. *The Hunting Apes: Meat Eating and the Origins of Human Behavior.* Princeton University Press, 1999. 245 pp. *Nature* 399, 653.

Brand-Miller, J.C. and Holt, S.H.A. (1998) Australian aboriginal plant foods: a consideration of their nutritional composition and health implications. *Nutrition Research Reviews* 11, 5–23.

Cordain, L. (1999) Cereal grains: humanity's double-edged sword. In: Simopoulos, A.P. (ed.) *Evolutionary Aspects of Nutrition and Health. World Review of Nutrition and Dietetics* 84, 19–73.

Cordain, L. (2002) *The Paleo Diet.* John Wiley and Sons, New York.

Cordain, L., Martin, C., Florant, G. and Watkins, B.A. (1998) The fatty acid composition of muscle, brain, marrow and adipose tissue in elk: evolutionary implications for human dietary lipid requirements. *World Review of Nutrition and Dietetics* 83, 225–226.

Cordain, L., Miller, J.B., Eaton, S.B., Mann, N., Holt, S.H.A. and Speth, J.D. (2000) Plant-animal subsistence ratios and macronutrient energy estimations in worldwide hunter-gatherer diets. *American Journal of Clinical Nutrition* 71, 682–692.

Crawford, M.A. (1968) Fatty-acid ratios in free-living and domestic animals. *Lancet* 1, 1329–1333.

Crawford, M.A. and Gale, M.M. (1969) Linoleic acid and linolenic acid elongation products in muscle tissue of *Syncerus caffer* and other ruminant species. *Biochemical Journal* 115, 25–27.

Diamond, J. (1997) *Guns, Germs and Steel. The Fates of Human Societies.* W.W. Norton and Co., New York.

Eaton, S.B. (1992) Humans, lipids, and evolution. *Lipids* 27, 814–820.

Eaton, S.B. (2006) The ancestral human diet: what was it and should it be a paradigm for contemporary nutrition? *Proceedings of the Nutrition Society* 65, 1–6.

Eaton, S.B. and Konner, M. (1985) Paleolithic nutrition: a consideration of its nature and current implications. *New England Journal of Medicine* 312, 283–289.

Eaton, S.B., Eaton III, S.B., Konner, M.J. and Shostak, M. (1996) An evolutionary perspective enhances understanding of human nutritional requirements. *Journal of Nutrition* 126, 1732–1740.

Eaton, S.B., Eaton III, S.B., Sinclair, A.J., Cordain, L. and Mann, N.J. (1998) Dietary intake of long-chain polyunsaturated fatty acids during the Paleolithic. In: Simopoulos, A.P. (ed.) *The Return of ω3 Fatty Acids into the Food Supply. I. Land-Based Animal Food Products and Their Health Effects. World Review of Nutrition and Dietetics* 83, 12–23.

Frassetto, L.A., Morris, R.C., Jr, Sellmeyer, D.E., Todd, K. and Sebastian, A. (2001) Diet, evolution and aging. The pathophysiological effects of the post-agricultural inversion of the potassium-to-sodium and base-to-chloride ratios in the human diet. *European Journal of Nutrition* 40, 200–213.

Gale, M.M., Crawford, M.A. and Woodford, M. (1969) The fatty acid composition of adipose and muscle tissue in domestic and free-living ruminants. *Biochemical Journal* 113, 6.

Hankins, O.G., Ellis, N.R. and Zeller, J.H. (1928) Some results of soft pork investigations. *United States Department of Agriculture (USDA) Agricultural Bulletin* 1492.

Jajoo, R., Song, L., Rasmussen, H., Harris, S.S. and Dawson-Hughes, B. (2006) Dietary acid-base balance, bone resorption, and calcium excretion. *Journal of the American College of Nutrition* 25, 224–230.

Larick, D.K. and Turner, B.E. (1989) Influence of finishing diet on the phospholipid composition and fatty acid profile of individual phospholipids in lean muscle of beef cattle. *Journal of Animal Science* 67, 2282–2293.

Logan, A.G. (2006) Dietary sodium intake and its relation to human health: a summary of the evidence. *Journal of the American College of Nutrition* 25, 165–169.

Meyer, H.H.D., Rowell, A., Streich, W.J., Stoffel, B. and Hofmann, R.R. (1998) Accumulation of polyunsaturated fatty acids by concentrate selecting ruminants. *Comparative Biochemistry and Physiology Part A* 120, 263–268.

Millward, D.J. (1999) Meat or wheat for the next millennium? *Proceedings of the Nutrition Society* 58, 209–210.

Nestle, M. (1999) Meat or wheat for the next millennium? Plenary lecture. Animal v. plant foods in human diets and health: is the historical record unequivocal? *Proceedings of the Nutrition Society* 58, 211–218.

O'Dea, K. (1991) Traditional diet and food preferences of Australian aboriginal hunter-gatherers. *Philosophical Transactions of the Royal Society London B* 334, 233–241.

Rosegrant, M.W., Leach, N. and Gerpacio, R.V. (1999) Meat or wheat for the next millennium? Plenary lecture. Alternative futures for world cereal and meat consumption. *Proceedings of the Nutrition Society* 58, 219–234.

Sebastion, A., Frassetto, L.A., Sellmeyer, D.E., Merriam, R.L. and Morris, R.C. (2002) Estimation of the net acid load of the diet of ancestral preagricultural *Homo sapiens* and their hominid ancestors. *American Journal of Clinical Nutrition* 76, 1308–1316.

Shorland, E.B. (1988) Is our knowledge of human nutrition soundly based? *World Review of Nutrition and Dietetics* 57, 126–213.

Simopoulos, A.P. (1998) Overview of evolutionary aspects of ω-3 fatty acids in the diet. In: Simopoulos, A.P. (ed.) The return of ω-3 fatty acids into the food supply. I. Land-based animal food products and their health effects. *World Review of Nutrition and Dietetics* 83, 1–11.

Sponheimer, M. and Lee-Thorp, J.A. (1999) Isotopic evidence for the diet of an early hominid, *Australopithecus africanus*. *Science* 283, 368–370.

Stanford, C.B. and Bunn, H.T. (eds) (2001) *Meat Eating and Human Evolution*. Oxford University Press, New York.

Widdowson, E.M. and Whiten, A. (eds) (1991) Foraging strategies and natural diet of monkeys, apes and humans. *Philosophical Transactions of the Royal Society London B* 334, 159–295.

Zoran, D.L. (2002) The carnivore connection to nutrition in cats. *Journal of the American Veterinary Medical Association* 221, 1559–1567.

16 Disorders and Unique Aspects of Energy Metabolism

A number of metabolic disorders have their basis in disturbances in energy metabolism. These include diabetes, metabolic syndrome and ketosis. Besides these, other aspects of energy metabolism discussed in this chapter include metabolic events in obesity and longevity. The 'thrifty gene' concept in humans is discussed.

Ketosis

Ketosis is a metabolic disease in which excessive quantities of ketone bodies (Chapter 12) are produced. It commonly occurs in starvation when body lipid is mobilized, and is a frequent condition in domestic ruminants (twin-lamb disease or pregnancy paralysis in sheep; ketosis and downer cow syndrome in dairy cattle). A critical factor in the development of ketosis is insufficiency of glucose for brain metabolism. Glucose is specifically required as an energy source by some tissues. For example, the brain and central nervous system require glucose, although ketone bodies can be used to some extent. The energy requirement of the brain under normal circumstances is met almost entirely from the metabolism of glucose. The **blood-brain barrier** limits the penetration of large molecules, such as lipids, into the brain. As a result, the brain depends on glucose to meet its very high energy needs.

One explanation for ketosis is the oxaloacetate shortage theory. The **oxaloacetate shortage theory of ketosis** is probably an over-simplification, but does provide for a meaningful explanation of the metabolic causes of ketosis in ruminants. In ruminants, carbohydrate-derived energy is absorbed not as glucose but as volatile fatty acids (VFAs), mainly acetate, propionate and butyrate. Of these, propionate is glucogenic while acetate and butyrate are ketogenic. Propionate is glucogenic because it is converted to succinate in the citric acid cycle. Each molecule of propionate which enters the cells yields

a net increase in oxaloacetate (OAA). OAA can be converted to pyruvate, which by reverse glycolysis can yield glucose. (The conversion of pyruvate to acetyl CoA is not reversible; thus the glucogenesis pathway begins with OAA.) Conversely, there is no net increase in OAA by metabolism of acetate and butyrate. Butyrate is converted to acetate. Every molecule of acetate that enters the citric acid cycle (also known as the **TCA cycle**) requires one OAA, and one OAA is produced at the end of each turn of the TCA cycle. Thus by catabolism of acetate, there can be no net synthesis of OAA.

Pregnancy disease in sheep occurs in late gestation, particularly in ewes with multiple fetuses. Multiple fetuses decrease feed intake of the ewe by reducing the rumen volume (Forbes, 1970); the fetuses take up a major portion of the abdominal cavity. Thus the late gestation ewe may not be able to eat enough to meet her energy requirements, so body lipid is mobilized. This produces a high yield of acetyl CoA. The brain specifically requires glucose as its fuel, and brain metabolism represents a major part of total energy expenditure. Also, glucose is the only fuel used by fetal tissues. Thus the ewe needs to synthesize glucose (glucogenesis) from OAA, to maintain blood glucose to support brain metabolism and fetal growth. Because of excess (above energy needs of the liver) mobilization of fatty acids, the liver is burdened with an excess of fatty acids and thus acetyl CoA. The excess acetyl CoA is converted to ketone bodies. When pregnancy disease occurs, the amount of OAA is insufficient to meet both of these requirements, so the brain suffers from lack of glucose, and there is an excess of ketones. The ewe goes into a coma from the brain's lack of glucose, and the expired air smells of acetone, due to the respiratory excretion of ketones. Treatment involves intravenous glucose administration. Prevention can involve increasing ruminal propionate production by feeding grain, which increases energy intake, and the molar proportion of propionate in total ruminal VFA production increases when grain replaces roughage. Multiple fetuses exacerbate ketosis in ewes by causing an increased fetal demand for glucose and a reduced feed intake by suppression of rumen volume. Similar metabolic events occur in high producing early-lactation dairy cows. They need to synthesize large amounts of glucose to synthesize lactose in the mammary gland, and they mobilize body fat because feed intake cannot support the high-energy demands of peak lactation.

Sheep and cattle that are adapted to very cold conditions may adjust their comfort zone (Chapter 17). The **lower critical temperature** is the environmental temperature below which an animal must expend extra metabolic energy to maintain body temperature. Webster *et al.* (1969) found that in sheep exposed to cold, the lower critical temperature dropped from −14°C in November to −35°C in March. They state, 'Cold-acclimated ewes, with a lower critical temperature of −35°C, might exhibit heat stress when brought into a building at any temperature above 0°C.' Webster *et al.* (1970) have shown that cold-acclimated cattle experience severe heat stress at 20°C. Heat stress results in reduced feed intake. Thus moving cold-acclimated ewes or cows into warm housing, which seems intuitively reasonable at calving or lambing, might actually induce ketosis (Karihaloo *et al.*, 1970) by inhibiting feed intake.

Ketosis in **dairy cattle** generally occurs in the early stage of lactation in cows in negative energy balance. Inciting factors include an inadequate post-parturient feed intake, high milk production and mobilization of body lipid to sustain energy needs, especially in cows with high body fat. There is a lack of carbohydrate precursors such as propionate and amino acids for incorporation of fats (as acetyl CoA) into the citric acid cycle, so ketone bodies are produced at greater rates. Ketosis is often secondary to other disorders that depress feed intake. Some feed supplements when fed during the transition period (just prior to and just after parturition) may reduce the incidence of ketosis. These include chromium (Besong *et al.*, 1996), Rumensin®, niacin (Jaster and Ward, 1990) and calcium propionate and propylene glycol (Stokes and Goff, 2001). Calcium propionate and propylene glycol function by increasing available propionate, which produces a net increase in gluconeogenesis and leads to an increase in insulin, which decreases lipolysis. Ketosis in dairy cattle and sheep is treated by intravenous administration of glucose, dexamethasone[1] and glucose precursors.

The events occuring in ketosis are shown in Fig. 16.1 and are as follows (the numbers apply to the reactions in Fig. 16.1):

1. There is a high demand for glucose (for brain metabolism and fetal growth in sheep; and lactose synthesis in dairy cattle).
2. Glucogenesis occurs by the reverse of glycolysis.
3. Acetyl CoA cannot be converted to pyruvate; the reaction by which pyruvate enters the TCA cycle is irreversible.
4. OAA is used to synthesize pyruvate, which in turn produces glucose.
5. A shortage of propionate from rumen fermentation limits OAA production.
6. Acetyl CoA concentrations are increased because body lipid is mobilized to meet energy demands. Excess fatty acids being mobilized causes fatty liver.
7. There is a shortage of glucose precursors (e.g. OAA) for both glucogenesis (4) and entrance of acetyl CoA into the TCA cycle (7).
8. Excess acetyl CoA is converted to ketone bodies, leading to excretion of acetone in the expired air (9).

Ketosis in dairy cattle is rarely fatal, while it is often fatal in pregnant ewes. Cows can reduce the metabolic need for glucose by decreasing milk secretion, but the ewe is unable to reduce the increasing glucose requirements of late-term fetuses. The conditions described above are referred to as **primary ketosis**, which is a pathological state arising from the unmet demand for a high rate of gluconeogenesis. **Secondary ketosis** often accompanies other disease states, occurring as a response to stress and lack of feed intake. These conditions stimulate lipid mobilization and a rise in blood ketones.

Diabetes

Diabetes mellitus (*diabetes* from Greek referring to excessive urination; *mellitus* from Greek referring to sugar in urine) is a metabolic disorder characterized by elevated concentrations of blood glucose (**hyperglycaemia**). There are four major categories of diabetes: (i) Type 1; (ii) Type 2; (iii) gestational; and (iv) secondary. The major ones, Type 1 and Type 2, will be the ones discussed here. Type 2 is the most common form; 90–95% of the diabetics in the USA have this type.

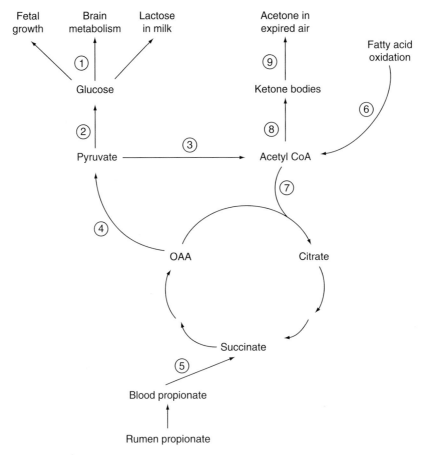

Fig. 16.1. Metabolic reactions involved in ketosis. See text for discussion of the numbered reactions.

Type 1 diabetes

This type occurs most often in childhood, and was formerly called juvenile-onset diabetes or insulin-dependent diabetes mellitus. Type 1 diabetes is an autoimmune disorder; the immune system produces antibodies that attack and destroy the insulin-producing β-cells of the pancreas. Loss of β-cells results in a lack of insulin production, leading to the onset of the signs of diabetes. These signs include extreme thirst, hunger, frequent urination and fatigue. These symptoms are all a result of elevated blood glucose.

Type 2 diabetes and insulin resistance

In humans, Type 2 diabetes occurs most frequently in middle-aged and older adults. Most people with this condition have normal or above normal

concentrations of blood insulin. Type 2 diabetes is caused by **insulin resistance**, which means that the body's cells cannot respond to insulin. Insulin functions in the transfer of glucose across cell membranes. Insulin binds to insulin receptors on the surface of tissue cell membranes, allowing glucose to enter the cells. Insulin resistance occurs when the cell receptors do not recognize or bind insulin. With insulin resistance, glucose uptake is impaired and hyperglycaemia results. Chronic hyperglycaemia damages blood vessels and nerves, sometimes leading to blindness and limb amputation. Some Type 2 patients respond to exogenous insulin, although insulin resistance does not imply a lack of the hormone. In these patients, a chronic over-stimulation of the pancreas to produce more insulin in response to hyperglycaemia may eventually cause the pancreatic β-cells to 'wear out'. Besides its role in diabetes, insulin resistance is also a major factor in the development of metabolic syndrome (this chapter), in both humans and equines.

The Glycaemic Index

Carbohydrates that are digested slowly and release glucose gradually may produce metabolic effects that are different from dietary carbohydrates which are digested rapidly. The **glycaemic index** measures the blood glucose response to a fixed amount of dietary carbohydrate compared to the same amount of a standard carbohydrate source (formerly glucose, but now white bread), and thus measures the blood-glucose-raising potential of foods. The blood-glucose area under the curve (see Fig. 15.1 in Chapter 15) in a glucose tolerance test is expressed as a percentage of the standard. The **glycaemic load**, which assesses the total glycaemic effect of the diet, is the product of the dietary glycaemic index and the total dietary carbohydrate (Jenkins *et al.*, 2002). The glycaemic index of cereal products is explained by their contents of slowly versus rapidly digested carbohydrates (Englyst *et al.*, 2003). Numerous factors affect the glycaemic index, including the nature of the starch, cooking and food processing methods, particle size, and the presence of fibre, lipid and proteins. The chemical nature of carbohydrates includes the type of monosaccharide (fructose and galactose have a lower glycaemic index than glucose), type of starch (amylopectin is digested more rapidly than amylose), and the presence of viscous non-starch polysaccharides (gums, β-glucans) which because of their viscosity reduce the rate of glucose absorption (Aston, 2006). Foods with an intact botanical structure (whole grains) are digested more slowly than those with processed, gelatinized starch (consistent with Shorland's nutritional distortion concept, see Chapter 15). Cooking, processing and refining all tend to increase the glycaemic index. Foods that contain **inulin** (polymerized fructose), such as Jerusalem artichokes, have a low glycaemic index because inulin is indigestible. Low glycaemic index foods, such as whole grains and unprocessed foods, tend to produce a gradual, continual absorption of glucose rather than a blood **glucose spike** that can occur with rapidly digested and absorbed carbohydrates. A glucose spike can trigger over-secretion of insulin, which may produce hypoglycaemia, triggering a metabolic response (glucagon, epinephrine secretion), which restores glucose homeostasis but also causes lipolysis and release of free fatty acids into the blood. Low glycaemic-load diets tend to attenuate or modulate rapid shifts in blood glucose and fatty acids, which has benefits in a wide variety of metabolic disorders (Jenkins *et al.*, 2002; Aston, 2006).

Foods with a high glycaemic index (70–99) include corn flakes, baked potato, croissant, candy; medium glycaemic index (56–69) foods include whole wheat products including bread, rice, sweet potato and table sugar; and low glycaemic index foods include most fruit and vegetables, pasta, legumes/pulses (e.g. beans and peas) and low carbohydrate foods (meat, fish, eggs, oils).

The starchy staples of many traditional diets were often foods that had low glycaemic indexes, such as pasta, wholegrain breads, rice, dried pulses (peas, beans, lentils). A classic case involves the **Pima Indians** of the US southwest and northern Mexico. Those in the USA had adopted a Western diet of processed foods, and have very high rates of diabetes and obesity. Pima Indians in Mexico retain a traditional lifestyle, and have a low incidence of these disorders. People who traditionally inhabited harsh environments with irregular food availability may have a **thrifty gene**(s) that allows them to survive famine and starvation, but also makes them susceptible to obesity when food is abundant.

Glucose tolerance is the ability of the body to regulate blood glucose after the administration of a test dose of glucose. Glucose tolerance is impaired in both Type 1 and Type 2 diabetes. In a normal glucose tolerance test, blood glucose returns to normal rapidly in a normal subject (see Fig. 15.1). In an individual with impaired glucose tolerance, the blood glucose rises to a high peak and returns to normal more slowly, because of impaired glucose uptake by the body tissues. In Type 1 diabetes, this is due to lack of insulin, while in Type 2 it is caused by insulin resistance.

The glycaemic index concept has been applied in **equine nutrition**. High glycaemic feeds are those rich in starch and fermentable sugars such as fructans. Kronfeld *et al.* (2005) have reviewed the topic. Examples of high glycaemic feeds are grains (maize, oats, wheat, barley), sweet feeds (containing molasses) and beet pulp. Low glycaemic feeds include lucerne, wheat bran and rice bran. A high glycaemic load may increase susceptibility to various disorders including gastrointestinal disturbances, laminitis and insulin resistance.

Metabolic Syndrome

Metabolic syndrome has been proposed as a disorder in humans characterized by impaired insulin sensitivity, hyperglycaemia, elevated blood triacylglycerol (TAG), abdominal obesity and hypertension (Shaw *et al.*, 2005). **Insulin resistance** refers to the lack of effect of insulin in stimulating glucose uptake by tissue cells, resulting in hyperinsulinaemia and hyperglycaemia. Similarly, normal effects of insulin on lipid metabolism are reduced, causing elevated blood TAG and HDL cholesterol concentrations. Metabolic syndrome increases risk of Type 2 diabetes and cardiovascular disease. Dietary factors may influence hyperinsulinaemia. For example, chili peppers (*Capsicum annum*) decrease postprandial (after eating) blood insulin concentrations, which may have a favourable effect on lowering insulin, obesity and cardiovascular disease (Ahuja *et al.*, 2006). A number of other herbs, cited by these authors, have similar effects.

Brand-Miller and Colagiuri (1999) proposed that widespread incidence of insulin resistance in modern humans is a reflection of the evolutionary history of humans as carnivores. Their hypothesis (the carnivore connection) proposes:

> that the selective force for insulin resistance was the low-carbohydrate, high-meat diet that prevailed in many parts of the world during the Ice Ages that spanned the last two million years of human evolution. In this environment, we argue that insulin sensitivity would have been a liability, compromising survival and reproductive performance.

Equine metabolic syndrome is a disorder in horses with similarities to human metabolic syndrome. Affected horses are obese, have insulin resistance and chronic laminitis, in the absence of usual inciting factors for laminitis. Affected horses are often grossly obese, with excessive accumulation of adipose tissue in the crest of the neck, over the rump and around the tail head. Treatment involves strict limitation of soluble carbohydrates in the diet. Grain feeding and pasture should be avoided, with the diet based on good quality grass hay (1–1.5% of body weight/day). The causes of laminitis in horses with equine metabolic syndrome are not well defined. Increased cortisol secretion caused by disturbances in fat metabolism may play a role in the predisposition to laminitis. Vick *et al.* (2007) uncovered an association between obesity, insulin sensitivity and inflammatory cytokines in horses. Elevated **inflammatory cytokines** such as tumour necrosis factor (TNFα) and interleukins have a direct role in development of obesity-associated insulin resistance. Vick *et al.* (2006) have also associated abnormal reproductive function in mares with obesity and insulin resistance.

Insulin resistance in horses has been reviewed by Kronfeld *et al.* (2005). Growing horses chronically adapted to high glycaemic-load diets (rich in sugars and starch) develop decreased insulin-mediated glucose metabolism (Treiber *et al.*, 2005). This decreased insulin sensitivity is compensated for by increased insulin secretion, which may increase the risk of metabolic disease. Adaptation by increased insulin secretion may maintain glucose homeostasis but may alter insulin signalling in other systems, increasing the risk of metabolic disorder (Treiber *et al.*, 2005). Dietary management involves reducing intake of fermentable carbohydrates (starch, sugars, fructans) and maintaining energy intakes with supplementary lipid (e.g. vegetable oil). Ponies that are predisposed to develop laminitis (prelaminitic metabolic syndrome) are insulin resistant and have exaggerated production of insulin in response to dietary fructans (Bailey *et al.*, 2007).

Hyperglycaemia is a common finding in horses with acute abdominal disease or colic (Hollis *et al.*, 2007). The cause of hyperglycaemia may reside in endocrine dysfunction and/or the release of pro-inflammatory cytokines.

Sucrose, Fructose and Metabolic Syndrome

Table sugar (sucrose) is widely added to processed foods. The availability of abundant amounts of sucrose is a recent development. Before the discovery of the Americas and the development of large-scale sugarcane production, most humans consumed virtually no sugar (Fig. 16.2), and very small amounts of honey. Beginning in the 1970s, **high fructose corn syrup** (HFCS) has become an extensively used sweetener.

The rapid increase in sucrose and HFCS consumption by humans has been paralleled by a rapid increase in '**diseases of Western civilization**' such as diabetes, coronary heart disease, obesity, hypertension, kidney disease and metabolic syndrome, suggesting a possible relationship between sugar consumption and these diseases (Bray, 2007; Johnson *et al.*, 2007). Several lines of evidence suggest that fructose, as half the sucrose molecule and the major component of HFCS, may be the

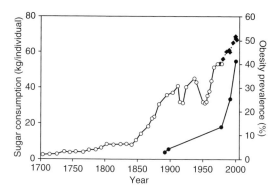

Fig. 16.2. Sugar intake per capita in the UK from 1700 to 1978 (○) and in the USA from 1975 to 2000 (■) compared to the obesity rates in the USA for non-Hispanic white males (•) (courtesy of R.J. Johnson and the *American Journal of Clinical Nutrition*).

component of concern. Fructose differs in several important ways from glucose. Fructose is absorbed from the gastrointestinal tract by a different mechanism than glucose. Glucose stimulates insulin secretion by the pancreas, but fructose does not. Fructose cannot enter most tissue cells, whereas glucose is taken up by all cells. Fructose is taken up by the liver, and can enter the metabolic pathway for glycerol synthesis (glycerol is the 'backbone' of fats – i.e. triacylglycerols). Fructose is metabolized in the liver by phosphorylation on the 1-position which bypasses the rate-limiting phosphofructokinase step. Thus fructose metabolism in the liver favours lipogenesis. The ADP formed from ATP after phosphorylation of fructose can be further metabolized to **uric acid**, raising blood uric acid levels. Besides causing gout, uric acid has numerous metabolic effects, including stimulating the release of inflammatory substances in vascular tissue. Elevated uric acid is a risk factor for such diseases as obesity, renal disease and cardiovascular diseases (Johnson *et al.*, 2007). Uric acid decreases endothelial nitric oxide concentration, which predisposes development of the metabolic syndrome, including hypertension, hypertriacylglycerolaemia and insulin resistance (Johnson *et al.*, 2007).

Fructose may cause **obesity** by several different mechanisms. Fructose may not cause the degree of satiety equivalent to that of a glucose-based meal, due to the inability of fructose to stimulate insulin and leptin and to inhibit ghrelin, all factors which affect the satiety centre in the brain (Johnson *et al.*, 2007). Fructose-induced elevation of plasma uric

acid reduces secretion of **adiponectin** from the adipocytes. Adiponectin acts with leptin to cause satiety. Fructose increases the synthesis of fatty acids and stimulates liver re-esterification of fatty acids from all sources (Parks *et al.*, 2008).

Thus there are good reasons to believe that the **diseases of Western civilization** are due in part to the high intakes of sucrose and fructose (from HFCS and well as from sucrose) in the modern diet. It is interesting that since widespread use of HFCS in soft drinks and processed foods has occurred, there has been an effective public relations campaign in the USA to reduce lipid consumption, but an 'obesity epidemic' has nevertheless developed. There is increasing concern that fructose is the major culprit (Bray, 2007).

Chromium – the Glucose Tolerance Factor

Chromium has been identified as an essential nutrient for humans and animals (Mertz, 1993). It is a component of the **glucose tolerance factor**, a complex containing trivalent chromium, nicotinic acid (niacin) and amino acids. The glucose tolerance factor potentiates the action of insulin in the uptake of glucose by cells. 'Glucose tolerance' refers to the ability of glucose to be taken up by cells. With impaired glucose tolerance, cellular uptake of glucose is subnormal and blood glucose levels are elevated (**hyperglycaemia**), as in the disease diabetes. Some cases of diabetes are responsive to supplemental chromium (Mertz, 1993). Because of its effect on insulin, chromium influences carbohydrate, fat and protein metabolism. Chromium is absorbed most effectively in an organic form, with chromium picolinate being the most common supplemented form. Picolinic acid is an organic acid derived from the vitamin niacin and the amino acid tryptophan (see Fig. 6.14 in Chapter 6). **Chromium picolinate** is approved as a feed additive for pigs. When fed to growing-finishing pigs, it increases leanness and reduces carcass fat (Kornegay *et al.*, 1997; Mooney and Cromwell, 1997).

In cattle, chromium supplementation has been of interest as a means of increasing the immunocompetence of stressed calves entering the feedlot (Mowat *et al.*, 1993; Chang *et al.*, 1995). Chromium supplementation has beneficial effects in reducing morbidity (illness) from pneumonia, shipping fever and other forms of respiratory disease. Van Heugten and Spears (1997) did not find an effect of chromium as chromium chloride, chromium picolinate or chromium nicotinic acid complex on the immune status of stressed pigs. Data that unequivocally show an immunostimulatory effect of chromium are lacking, but it is documented that under stressful conditions there is increased loss of chromium in the urine (Van Heugten and Spears, 1997). Kegley *et al.* (1997) found that supplemental chromium improved the growth rate of steers that were stressed by transportation but did not have any effect on immune responses, suggesting other modes of action may be involved.

Caloric Restriction and Longevity

In the 1930s, McCay *et al.* (1935) at Cornell University reported that growing rats fed a severely restricted allotment of food, sufficient to cause growth to cease, had elongated lifespans. When they were older than the normal lifespan of rats, they were still capable of growing and nearly reaching normal body size. This study was the first major research which demonstrated that caloric restriction retards ageing and extends median and maximal lifespan (Heilbronn and Ravussin, 2003). Since the work of McCay *et al.*, similar findings have been reported for a variety of species including rats, mice, fish, flies, worms and yeast. A 25% diet restriction of dogs resulted in increased lifespan in a two-decade study (Lawler *et al.*, 2008). Large animals tend to live longer than small animals, a relationship which correlates with metabolic rate. The naked (African) mole rat (see Chapter 18) has an extraordinarily long maximum lifespan exceeding 28 years (Hulbert *et al.*, 2007; Buffenstein, 2008). Mole rats in captivity live over nine times as long as similar sized mice. They show no decline in fertility even into the third decade of life, and have never been observed to develop neoplasms (Buffenstein, 2008). Compared to other animals of similar size, such as sheep and pigs, humans also have an extremely long lifespan.

Cellular metabolism inevitably produces peroxides and other oxidants (see Chapter 13). One theory to account for the longevity response to caloric restriction is that the reduced rate of metabolism caused by energy restriction results in a lower production of **reactive oxygen species** (**ROS**) which are linked to tissue damage (the oxidative-stress theory of ageing). Reducing metabolic rate by using caloric restriction may reduce oxygen consumption,

which could reduce ROS such as superoxide radicals, hydrogen peroxide and other oxidants, potentially increasing lifespan (Heilbronn and Ravussin, 2003). The species-specific fatty acid composition of cell membranes may influence the susceptibility of animals to oxidative damage (Hulbert *et al.*, 2007).

Ageing is associated with a general decline in the vitality of cells, tissues and organs, as well as with cognitive decline and age-related disorders associated with brain pathology (Milgram *et al.*, 2007). Much of the ageing process may be a consequence of oxidative damage to mitochondria. There is evidence that mitochondrial decay can be delayed by dietary supplements of α-lipoic acid and acetyl-L-carnitine (Milgram *et al.*, 2007). Lipoic acid functions in the formation of acetyl CoA while carnitine (see Fig. 12.4 in Chapter 12) functions in the transport of activated long-chain fatty acids across the mitochondrial membrane (see Chapter 12).

There is evidence that a class of proteins, called **sirtuins**, may have a role in the mode of action of caloric restriction on increasing longevity (Wood *et al.*, 2004). Certain dietary phenolics such as resveratrol (found in grape skins and red wine) appear to activate sirtuins. The effects of caloric restriction on longevity of humans are unknown, although there is some evidence of such an effect in monkeys (Heilbronn and Ravussin, 2003). A long-term trial in humans (Comprehensive Assessment of Long-Term Effects of Reducing Intake of Energy), funded by the National Institute of Aging, is in progress.

Should our eating habits be more like those of feedlot steers and broiler chickens or like those of range cattle and wild pigs? There is considerable evidence that there is genetic control of the ageing process, with tissue cells capable of a finite number of cell divisions. This 'biological clock' seems to operate by a shortening of the chromosomes each time a cell divides, until a critical length of the **telomere** (non-gene end section of chromosomes) is reached (de Lange, 1998). When the rate of metabolism is slowed by undernutrition, the **ageing process** is retarded because of the slower rate of cell division. In simple terms, we have a finite amount of metabolism possible before a genetic programme causes the system to self-destruct. A fast rate of metabolism uses up the allotted metabolic capacity more quickly, whereas a slow metabolic rate prolongs it (the rate-of-living theory of ageing). In a review of this subject, Lynn and Wallwork (1992, p.1917) stated, 'Rate of living, i.e. metabolic rate, is proportional to rate of ageing, i.e. rate of degenerative cell destruction.'

The Western-style low fibre diet, with a high density of protein and energy from meat, milk, vegetable oils, sugar and so on, supports a very rapid growth rate. Children fed a typical Western diet grow faster, reach puberty quicker, and are taller and heavier as adults than those in developing countries consuming a higher fibre, lower energy diet based on complex carbohydrates (rice, cassava) with less or no animal protein. Maximizing the growth rate of humans is not necessarily the best strategy for optimizing longevity and freedom from degenerative diseases. Perhaps the same is true for companion animals and horses, for whom longevity is a desired quality.

The Thyroid Hormones – Major Integrators of Metabolism

The thyroid gland produces several **thyroid hormones** (**THs**) that have many important roles in virtually all aspects of animal metabolism. The major THs are **thyroxine** (**T4**), also referred to as tetraiodothyronine, and **triiodothyronine** (**T3**)

(Fig. 16.3). T4 is synthesized in the thyroid gland, and released into the circulation. T4 is converted into the metabolically active form, T3, in the tissues.

A large iodine-containing (iodinated) glycoprotein called **thyroglobulin** is the precursor of T4. Inorganic iodine, the iodide ion (I^-) is taken up by the thyroid, linked to a Na^+-K^- ATPase-dependent I^- transporter. The activity of this transporter is controlled by **thyroid-stimulating hormone** (**TSH**) produced in the pituitary gland. TSH release in turn is controlled by **thyrotropin releasing hormone** (**TRH**) produced in the pituitary gland. Thus TH synthesis and secretion are finely regulated by a negative feedback system, the hypothalamic/pituitary/thyroid axis (Yen, 2001).

In the thyroid gland, I^- is oxidized by the action of a peroxidase utilizing hydrogen peroxide, (H_2O_2), and incorporated into the thyroglobulin molecule. This synthesis involves the production of diiodothyronines (DITs) by reaction of iodide with tyrosine; two DITs react together within the thyroglobulin molecule to form T4 (Fig. 16.3). After stimulation with TSH, thyroglobulin is hydrolysed into its constituent amino acids, including T4 and T3.

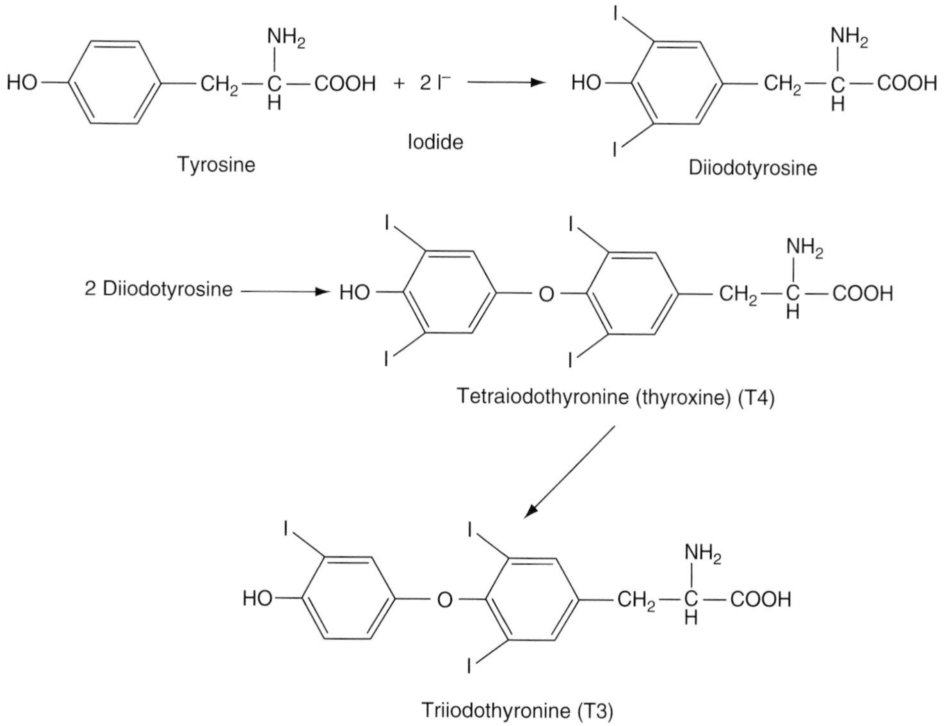

Fig. 16.3. Synthesis of thyroid hormones (T3 and T4) from the amino acid tyrosine.

Selenium is a component of three selenoenzymes involved in activation and metabolism of THs, the iodothyronine deiodinases. For example, a **deiodinase** is required for conversion of T4 to T3. Unique features of THs are that they have the same molecular structure in all organisms, and that they are absorbed intact in the digestive tract, and so can be obtained exogenously. In carnivores, THs are obtained from the consumption of prey, in addition to endogenous synthesis. Although THs are synthesized enzymatically in the thyroid, T4 can be readily formed without enzymatic involvement. For example, casein can be treated with iodine to form **iodinated casein**, which when fed to animals releases THs in the gut. A feed additive (Protamone®) containing iodinated casein has been used to improve growth and milk production.

Numerous plants contain thyroid inhibitors, or **goitrogens**. Plants in the cabbage family (genus *Brassica*) are particularly noteworthy for their goitrogenic activity (Cheeke, 1998). Brassicas contain sulfur-containing compounds called glucosinolates. Derivatives of **glucosinolates**, such as thiocyanates and isothiocyanates, are goitrogens. These compounds inhibit the uptake of iodine by the thyroid. The shortage of iodine in the gland impairs production of THs, causing the thyroid gland to enlarge (**goitre**). Causes of goitre include either a dietary deficiency of iodine, presence of goitrogens or a combination of both.

THs are released into the blood as a result of a three-step hormonal relay: (i) TRH is released from the hypothalamus; (ii) this induces the release of TSH by the pituitary gland; and (iii) TSH stimulates TH release from the thyroid gland into the blood. THs are transported in the circulatory system in association with plasma proteins, including thyroxine-binding globulin (TBG), serum albumin and transthyretin. Transthyretin also transports retinoic acid, a form of vitamin A that shares with TH some of the same roles in embryonic development. A somewhat crude estimate of total blood TH is **protein-bound iodine** (PBI), which is determined by measuring the iodine content of precipitated plasma proteins.

The metabolic actions of THs involve gene regulation. **Thyroid hormone receptor-associated proteins** (TRAPs) bind TH to specific DNA sequences, resulting in T3-regulated transcription (Yen, 2001), inducing enzyme synthesis. Examples include enzymes involved in energy metabolism, such as acetyl CoA carboxylase, malic enzyme, glucose-6-

phosphate dehydrogenase, fatty acid synthase and other lipogenic enzymes (Yen, 2001). TH also regulates the synthesis and secretion of several pituitary hormones, such as growth hormone. While most of the effects of T3 are mediated by TH regulation of target gene transcription in the nucleus, there are some non-genomic effects of TH (Yen, 2001). For example, T3 enhances uptake of sugars by tissues by a direct effect on membrane transport systems. Another non-genomic effect is the stimulation of Ca^{++}-ATPase production in cell membranes, increasing oxidative phosphorylation in mitochondria, increasing heat production (metabolic rate).

Crockford (2003, 2006) has advanced a unique hypothesis to explain **evolutionary processes**, including animal domestication. The THs are essential regulators of many biological processes beginning with the earliest stages of embryonic growth, and continuing throughout the entire postnatal period, including reproductive functions and the behavioural and physiological responses to stress. Crockford (2006) hypothesizes that species-specific rhythms in TH secretion, in a pulsatile manner, control developmental events, and can explain rapid evolutionary changes, such as the conversion of wolves to dogs in the domestication process. Her theory states that the biological mechanism responsible for generating new species – reproductively isolated descendant populations with a distinctive suite of well-coordinated traits – involves selection for particular variants of TH production patterns that occur naturally within ancestral species (Crockford, 2003).

Crockford (2006), in presenting her theory of thyroid-induced evolution, summarized the physiological effects of THs, concluding that 'the range of body functions influenced or controlled by thyroid hormones is truly staggering'. Some of these listed by Crockford (2006) are:

1. THs control brain and body growth of the embryo, beginning just after conception. During fetal development, TH is initially supplied by maternal transport across the placenta, and later by the developing fetal thyroid gland. During fetal development, severely deficient concentrations of maternal THs (usually from iodine deficiency) cause profound mental retardation (cretinism); mild TH insufficiency can cause detectable brain defects.
2. THs control the rate of metabolism, including carbohydrate and fat metabolism and the rate of oxidative reactions.

3. TH regulates hair growth and colour, including both initial growth of hair and seasonal changes, such as annual moults. The pattern of hair pigmentation (e.g. piebalding) is determined during fetal development. One of the colour-producing genes that operates in melanocytes is **melanocyte-stimulating hormone** (MSH), which is dependent on TH.

4. TH controls metamorphosis (e.g. conversion of tadpoles to frogs), certain body form changes in fish and hibernation.
5. THs are involved in regulating reproduction.
6. TH synchronizes the body's response to stress and behavioural responses to psychological stresses such as fear of predators.

Questions and Study Guide

1. Dosing of dairy cattle affected with ketosis with a solution of sodium acetate is not an effective treatment. Why not?
2. Ewes with pregnancy disease have a higher mortality rate than dairy cows with ketosis. Why?
3. Explain the metabolic events that could cause a cold-adapted pregnant ewe to develop ketosis when penned up in a warm barn.
4. What is the glycaemic index? How can it be used in the feeding of horses?
5. What is meant by the 'thrifty gene hypothesis'?
6. How is a glucose tolerance test conducted?
7. What is equine metabolic syndrome? How are horses with this condition managed?
8. In what ways does the metabolism of fructose differ from glucose metabolism?
9. What is the glucose tolerance factor?
10. What is the apparent relationship between caloric intake and longevity? What is the relevance of this relationship to the contemporary American diet?
11. How is selenium involved in activities of the thyroid gland?

Note

[1] Dexamethasone is a synthetic glucocorticoid hormone with potent glucogenic effects.

References

Ahuja, K.D.K., Robertson, I.K., Geraughty, D.P. and Ball, M.J. (2006) Effects of chili consumption on postprandial glucose, insulin, and energy metabolism. *American Journal of Clinical Nutrition* 84, 63–69.

Aston, L.M. (2006) Glycaemic index and metabolic disease risk. *Proceedings of the Nutrition Society* 65, 125–134.

Bailey, S.R., Menzies-Gow, N.J., Harris, P.A., Habershon-Butcher, J.L., Crawford, C., Berhane, Y., Boston, R.C. and Elliott, J. (2007) Effect of dietary fructans and dexamethasone administration on the insulin response of ponies predisposed to laminitis. *Journal of the American Veterinary Medical Association* 231, 1365–1373.

Besong, S.J., Jackson, J., Trammel, S. and Amaral-Phillips, D. (1996) Effect of supplemental chromium picolinate on liver triglycerides, blood metabolites, milk yield and milk composition in early lactation cows. *Journal of Dairy Science* 79(Supplement 1), 196 (Abstract).

Brand-Miller, J.C. and Colagiuri, S. (1999) Evolutionary aspects of diet and insulin resistance. In: Simopoulos, A.P. (ed.) *Evolutionary Aspects of Nutrition and Health. Diet, Exercise, Genetics and Chronic Disease.*

World Review of Nutrition and Dietetics, Karger, Basel, Switzerland, pp. 75–105.

Bray, G.A. (2007) How bad is fructose? *American Journal of Clinical Nutrition* 86, 895–896.

Buffenstein, R. (2008) Negligible senescence in the longest living rodent, the naked mole-rat: insights from a successfully aging species. *Journal of Comparative Physiology B* 178, 439–445.

Chang, X., Mowat, D.N. and Mallard, B.A. (1995) Supplemental chromium and niacin for stressed feeder calves. *Canadian Journal of Animal Science* 75, 351–358.

Cheeke, P.R. (1998) *Natural Toxicants in Feeds, Forages, and Poisonous Plants*. Prentice Hall, Upper Saddle River, New Jersey.

Crockford, S.J. (2003) Thyroid rhythm phenotypes and hominid evolution: a new paradigm implicates pulsatile hormone secretion in speciation and adaptation changes. *Comparative Biochemistry and Physiology* 135A, 105–129.

Crockford, S.J. (2006) *Rhythms of Life. Thyroid Hormone and the Origin of Species*. Trafford Publishing, Victoria, British Columbia, Canada.

de Lange, T. (1998) Telomeres and senescence: ending the debate. *Science* 279, 334–335.

Englyst, K.N., Vinoy, S., Englyst, H.N. and Lang, V. (2003) Glycaemic index of cereal products explained by their content of rapidly and slowly available glucose. *British Journal of Nutrition* 89, 329–339.

Forbes, J.M. (1970) Voluntary food intake of pregnant ewes. *Journal of Animal Science* 31, 1222–1227.

Heilbronn, L.K. and Ravussin, E. (2003) Calorie restriction and aging: review of the literature and implications for studies in humans. *American Journal of Clinical Nutrition* 78, 361–369.

Hollis, A.R., Boston, R.C. and Corley, K.T.T. (2007) Blood glucose in horses with acute abdominal disease. *Journal of Veterinary Internal Medicine* 21, 1099–1103.

Hulbert, A.J., Pamplona, R., Buffenstein, R. and Buttemer, W.A. (2007) Life and death: metabolic rate, membrane composition, and life span of animals. *Physiological Reviews* 87, 1175–1213.

Jaster, E.H. and Ward, N.E. (1990) Supplemental nicotinic acid or nicotinamide for lactating dairy cows. *Journal of Dairy Science* 77, 2880–2889.

Jenkins, D.J.A., Kendall, C.W.C., Augustin, L.S.A., Franceschi, S., Hamidi, M., Marchie, A., Jenkins, A.L. and Axelsen, M. (2002) Glycemic index: overview of implications in health and disease. *American Journal of Clinical Nutrition* 76(Supplement), 266S–273S.

Johnson, R.J., Segal, M.S., Sautin, Y., Nakagawa, T., Feig, D.I., Kang, D.-H., Gersch, M.S., Benner, S. and Sanchez-Lozada, L.G. (2007) Potential role of sugar (fructose) in the epidemic of hypertension, obesity and the metabolic syndrome, diabetes, kidney disease, and cardiovascular disease. *American Journal of Clinical Nutrition* 86, 899–906.

Karihaloo, A.A., Webster, A.J.F. and Combs, W. (1970) Effects of cold, acute starvation and pregnancy on some indices of energy metabolism in Lincoln and Southdown sheep. *Canadian Journal of Animal Science* 50, 191–198.

Kegley, E.B., Spears, J.W. and Brown, T.T., Jr (1997) Effect of shipping and chromium supplementation on performance, immune response, and disease resistance of steers. *Journal of Animal Science* 75, 1956–1964.

Kornegay, E.T., Wang, Z., Wood, C.M. and Lindemann, M.D. (1997) Supplemental chromium picolinate influences nitrogen balance, dry matter digestibility, and carcass traits in growing-finishing pigs. *Journal of Animal Science* 75, 1319–1323.

Kronfeld, D.S., Treiber, K.H., Hess, T.M. and Boston, R.C. (2005) Insulin resistance in the horse: definition, detection, and dietetics. *Journal of Animal Science* 83(E. Supplement), E22–E31.

Lawler, D.F., Larson, B.T., Ballam, J.M., Smith, G.K., Biery, D.N., Evans, R.H., Greeley, E.H., Segre, M., Stowe, H.D. and Kealy, R.D. (2008) Diet restriction and ageing in the dog: major observations over two decades. *British Journal of Nutrition* 99, 793–805.

Lynn, W.S. and Wallwork, J.C. (1992) Does food restriction retard aging by reducing metabolic rate? *Journal of Nutrition* 122, 1917–1918.

McCay, C.M., Crowel, M.F. and Maynard, L.A. (1935) The effect of retarded growth upon the length of the life span and upon the ultimate body size. *Journal of Nutrition* 10, 63–79.

Mertz, W. (1993) Chromium in human nutrition: a review. *Journal of Nutrition* 123, 626–633.

Milgram, N.W., Araujo, J.A., Hagen, T.M., Treadwell, B.V. and Ames, B.N. (2007) Acetyl-L-carnitine and α-lipoic acid supplementation of aged beagle dogs improves learning in two landmark discrimination tests. *FASEB Journal* 21, 3756–3762.

Mooney, K.W. and Cromwell, G.L. (1997) Efficacy of chromium picolinate and chromium chloride as potential carcass modifiers in swine. *Journal of Animal Science* 75, 2661–2671.

Mowat, D.N., Chang, X. and Yang, W.Z. (1993) Chelated chromium for stressed calves. *Canadian Journal of Animal Science* 73, 49–55.

Parks, E.J., Skokan, L.E., Timlin, M.T. and Dingfelder, C.S. (2008) Dietary sugars stimulate fatty acid synthesis. *Journal of Nutrition* 138, 1039–1046.

Shaw, D.I., Hall, W.L. and Williams, C.M. (2005) Metabolic syndrome: what is it and what are the implications? *Proceedings of the Nutrition Society* 64, 349–357.

Stokes, S.R. and Goff, J.P. (2001) Evaluation of calcium propionate and propylene glycol administered into the esophagus of dairy cattle at calving. *The Professional Animal Scientist* 17, 115–122.

Treiber, K.H., Boston, R.C., Kronfeld, D.S., Staniar, W.B. and Harris, P.A. (2005) Insulin resistance and compensation in thoroughbred weanlings adapted to high-glycemic meals. *Journal of Animal Science* 83, 2357–2364.

Van Heugten, E. and Spears, J.W. (1997) Immune response and growth of stressed weanling pigs fed diets supplemented with organic or inorganic forms of chromium. *Journal of Animal Science* 75, 409–416.

Vick, M.M., Sessions, D.R., Murphy, B.A., Kennedy, E.K., Reedy, S.E. and Fitzgerald, B.P. (2006) Obesity is associated with altered metabolic and reproductive activity in the mare: effects of metformin on insulin sensitivity and reproductive cyclicity. *Reproduction, Fertility and Development* 18, 609–614.

Vick, M.M., Adams, A.A., Murphy, B.A., Sessions, D.R., Horohov, D.W., Cook, R.F., Shelton, B.J. and Fitzgerald, B.P. (2007) Relationships among inflammatory cytokines, obesity, and insulin sensitivity in the horse. *Journal of Animal Science* 85, 1144–1155.

Webster, A.J.F., Hicks, A.M. and Hays, F.L. (1969) Cold climate and cold temperature changes in the heat production and thermal insulation of sheep. *Canadian Journal of Physiology and Pharmacology* 47, 553–562.

Webster, A.J.F., Chlumecky, J. and Young, B.A. (1970) Effects of cold environments on the energy exchanges of young beef cattle. *Canadian Journal of Animal Science* 50, 89–100.

Wood, J.G., Rogina, B., Lavu, S., Howitz, K., Helfand, S.L., Tatar, M. and Sinclair, D. (2004) Sirtuin activators mimic caloric restriction and delay ageing in metazoans. *Nature* 430, 686–689.

Yen, P.M. (2001) Physiological and molecular basis of thyroid hormone action. *Physiological Reviews* 81, 1097–1142.

17 Feeding Behaviour and Regulation of Feed Intake

Feeding Behaviour

Feeding behaviour and digestive tract physiology in animals are closely interrelated. The feeds normally consumed by animals are those they are capable of digesting. There are three major types of animal feeding behaviour: (i) carnivorous; (ii) omnivorous; and (iii) herbivorous. **Carnivores**, such as cats, are adapted to a meat-based diet and require a high-quality, highly digestible source of nutrients. Carnivores (mammalian, avian, reptilian) have simple digestive tracts with little microbial activity. They may require certain nutrients, such as pre-formed vitamin A, ω-3 fatty acids and taurine, that in the wild can be obtained only from consumption of meat. At the other end of the spectrum, herbivores are animals that normally consume only plant material and have a more complex digestive tract with symbiotic microbial activity that permits the digestion of plant fibre. Herbivores include the ruminants, such as cattle, and non-ruminant herbivores, such as horses and rabbits. **Omnivores** are animals that are less fastidious in their feeding behaviour and consume a wide variety of animal and plant foods. Pigs, poultry and humans are examples.

Ruminant animals vary considerably in their feeding strategies. Hofmann (1973, 1989), in a classic study of the stomach anatomy and function of African wild ruminants, classified ruminants into three groups based on feeding strategy: (i) concentrate selectors; (ii) bulk and roughage eaters; and (iii) intermediate feeders (see Chapter 3). **Concentrate selectors** (browsers) select the more nutritious low fibre parts of herbage such as leaves, fruit and other soft, succulent plant parts. This material can be rapidly fermented, and much of the plant cell contents fraction is absorbed directly without fermentation. Concentrate selectors (Fig. 17.1) have a stomach anatomy adapted to the use of low fibre forage. They have a relatively small rumen and a small omasum that can become impacted readily with poor-quality fibrous herbage. The reticular groove is well developed, allowing high quality feed to bypass rumen fermentation. Examples of concentrate selectors are the moose, giraffe and many species (but not all) of deer. These animals tend to nibble fastidiously on a wide variety of plants and plant parts and often occupy ecological niches unavailable to grazing ruminants.

Concentrate-selector ruminants are sometimes difficult to maintain in zoo exhibits, because of a number of diet-related problems such as **chronic wasting disease**. Moose, the second largest ruminant concentrate selector, are rarely exhibited in zoos because of premature mortality (Shochat et al., 1997). 'Moose wasting syndrome complex' is the cause of many mortalities (Clauss et al., 2002). Moose are unable to survive on a diet of grass hay (Clauss et al., 2002). Giraffes, the largest concentrate selector, also have a number of problems, including wasting disease and high mortality. Small concentrate-selector ruminants, such as duikers, experience high mortality from chronic wasting disease, rumen hypomotility syndrome, bloat and rumenitis (Willette et al., 2002). Dierenfeld et al. (2002) reviewed dietary requirements of captive duikers. In the wild, duikers are frugivorous (fruit eaters), consuming a diet with moderate fibre and protein, and low starch. The relative proportions of sugar and starch in their natural diets (2–15 times more sugar than starch) is the opposite of that found on many commercially available grains and by-product feeds (Dierenfeld et al., 2002). Colobine monkeys, which have a multi-chambered stomach with fermentation, have some of the same problems as concentrate-selector ruminants in dealing with zoo diets (Tovar et al., 2005). They have a preference for browse that is relatively low in fibre content.

In contrast, **bulk and roughage eaters**, such as cattle, are grazing animals, with large rumens

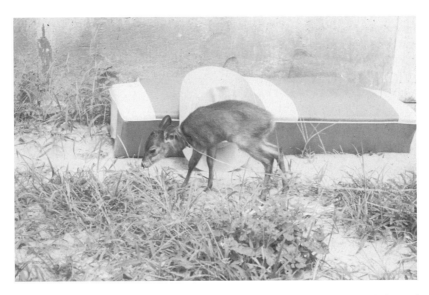

Fig. 17.1. The red duiker, an example of a small concentrate-selector ruminant. Note size in relation to the hat behind the animal.

adapted to the intake of large amounts of low-energy fibrous feeds. Rumination is pronounced. The omasum is highly developed, retaining fibrous feed in the rumen to maximize fibre digestion. **Intermediate feeders**, such as sheep and goats, share feeding and digestive strategies of both the concentrate selectors and the grazers. They are very adaptable to varying environments and habitats. Sheep graze on grass, but they will also extensively utilize shrubs and forbs. Their feeding behaviour is much more selective than that of cattle. Goats will graze on grass, but prefer browse.

An appreciation of these differences is desirable when dealing with domestic ruminants and vital when dealing with wild animals. Differences in digestive physiology and feeding strategy explain why winter feeding of deer with hay may produce mortality, or why the proper selection of forage for feeding giraffes or duikers in a zoo will determine whether they will survive.

While the three anatomical categories of ruminants described by Hofmann (1989) correlate well with feeding behaviour, it appears from studies to test Hofmann's hypotheses that the differences in nutritional ecology of ruminants relate more to feeding behaviour and diet selection than to anatomical differences in stomach anatomy (Gordon and Illius, 1994, 1996; Robbins *et al.*, 1995). However, testing of these hypotheses has led to

much greater understanding of ruminant evolution, behaviour and ecology of herbivore communities (Robbins *et al.*, 1995), as discussed in Chapter 3. In fact, Hofmann's descriptions of ruminants have largely been validated (Chapter 3).

Factors Affecting Feed Intake

The regulation of feed intake and appetite is a complex subject. This section emphasizes the properties of feeds affecting feed intake. More detailed information can be obtained in the reviews of Forbes (1986a, b; 1996) and the National Research Council (1987). A symposium on controls of feeding in farm animals, with separate review articles on pigs, horses, sheep and cattle, was published in the *Journal of Animal Science* (59:1345–1380, 1984). A series of review articles on the regulation of voluntary forage intake of ruminants was published in the *Journal of Animal Science* (74:3029–3081, 1996).

Maximal feed intake can be achieved only with free choice water available. When water is restricted, feed intake is reduced. If a group or pen of animals goes off feed, the first thing to check is the water supply. Large amounts of water are required to moisten food in the gut, especially in herbivores. Ingredients with high water-absorbing properties, such as bran, increase the water requirements.

Palatability and feed preference

Palatability is a determinant of feed intake. **Palatability** is the summation of the taste, olfactory and textural characteristics of a feedstuff that determine its degree of acceptance. Taste is a major component of the palatability complex. The major **taste responses** are sweet, salty, bitter and acid. A fifth taste sensation has been recognized, called umami (Japanese meaning savoury deliciousness). The umami taste, which is the taste of glutamate, is considered to represent the taste for dietary protein (Luscombe-Marsh *et al.*, 2007). Virtually all animals except strict carnivores show a preference for the sweet taste (sweet tooth). The sweet taste is recognized by a taste bud receptor composed of the products of two genes. In the domestic cat and others such as the tiger and cheetah, one of the genes is not functional and is not expressed (Li *et al.*, 2009). Thus the cat cannot taste sweet stimuli. Probably because of its strict carnivorous diet, selection pressure to maintain a functional receptor was relaxed. Molasses and to a lesser extent sucrose are used in feeds for many species as sources of sweet taste to increase palatability. Most animals also show a pronounced appetite for salt. This is particularly true of herbivores. Animals show quite divergent responses to bitterness. Generally the herbivorous species are quite tolerant of bitter substances because many of the secondary compounds in plants, such as alkaloids and glycosides, are bitter. Herbivores that are intolerant of bitterness are not likely to find anything acceptable to eat, which promotes either rapid evolution of tolerance to bitter substances or extinction! Dietary fat is a positive preference factor for most animals. The attraction for sweet taste (sugars) and fat is of obvious evolutionary benefit, attracting animals to feeds that are rich in energy. While a 'sweet tooth' was of obvious benefit to pre-modern humans, it has become a liability today. It is probable that nobody became obese when attracted to the sweet taste of fruit; in the modern world, the widespread occurrence of sucrose in processed foods (Shorland's nutritional distortion concept, see Chapter 15) attracts people to unhealthy, obesity-causing foods. Other palatability factors for various species include size, shape, smell, colour and movement. For example, baby frogs are attracted to movement, and in frog farms they must be fed moving food (e.g. fly larvae) for them to learn to eat. Palatability of foods for humans relates to both nutritional need and a hedonistic need-free

stimulation of appetite (Yeomans *et al.*, 2004). Thus a preference for sweet tastes when hungry may be an expression of caloric needs, while salt deprivation may enhance palatability of salty tastes. The neural systems underlying the need-free stimulation of appetite and the homeostatic controls relating to biological nutrient need are separate, involving distinctly different brain structures and neurochemicals (Yeomans *et al.*, 2004).

Most domestic animals are **generalist feeders** and are quite tolerant of a wide array of divergent tastes and feed textures. Lack of palatability of feeds is not usually a major problem. Specialist feeders are animals that eat only a narrow range of feeds. Many insects are **specialist feeders** and feed only on a particular plant species. Koalas and pandas are examples of mammalian specialist feeders; they will eat only a few species of eucalyptus (koalas) and bamboo (pandas). These animals are difficult to feed and exhibit in zoos because of their specialist feeding behaviour.

Knowledge of species differences in feed preferences and taste responses can be useful in developing and employing feed flavours. For example, many cats respond favourably to the herb catnip (*Nepeta cataria*), whereas rabbits are attracted to thyme (*Thymus vulgaris*). Anise seed or oil is often used as a feed flavour or attractant, as are garlic and onion for carnivores.

Feed preferences are often evaluated in a two-choice self-selection test. Results from such evaluations must be interpreted with caution. A particular ingredient may appear unpalatable to animals when it is presented in a choice situation, but, if they are not given a choice, they may consume it readily.

The major distinction between **hunger** and palatability is that calories satisfy hunger, but appetite (the desire to repeat a pleasant feeling) can only be satisfied by palatability (Tovar *et al.*, 2005).

Secondary compounds, feeding strategies and palatability

Secondary compounds in plants are those compounds that are not involved in the primary processes of cellular metabolism, but have secondary roles, such as in chemical defences. Examples of secondary compounds include a wide variety of toxic substances such as alkaloids, cyanogenic compounds, phyto-oestrogens, tannins, toxic amino acids and other plant toxins. These compounds help protect plants against being eaten and thus serve as a form of chemical defence against predators, which include bacteria, viruses, insects and mammalian herbivores. Thus, in crop and forage plants, there must be a balance between having sufficient chemical defences to survive attacks by insects and other pests but not be so strongly protected that they are highly unpalatable or toxic to livestock. Differences in palatability of various forages can be explained largely by their contents of secondary compounds or, in some cases, by the presence of physical defences, such as prickliness or coarseness. It is very difficult to maintain a mixture of highly palatable and less palatable forage species in a pasture; the palatable plants will be overgrazed and killed out while the underutilized plants will become mature and even more unpalatable (Provenza *et al.*, 2003). Rotational grazing systems with high stocking density help to prevent selective grazing.

As plants have evolved chemical and physical defences, herbivores have developed means of surmounting them. This is most obvious in the insect world because of the short-generation interval. Many insects, having developed the enzymatic capacity to detoxify plant toxins, are specialist feeders and feed only on plants containing the particular toxin to which they are adapted. The toxins act as attractants and feeding stimulants. In some cases, the plant toxins actually become essential metabolites for the insect and may be used in the synthesis of pheromones. As herbivores surmount the plant chemical defences, the plants often chemically modify the toxin to overcome the herbivores' metabolic adaptations. These interactions are known as **coevolution**. These continual changes in plant and herbivore enzymatic activity represent a coevolutionary arms race! Examples of mammalian adaptations to surmount plant defences include the enzymatic resistance of sheep and goats to many poisonous plants (Cheeke, 1998), and the ability of the elephant, rhinoceros and the goat to munch contentedly on twigs that are armed with vicious thorns and spines (Cooper and Owen-Smith, 1986).

The effect of secondary compounds on diet selection and feed intake of wild animals is an active area of research. Chemical factors influencing palatability are nutrients, fibre or secondary compounds. Soluble carbohydrates are probably the main nutrient category involved. Although there often is an association between protein content and palatability, Cooper *et al.* (1988) suggest that animals do not have taste receptors for protein, but

because leaf protein concentration is largely chloroplastic, high concentrations of leaf protein are correlated with high photosynthetic rates and, thus, high soluble carbohydrates.

Many secondary compounds in plants are bitter or otherwise unpleasant tasting. Alkaloids and glycosides are often bitter, while phenolic compounds such as tannins are astringent. Sheep and goats and other concentrate-selector herbivores are more tolerant of bitter substances than are grazers such as cattle and horses (Cheeke, 1998). Many wild herbivores (e.g. deer) have **tannin-binding salivary proteins** rich in the amino acid proline that bind with tannins and reduce their toxic and astringent effects (Austin *et al.*, 1989). This phenomenon is a metabolic adaptation that permits many browsers to utilize chemically protected plants (McArthur *et al.*, 1995). The salivary tannin-binding proteins from herbivorous mammals have different abilities to bind various tannins. Salivary proteins from generalists, like the black bear and mule deer, bind several different types of tannin (Hagerman and Robbins, 1993). Salivary proteins from specialist feeders, such as the moose and beaver, bind only the tannin most characteristic of their preferred diet (aspen, birch, willow and alder for beaver; aspen, birch, willow and mountain ash for moose). The omnivorous black bear produces salivary proteins that bind all types of tannins. Thus the specificity of tannin-binding salivary proteins is correlated with an animal's feeding preferences (Hagerman and Robbins, 1993). There are even geographical differences: Scandinavian and North American moose differ in their salivary tannin-binding proteins (Juntheikki, 1996). Some species (e.g. roe deer) actually prefer tannins (Clauss *et al.*, 2003). The black rhinoceros, a browser, has higher concentrations of salivary tannin-binding proteins than the white rhino, a grazer (Clauss *et al.*, 2005). Clauss (2003) has compiled a list of animals with demonstrated salivary tannin-binding proteins (Table 17.1).

Small herbivores such as rabbits, voles and lemmings characteristically undergo **population cycles**. A classic example is the snowshoe hare of Arctic regions. **Snowshoe hares** have a cycle of about 10 years, in which the population rises to a peak, and then crashes to a very low level. Numbers rebuild over the next 10-year cycle. This population cycle seems to involve a complex interaction of predators and plant secondary compounds (Krebs *et al.*, 2001). The numbers of the main predator of

Table 17.1. Animals with documented salivary tannin-binding proteins (adapted from Clauss, 2003).

Species
Swamp wallaby (*Wallabia bicolor*)
Pademelon (*Thylogale thetis*)
Human (*Homo sapiens*)
Mouse (*Mus musculus*)
Rat (*Rattus norvegicus*)
Root vole (*Microtus oeconomus*)
Beaver (*Castor canadensis*)
Pika (*Ochotona princeps*)
Rabbit (*Oryctolagus cuniculus*)
Mountain hare (*Lepus timidus*)
Black bear (*Ursus americanus*)
Black rhinoceros (*Diceros bicornis*)
Camel (*Camelus dromedarius*)
Roe deer (*Capreolus capreolus*)
White-tailed deer (*Odocoileus virginianus*)
Mule deer (*Odocoileus hemionus*)
Moose (*Alces alces*)

snowshoe hares, the Canada lynx, follow, with a slight time lag, the rise and fall of snowshoe hare numbers. However, plant chemistry also plays a role in the hare cycle. Many studies have shown that as the browsing intensity on Arctic trees and shrubs increases with increasing hare numbers, the plants respond by increasing their synthesis of feeding deterrents and toxins, mostly of a phenolic nature. The concentrations of the **plant secondary compounds** are higher in juvenile plant tissues, such as suckers from root and stump sprouts, that is, the regrowth of browsed-upon plants. Some of the plant secondary compounds are feeding deterrents, and some inhibit digestibility. Thus as the hare population increases, the available winter browse becomes increasingly chemically defended and unpalatable and indigestible to hares. In conjunction with the higher predator numbers, these environmental pressures cause a crash in the hare population. The decreased herbivory results in a relaxation of the plant synthesis of chemical defences, so the small hare population at the low point of the cycle can recover quickly. The plant chemicals involved, which are mainly phenolics, have been reviewed by Bryant *et al.* (1991) and Krebs *et al.* (2001). The subject of plant chemical defences against mammalian herbivory is covered in detail in Palo and Robbins (1991).

Another example involves beavers. When aspen trees are cut down by beavers, the new shoots arising from the stumps are rich in phenolic compounds, which the beavers then avoid (Basey *et al.*, 1988). Rather than clear-cutting forests, beavers select trees with low concentrations of phenolics, and trees they have cut can regenerate if they increase their chemical protection. Eventually, when most of the trees in an area are well defended chemically, the beavers move to a new habitat, beginning the cycle again. The current annual growth of many woody species contains higher concentrations of defensive chemicals than does older growth, which is reflected in the pattern of herbivory (Bryant *et al.*, 1992).

Most animals consuming browse are generalist feeders, although there are some **specialist feeders**. An example is the **pygmy rabbit**, which has an obligate dietary relationship with terpene-containing sagebrush. In this species, most of the terpenes in sagebrush are volatilized during mastication (White *et al.*, 1982). **Australian marsupials** which feed on *Eucalyptus* foliage are specialist feeders. Examples include the koala and the greater glider. These specialist feeders have high liver oxidative enzyme capacity, and excrete highly oxidized metabolites of the *Eucalyptus* monoterpenes (McLean *et al.*, 2003). Specialists tend to detoxify plant defensive chemicals differently than generalists (Dearing *et al.*, 2000). Generalists must detoxify low to moderate levels of a variety of plant chemicals, while specialists evolve detoxification mechanisms best suited to the chemicals characteristic of their specialist diet. Generalist herbivores (most herbivores) tend to choose mixed diets to minimize the toxic effects of plant secondary compounds (Iason, 2005). Generalists eat more when presented with a choice of foods with different plant secondary compounds added than when they are offered no choice or a diet containing only one of the plant secondary compounds (Villalba *et al.*, 2004).

Many plants respond to herbivory by increasing their physical or chemical defences. Examples of physical defences are **spines and thorns**. For example, the thorns on *Acacia* trees browsed by goats are longer than those on trees protected against goat browsing (Young, 1987). The main effect of thorns and spines is to restrict bite sizes by browsing herbivores, tending to decrease herbivory pressure on the spine-defended plant (Cooper and Owen-Smith, 1986). Some animals, such as goats, black rhinos and elephants, overcome these physical defences by hard mouth parts that are largely unaffected by spines and thorns (Fig. 17.2). Others, such as impala and giraffes, have a delicate browsing technique that allows them to avoid thorns (Cooper and Owen-Smith, 1986). Pointed muzzles and mobile lips (Fig. 17.3) are adaptations for feeding on thorny vegetation (Myers and Bazely, 1991).

Another physical defence of plants is the **silica** deposited in the cell walls of many grass species. It may act as a 'varnish' on cell walls to reduce accessibility of rumen microbes to the cell contents, and it contributes to the physical roughness or harshness of many grass species. This may have negative effects on palatability of grasses to grazing animals (Shewmaker *et al.*, 1989). Silica in forages is also important as a cause of urinary calculi formation and rapid tooth wear.

Trees exposed to herbivory may release **ethylene** gas, which stimulates adjacent trees to increase their synthesis of defensive phenolic compounds. This chemical communication between plants has been termed 'talking trees' (Baldwin and Schultz, 1983; Fowler and Lawton, 1985). Furstenberg and Van Hoven (1994) in South Africa reported that browsing of *Acacia* trees by giraffes resulted in an increase in the tannin content of the foliage within 2–10 min of initiation of browsing, causing the tree's foliage to become less palatable. A mechanism by which

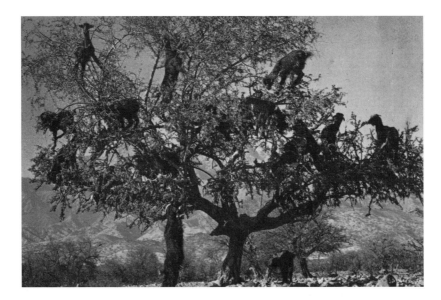

Fig. 17.2. Goats can even climb trees to obtain browse.

(a)

(b)

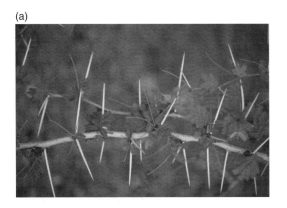

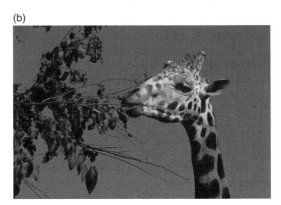

Fig. 17.3. (a) Spines on *Acacia* trees in Africa. (b) Pointed muzzles, long tongues and mobile lips are adaptations for feeding on thorny vegetation, such as the *Acacia* which are browsed upon by giraffes.

such a rapid change in tannin content could occur might be that quinones produced by the action of polyphenoloxidases on phenolics might be more toxic and be a greater deterrent to feeding than the original phenolics (Lowry *et al.*, 1996). Tissue maceration caused by browsing would activate polyphenoloxidase activity. Not only did the trees browsed by giraffes show a rise in tannin content and lowered palatability, adjacent non-browsed *Acacia* trees also showed a marked increase in tannin content in the same time period of 2–10 min (Furstenberg and Van Hoven, 1994).

Toxin metabolism often results in the formation of organic acids which are excreted as salts of ammonium, sodium or other cations. Foley *et al.* (1995) have proposed that acidosis induced by metabolism of plant toxins may contribute to disturbances in **acid–base balance** and nutrient retention. For example, generation of calcium ions from the skeletal system and ammonium ions from muscle tissue to buffer organic acids may lead to nutritional and physiological problems. These reactions could be particularly important when animals are consuming nutrient-poor, toxin-rich plants, such as the winter diets of bark and twigs of Arctic hares, or the *Eucalyptus* foliage consumed by marsupials such as the koala (Foley *et al.*, 1995). Freeland *et al.* (1985) demonstrated that diets containing hydrolysable or condensed tannins caused sodium depletion in herbivores, and suggested that chemical defences of plants exert their effects by causing mineral depletion and deficiency in herbivores varying in size from moose to meadow voles. Iason and Palo (1991) found that dietary birch-twig phenolics cause severe sodium losses in European hares (grazers) but not in mountain hares (browsers). They suggested that browsers might have adapted to phenolic-rich diets by metabolic regulation of sodium balance. Some northern rodents and lagomorphs dependent on hindgut digestion of bark and other nutrient-poor fibrous materials are able to maintain high levels of minerals in the hindgut by efficient mechanisms of mineral absorption and retention via coprophagy and caecotrophy (Staaland *et al.*, 1995).

Preferences for certain forages may involve the absence of unpalatable secondary compounds, or the presence of palatable components such as sugars or amino acids. However, Mayland *et al.* (2000) found that grazing preferences of cattle for tall fescue cultivars were not related to malate, citrate or amino acid concentrations among cultivars.

Afternoon forage is higher in photosynthate (sugars) than morning forage, and thus may be more palatable (Huntington and Burns, 2007).

Detoxification of plant secondary compounds utilizes energy- and protein-requiring enzymatic processes in the liver. When animals consume more energy and protein, they can eat more of foods that contain toxins. In contrast, they eat less food with toxins when levels of nutrients such as sodium are low (Freeland and Choquenot, 1990). According to Provenza and Villalba (2006) and Provenza *et al.* (2003), feeding decisions depend on an animal's ability to detoxify plant toxins. A herbivore that can detoxify a toxin quickly should be able to eat more. This was demonstrated by Marsh *et al.* (2005) with brushtail possums. Possums supplemented with glycine, which conjugates benzoic acid, eat more diet with benzoic acid than unsupplemented animals. Provenza and Villalba (2006) and Provenza *et al.* (2003) contend that animals possess **nutritional wisdom** which allows them to consume an optimal balance of nutrients and toxins. The selection process may be mediated by a homeostatic regulation of a state of well-being (e.g. excessive consumption of a toxin induces a state of nausea or distress).

Dietary energy level

If feeds are sufficiently palatable to be readily consumed, the main dietary factor that controls voluntary feed intake is dietary energy concentration. A long-standing maxim in animal nutrition is that animals eat to satisfy their energy requirements. The amount of feed consumed is regulated so as to provide a constant intake of digestible energy. If a low energy diet is used, feed intake is high, whereas with a high energy diet, feed intake is reduced. The energy intake is about the same in each case. This is illustrated in Fig. 17.4 and Table 17.2. The lower limit of this relationship is when **gut capacity** is reached and the animal cannot consume enough feed to meet its energy requirements; thus its performance is reduced. The relationship between dietary energy level and feed intake is well illustrated in the data of Wood (1964) for rats (Table 17.2). As the dietary energy concentration was increased, feed intake decreased but the animals consumed about the same total daily dietary energy. Dietary protein concentration was expressed as milligrams of crude protein per kcal of dietary energy. Thus when the animals had consumed

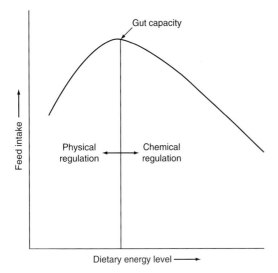

Fig. 17.4. The relationship between feed intake and dietary energy level. Animals eat to meet their energy requirements. Feed intake declines at very low dietary energy levels because a low energy diet is very high in fibre and gut capacity becomes limiting; the animal simply can't eat enough of a very low energy diet to meet its energy needs. This portion of the graph would apply primarily to ruminants fed very low quality roughages such as straw.

sufficient feed to meet their energy requirements, they had also met their protein requirements.

Because of this relationship, there is no specific energy concentration per pound or kilogram of diet required in diets for livestock. The requirement is best expressed in kilocalories per animal per day. Above the energy concentration at which gut capacity becomes limiting, animals can adjust their voluntary intake to consume the required amount of kilocalories. This regulation is largely accomplished by concentrations of blood metabolites. In non-ruminants, **blood glucose** is the principal regulator of feed intake. When glycogen reserves are depleted and blood glucose concentration begins to fall, the appetite centre in the brain initiates neural activity to produce sensations of hunger, stimulating feed intake. In ruminants, blood concentrations of VFAs fulfill this role (Illius and Jessop, 1996). Control of intake by effects of blood metabolites on the appetite centre is known as **chemostatic regulation** of feed intake. At the molecular level, it appears that a number of neuropeptides are involved in the function of the appetite centre (Baile and McLaughlin, 1987). The opioid peptides, such as β-endorphin, stimulate feed intake, whereas cholecystokinin (CCK) inhibits feed intake. Because CCK is a gastrointestinal hormone as well as one that is released in the brain, there may be a connection between gastrointestinal tract release of CCK and development of satiety. Opioid receptors in the brain are implicated in long-term feed intake regulation (Obese *et al.*, 2007). Opioid agonists stimulate, while opioid antagonists attenuate feed intake.

A variety of gastrointestinal hormones, such as CCK, glucagon-like peptide 1 and peripheral hormone peptide YY, have effects on feed intake by promoting satiety. A newly discovered hormone, **ghrelin**, has the opposite effect and promotes an increase in feed intake. Ghrelin is produced in the stomach of non-ruminants, and in the abomasal and ruminal tissues of ruminants. It is a peptide hormone that stimulates feed intake by signalling the release of anabolic neuropeptides from the hypothalamus. Ghrelin appears to serve as a metabolic signal to alter energy intake of cattle (Wertz-Lutz *et al.*, 2006). The name ghrelin is derived from growth-hormone-releasing peptide. Propionate is a

Table 17.2. The relationship between diet caloric density and protein/kcal ratio on daily feed intake of the weanling rat (Wood, 1964).

Dietary protein concentration (mg crude protein/kcal dietary energy)	Caloric density (kcal dietary energy/kg diet)				
	2000	3000	4000	5000	5700
30	21.9[a] (43.8)[b]	12.9 (38.7)	11.9 (47.6)	8.4 (42.0)	7.8 (44.5)
45	20.1 (40.2)	14.9 (44.7)	12.0 (48.0)	9.2 (46.0)	7.6 (43.3)
60	19.7 (39.4)	14.1 (42.3)	10.4 (41.6)	9.3 (46.5)	6.9 (39.3)
75	19.4 (38.8)	12.2 (36.6)	10.5 (42.0)	9.2 (46.0)	7.2 (41.0)

[a]Daily feed intake (g).
[b]Daily dietary energy intake (kcal).

major satiety signal in ruminants, by way of its concentration in the liver (Allen *et al.*, 2009). It has been proposed that feed intake in ruminants is controlled by a signal from the liver to the brain that is stimulated by the oxidation of metabolic fuels such as propionate (Allen *et al.*, 2009). This is known as the hepatic oxidation theory of the control of feed intake.

Insulin and the hormone **leptin** help to regulate long-term energy balance. Leptin is produced by the adipose tissue, and serves to communicate to the brain the status of adipose tissue deposits. Increased body fat causes leptin and insulin concentrations to increase, which causes the brain to release catabolic neuropeptides which suppress feed intake. Decreased adiposity causes blood leptin and insulin to decrease, which stimulates release of anabolic neuropeptides and increased feed intake. **Adiponectin** is a polypeptide hormone secreted exclusively by adipose tissue into the blood. It has similar and complementary action to leptin, and may have a role in reducing metabolic derangements that cause diabetes, obesity, atherosclerosis and non-alcoholic fatty liver disease.

With most practical diets fed to pigs and poultry in the industrialized countries, the energy concentration of the diet is above the level at which gut capacity limits feed intake. In developing countries, use of ingredients such as rice bran may result in diets that are too low in digestible energy to support maximal performance. With ruminant animals, forage-based diets are too low in digestible energy to meet the energy requirements for maximal growth and lactational performance. This fact is why the beef feedlot industry and high-concentrate feeding of dairy cattle have developed in North America and Europe. When grain resources are abundant, high concentrate diets for ruminants are economically more attractive than forage-based systems because of the much higher productivity obtained. With the increasing competition for feed grains from biofuel (ethanol) production, high concentrate diets for ruminants may become less economically feasible than forage-based systems.

Because of the relationship between dietary energy concentration and feed intake, the feed-conversion efficiency is largely dependent on the energy density of the feed. Feed efficiency is commonly expressed as the amount of feed required per unit of live weight gain. Also, because of the energy density-feed intake relationship, for maximal precision in diet formulation, it is desirable to express nutrient requirements on a per kilocalorie basis. Thus, regardless of the amount of feed required to meet the energy requirement, the requirements for other nutrients would automatically be met as well. On a percentage basis, the optimal percentage of crude protein, for example, would be high in a high energy diet and lower in a low energy diet.

In ruminants, the break-off point – where gut capacity ceases to limit feed intake and intake is regulated by chemostatic means – is at an energy density approximately at the change from a roughage-based diet to a concentrate diet (Fig. 17.4), corresponding to a dry-matter digestibility of approximately 66–69%. As forage quality declines, so does feed intake, largely as a result of a reduced rate of digestion leading to a longer retention time in the rumen for poor-quality roughages. Ruminants fed high grain diets (2.7–3.3 Mcal/kg dry matter) eat to maintain constant energy intake (Krehbiel *et al.*, 2009).

Ketelaars and Tolkamp (1996) have proposed that the unifying factor relating energy metabolism and feed intake is the efficiency of oxygen utilization. Voluntary energy intake corresponds to the feed consumption level at which oxygen efficiency (net energy yield per litre of oxygen consumed) is maximum.

Protein and amino acid concentrations

Dietary energy density has a much greater impact on voluntary feed intake than does dietary protein status. Nevertheless, protein intake in growing animals is subject to some regulation (Henry, 1985). The growing pig, for example, has the ability to preferentially select diets adequate in essential amino acids over amino-acid-deficient diets (Henry, 1987). Baby pigs are able to discriminate among diets varying in methionine content, and prefer a diet balanced for methionine over a methionine-deficient diet (Roth *et al.*, 2006). Plasma concentrations of certain amino acids (e.g. lysine and tryptophan) provide signals for release of neurotransmitters, such as serotonin in the brain, that play a role in feed-intake regulation.

The provision of bypass protein to ruminants fed low quality roughages increases feed intake. Part of the response in growing animals may be that bypass protein provides amino acids in which microbial protein is deficient, thus increasing growth rate, which in turn will increase feed intake.

However, there is a specific effect of bypass protein on feed intake in addition to effects it might have on improved absorbed nutrient balance. The effect of bypass protein on enhancing roughage intake seems to be facilitation of greater fill, perhaps affecting the set point at which rumen distention causes cessation of intake (Ndlovu and Buchanan-Smith, 1987). The effect of bypass protein on stimulating feed intake is greater with tropical than temperate roughages. Supplementation with bypass energy sources, such as rice polishings, improves growth performance of animals fed low quality roughages without affecting roughage intake (Preston, 1982). Supplementation of low quality roughage (grass hay) with rumen degradable protein also increases feed intake and digestibility (Arroquy *et al.*, 2004).

Ruminants may have the ability to select a diet of adequate nitrogen content when grazing. Sheep and goats graze more selectively than cattle and, under conditions of poor quality pasture, may be better able to select a diet of adequate nitrogen content than cattle.

Minerals

Animals have a well-recognized appetite for salt (sodium chloride). This salt appetite is often triggered by low contents of sodium relative to potassium in plants, as well as frank sodium deficiency in forages. Sodium and potassium are two of the major blood electrolytes. A sodium-to-potassium imbalance may disturb blood electrolyte balance; therefore, the animal is attracted to sources of the deficient mineral. Diets of herbivores tend to be high in potassium relative to sodium.

Ruminants have a pronounced ability to conserve sodium. The rumen acts as a sodium storehouse. When sodium-deficient diets are consumed, rumen sodium is drawn upon to counteract blood sodium depletion, and potassium, which is abundant in grass, replaces sodium in saliva. These mechanisms allow ruminants to adapt to the large sodium-deficient areas of the world, which include most non-coastal land areas. Northern ruminants, such as moose, eat large amounts of sodium-containing aquatic plants during a 3-month season and draw on the rumen sodium pool during the rest of the year (Botkin *et al.*, 1973). While aquatic plants are richer than terrestrial plants in sodium, they often have high concentrations of toxic heavy metals such as cadmium (Ohlson and

Staaland, 2001). Reindeer and moose are often in negative sodium balance during winter, so that availability of sodium-rich vegetation in spring and early summer may be critical. Ohlson and Staaland (2001) suggest that winter migrations of large herbivores from inland to coastal areas may be partly driven by a physiological need for sodium.

Sheep grazing on forages with a high salt content (e.g. *Atriplex* spp. or saltbrush) produce lambs which as adults can excrete salt more rapidly, drink less water and maintain feed intake when given a high dose of salt compared to the offspring of ewes fed a diet with lower salt concentrations (Chadwick *et al.*, 2009). There is a reduction in plasma rennin activity in the salt-adapted sheep. Rennin is the rate-limiting step in the rennin-angiotensin system that is involved in the control of salt balance by the kidney.

A presumed example of **nutritional wisdom** is evident in the results of Sanders and Jarvis (2004) with band-tailed pigeons. During the nesting season in western Oregon, the pigeons consume a diet made up almost exclusively of red elderberries (*Sambucus racemosa*), blue elderberries (*Sambucus cerulea*) and cascara (*Rhamnus purshiana*). It had been observed for many years that the pigeons congregate at mineral sites, including Pacific Ocean beaches, and consume mineral deposits (Fig. 17.5). It was generally assumed that the birds were using these sites as sources of calcium to support the calcium needs for egg shell formation and production of 'crop milk' (Sanders and Jarvis, 2004). However, mineral analysis of the berries (Table 17.3) reveals extremely high potassium concentrations relative to sodium content. Absorption and retention of sodium can be reduced by excessive potassium intake. Salt (sodium) appetite in many species is often associated with high potassium:sodium ratios in plant foods. Thus it is likely that as a result of dependence on elder and cascara berries during the nesting season, the band-tailed pigeons seek a source of sodium to overcome the negative effects of potassium loading (Sanders and Jarvis, 2004), and thus use mineral seeps extensively. The physiological driving force may be homeostatic mechanisms to correct cationic electrolyte imbalance.

Many herbivores utilize mineral licks as sources of sodium. Holdo *et al.* (2002) reported data in elephants similar to the pigeon data of Sanders and Jarvis (2004). Forage used by African elephants

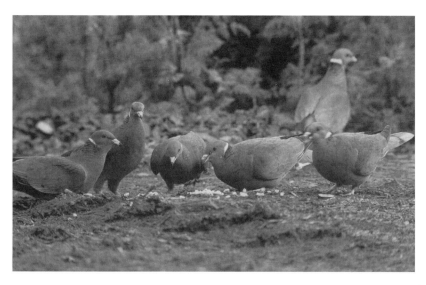

Fig. 17.5. Band-tailed pigeons consuming soil at a mineral (salt) site (courtesy of T.A. Sanders, United States Fish and Wildlife Service, Portland, Oregon, USA).

Table 17.3. Sodium, calcium and potassium contents (mg/kg dry matter) of berries consumed by band-tailed pigeons (Sanders and Jarvis, 2004).

Nutrient	Source of berries		
	Red elder	Cascara	Blue elder
Calcium	1,960	2,290	2,220
Potassium	26,980	12,470	19,690
Sodium	254	20	73
K:Na ratio	106	624	270

contained 20–580 mg/kg of sodium and 1190–36090 mg/kg of potassium (Holdo *et al.*, 2002). Elephants consumed mineral licks rich in sodium to overcome the sodium:potassium imbalance. They also utilized vegetation on termite mounds preferentially (Holdo and McDowell, 2004), although the trees growing on termite mounds were not higher in sodium. Fashing *et al.* (2006) observed that colobus monkeys in Kenya travelled far outside their home ranges to forage on rare foods which contained exceptionally high sodium concentrations.

Desert vegetation often has a high sodium content. **Halophytes** (salt-loving plants) are able to take up saline water and sequester the sodium salts in some way. Saltbrush (*Atriplex* spp.), for example, concentrates sodium chloride in the cells of the outer tissues of the leaves. As these cells accumulate salt, they burst, depositing salt crystals on the leaf surface (Mares *et al.*, 1997). The salt crystals shade the plant from direct sunlight and function as a deterrent to herbivory. Various desert animals are able to successfully feed on halophytes. Kangaroo rats, for example, have highly specialized kidneys that produce very concentrated urine. The chisel-toothed kangaroo rat uses its incisors to peel off the outer salt layer of *Atriplex* leaves (Mares *et al.*, 1997). Small desert rodents in various parts of the world have similar adaptations to allow consumption of halophytes.

Tree bark may serve as a source of supplementary minerals for arboreal folivores including primates, squirrels and marsupials. Stephens *et al.* (2006) found that the mineral content of bark of trees that arboreal marsupials consumed was higher than for trees for which bark was not consumed. They concluded that tree bark was an important source of calcium and phosphorus for these animals.

Forage composition

In ruminants, forage quality and composition influence feed intake. A major factor regulating forage intake is the **neutral detergent fibre** (NDF) and its digestibility. The NDF seems to be the major component limiting rumen fill. Van Soest (1994) used the following analogy (**the skyscraper theory**) to illustrate this effect:

> The effect [of NDF breakdown] may be compared to the demolition of a tall city skyscraper; the contents of the rooms, non-bearing walls, plaster, doors and furniture can be expelled without altering the volume of the building. Only when the wrecking ball smashes the structure does its effective volume decrease.

In the rumen, only when the NDF is digested is its effect on rumen fill eliminated (Allen, 1996). Lippke (1986) confirmed this relationship with cattle; the intake of forage was regulated by the intake of indigestible NDF. When given a choice, cattle selected a diet that maximized digestible organic matter intake. The NDF content is highly correlated with rumination or chewing time. Both the initial volume of the feed and the amount of chewing required to reduce its volume have a role in the fill effect. Because both the chewing time and the feed volume are correlated with NDF content, the NDF is probably the best estimator of forage quality. Some ingredients, such as finely ground cottonseed hulls and soybean hulls, have a high NDF content but stimulate little rumination because of their small particle size. Therefore, for these ingredients, NDF may not be a good estimator of potential feed intake and forage quality.

In dairy cattle nutrition, there is an increasing tendency to use NDF requirement figures in ration formulation to optimize the roughage intake for proper rumen fermentation and milk fat production. Another approach is that of French researchers (Jarrige et al., 1986), who have developed a 'fill unit' system to estimate the **ingestibility** of forages and forage-concentrate diets. Separate fill units were developed for sheep and cattle. The system proposed that the fill unit value of a forage is a unique characteristic, just like its protein or energy content, and that animals consume a fixed amount of fill units rather than a fixed amount of dry matter. Fill units can be entered into computer programs for diet formulation. Although undoubtedly numerous refinements will be needed, this or a similar system will be very useful in estimating feed intake and thus providing nutrients in the amount needed per animal per day, rather than simply as a percentage of diet.

In the USA, the concept of **effective NDF (eNDF)** has been developed to measure NDF that contributes to rumen fill. The eNDF is determined by subtracting from total NDF the NDF fraction that passes through a 1 mm screen (Van Soest, 1994). The eNDF concept, also known as physically effective NDF (peNDF), has been reviewed by Yang and Beauchemin (2006). The eNDF is related not only to rumen fill but also to **chewing time**. Increased chewing activity as a result of increased eNDF can increase ruminal pH (via increased salivary secretion) and help minimize ruminal acidosis in dairy cows. Lammers et al. (1996) developed a practical device, the Penn State Particle Separator, for routine on-farm use to measure the eNDF of forages and total mixed rations.

The water content of forages can sometimes influence intake. Gallavan et al. (1989) found that the low dry-matter content of lush wheat pasture limited the dry-matter intake of sheep to below maintenance. A minimum dry-matter content of 17% was required for sheep to consume their maintenance requirements, and a dry-matter content of 28–30% was required for optimal growth. Intracellular water of forages can limit intake through a bulk effect because of the time period required for its release in the rumen and subsequent absorption.

The **water-holding capacity** of feedstuffs may affect feed intake. Feeds with high water-holding capacity include wheat bran, beet pulp, lucerne meal and grains (e.g. wheat). In a comparison of 23 wheat samples in diets for broilers, Pirgozliev et al. (2003) reported that feed intake was negatively correlated with water-holding capacity of the wheat.

Environmental temperature

The environmental temperature has an important influence on feed intake. The metabolic rate of an animal is at a minimum in the **comfort zone** (Fig. 17.6), also known as the **zone of thermoneutrality**. As environmental temperatures decrease below the comfort zone, an increase in metabolic rate is necessary to maintain body temperature. Thus feed intake increases as environmental temperature decreases. It is difficult to quantify these relationships (e.g. to indicate that with a 10°C decrease in environmental temperature the feed intake will increase by a certain percentage) because of the involvement of other factors, such as humidity and wind velocity. Kennedy et al. (1986) discussed some of the complexities in ruminants. In cold environments, digestibility is reduced because passage rate through the rumen is increased. The **heat of rumen fermentation** is a negative factor for an animal in the comfort zone but is beneficial at low environmental temperatures. Roughages, which

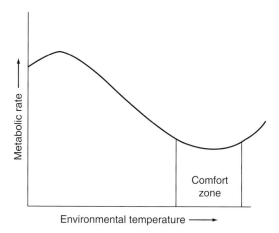

Fig. 17.6. Metabolic rate (and consequently feed intake) is at a minimum in the environmental temperature range where the animal does not need to employ cooling or heating mechanisms (the comfort zone). At low temperatures, metabolic rate is increased to maintain body temperature, so feed intake is also increased.

produce a high amount of heat of fermentation, have a higher net energy value at lower than at higher temperatures. This is due partly to the greater ruminal heat of fermentation and partly to the heat increment associated with acetate catabolism, the VFA produced in greatest proportion with high roughage diets. At temperatures above the comfort zone, there is also an increase in metabolic rate, caused by the employment of heat-dissipating actions such as panting.

Hormonal changes influence winter feed intake. During a period of exposure to cold, the comfort zone is lowered by alterations in the output of such hormones as thyroxine. The winter hair coat also provides insulation to reduce energy requirements. Wild ungulates, such as deer, accumulate large amounts of body fat in the summer and have a very low feed intake in the winter, surviving on body-fat stores. Domestic ruminants appear to have vestiges of this photoperiod-controlled feed intake pattern (Kennedy *et al.*, 1986).

Wild ruminants resemble their domesticated counterparts in digestive physiology and nutritional requirements. Ruminants native to temperate and Arctic areas often show a marked **seasonal variation in feed intake**, corresponding to patterns of seasonal availability of feed. Deer, for example, have a high feed intake in the summer and accumulate large fat deposits. In the winter, they may go for many days without eating, meeting their energy

needs by mobilization of body fat (Wood *et al.*, 1962). This **periodicity in feed intake** is even observed in captive animals with free access to feed (Parker *et al.*, 1993; Freudenberger *et al.*, 1994) and seems to be photoperiodically regulated (Louden, 1994; Morgan and Mercer, 1994; Adam *et al.*, 1996). In males, there is a second period of **voluntary hypophagia** (lack of feed intake) associated with the autumn mating season or rut. It is correlated with testosterone concentrations (West and Nordan, 1976; McMillin *et al.*, 1980) that show seasonal variations (Whitehead and McEwan, 1973). Hypophagia during the rut period may be an adaptive feature helping to ensure reproductive success.

Seasonal changes in feed intake are accompanied by changes in the gut. With hypophagia, there is a reduction in the rumen microbial population, particularly of cellulose digesters. Microbial changes are followed by alterations in the rumen mucosa, with seasonal variation in the volume and absorptive surface of rumen papillae. Winter starvation of browsers and intermediate feeders is primarily a consequence of the lack of cellulolytic rumen microbes (Hofmann, 2000). Musk oxen may lose 40% of their body mass during winter. Their rumen papillae recover rapidly in summer, allowing rapid and maximal absorption of nutrients.

Seasonal hyperphagia (high feed intake) during summer and autumn does not reduce the digestive efficiency in an Arctic grazer, the musk ox (Peltier *et al.*, 2003; Barboza *et al.*, 2006). Seasonal increases in digestive and metabolic functions allow musk oxen to rapidly accumulate energy and other nutrients in body tissue during the short season of plant growth. This strategy compensates for the foraging limitations and increased costs of thermoregulation and mobility during the harsh winter season.

Seasonal changes in physiology and behaviour such as seasonality in breeding, voluntary feed intake and so on are regulated by **photoperiod**, which is a highly predictable environmental cue (Morgan and Mercer, 1994). The hormone **melatonin** is synthesized by the **pineal gland** (located in the epithalamus of the brain) in a precisely regulated pattern, with the neural transmission of a signal from the retina of the eye to the pineal gland. During the day, low levels of melatonin synthesis and secretion occur. At night, melatonin synthesis and blood melatonin levels are increased in direct proportion to the length of the dark period. Thus, winter and summer photoperiods are reflected in long- and short-duration melatonin signals, respectively.

The **annual cycles** in reproductive behaviour and feed intake in wild ruminants have evolved via adaptation mechanisms to ensure reproductive success and winter survival. Deer and other temperate ruminants have a number of other physiologic adaptations to enhance their likelihood of winter survival besides the accretion of large fat deposits in the summer. The fasting metabolic rate of white-tailed deer is 30–40% lower in winter than in summer (McMillin *et al.*, 1980), reducing winter energy requirements. Heart rates and body temperature are also lower in winter. These changes seem to be mediated by thyroid hormones (McMillin *et al.*, 1980). Physical activity may be markedly reduced. In **tropical deer**, seasonal patterns of growth, voluntary feed intake and plasma hormone concentrations do occur, but they are less pronounced than in temperate deer species (Semiadi *et al.*, 1995). Such variability may be important in overall health and body condition of captive hoof-stock, but consequences have not been examined in detail in zoo collections. Similar animal responses may be seen *in situ*, even at equatorial latitudes, if one considers seasonality in terms of forage or prey quality and quantities in relation to rainy versus dry environmental conditions. There is evidence of seasonality of feed intake in domestic ruminants such as sheep (Iason *et al.*, 2000).

Supplemental feeding of big game animals is often necessary for a variety of reasons, including emergency feeding during unusually severe winters and enticing wild animals away from haystacks or other sources of privately owned feed. Such feeding is especially important with elk in the western USA. Artificial feeding of deer and elk has been reviewed by Dean (1980). Good-quality lucerne hay is satisfactory to entice moose and elk to feeding stations. Deer may suffer **rumen and omasum impaction** when fed poor-quality lucerne hay or other fibrous feed. Deer should be fed a pelleted concentrate diet containing grain, plant protein supplement and lucerne meal.

Under conditions of high environmental temperature, the **heat increment** of feeds becomes important. The heat increment is the extra heat production that arises from the metabolism of nutrients. It is highest for protein and corresponds to the extra metabolism (operation of the urea cycle in the liver) required to deaminate amino acids and convert the ammonia to urea when amino acids are used as an energy source. Thus,

under conditions of high temperatures, the dietary protein level may need to be reduced. Under conditions of cold environmental temperatures, the percentage of dietary protein can also be lowered because feed intake is increased. Because the heat increment is lowest for fat, it is desirable to increase the dietary fat content under conditions of high environmental temperatures.

The heat increment includes the heat of rumen fermentation. It is useful at temperatures below the comfort zone and detrimental at high environmental temperatures. The heat of fermentation is higher with high roughage diets than with concentrates.

Preston and Leng (1987) suggest that one of the reasons imported breeds of livestock, such as the Holstein cow, often perform poorly when introduced into the tropics is because they have a higher basal metabolic rate (BMR) than indigenous breeds. With the lower feed intake characteristic of hot environments, the imported breeds use a greater fraction of energy intake for maintenance and thus have less available for production. The higher BMR, producing more heat to be dissipated, also contributes to a greater sensitivity to heat stress.

Metabolic imbalance can reduce feed intake by way of **thermogenic effects**. In ruminants, an excess of C2-energy sources (acetate and butyrate) relative to gluconeogenic precursor (propionate) leads to increased heat production from disposal of the excess C2 sources. Increased carbohydrate metabolism is necessary to produce the extra oxaloacetic acid (OAA) necessary for incorporation of C2 (acetate) into the citric acid cycle. The feed intake is reduced in response to this thermogenic effect, particularly in hot climates (Preston and Leng, 1987). As mentioned earlier, the thermogenic effect of acetate is useful under cold conditions.

Pregnancy and lactation

Voluntary feed intake shows characteristic changes in pregnancy and lactation. In late gestation, feed intake decreases, perhaps an effect of the high levels of circulating oestrogens at that time that may alter metabolism to reduce energy requirements (Forbes, 1986a). Also, the increasing size of the fetus or fetuses takes up an increasing volume of the abdominal cavity, so that in ewes with multiple fetuses, for instance, the **rumen volume** is substantially reduced in late pregnancy (Forbes, 1970). Also, there is an increase in rate of passage of digesta through the rumen as pregnancy progresses, that is probably caused by an increase in rumination time, which would increase the rate of breakdown of feed particles (Forbes, 1970).

During peak lactation, feed intake is very high, to support high levels of milk production. In dairy cattle, the peak in feed intake is reached after peak lactation occurs, so body reserves are mobilized during this period. In ruminants, rapid rates of utilization of VFAs for synthesis of milk may reduce blood VFA levels, reducing the negative feedback on chemoreceptors in the appetite centre, partially accounting for the increased feed intake during lactation.

Learning and conditioning

Animals often exhibit neophobia, a reluctance to accept a new food. Such a reaction can have practical implications. Where supplemental feeding of livestock is required under drought conditions, grain or pellets may be the least expensive and most convenient sources of emergency feed. However, sheep that have never eaten these feeds may not recognize them as feed and may starve. Chapple *et al.* (1987) found that it took sheep several weeks to overcome fear of the feed trough and supplementary wheat, and then a period was needed to learn to eat, chew and swallow wheat. The learning process was accelerated if there were some experienced animals in the flock. Animals that have learned to eat a novel feed at a young age will readily accept it again even after a several-year lack of exposure to it.

Livestock can be trained to avoid poisonous plants, such as larkspur, by a process of aversive conditioning (Ralphs *et al.*, 1988; Lane *et al.*, 1990). If cattle are fed larkspur and then dosed with lithium chloride, they associate the temporary discomfort induced by the lithium chloride with the larkspur and avoid the plant in the future. Various feed additives such as monensin (Baile *et al.*, 1979) and urea may cause a temporary feed aversion, which is overcome during an adaptation period.

Metabolic body size

Common experience indicates that the feed intake of animals does not vary directly with body size. The smallest mammal, the shrew, weighs approximately 1–6 g and eats its body weight in food daily. It has an intense rate of metabolism and eats voraciously just to keep alive. A shrew can die of starvation after as little as 3 h without food. It is evident that the larger an animal is, the less feed it consumes per unit of body weight. Obviously, an elephant does not consume its body weight in feed each day. This relationship (Fig. 17.7) was one of great interest to animal scientists for much of the 20th century. Two of the most active researchers were Samuel Brody of the University of Missouri and Max Kleiber of the University of California. Their contributions were summarized in two classic books (Kleiber, 1961; Brody, 1964) dealing with bioenergetics and its relationship to body size.

Brody conducted calorimetric experiments with animals ranging in size from mice to elephants and found that the metabolic rate (hence energy requirements and feed intake) of animals per unit of body weight decreased as body size increased. When body weight doubled, **basal metabolic rate (BMR)** increased by only 73%. Brody derived an equation relating BMR to body size:

$$\text{BMR (kcal/day)} = 70.5 \, W^{0.734}$$

The BMR is the lowest rate of metabolism (expressed as heat production) of an animal under conditions of complete rest, in a thermoneutral environment and in a fasting state. 'W' is body weight in kg.

Kleiber conducted similar research and arrived at the exponent of 0.75. Brody and Kleiber debated for years as to which exponent was correct! In reality, the relationship is influenced by other factors such as body surface area, species differences in endocrine regulation of metabolic rate, and age, so that there is no 'best' exponent. The exponent 0.75 has become accepted as the most suitable figure for general use; the body weight raised to the 3/4 power ($W^{0.75}$) is known as **metabolic body size**. Recent research (West *et al.*, 2002) has shown that the 0.75 exponent applies to cold-blooded animals, plants and even to intracellular organelles and molecules (mitochondria, respiratory chain complex). Kleiber, in his classic book *The Fire of Life* (1961), illustrated the effect of body size on feed intake by comparing the utilization of 1 t of hay by 1300 lb of either cattle or rabbits (Fig. 17.8). The higher daily feed intake of smaller animals (e.g. sheep, rabbits) is compensated for by higher productivity (e.g. gain per day). However, for animals kept under maintenance conditions, feed requirements are greater for small animals (e.g. sheep) than for an equivalent mass of larger animals (e.g. cattle). Thus the smaller the body weight, the greater the importance of keeping animals in a productive state.

Metabolic rate can be estimated by measuring parameters that reflect the metabolic events

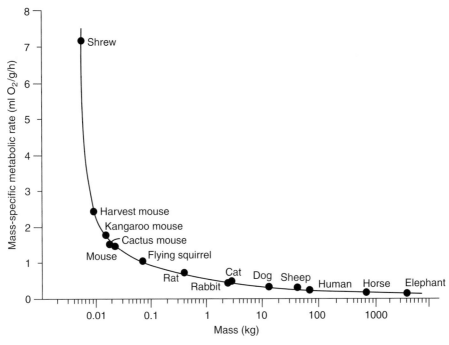

Fig. 17.7. The relationship between basal metabolic rate (BMR) and body weight. (From Schmidt-Nelson, 1997.)

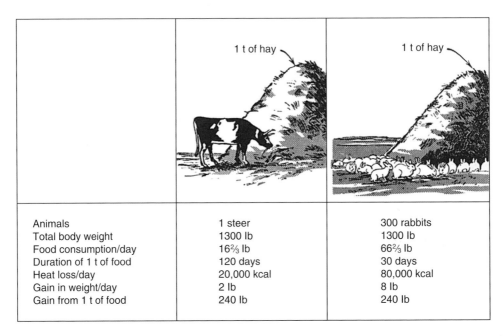

Animals	1 steer	300 rabbits
Total body weight	1300 lb	1300 lb
Food consumption/day	16⅔ lb	66⅔ lb
Duration of 1 t of food	120 days	30 days
Heat loss/day	20,000 kcal	80,000 kcal
Gain in weight/day	2 lb	8 lb
Gain from 1 t of food	240 lb	240 lb

Fig. 17.8. The effect of body size on feed utilization. Small animals have higher feed intake per unit of body weight than large animals (from Kleiber, 1961; courtesy of John Wiley and Sons, Inc.).

occurring in the tissues. Oxygen consumption can be measured using either respiration chambers or facemasks connected to an oxygen source. Metabolism is basically the summation of oxidation reactions. Output of carbon dioxide directly reflects oxidative activity. Heat production, a by-product of oxidative reactions, can also be measured. For free-ranging animals, equipped with monitoring devices, heart rate correlates directly with energy expenditure (Brosh, 2007).

Metabolic body size is widely used in animal nutrition research, particularly for interspecies comparisons of feed intake (e.g. sheep versus cattle). A typical example is the data of Reid *et al.* (1988) shown in Table 17.4. On a metabolic size basis, the intake by cattle of temperate (C3) grasses and legumes and tropical (C4) grasses was greater than for sheep, indicating the greater capacity for forage intake of grazers (cattle) over intermediate feeders (sheep).

The **surface area** of animals shows a similar relationship with metabolic rate as does body weight, which has led to theories suggesting that metabolic rate is a function of ability to dissipate heat to the environment (Kleiber, 1961). Zoologists refer to **Bergmann's rule**, which asserts that within a species the body mass increases with latitude and colder climate. An advantage would be that larger animals radiate less heat per unit of mass than small animals, which would provide an advantage in thermoregulation under cold conditions. Bergmann's rule is vigorously denounced by some scientists (e.g. Geist, 1987, 1990) and defended by others (e.g. Paterson, 1990).

Other factors

Many other factors, often in combination with some of the items mentioned above, may influence feed intake. Smell is very important. Sometimes animals will reject a diet or a forage without even tasting it, suggesting that olfactory cues are involved. Grazing animals will not graze in the immediate area of manure droppings (Fig. 17.9), but if the grass around the dung is cut and taken to

Table 17.4. Forage intake of sheep and cattle consuming temperate and tropical forages, expressed on a metabolic size basis (adapted from Reid *et al.*, 1988).

Forage fraction intake (g/kg $W^{0.75}$)	C3 Grasses	C3 Legumes	C4 Grasses
Dry matter			
Sheep	71.4	90.7	65.7
Cattle	89.0	94.8	90.0
Neutral detergent fibre (NDF)			
Sheep	40.8	43.7	48.6
Cattle	58.1	48.6	66.7

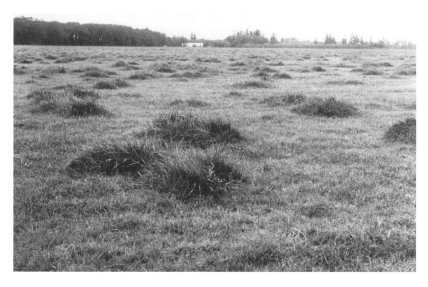

Fig. 17.9. Uneaten grass growing on dung spots in a cattle pasture. Animals avoid grazing forage growing on dung spots from their own species but will consume it from dung spots from other species. Thus, mixed animal species grazing (e.g. sheep and cattle) can improve forage utilization.

an animal, it will be readily consumed (Marten, 1978). This behaviour is probably beneficial in reducing exposure to internal parasites. Specific volatile chemicals in cattle faeces deter cattle from grazing forage near their faeces for about 30 days (Dohi *et al.*, 1991). Urine patches are avoided for only a few days (Sporndly, 1996). Some animals, such as horses, establish dunging areas in a pasture; such areas may occupy up to 25% of the total area (Archer, 1978). Harrowing pastures helps to spread out the dung piles and reduce the area of uneaten forage. Mixed grazing can also be used; animals avoid manure only from their own species.

Fatigue can limit feed intake. Ruminants consuming coarse forages may become fatigued in seeking, ingesting, chewing and ruminating feed (Preston and Leng, 1987; McLeod and Smith, 1989). **Rumination time** is directly related to plant cell wall content. Sheep and cattle have a maximum rumination time of approximately 10 h/day and cannot be forced to ruminate beyond this limit (Van Soest, 1994). Small ruminants, such as sheep and goats, must ruminate fibrous feeds to a smaller particle size than cattle for the indigestible fibre to exit the rumen through the smaller omasal orifice. Therefore, rumination may be a more limiting factor for the smaller ruminants. Horses can, if necessary, graze almost continuously.

Illness (sickness behaviour) that involves activation of the immune system results in loss of appetite. This is a consequence of the metabolic actions of various **cytokines**, such as interleukins and tumour necrosis factor. The actions of inflammatory cytokines are discussed in Chapter 24.

Predicting Feed Intake

Prediction of feed intake is very important in meeting nutrient requirements of animals. Ideally, diets are to be formulated and fed so as to precisely meet an individual animal's nutrient requirements. This is done with dairy cattle, where feed intake can be individually regulated and adjusted according to the lactational potential and performance of the cow. Computer modelling is used to account for factors affecting feed intake, and it provides equations for predicting intake and digestibility. Prediction of intake and digestibility for ruminants has been reviewed by Mertens (1987) and the National Research Council (1987). These sources should be consulted for more information.

Feed intake is readily measured in pen-fed animals. Feed intake measurements are a normal component of feeding trials. If the unconsumed feed (orts) is appreciably different from the offered feed, then in experimental work the orts should be analysed and a correction of nutrient intake calculated. For example, if the animals are selectively sorting out an unpalatable component, then the measured nutrient intake will not be the same as the actual feed intake. Measurement of feed intake of grazing animals is more difficult. A common procedure is to surgically prepare selected animals with an oesophageal fistula. When feed intake is to be measured, a collection bag is attached to the animal, with the consumed feed going into the bag rather than into the rumen. The bag contents (extrusa) can be analysed for botanical composition and nutrient content.

Questions and Study Guide

1. Why are moose rarely exhibited in zoos?
2. What are the five major taste responses?
3. What are some examples of specialist feeders?
4. Why don't cats have a sweet tooth?
5. What are 'secondary compounds' in plants?
6. Deer often feed on tannin-containing plants. What adaptation renders them tolerant of tannins?
7. What is the relationship between plant chemistry and population cycles of small animals such as snowshoe hares?
8. When Europeans arrived in North America, there were millions of beavers present. Why was it that these animals did not 'clear-cut' the entire continent?

9. How do generalist feeders differ from specialist feeders in their abilities to detoxify plant secondary compounds?
10. What are 'talking trees'?
11. Discuss the concept of nutritional wisdom.
12. Compare physical and chemical regulation of feed intake.
13. In the data of Table 17.4, why was the NDF intake for sheep higher with C4 grass than with the other forages, even though the feed intake was lowest with this forage?
14. What are some animal adaptations to the consumption of halophytes?

Continued

Questions and Study Guide Continued.

15. What is the 'skyscraper theory'? What is its relationship to regulation of feed intake in cattle?
16. What is the zone of thermal neutrality?
17. Do deer and musk oxen have higher or lower feed intakes in winter or summer? Why?
18. Why does the voluntary feed intake of pregnant sheep often decrease during late gestation?
19. What is metabolic body size?
20. According to the National Research Council, the daily requirements for maximum growth of a young pig are 6460 kcal dietary energy, 285 g crude protein and 14.3 g lysine/day. Assume you have two diets: one with 2700 kcal dietary energy/kg and one with 3800 kcal dietary energy/kg. Calculate the following for each diet:
    (i) Expected daily feed intake;

(ii) Optimal percentage of protein and lysine in each diet;
(iii) Optimal protein/kcal and lysine/kcal ratios, expressed as mg/kcal;

What advantage, if any, is there to expressing nutrient requirements on a per kcal basis rather than as percentage of diet?

21. What is the highest possible energy level you could achieve in a diet? For example, could you formulate a diet that contained 12,000 kcal dietary energy/kg? What ingredients would you use to achieve this energy level?
22. Refer to data in Table 17.5. How do you explain the decline in carcass lipid content as the protein/kcal ratio increases? Also explain why the percentage of the carcass lipid content increases as caloric density increases.

Table 17.5. The effect of dietary protein/kcal ratio on carcass lipid content (%) of weanling rats (Wood, 1964).

Dietary protein concentration (mg crude protein/kcal dietary energy)	Caloric density (kcal dietary energy/kg diet)				
	2000	3000	4000	5000	5700
30	12.2[a]	15.2	18.9	16.7	19.8
45	8.2	10.2	12.0	12.5	11.9
60	6.1	7.9	9.9	10.8	10.8
75	4.1	6.0	9.5	10.1	12.3

[a]Carcass lipid (%).

References

Adam, C.L., Kyle, C.E. and Young, P. (1996) Seasonal patterns of growth, voluntary feed intake and plasma concentrations of prolactin, insulin-like growth factor-1, LH and gonadal steroids in male and female pre-pubertal red deer (*Cervus elaphus*) reared in either natural photoperiod or constant daylight. *Animal Science* 62, 605–613.

Allen, M.S. (1996) Physical constraints on voluntary intake of forages by ruminants. *Journal of Animal Science* 74, 3063–3075.

Allen, M.S., Bradford, B.J. and Oba, M. (2009) The hepatic oxidation theory of the control of feed intake and its application to ruminants. *Journal of Animal Science* 87, 3317–3334.

Archer, M. (1978) Further studies on palatability of grasses to horses. *Journal of British Grassland Society* 33, 239–243.

Arroquy, J.I., Cochran, R.C., Villarreal, M., Wickersham, T.A., Llewellyn, D.A., Titgemeyer, E.C., Nagaraja, T.G., Johnson, D.E. and Gnad, D. (2004) Effect of level of rumen degradable protein and type of supplemental non-fiber carbohydrate on intake and digestion of low-quality grass hay by beef cattle. *Animal Feed Science and Technology* 115, 83–99.

Austin, P.J., Suchar, L.A., Robbins, C.T. and Hagerman, A.E. (1989) Tannin-binding proteins in saliva of deer and their absence in saliva of sheep and cattle. *Journal of Chemical Ecology* 15, 1335–1347.

Baile, C.A. and McLaughlin, C.L. (1987) Mechanisms controlling feed intake in ruminants: a review. *Journal of Animal Science* 64, 915–922.

Baile, C.A., McLaughlin, C.L., Potter, E.L. and Chalupa, W. (1979) Feeding behavior changes of cattle during introduction of monensin with roughage or concentrate diets. *Journal of Animal Science* 48, 1501–1508.

Baldwin, S.E. and Schultz, J.C. (1983) Rapid changes in tree leaf chemistry induced by damage: evidence for communication between plants. *Science* 221, 277–279.

Barboza, P.S., Peltier, T.C. and Forster, R.J. (2006) Ruminal fermentation and fill change with season in an Arctic grazer: responses to hyperphagia and hypophagia in muskoxen (*Ovibos moschatus*). *Physiological and Biochemical Zoology* 79, 497–513.

Basey, J.M., Jenkins, S.H. and Busher, P.E. (1988) Optimal central-place foraging by beavers: tree-size selection in relation to defensive chemicals of quaking aspen. *Oecologia* 76, 278–282.

Botkin, D.B., Jordan, P.A., Dominski, A.S., Lowendorf, H.S. and Hutchinson, G.E. (1973) Sodium dynamics in a northern ecosystem. *Proceedings of the National Academy of Sciences, USA* 70, 2745–2748.

Brody, S. (1964) *Bioenergetics and Growth*. Hafner, New York.

Brosh, A. (2007) Heart rate measurements as an index of energy expenditure and energy balance in ruminants: a review. *Journal of Animal Science* 85, 1213–1227.

Bryant, J.P., Danell, K., Provenza, F., Reichardt, P.B. and Clausen, T.A. (1991) Effects of mammal browsing on the chemistry of deciduous woody plants. In: Tallamy, D.W. and Raupp, M.J. (eds) *Phytochemical Induction by Herbivores*. John Wiley & Sons, Chichester, Sussex, UK, pp. 293–323.

Bryant, J.P., Reichardt, P.B. and Clausen, T.P. (1992) Chemically mediated interactions between woody plants and browsing mammals. *Journal of Range Management* 45, 18–24.

Chadwick, M.A., Vercoe, P.E., Williams, I.H. and Revell, D.K. (2009) Programming sheep production on saltbush: adaptations of offspring from ewes that consumed high amounts of salt during pregnancy and early lactation. *Animal Production Science* 49, 311–317.

Chapple, R.S., Wodzicka-Tomaszewska, M. and Lynch, J.J. (1987) The learning behavior of sheep when introduced to wheat. II. Social transmission of wheat feeding and the role of the senses. *Applied Animal Behaviour Science* 18, 163–172.

Cheeke, P.R. (1998) *Natural Toxicants in Feeds, Forages, and Poisonous Plants*. Prentice Hall, Upper Saddle River, New Jersey.

Clauss, M. (2003) Tannins in the nutrition of wild animals. A review. In: Fidgett, A., Clauss, M., Ganslosser, U., Hatt, J.-M. and Nijboer, J. (eds) *Zoo Animal Nutrition*, Vol. 2. Filander Verlag, Fürth, Germany, pp. 53–89.

Clauss, M., Kienzle, E. and Wiesner, H. (2002) Importance of the wasting syndrome complex in captive moose (*Alces alces*). *Zoo Biology* 21, 499–506

Clauss, M., Lason, K., Gehrke, J., Lechner-Doll, M., Fickel, J., Grune, T. and Streich, W.J. (2003) Captive roe deer (*Capreolus capreolus*) select for low amounts of tannic acid but not quebracho: fluctuation of preferences and potential benefits. *Comparative Biochemistry and Physiology* 136, 369–382.

Clauss, M., Gehrke, J., Hatt, J.-M., Dierenfeld, E.S., Flach, E.J., Hermes, R., Castell, J., Streich, W.J. and Fickel, J. (2005) Tannin-binding salivary proteins in three captive rhinoceros species. *Comparative Biochemistry and Physiology* 140, 67–72.

Cooper, S.M. and Owen-Smith, N. (1986) Effects of plant spinescence on large mammalian herbivores. *Oecologia* 68, 446–455.

Cooper, S.M., Owen-Smith, N. and Bryant, J.P. (1988) Foliage acceptability to browsing ruminants in relation to seasonal changes in the leaf chemistry of woody plants in a South African savanna. *Oecologia* 75, 336–342.

Dean, R.E. (1980) The nutrition of wild ruminants. In: Church, D.C. (ed.) *Digestive Physiology and Nutrition of Ruminants*, Vol. 3. O & B Books, Corvallis, Oregon, pp. 278–305.

Dearing, M.D., Mangione, A.M. and Karasov, W.H. (2000) Diet breadth of mammalian herbivores: nutrient versus detoxification constraints. *Oecologia* 123, 397–405.

Dierenfeld, E.S., Mueller, P.J. and Hall, M.B. (2002) Duikers: native food composition, micronutrient assessment, and implications for improving captive diets. *Zoo Biology* 21, 185–196.

Dohi, H., Yamada, A. and Entsu, S. (1991) Cattle feeding deterrents emitted from cattle feces. *Journal of Chemical Ecology* 17, 1197–1203.

Fashing, P.J., Dierenfeld, E.S. and Mowry, C.B. (2006) Influence of plant and soil chemistry on food selection, ranging patterns, and biomass of *Colobus guereza* in Kakamega Forest, Kenya. *International Journal of Primatology* 28, 673–703.

Foley, W.J., McLean, S. and Cork, S.J. (1995) Consequences of biotransformation of plant secondary metabolites on acid–base metabolism in mammals – a final common pathway? *Journal of Chemical Ecology* 21, 721–743.

Forbes, J.M. (1970) Voluntary food intake of pregnant ewes. *Journal of Animal Science* 31, 1222–1227.

Forbes, J.M. (1986a) The effects of sex hormones, pregnancy, and lactation on digestion, metabolism, and voluntary food intake. In: Milligan, L.P., Grovum, W.L. and Dobson, A. (eds) *Control of Digestion and Metabolism in Ruminants*. Prentice-Hall, Englewood Cliffs, New Jersey, pp. 420–435.

Forbes, J.M. (1986b) *The Voluntary Food Intake of Farm Animals*. Butterworths, London.

Forbes, J.M. (1996) Integration of regulatory signals controlling forage intake in ruminants. *Journal of Animal Science* 74, 3029–3035.

Fowler, S.V. and Lawton, J.H. (1985) Rapidly induced defenses and talking trees; the devil's advocate position. *American Naturalist* 126, 181–195.

Freeland, W.J., Calcott, P.H. and Geiss, D.P. (1985) Allelochemicals, minerals and herbivore population size. *Biochemical Systematics and Ecology* 13, 195–206.

Freeland, W.J. and Choquenot, D. (1990) Determinants of herbivore carrying capacity: plants, nutrients, and *Equus asinus* in northern Australia. *Ecology* 71, 589–597.

Freudenberger, D.O., Toyakawa, K., Barry, T.N., Ball, A.J. and Suttie, J.M. (1994) Seasonality in digestion and rumen metabolism in red deer (*Cervus elaphus*) fed on a forage diet. *British Journal of Nutrition* 71, 489–499.

Furstenberg, D. and Van Hoven, W. (1994) Condensed tannin as anti-defoliate agent against browsing by giraffe (*Giraffa camelopardalis*) in the Kruger National Park. *Comparative Biochemistry and Physiology* 107A, 425–431.

Gallavan, R.H., Jr, Phillips, W.A. and Von Tungeln, D.L. (1989) Forage intake and performance of yearling lambs fed harvested wheat forage. *Nutrition Reports International* 39, 643–648.

Geist, V. (1987) Bergmann's rule is invalid. *Canadian Journal of Zoology* 65, 1035–1038.

Geist, V. (1990) Bergmann's rule is invalid: a reply to J.D. Paterson. *Canadian Journal of Zoology* 68, 1613–1615.

Gordon, I.J. and Illius, A.W. (1994) The functional significance of the browser-grazer dichotomy in African ruminants. *Oecologia* 98, 167–175.

Gordon, I.J. and Illius, A.W. (1996) The nutritional ecology of African ruminants: a reinterpretation. *Journal of Animal Ecology* 65, 18–28.

Hagerman, A.E. and Robbins, C.T. (1993) Specificity of tannin-binding salivary proteins relative to diet selection by mammals. *Canadian Journal of Zoology* 71, 628–633.

Henry, Y. (1985) Dietary factors involved in feed intake regulation in growing pigs: a review. *Livestock Production Science* 12, 339–354.

Henry, Y. (1987) Self-selection by growing pigs of diets differing in lysine content. *Journal of Animal Science* 65, 1257–1265.

Hofmann, R.R. (1973) *The Ruminant Stomach*. East African Literature Bureau, Nairobi, Kenya.

Hofmann, R.R. (1989) Evolutionary steps of ecophysiological adaptation and diversification of ruminants: a comparative view of their digestive system. *Oecologia* 78, 443–457.

Hofmann, R.R. (2000) Functional and comparative digestive system anatomy of Arctic ungulates. *Rangifer* 20, 71–81.

Holdo, R.M. and McDowell, L.R. (2004) Termite mounds as nutrient-rich food patches for elephants. *Biotropica* 36, 231–239.

Holdo, R.M., Dudley, J.P. and McDowell, L.R. (2002) Geophagy in the African elephant in relation to availability of dietary sodium. *Journal of Mammology* 83, 652–664.

Huntington, G.B. and Burns, J.C. (2007) Afternoon harvest increases readily fermentable carbohydrate con-centration and voluntary intake of gamagrass and switchgrass baleage by beef steers. *Journal of Animal Science* 85, 276–284.

Iason, G. (2005) Symposium on 'Plants as animal foods: a case of catch 22?' The role of plant secondary metabolites in mammalian herbivory: ecological perspectives. *Proceedings of the Nutrition Society* 64, 123–131.

Iason, G.R. and Palo, R.T. (1991) Effects of birch phenolics on a grazing and a browsing mammal: a comparison of hares. *Journal of Chemical Ecology* 17, 1733–1743.

Iason, G.R., Sim, D.A. and Gordon, I.J. (2000) Do endogenous seasonal cycles of food intake influence foraging behaviour and intake by grazing sheep? *Functional Ecology* 14, 614–622.

Illius, A.W. and Jessop, N.S. (1996) Metabolic constraints on voluntary intake in ruminants. *Journal of Animal Science* 74, 3052–3062.

Jarrige, R., Demarquilly, C., Dulphy, J.P., Hoden, A., Robelin, J., Beranger, C., Geay, Y., Journet, M., Malterre, C., Micol, D. and Petit, M. (1986) The INRA 'fill unit' system for predicting the voluntary intake of forage-based diets in ruminants: a review. *Journal of Animal Science* 63, 1737–1758.

Juntheikki, M.-R. (1996) Comparison of tannin-binding proteins in saliva of Scandinavian and North American moose (*Alces alces*). *Biochemical Systematics and Ecology* 24, 595–601.

Kennedy, P.M., Christopherson, R.J. and Milligan, L.P. (1986) Digestive responses to cold. In: Milligan, L.P., Grovum, W.L. and Dobson, A. (eds) *Control of Digestion and Metabolism in Ruminants*. Prentice-Hall, Englewood Cliffs, New Jersey, pp. 285–306.

Ketelaars, J.J.M.H. and Tolkamp, B.J. (1996) Oxygen efficiency and the control of energy flow in animals and humans. *Journal of Animal Science* 74, 3036–3051.

Kleiber, M. (1961) *The Fire of Life: An Introduction to Animal Energetics*. Wiley, New York.

Krebs, C.J., Boonstra, R., Boutin, S. and Sinclair, A.R.E. (2001) What drives the 10-year cycle of snowshoe hares? *BioScience* 51, 25–35.

Krehbiel, C.R., Cranston, J.J. and McCurdy, M.P. (2009) An upper limit for caloric density of finishing diets. *Journal of Animal Science* 84, E34–E49.

Lammers, B.P., Buckmaster, D.R. and Heinrichs, A.J. (1996) A simple method for the analysis of particle sizes of forage and total mixed rations. *Journal of Dairy Science* 79, 922–928.

Lane, M.A., Ralphs, M.H., Olsen, J.D., Provenza, F.D. and Pfister, J.A. (1990) Conditioned taste aversion: potential for reducing cattle loss to larkspur. *Journal of Range Management* 43, 127–131.

Li, X., Li, W., Wang, H., Cao, J., Maehashi, K., Huang, L., Bachmanov, A.A., Reed, D.R., Legrand-Defretin, V., Beauchamp, G.K. and Brand, J.G. (2009) Pseudogenization of a sweet-receptor gene accounts for cats' indifference toward sugar. Available at: www.plosgenetics.org/article/info:doi/10.1371/journal.pgen.001003 (accessed 2 February 2010).

Lippke, H. (1986) Regulation of voluntary intake of ryegrass and sorghum forages in cattle by indigestible neutral detergent fiber. *Journal of Animal Science* 63, 1459–1468.

Louden, A.S.I. (1994) Photoperiod and the regulation of annual and circannual cycles of food intake. *Proceedings of the Nutrition Society* 53, 495–507.

Luscombe-Marsh, N.D., Smeets, A.J.P.G. and Westerterp-Plantenga, M.S. (2007) Taste sensitivity for monosodium glutamate and an increased liking of dietary protein. *British Journal of Nutrition* 99, 904–908.

Lowry, J.B., McSweeney, C.S. and Palmer, B. (1996) Changing perceptions of the effect of plant phenolics on nutrient supply in the ruminant. *Australian Journal of Agricultural Research* 47, 829–842.

Mares, M.A., Ojeda, R.A., Borghi, C.E., Giannoni, S.M., Diaz, G.B. and Braun, J.K. (1997) How desert rodents overcome halophytic plant defenses. *BioScience* 47, 699–704.

Marsh, K.J., Wallis, I.R. and Foley, W.J. (2005) Detoxification rates constrain feeding in common brushtail possums (*Trichosurus vulpecula*). *Ecology* 86, 2946–2954.

Marten, G.C. (1978) The animal–plant complex in forage palatability phenomena. *Journal of Animal Science* 46, 1470–1477.

Mayland, H.F., Martin, S.A., Lee, J. and Shewmaker, G.E. (2000) Malate, citrate, and amino acids in tall fescue cultivars: relationship to animal preference. *Agronomy Journal* 92, 206–210.

McArthur, C., Sanson, G.D. and Beal, A.M. (1995) Salivary proline-rich proteins in mammals: roles in oral homeostasis and counteracting dietary tannin. *Journal of Chemical Ecology* 21, 663–691.

McLean, S., Brandon, S., Davies, N.W., Boyle, R., Foley, W.J., Moore, B. and Pass, G.J. (2003) Glucuronuria in the koala. *Journal of Chemical Ecology* 29, 1465–1477.

McLeod, M.N. and Smith, B.R. (1989) Eating and ruminating behaviour in cattle given forages differing in fibre content. *Animal Production* 48, 503–511.

McMillin, J.M., Seal, U.S. and Karns, P.D. (1980) Hormonal correlates of hypophagia in white-tailed deer. *Federation Proceedings* 39, 2964–2968.

Mertens, D.R. (1987) Predicting intake and digestibility using mathematical models of ruminal function. *Journal of Animal Science* 64, 1548–1558.

Morgan, P.J. and Mercer, J.G. (1994) Control of seasonality by melatonin. *Proceedings of the Nutrition Society* 53, 483–493.

Myers, J.H. and Bazely, D. (1991) Thorns, spines, prickles, and hairs: are they stimulated by herbivory and do they deter herbivores? In: Tallamy, D.W. and Raupp, M.J. (eds) *Phytochemical Induction by Herbivores*. John Wiley & Sons, Chichester, Sussex, UK.

National Research Council (1987) *Predicting Feed Intake of Food-Producing Animals*. National Academy Press, Washington, DC.

Ndlovu, L.R. and Buchanan-Smith, J.G. (1987) Alfalfa supplementation of corncob diets for sheep: effect of ruminal or postruminal supply of protein on intake, digestibility, digesta passage and liveweight changes. *Canadian Journal of Animal Science* 67, 1075–1082.

Obese, F.Y., Whitlock, B.K., Steele, B.P., Buonomo, F.C. and Sartin, J.L. (2007) Long-term feed intake regulation in sheep is mediated by opioid receptors. *Journal of Animal Science* 85, 111–117.

Ohlson, M. and Staaland, H. (2001) Mineral diversity in wild plants: benefits and bane for moose. *OIKOS* 94, 442–454.

Palo, R.T. and Robbins, C.T. (eds) (1991) *Plant Defenses Against Mammalian Herbivory*. CRC Press, Boca Raton, Florida.

Parker, K.L., Gillingham, M.P., Hanley, T.A. and Robbins, C.T. (1993) Seasonal patterns in body mass, body composition, and water transfer rates of free-ranging and captive black-tailed deer (*Odocoileus hemionus sitkensis*) in Alaska. *Canadian Journal of Zoology* 71, 1397–1404.

Paterson, J.D. (1990) Comment – Bergmann's rule is invalid: a reply to V. Geist. *Canadian Journal of Zoology* 68, 1610–1612.

Peltier, T.C., Barboza, P.S. and Blake, J.E. (2003) Seasonal hyperphagia does not reduce digestive efficiency in an Arctic grazer. *Physiological and Biochemical Zoology* 76, 471–483.

Pirgozliev, V.R., Birch, C.L., Rose, S.P., Kettlewell, P.S. and Bedford, M.R. (2003) Chemical composition and the nutritive quality of different wheat cultivars for broiler chickens. *British Poultry Science* 44, 464–475.

Preston, T.R. (1982) Nutritional limitations associated with the feeding of tropical forages. *Journal of Animal Science* 54, 877–884.

Preston, T.R. and Leng, R.A. (1987) *Matching Ruminant Production Systems with Available Resources in the Tropics and Sub-Tropics*. Penambul Books, Armidale, Australia.

Provenza, F.D. and Villalba, J.J. (2006) Foraging in domestic herbivores: linking the internal and external milieu. In: Bels, V.L. (ed.) *Feeding in Domestic Vertebrates: From Structure to Function*. CAB International, Wallingford, Oxon, UK, pp. 210–240.

Provenza, F.D., Villalba, J.J., Dziba, L.E., Atwood, S.B. and Banner, R.E. (2003) Linking herbivore experience, varied diets, and plant biochemical diversity. *Small Ruminant Research* 49, 257–274.

Ralphs, M.H., Olsen, J.D., Pfister, J.A. and Manners, G.D. (1988) Plant–animal interactions in larkspur poisoning in cattle. *Journal of Animal Science* 66, 2334–2342.

Reid, R.L., Jung, G.A. and Thayne, W.V. (1988) Relationships between nutritive quality and fiber components of cool season and warm season forages: a retrospective study. *Journal of Animal Science* 66, 1275–1291.

Robbins, C.T., Spalinger, D.E. and van Hoven, W. (1995) Adaptation of ruminants to browse and grass diets: are anatomical based browser-grazer interpretations valid? *Oecologia* 103, 208–213.

Roth, F.X., Meindl, C. and Ettle, T. (2006) Evidence of a dietary selection for methionine by the piglet. *Journal of Animal Science* 84, 379–386.

Sanders, T.A. and Jarvis, R.L. (2004) Do band-tailed pigeons seek a calcium supplement at mineral sites? *The Condor* 102, 855–863.

Schmidt-Nelson, K. (1997) *Animal Physiology. Adaption and Environment.* Cambridge University Press, Cambridge, UK.

Semiadi, G., Barry, T.N. and Muir, P.D. (1995) Comparison of seasonal patterns of growth, voluntary feed intake and plasma hormone concentrations in young sambar deer (*Cervus unicolor*) and red deer (*Cervus elaphus*). *Journal of Agricultural Science* 125, 109–124.

Shewmaker, G.E., Mayland, H.F., Rosenau, R.C. and Asay, K.H. (1989) Silicon in C-3 grasses: effects on forage quality and sheep preference. *Journal of Range Management* 42, 122–127.

Shochat, E., Robbins, C.T., Parish, S.M., Young, P.B., Stephenson, T.R. and Tamayo, A. (1997) Nutritional investigations and management of captive moose. *Zoo Biology* 16, 479–494.

Sporndly, E. (1996) The effect of fouling on herbage intake of dairy cows on late season pasture. *Acta Agriculturae Scandinavica* 46(A), 144–153.

Staaland, H., White, R.G. and Kortner, H. (1995) Mineral concentrations in the alimentary tract of northern rodents and lagomorphs. *Comparative Biochemistry and Physiology* 112A, 619–627.

Stephens, S.A., Salas, L.A. and Dierenfeld, E.S. (2006) Bark consumption by the painted ringtail (*Pseudochirulus forbesi larvatus*) in Papua New Guinea. *Biotropica* 38, 617–624.

Tovar, T.C., Moore, D. and Dierenfeld, E. (2005) Preferences among four species of local browse offered to *Colobus guereza kikuyuensis* at the Central Park Zoo. *Zoo Biology* 24, 267–274.

Van Soest, P.J. (1994) *Nutritional Ecology of the Ruminant.* Cornell University Press, Ithaca, New York.

Villalba, J.J., Provenza, F.D. and GouDong (2004) Experience influences diet mixing by herbivores: implications for plant biochemical diversity. *Oikos* 107, 100–1009.

Wertz-Lutz, A.E., Knight, T.J., Pritchard, R.H., Daniel, J.A., Clapper, J.A., Smart, A.J., Trenkle, A. and Beitz, D.C. (2006) Circulating ghrelin concentrations fluctuate relative to nutritional status and influence feeding behavior in cattle. *Journal of Animal Science* 84, 3285–3300.

West, G.B., Woodruff, W.H. and Brown, J.H. (2002) Allometric scaling of metabolic rate from molecules and mitochondria to cells and mammals. *Proceedings of the National Academy of Sciences, USA* 99, 2473–2478.

West, N.O. and Nordan, H.C. (1976) Hormonal regulation of reproduction and the antler cycle in the male Columbian black-tailed deer (*Odocoileushemionus hemionus columbianus*). Part I. Seasonal changes in the histology of the reproductive organs, serum testosterone, sperm production, and the antler cycle. *Canadian Journal of Zoology* 54, 1617–1636.

White, S.M., Welch, B.L. and Flinders, J.T. (1982) Monoterpenoid content of pygmy rabbit stomach ingesta. *Journal of Range Management* 35, 107–109.

Whitehead, P.E. and McEwan, E.H. (1973) Seasonal variation in the plasma testosterone concentration of reindeer and caribou. *Canadian Journal of Zoology* 51, 651–658.

Willette, M.M., Norton, T.L., Miller, C.L. and Lamm, M.G. (2002) Veterinary concerns of captive duikers. *Zoo Biology* 21, 197–207.

Wood, A.J. (1964) Early weaning and growth of the pig. In: *Proceedings of the Sixth International Congress on Nutrition.* E&S Livingstone, Edinburgh, pp. 89–99.

Wood, A.J., Cowan, I.McT. and Nordan, H.C. (1962) Periodicity of growth in ungulates as shown by deer of the genus *Odocoileus. Canadian Journal of Zoology* 40, 593–603.

Yang, W.Z. and Beauchemin, K.A. (2006) Physically effective fiber: method of determination and effects on chewing, ruminal acidosis, and digestion by dairy cows. *Journal of Dairy Science* 89, 2618–2633.

Yeomans, M.R., Blundell, J.E. and Leshem, M. (2004) Palatability: response to nutritional need or need-free stimulation of appetite? *British Journal of Nutrition* 92(Suppl. 1), S3–S14.

Young, T.P. (1987) Increased thorn length in *Acacia depranolobium* – an induced response to browsing. *Oecologia* 71, 436–438.

PART VI
Structural Features

This part covers structural features of the body, such as the skeletal system, cell membranes, connective tissue (extracellular matrix), the integument (skin, hooves, hair and feathers) including skin and hair/feather pigmenting agents such as carotenoids. Functions of a major carotenoid, vitamin A, are discussed.

Part Objectives

1. To discuss the roles of calcium, phosphorus and vitamin D in bone metabolism and to describe deficiency states of these nutrients. Roles of other nutrients in bone growth, such as vitamin K, vitamin C, vitamin A, copper and manganese are also considered.
2. To discuss bone growth disorders, such as perosis, cage layer fatigue and tibial dyschondroplasia in poultry, and developmental orthopedic diseases in horses.
3. To discuss the metabolic causes of nutritional secondary hyperparathyroidism in horses and big cats (e.g. lions, tigers, cheetahs).
4. To discuss hair growth and nutritional factors that affect it.
5. To discuss achromatrichia, or lack of hair pigmentation, and the roles of various nutrients such as iron, copper and biotin.
6. To discuss nutritional effects on hoof and foot health, including roles of nutrients such as biotin.
7. To discuss causes of laminitis (founder) in horses and other animals.
8. To describe the functions of cell membranes and collagens (extracellular matrix) in the structure of the body.
9. To describe the effects of carotenoids on pigmentation of skin and feathers.
10. To discuss the other metabolic roles of carotenoids, especially as sources of vitamin A, and to discuss the metabolic roles of vitamin A in vision.
11. To describe vitamin A toxicity syndromes.

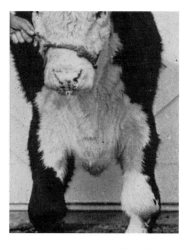

Rickets (above) involves deficiencies of calcium, phosphorus and/or vitamin D.

18 The Skeletal System: Calcium, Phosphorus and Vitamin D

Calcium, Phosphorus and Vitamin D

The requirements and metabolism of calcium, phosphorus and vitamin D are closely interrelated; therefore, they will be discussed together. Bone mineral consists mainly of tricalcium phosphate and other salts of these two minerals. Approximately 99% of the calcium and 80% of the phosphorus in the animal body occur in the bones and teeth. **Phosphorus** is very important in cellular metabolism; many of the intermediates of carbohydrate metabolism are phosphorylated (e.g. glucose-6-phosphate, fructose-1,6-diphosphate and phosphoglyceric acid). The central compound in energy metabolism, adenosine triphosphate (ATP), is a phosphorylated compound. DNA and RNA contain phosphorylated pentose sugars. Thus, reactions involving phosphorus are crucial to animal metabolism. Increasingly, calcium is being found to be involved in processes of energy metabolism as well. For example, calcium activates a regulatory protein, calmodulin, which activates ion channels and numerous enzymes. A number of critical metabolic enzymes are regulated by calcium and/or phosphorylation, including glycogen synthase, pyruvate kinase, pyruvate carboxylase, glycerol-3-phosphate dehydrogenase and pyruvate dehydrogenase.

Calcium and/or phosphorus deficiency symptoms reflect the metabolic functions of these nutrients as well as **vitamin D**. Vitamin D functions in calcium and phosphorus absorption and in bone mineralization. In growing animals, the primary sign of deficiency of calcium, phosphorus and/or vitamin D, is rickets. **Rickets** is characterized by spongy, poorly mineralized bones, leading to lameness, fractures, misshapen bones and death. In adults, bone demineralization occurs with a deficiency of calcium, phosphorus and/or vitamin D. This condition is known as **osteomalacia** (adult rickets). **Osteoporosis** is a bone disorder in which the bone mass decreases, although its mineral composition is normal. Osteoporosis is common in elderly women.

Acute metabolic calcium deficiency causes an impairment of nerve and muscle function because of the role of calcium in the transmission of nerve impulses to muscle (neuromuscular junction). This situation results when serum calcium concentrations are depressed (**hypocalcaemia**). Hypocalcaemia does not usually develop from a simple dietary deficiency of calcium, but from impaired calcium mobilization from bone. Hypocalcaemia is common in dairy cattle; it is referred to as **milk fever** or **parturient paresis**. It occurs most frequently soon after lactation begins, because of a hormonal insufficiency coupled with a high calcium demand for lactation. Normally, bone mineral is mobilized to meet the high calcium requirement of lactation. Mobilization of bone mineral is stimulated by various hormones, especially **parathyroid hormone** (PTH). It is often considered desirable to 'prime' dry cows on a low calcium diet to stimulate endocrine activity so that when lactation begins a high rate of mobilization of bone calcium can occur as a result of increased PTH secretion. The bone mineral is replenished during the dry (non-lactating) period. Electrolyte balance is also important in prevention of milk fever, and is discussed in Chapter 21.

Signs of milk fever include incoordination and staggers, followed by collapse, with the head bent over on the flank. Treatment involves intravenous administration of calcium. Cows usually recover rapidly following treatment, but may require additional calcium administration. Oxalate poisoning (this chapter), which causes hypocalcaemia, produces similar signs as milk fever.

Phosphorus deficiency of livestock is relatively common in many tropical parts of the world where soil phosphorus contents are low. Such conditions are prevalent in parts of South America (e.g. the savannahs of Colombia, Venezuela and Brazil) where the soils are acid and infertile.

Phosphorus-deficient grazing animals often have a depraved appetite (pica) and consume wood, bones and so on. Death from botulism may occur from bone chewing. Deficiencies severe enough to cause pica rarely occur in the USA. Less obvious phosphorus inadequacy may impair **reproductive performance**; cattle may not have normal oestrous cycles and may not experience oestrus or heat periods (Karn, 2001). Thus, conception rates are low and calving intervals are extended. In parts of the tropics, cows may not produce a calf more often than once every 2 or 3 years or may not even come into oestrus because of severe phosphorus deficiency. Phosphorus nutrition of grazing cattle has been reviewed by Karn (2001).

The utilization of calcium and phosphorus is influenced by the relative amounts of each in the diet. A high ratio of phosphorus to calcium may cause **nutritional secondary hyperparathyroidism** (**NSHP**; discussed in this chapter).

Vitamin D is aptly known as 'the sunshine vitamin'. It is formed by the irradiation of sterols in plants and in the skin of animals. Vitamin D occurs in two major forms: (i) vitamin D_2 (ergocalciferol); and (ii) vitamin D_3 (cholecalciferol). **Ergocalciferol** is activated plant sterol; **cholecalciferol** is activated animal sterol. They differ slightly in chemical structure; vitamin D_2 has a double bond in the side chain (Fig. 18.1). Dietary sources of vitamin D include hay and other sun-cured forage and fish-liver oils. In contrast to their vitamin A activity, plants contain vitamin D activity only after the plant cells have died and been exposed to sunlight. Thus, for animals on green pasture, the only sources of vitamin D would be dead plant leaves and exposure to sunlight. Hay that is green in colour, which can be an excellent source of vitamin A activity, may be low in vitamin D.

Animals kept in total confinement, as is the case in modern pig and poultry facilities, are not exposed to sunlight and will require a dietary source of vitamin D. Grazing animals exposed to sunlight normally do not require supplementation with vitamin D. In the winter in northern climates, the amount and intensity of sunlight is often too low for adequate synthesis of vitamin D in the skin, and provision of a supplement is advisable. Smith and Wright (1984) in the UK demonstrated that the level of metabolically active vitamin D in the blood of sheep decreased drastically in the winter months and that supplementation with the vitamin was advisable. The rapid decline in blood levels in the autumn suggested that vitamin D stores are rapidly depleted, at least in sheep.

In all animals, vitamin D_2 is converted to D_3, with D_3 being the metabolically active form. The efficiency of conversion is very low in poultry. Vitamin D plays an important role in calcium metabolism, being involved in the regulation of calcium absorption and bone mineralization. The **metabolically active form** of the vitamin is 1,25-dihydroxycholecalciferol (1,25-OHD$_3$), which is formed by the addition of two hydroxyl (–OH) groups to D_3. The first hydroxylation takes place in the liver to produce 25-OHD$_3$. This compound is then secreted into the blood. In the kidney, it is converted to 1,25-OHD$_3$ (calcitriol), which in turn is secreted into the blood. It acts like a hormone in regulating calcium absorption and bone mineralization. The rate of formation of 1,25-OHD$_3$ is regulated by **PTH** that, in turn, is regulated by the serum calcium concentration. Thus, when there is a need for more calcium, calcium absorption is increased by 'turning on' 1,25-OHD$_3$ formation. Major metabolic forms and metabolism of vitamin D are shown in Fig. 18.2.

Although commonly classified as a vitamin, vitamin D actually functions as a **steroid hormone**. It meets the criteria for a hormone, outlined in Chapter 1. The hormonal form is the hydroxylated compound, 1,25-OHD$_3$. It is produced in a gland (the kidney) and is transported by the blood to the target tissue (the intestine). Its formation and secretion are controlled by a feedback mechanism (blood calcium concentration).

The 25-OHD$_3$ and 1,25-OHD$_3$ metabolites have useful applications in human and animal medicine. In humans, non-vitamin-D-responsive rickets is caused by a genetic lack of enzymatic formation of 1,25-OHD$_3$ in the kidney. The direct administration of the metabolite overcomes this barrier. Similarly, in patients with kidney failure, serious bone disease occurs due to lack of 1,25-OHD$_3$. This vitamin D metabolite can now be administered directly to alleviate the condition. In dairy cattle, administration of vitamin D metabolites prepartum protects against milk fever (Gast *et al.*, 1979). The 1-hydroxycholecalciferol form of vitamin D is less costly to synthesize than the 1,25-OHD$_3$ and is as effective in improving calcium and phosphorus utilization in chicks (Biehl and Baker, 1997) and pigs (Biehl and Baker, 1996).

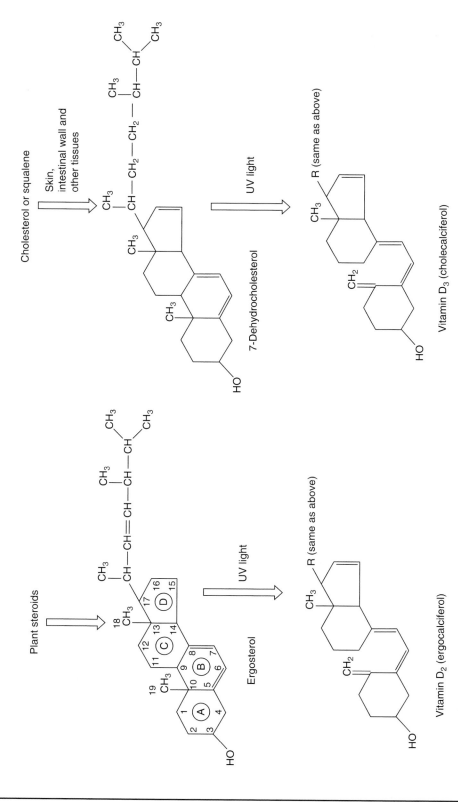

Fig. 18.1. Structures of vitamin D_2 and vitamin D_3. The difference between them is that vitamin D_2 has a double bond in the side chain.

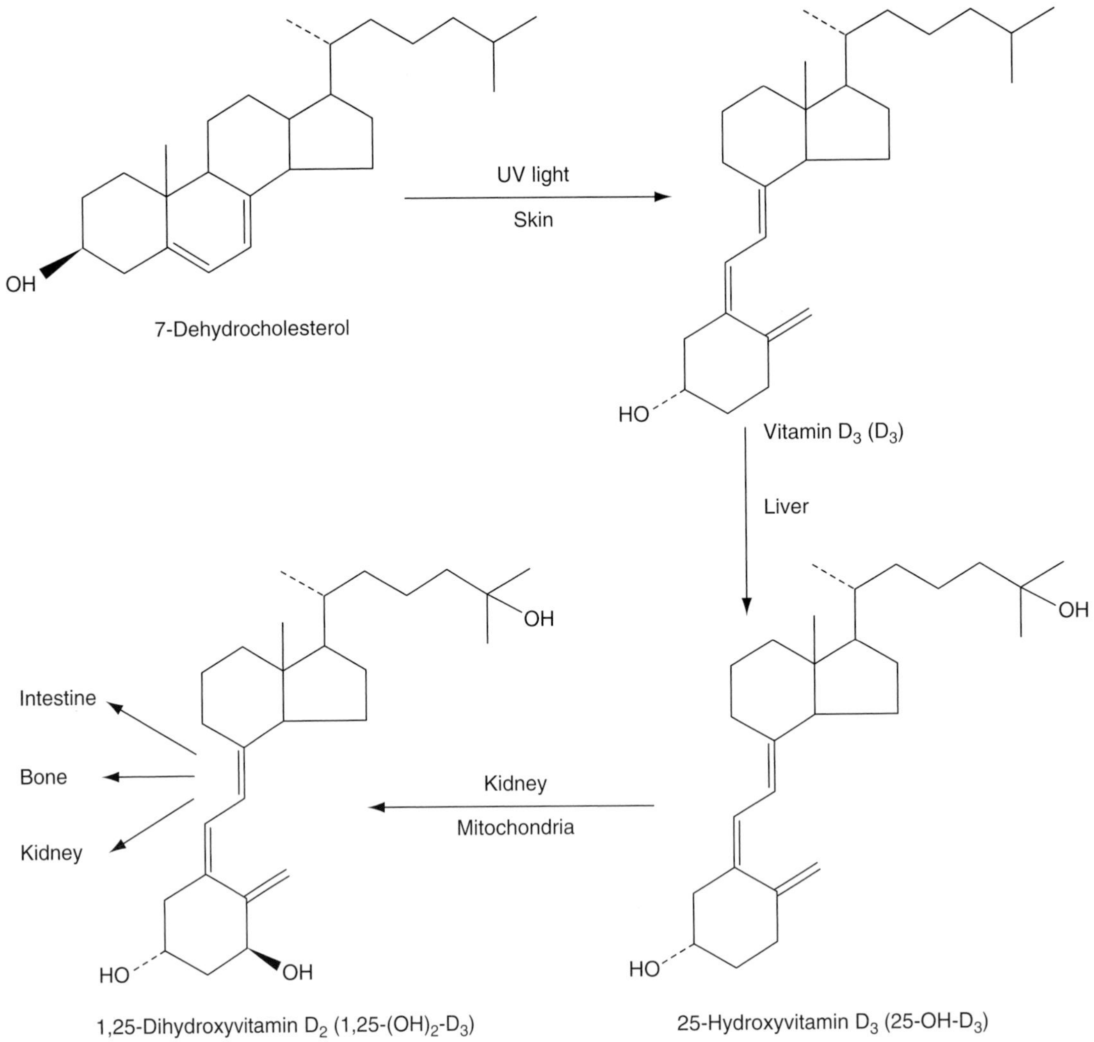

Fig. 18.2. Metabolism of vitamin D₃ to produce a steroid hormone, 1,25-dihydroxyvitamin D₃.

These vitamin D metabolites increase the utilization of phytate phosphorus, apparently by enhancing intestinal phytase activity (Biehl and Baker, 1997).

An interesting application of vitamin D is its use to improve **meat tenderness** (Foote *et al.*, 2004). Administration of 25-OHD₃ to beef steers prior to slaughter increases the calcium content of the muscle, which activates enzymes called **calpains**, which promote post-mortem tenderness.

The presence of mycotoxins such as aflatoxin in the diet increases the vitamin D requirement. This mycotoxin effect has been of practical importance

in poultry. Aflatoxin impairs vitamin D absorption, and its hepatotoxic effects may interfere with the formation of 25-OHD₃ in the liver (Edwards, 1990).

The major physiological role of vitamin D is to regulate the absorption of calcium from the intestine by regulating the mucosal synthesis of **calcium-binding protein** (calbindin). There are some interesting differences among species in vitamin D regulation of calcium absorption, reflecting evolutionary background. For example, **llamas** have a high dietary vitamin D requirement because in their native habitat at high elevations in the

Andes, they are exposed to intense solar radiation (Van Saun *et al.*, 1996). Thus, they evolved in a situation where inefficient vitamin D synthesis in the skin was not a problem because of the abundant UV radiation. At the other extreme, the **African mole rat** spends its entire life underground and is never exposed to sunlight. In this species, calcium is passively absorbed in an efficient, non-vitamin-D-dependent process, so they have no dietary requirement for vitamin D (Pitcher *et al.*, 1992; Pitcher and Buffenstein, 1994, 1995), although mole rats are capable of synthesizing vitamin D from sunlight and can convert the vitamin to the active 1,25-OHD_3 metabolite (Pitcher *et al.*, 1994). **New World primates**, such as marmosets and tamarins, have very high vitamin D requirements, because they have high exposure to solar radiation in their habitat in the tree canopy in equatorial regions. In contrast, **New World rodents**, such as pacas and agoutis, that live on the dark forest floor have very low vitamin D requirement and are very efficient in calcium absorption (Kenny *et al.*, 1993). **Mixed species exhibits** in zoos are becoming increasingly popular. At the Denver Zoo, an exhibit was established with New World primates and two rodent species, pacas and agoutis (Kenny *et al.*, 1993). All animals had access to one diet, which was formulated to meet the requirements of the primates. After several months, paca and agouti mortalities occurred, with extensive soft tissue calcification. Death occurred from kidney failure. The pathological lesions were typical of classic vitamin D toxicity. **New World rodents**, which inhabit the dark forest floor, have evolved physiology that is very efficient in absorbing calcium and phosphorus, with a very low requirement of vitamin D. **New World monkeys**, on the other hand, live in the forest canopy with extensive exposure to solar radiation, so they have evolved with abundant tissue levels of vitamin D. Therefore they have a high dietary requirement when appropriate light sources are not available, whereas the rodents have a very low requirement. The dietary concentration of vitamin D required for the primates is a lethal toxic dose for pacas and agoutis. These differences are important in zoo animals. In animals that have evolved under conditions of high exposure to UV light, the dietary vitamin D requirement is high in the absence of exposure to high intensity of solar radiation. In contrast, animals that have evolved under conditions of low exposure to UV light

have low, or, in some cases, no dietary vitamin D requirement (e.g. rabbits, mole rats, cave-roosting fruit bats). In studies with various lizards, it appears that photoconversion of skin precursors to active metabolites of vitamin D is species-, temperature- and wavelength-dependent (Allen *et al.*, 1999; Ferguson *et al.*, 2002; Nijboer *et al.*, 2003).

Excretion of Calcium

In most species, calcium absorption is regulated by need, via the 1,25-OHD_3 (vitamin D) pathway, ultimately controlled by the serum calcium concentration. Serum calcium is homeostatically regulated by the actions of **PTH** (in response to hypocalcaemia) and **calcitonin** (in response to hypercalcaemia). Calcitonin is produced in the thyroid gland. Excess dietary calcium is not absorbed in most species and is excreted in the faeces. Urinary excretion is not a major pathway of calcium loss in most species. There are some exceptions to the pattern, discussed below.

Schmidt-Nielsen (1964) reviewed physiological adaptations of desert animals. He noted that pack rats (*Neotoma* spp.) excrete large amounts of urinary calcium. He commented:

The interest in calcium excretion in the pack rat began with the observation that urine samples from recently trapped animals contained such large amounts of a white precipitate that the urine looked like heavy cream. Frequently, the urine was also strongly coloured, orange, or even rust coloured or deep red. If pack rats were given cactus and grain to eat in the laboratory, their urine contained the white precipitate, but white rats on the same diet had a clear yellow urine.

Cheeke and Amberg (1973) observed very similar results in rabbits. Rabbits (both domestic and wild) often have urine loaded with a white precipitate, and the urine liquid portion is usually deeply pigmented orange, deep red or almost black. Cheeke and Amberg (1973) compared rats and rabbits fed a very high dietary calcium content (10% calcium carbonate). The rats excreted little calcium in the urine, which was clear yellow, while in rabbits the urinary calcium was very high (Table 18.1). The urine of the rabbits was thick and creamy (Fig. 18.3), and almost solid in some cases, as well as being very orange or red. Thus it appears that in pack rats and rabbits, regulation of calcium absorption by vitamin D does not occur or is very imprecise. The blood

Table 18.1. Comparative urinary excretion of calcium, phosphorus and magnesium by rats and rabbits fed high-calcium (10% $CaCO_3$) diets (Cheeke and Amberg, 1973).

	Amount in urine (% of amount ingested)	
Mineral	Rabbits	Rats
Ca	59.0	2.0
P	6.0	1.6
Mg	55.2	15.9

calcium concentration in rabbits is not as closely regulated homeostatically as in other species. Chapin and Smith (1967) noted that the serum calcium concentration in rabbits increases in direct proportion to dietary calcium content. Thus the high urinary excretion of calcium may simply reflect the high blood concentrations. It appears that all lagomorphs (rabbits and hares) are very efficient absorbers of calcium, excreting the excess in the urine. High urinary calcium has been observed in pikas (Broadbooks, 1965), jackrabbits (Nagy *et al.*, 1976) and mountain hares (Pehrson, 1983).

Clauss *et al.* (2007) observed that the black rhinoceros has a high digestibility coefficient for calcium. According to Clauss *et al.* (2007):

> The fact that most hindgut fermenting herbivores absorb more Ca from the gut than necessary to meet their requirements, and excrete the surplus in their urine, has not been explained satisfactorily. One

potential explanation could be that Ca needs to be absorbed from the ingesta in the small intestine in large quantities to ensure P availability both in the small intestine and in the hindgut. Phosphorus is a major component of bacterial dry matter and therefore a limiting factor for bacterial growth and action.

Bone Growth and Metabolism

Bones serve as the structural components of the skeletal system and are also storehouses of minerals, especially calcium and phosphorus, which can be mobilized as needed. Bone is in a continuous state of formation and mobilization – it is in a dynamic state, also known as **remodelling**. Two types of cells, osteoblasts and osteoclasts, are important in the remodelling process. **Osteoblasts** function in bone formation, while **osteoclasts** are responsible for bone mobilization. There are two types of bone: (i) dense cortical bone; and (ii) spongy trabecular bone.

Bone consists of an organic matrix that becomes mineralized. The organic matrix is cartilage, consisting primarily of the protein collagen. The growth of bone in length occurs at the junction of the epiphysis and diaphysis (Fig. 18.4). As the cartilage grows, bone mineral is deposited to form bone. When the cartilage ceases growing and is replaced by mineralized bone, the epiphysis and diaphysis unite and bone growth ceases. In vitamin D deficiency, the **proliferative zone of cartilage** grows normally, but does not become mineralized. The proliferative zone becomes wider (Fig. 18.5).

(a)

(b)

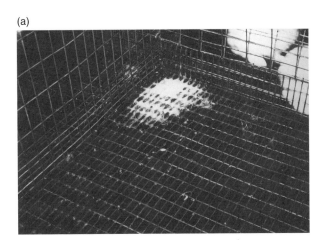
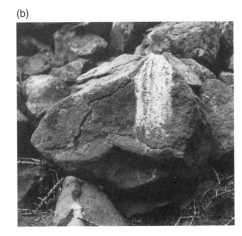

Fig. 18.3. Rabbits excrete calcium in the urine. (a) Thick white precipitate of calcium carbonate deposited on the floor of a rabbit cage. (b) Pika urine patches on rocks, illustrating the high urinary calcium excretion of this species.

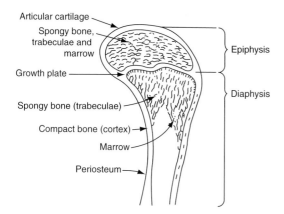

Chapter 18

Articular cartilage
Spongy bone, trabeculae and marrow
Growth plate
Spongy bone (trabeculae)
Compact bone (cortex)
Marrow
Periosteum
Epiphysis
Diaphysis

Fig. 18.4. A longitudinal section of a growing long bone. Growth in length occurs at the epiphysis-diaphysis junction.

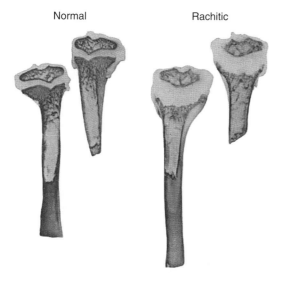

Normal   Rachitic

Fig. 18.5. In vitamin D-deficient rickets, the growth of the cartilage at the epiphysis-diaphysis junction continues normally, but does not become mineralized, so the proliferative zone of cartilage becomes wider (courtesy of Pfizer, Inc.).

Signs of rickets occur. The bones are weak and deformed. Signs of **rickets** in livestock include decreased growth, stiffness of gait, misshapen legs, enlarged and painful joints and an arched back (humpback).

Vitamin K has a role in bone metabolism. Vitamin K is required for the synthesis of a number of proteins containing **gamma-carboxyglutamic acid (GLA)**. In these proteins, vitamin K is involved, as a vitamin K-dependent carboxylase, in the carboxylation of glutamic acids to form a calcium-binding site. This is similar to the role of vitamin K in blood clotting, in the conversion of prothrombin to thrombin (see 'Blood Clotting and Vitamin K' in Chapter 21). There are three GLA proteins in bone; the major one is **osteocalcin**. Although its role in bone formation has not been conclusively identified, osteocalcin is believed to function in bone mineralization. Besides GLA, osteocalcin also contains hydroxyproline, so its synthesis is dependent on both vitamins K and C (vitamin C functions in hydroxylation of proline). In addition, its synthesis is induced by vitamin D.

The organic matrix of bone can be influenced by nutrient deficiencies. Proline and lysine are hydroxylated *in situ* in collagen, facilitating hydrogen bonding within the collagen molecule to provide structural rigidity. **Vitamin C** is required for the enzymes involved: proline hydroxylase and lysyl oxidase. **Copper** is a component of lysyl oxidase. **Manganese** deficiency causes abnormal bone growth and skeletal abnormalities. Manganese activates enzymes involved in the synthesis of chondroitin sulfate side chains of proteoglycan molecules. **Proteoglycans** are glycoprotein components of the cell matrix, and are present in cartilage. Some proteoglycans bind to collagen. Proteoglycans include chondroitin sulfate and hyaluronic acid; they contribute to the compressability of cartilage.

Vitamin A has a role in normal bone growth, via effects on the osteoclasts and osteoblasts of the epithelial cartilage. The bones are altered in shape during growth in vitamin A deficiency. Blindness in vitamin A-deficient calves may result from a constriction of the optic nerve caused by a narrowing of the bone canal through which it passes (Fig. 18.6).

Bone Growth Disorders

Leg abnormalities are a problem in poultry, especially in birds kept on wire. **Perosis** or slipped tendon (Fig. 18.7) is caused by deficiencies of choline and manganese. Perosis is due to an abnormality of the joint in the long bones of the leg, causing the tendon to slip and pull the leg sideways. **Cage layer fatigue** is a type of osteoporosis that involves excessive mobilization of calcium from the leg bones, which causes the birds to have difficulty standing and broken bones. It is primarily a problem with layers kept in wire cages at high stocking density. Lack of exercise is probably

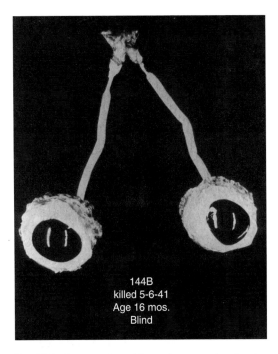

Fig. 18.6. Degeneration of the optic nerve of a vitamin A-deficient calf, resulting in blindness.

144B
killed 5-6-41
Age 16 mos.
Blind

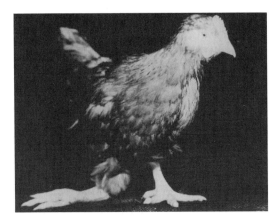

Fig. 18.7. Perosis or slipped tendon (courtesy of University Books, Guelph, Canada).

a contributing factor. At the end of the laying cycle, many layers have broken bones. Nutritional factors are no doubt involved, relating to calcium, phosphorus and vitamin D. However, supplementation with these nutrients does not prevent osteoporosis (Rennie *et al.*, 1997). Genetic factors may be involved as well.

Another leg disorder seen in broilers is **tibial dyschondroplasia (TD)** in which there is abnormal formation of cartilage in the long bones. The cartilage forms a thickened layer below the epiphyseal plate. The lesion arises from the failure of growth plate chondrocytes to differentiate (Rennie and Whitehead, 1996). Dietary electrolyte balance and dietary alterations that affect acid–base or cation–anion balance have a role in TD (Hulan *et al.*, 1987). High dietary chloride provokes an increased incidence (Edwards and Veltmann, 1983). Dietary zeolite has been shown to reduce the incidence and severity of TD (Ballard and Edwards, 1988), apparently by facilitating calcium utilization. High levels of vitamin A were reported by Jensen *et al.* (1983) to increase leg disorders, but this result was not confirmed by Ballard and Edwards (1988). Edwards (1984) found that a diet low in calcium and high in phosphorus and chloride, produced a high incidence of TD in broilers. Supplementation of high phosphorus diets with calcium reduces the incidence of TD (Edwards and Veltmann, 1983).

Edwards (1990) suggested that TD may be a manifestation of the inability of the rapidly growing broiler to convert vitamin D_3 to $1,25\text{-}(OH)_2D_3$ adequately for maximal calcium absorption and bone formation. Dietary supplementation with active **vitamin D metabolites** such as $1\text{-}(OH)D_3$, $25\text{-}(OH)D_3$, and $1,25\text{-}(OH)_2D_3$ is effective in preventing TD (Elliot *et al.*, 1995; Rennie and Whitehead, 1996). The $25\text{-}(OH)D_3$ metabolite is about ten times as toxic as vitamin D_3 to broilers (Yarger *et al.*, 1995), and should, therefore, be used prudently in diet formulation. The $25\text{-}(OH)D_3$ is especially effective in preventing TD when the dietary calcium concentration is below 0.85% (Ledwaba and Roberson, 2003).

Mycotoxins play a role in other leg disorders of poultry. A frequent cause of rickets in young poultry is calcium deficiency induced by aflatoxins. Aflatoxins cause liver damage and reduced bile secretion. Bile is necessary for the absorption of fat-soluble vitamins such as vitamin D. Aflatoxin reduces vitamin D absorption and the liver damage impairs formation of $25\text{-}OHD_3$ in the liver. Another mycotoxin, fusarochromanone, has been implicated as a causative agent of TD in broilers (Wu *et al.*, 1990).

Ratites (ostriches, emu and other large flightless birds) are susceptible to leg weakness problems. When fed high energy diets, young ratites may have excessive weight gain that causes great stress on the legs, which may become bowed or misshapen. Therefore, young ratites should be raised on pasture if possible, with limited exposure to concentrate feeds.

Bone development disorders are of major concern in young **horses**. This concern is particularly true in the thoroughbred racing industry (Fig. 18.8). Horses with abnormal bone development will not reach their racing potential and are susceptible to injury. The term **developmental orthopaedic diseases (DOD)** is used to describe a complex of bone disorders, including **osteochondrosis (OCD)**, physitis, contracted tendons, cervical vertebral malformation (wobbler syndrome) and similar abnormalities. OCD is a disease of the growth cartilage at articular or epiphyseal growth regions. It may occur at the growth plate (physis) or in developing the articular cartilage of joints. In the final stages of bone formation, the cartilage cells at the growth plate degenerate and the region is invaded

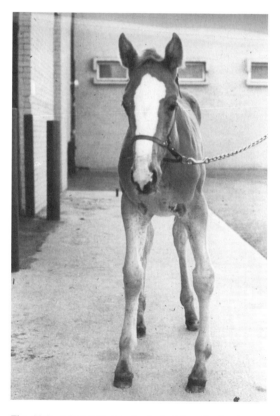

Fig. 18.8. A foal with angular limb deformity due to nutritional imbalance (courtesy of N.F. Cymbaluk, University of Saskatchewan, Saskatchewan, Canada).

by osteoprogenitor cells that initiate mineralization of the bone matrix. Disruption of this process results in thickening of the cartilage, inadequate mineralization, weak joints, fractures and pain. Extra bone is formed on the sides of the joints, giving a swollen appearance. **Physitis** is another term for this condition, meaning inflammation of the physis (growth plate). Contracted tendons cause a flexure of the leg (knuckling) and may be a secondary effect of OCD.

Feeding and nutrition influence the DOD syndrome. The most common cause is overfeeding young horses, coupled with lack of exercise. A high-energy intake promotes rapid growth; body weight increase may exceed the rate of normal bone development (Thompson *et al.*, 1988b). Excess energy or protein intake may modify blood hormone concentrations (e.g. insulin or thyroxine), which in turn may influence bone growth (Glade *et al.*, 1984). Contracted tendons are particularly likely to occur with overfeeding following a period of nutrient restriction. Nutrient imbalance is an important factor in DOD. Protein intake must be adequate because the cartilaginous matrix of bone is proteinaceous. When high energy diets are used, the protein content must be increased to maintain the optimal protein:energy ratio (Thompson *et al.*, 1988b). Savage *et al.* (1993) fed a control diet that contained digestible energy at the National Research Council's recommended level and a diet containing 129% of the recommended energy level for foals 2.5–6.5 months of age for 16–18 weeks. Eleven of the 12 foals on the high digestible energy diet developed multiple **dyschondroplastic (DCP)** (i.e. OCD) lesions. Only one of the foals fed the control diet developed DCP lesions. There were no differences in growth rates between the treatments. The authors suggest there may be an association between high digestible energy and the high incidence of DCP. Schryver *et al.* (1987) studied the effect of excess dietary protein (20% crude protein in the diet) on calcium metabolism and bone growth. This high content of protein had no effect on these parameters when compared to animals fed the recommended protein level, suggesting that National Research Council recommendations for protein are adequate.

The dietary **calcium:phosphorus ratio** is of particular importance in bone growth and development. Excess phosphorus and low calcium is the common situation when animals are overfed grain and given limited amounts of poor quality hay.

Although excess calcium is well tolerated if adequate phosphorus is present, there is some concern that high calcium intakes may have an adverse effect on bone development (Cymbaluk *et al.*, 1989). The optimal ratio of calcium to phosphorus is 1:1 to 2:1. Because of the high calcium content of lucerne and the variable, and sometimes low, calcium content of grass and cereal hays (Cymbaluk and Christensen, 1986), lucerne and grass hays should not be used interchangeably, particularly for young horses, without considering the effect on the balance of calcium and phosphorus. Adequate trace minerals are necessary for proper bone mineralization of horses. Copper, zinc, iron, manganese, cobalt and iodine are critical for bone mineralization (Ott and Asquith, 1995). Thompson *et al.* (1988a) studied the use of creep diets for foals and reported that when a creep diet provided the nutrient levels recommended by the National Research Council, growth rate and skeletal growth were increased with no detrimental effect on bone quality.

Developmental bone disorders also occur in **large breed dogs**. Large breed dogs should be fed so as to prevent rapid growth. Diets that promote a slow growth rate and normal skeletal development are preferred. If large dogs grow at a maximal rate, skeletal diseases such as OCD and hip dysplasia can develop.

Nutritional Secondary Hyperparathyroidism (NSHP)

A dietary calcium-phosphorus imbalance can result in **NSHP**. A low ratio of dietary calcium to phosphorus causes high blood phosphorus and low blood calcium concentrations. Both of these states cause the parathyroid gland to increase its secretion of **PTH**. PTH stimulates urinary phosphorus excretion and mobilization of calcium and phosphorus from bone (Fig. 18.9). On a chronic basis, with a prolonged inadequate calcium:phosphorus ratio, the continuous mobilization of bone mineral results in the bones becoming demineralized and fibrotic. The frontal bones of the face and the leg bones are particularly affected, especially in horses. The demineralized, fibrotic bone enlarges and is referred to as 'big head' in horses. In the past, it was called Miller's disease. When farmers hauled their grain to flour mills with horse-drawn wagons, the horses were often fed bran or other wheat milling by-products at the mill. If they were used on a regular

basis for this purpose, they frequently developed NSHP.

Various **tropical grasses** contain soluble oxalates (Fig. 18.10) in sufficient concentration to induce calcium deficiency in grazing animals. These include buffel grass (*Cenchrus ciliaris*), pangolagrass (*Digitaria decumbens*), setaria (*Setaria sphacelata*) and kikuyugrass (*Pennisetum clandestinum*). Numerous problems have been noted with these grasses in Australia, primarily with horses. **Oxalates** react with calcium to produce insoluble calcium oxalate, reducing calcium absorption. This leads to a disturbance in the absorbed calcium:phosphorus ratio, resulting in mobilization of bone mineral to alleviate the hypocalcaemia. Prolonged mobilization of bone mineral results in **NSHP** or osteodystrophy fibrosa (Fig. 18.11), in horses consuming

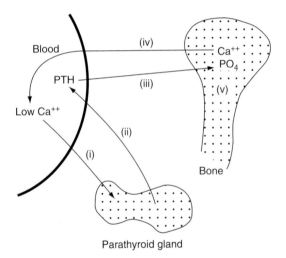

Parathyroid gland

Fig. 18.9. Metabolic events in the development of NSHP. (i) Low blood calcium stimulates the parathyroid gland; (ii) the parathyroid gland produces more parathyroid hormone (PTH); (iii) PTH stimulates mobilization of calcium and phosphorus from bone; (iv) serum calcium is increased; (v) the bone becomes demineralized and fibrotic.

Oxalic acid   Calcium oxalate

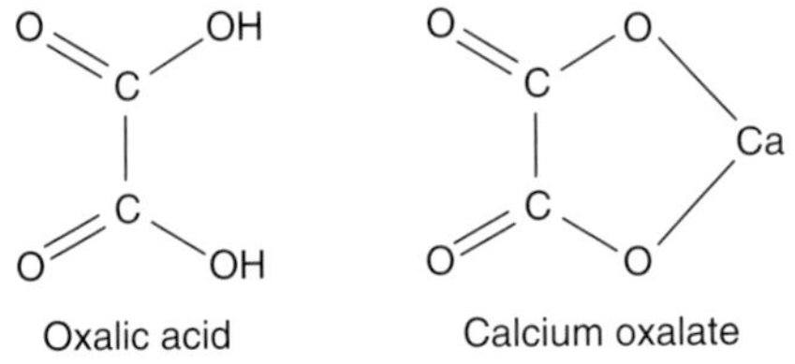

Fig. 18.10. Structures of oxalates occurring in plants.

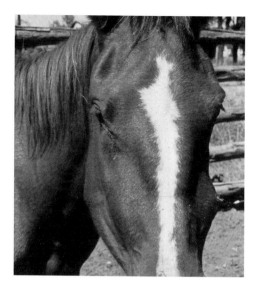

Fig. 18.11. NSHP or osteodystophy fibrosa ('big head') in a horse that had been grazing on tropical grass pasture species which are high in oxalate and low in calcium (courtesy of R.A. McKenzie, Department of Primary Industries, Queensland, Australia).

these tropical grasses (Blaney *et al.*, 1981a,b, 1982; McKenzie *et al.*, 1981). Cattle and sheep are less affected because of degradation of oxalate in the rumen (Allison *et al.*, 1981). However, cattle

mortalities from oxalate poisoning due to acute hypocalcaemia have occurred on setaria pastures (Jones *et al.*, 1970) and sheep have been poisoned while grazing buffel grass (McKenzie *et al.*, 1988).

Amounts of 0.5% or more soluble oxalate in forage grasses may induce NSHP in horses, whereas 2% or more soluble oxalate can lead to acute toxicosis in ruminants (McKenzie *et al.*, 1988). The oxalate content of grasses is highest under conditions of rapid growth with concentrations as high as 6% or more of dry weight.

Many nutritional problems with big cats (e.g. lions, tigers, cheetahs) have occurred in zoos, particularly with imbalances in calcium and phosphorus, and were among the first published reports of nutrient imbalance over a century ago (Dierenfeld, 1997). Diets high in meat may induce **juvenile osteoporosis** (NSHP) unless adequate calcium supplementation is provided in the diet (Van Rensburg and Lowry, 1988). In this disorder, the head and paws are enlarged and the skeletal system is soft and decalcified (Fig. 18.12). Although less prevalent in zoos that feed appropriately balanced meat-based diets, or commercial formulations, bone density issues are still a common health problem for large felids as well as rapidly growing carnivorous bird species such as storks. Each kilogram of raw meat fed must be supplemented with 5 g of calcium carbonate and 10 g of dicalcium phosphate

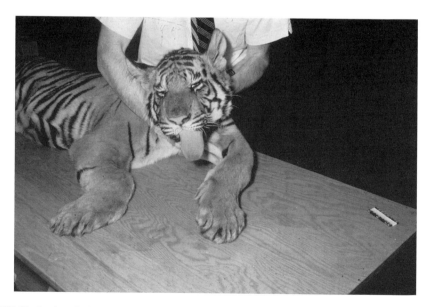

Fig. 18.12. NSHP of a tiger fed meat causing a calcium-to-phosphorus imbalance (courtesy of J. Krook, Cornell University, New York, USA).

(Ullrey and Bernard, 1989), along with appropriate vitamins; this can also be accomplished through the use of commercial supplements. In the wild, carnivores consume small bones of prey, maintaining an adequate calcium-to-phosphorus balance. Bones for chewing should be provided to captive big cats at least once a week to prevent dental plaque and calculus (Ullrey and Bernard, 1989).

Questions and Study Guide

1. What are the differences among rickets, osteomalacia and osteoporosis?
2. What is the role of the parathyroid hormone in the prevention of milk fever in dairy cattle?
3. When serum calcium concentration decreases, what homeostatic mechanisms return it to the normal range?
4. Vitamin D is often referred to as a steroid hormone. Explain.
5. Dietary aflatoxin may cause signs of rickets in poultry. Explain.
6. The African mole rat spends its entire life below ground and is never exposed to sunlight. Why does it not show signs of vitamin D deficiency?
7. The urine of rabbits is often white in colour. Why?
8. What is meant by the term 'bone remodelling'?
9. In what part of the growing bone does mineralization occur?
10. How is vitamin K involved in bone growth?
11. A vitamin C deficiency causes skeletal deformities. Why?
12. What is cage layer fatigue?
13. What causes bone development disorders in horses, ostriches and dogs?
14. Explain why horses can develop 'big head' and lameness when grazing on tropical grass pastures.

References

Allen, M.E., Chen, T.C., Holick, M.F. and Merkel, E. (1999) Evaluation of vitamin D status of the green iguana (*Iguana iguana*): oral administration vs. UVB exposure. In: Holick, M.F. and Jung, E.G. (eds) *Biologic Effects of Light*. Kluwer, Boston, pp. 99–101.

Allison, M.J., Cook, H.M. and Dawson, K.A. (1981) Selection of oxalate-degrading rumen bacteria in continuous cultures. *Journal of Animal Science* 53, 810–816.

Ballard, R. and Edwards, H.M., Jr (1988) Effects of dietary zeolite and vitamin A on tibial dyschondroplasia in chickens. *Poultry Science* 67, 113–119.

Biehl, R.R. and Baker, D.H. (1996) Efficacy of supplemental 1-α-hydroxycholecalciferol and microbial phytase for young pigs fed phosphorus- or amino acid-deficient corn-soybean meal diets. *Journal of Animal Science* 74, 2960–2966.

Biehl, R.R. and Baker, D.H. (1997) Utilization of phytate and nonphytate phosphorus in chicks as affected by source and amount of vitamin D₃. *Journal of Animal Science* 75, 2986–2993.

Blaney, B.J., Gartner, R.J.W. and McKenzie, R.A. (1981a) The effects of oxalate in some tropical grasses on the availability to horses of calcium, phosphorus and magnesium. *Journal of Agricultural Science* 97, 507–514.

Blaney, B.J., Gartner, R.J.W. and McKenzie, R.A. (1981b) The inability of horses to absorb calcium from calcium oxalate. *Journal of Agricultural Science* 97, 639–641.

Blaney, B.J., Gartner, R.J.W. and Head, T.A. (1982) The effects of oxalate in tropical grasses on calcium, phosphorus and magnesium availability to cattle. *Journal of Agricultural Science* 99, 533–546.

Broadbooks, H.E. (1965) Ecology and distribution of the pikas of Washington and Alaska. *American Midland Naturalist* 73, 299–335.

Chapin, R.E. and Smith, S.E. (1967) Calcium requirement of growing rabbits. *Journal of Animal Science* 26, 67–71.

Cheeke, P.R. and Amberg, J. (1973) Comparative calcium excretion by rats and rabbits. *Journal of Animal Science* 37, 450–454.

Clauss, M., Castell, J.C., Kienzle, E., Schramel, P., Dierenfeld, E.S., Flach, E.J., Behlert, O., Streich, W.J., Hummel, J. and Hatt, J.-M. (2007) Mineral absorption in the black rhinoceros (*Diceros bicornis*) as compared with the domestic horse. *Journal of Animal Physiology and Animal Nutrition* 91, 193–204.

Cymbaluk, N.F. and Christensen, D.A. (1986) Nutrient utilization of pelleted and unpelleted forages by ponies. *Canadian Journal of Animal Science* 66, 237–244.

Cymbaluk, N.F., Christison, G.I. and Leach, D.H. (1989) Nutrient utilization by limit- and *ad libitum*-fed growing horses. *Journal of Animal Science* 67, 414–425.

Dierenfeld, E.S. (1997) Captive wild animal nutrition: a historical perspective. *Proceedings of the Nutrition Society* 56, 989–999.

Edwards, H.M., Jr (1984) Studies on the etiology of tibial dyschondroplasia in chickens. *Journal of Nutrition* 114, 1001–1013.

Edwards, H.M., Jr (1990) Efficacy of several vitamin D compounds in the prevention of tibial dyschondroplasia in broiler chickens. *Journal of Nutrition* 120, 1054–1061.

Edwards, H.M., Jr and Veltmann, J.R., Jr (1983) The role of calcium and phosphorus in the etiology of tibial dyschondroplasia in young chicks. *Journal of Nutrition* 113, 1568–1575.

Elliot, M.A., Roberson, K.D., Rowland III, G.N. and Edwards, H.M., Jr (1995) Effect of dietary calcium and 1,25-dihydroxycholecalciferol on the development of tibial dyschondroplasia in broilers during the starter and grower periods. *Poultry Science* 74, 1495–1505.

Ferguson, G.W., Gehrmann, W.H., Chen, T.C., Dierenfeld, E.S. and Holick, M.F. (2002) Effects of artificial ultraviolet light exposure on reproductive success of the female panther chameleon (*Furcifer pardalis*) in captivity. *Zoo Biology* 21, 525–537.

Foote, M.R., Horst, R.L., Huff-Lonergan, E.J., Trenkle, A.H., Parrish, F.C., Jr and Beitz, D.C. (2004) The use of vitamin D_3 and its metabolites to improve beef tenderness. *Journal of Animal Science* 82, 242–249.

Gast, D.R., Horst, R.L., Jorgensen, N.A. and DeLuca, H.F. (1979) Potential use of 1,25-dihydroxycholecalciferol for prevention of parturient paresis. *Journal of Dairy Science* 62, 1009–1013.

Glade, M.J., Gupta, S. and Reimers, T.J. (1984) Hormonal responses to high and low planes of nutrition in weanling thoroughbreds. *Journal of Animal Science* 59, 658–665.

Hulan, H.W., Simons, P.C.M., Van Schagen, P.J.W., McRae, K.B. and Proudfoot, F.G. (1987) Effect of dietary cation–anion balance and calcium content on general performance and incidence of leg abnormalities of broiler chickens. *Canadian Journal of Animal Science* 67, 165–177.

Jensen, L.S., Fletcher, D.L., Lilburn, M.S. and Akiba, Y. (1983) Growth depression in broiler chicks fed high vitamin A levels. *Nutrition Reports International* 28, 171–179.

Jones, R.J., Seawright, A.A. and Little, D.A. (1970) Oxalate poisoning in animals grazing the tropical grass *Setaria sphacelata*. *Journal of the Australian Institute of Agricultural Science* 36, 41–43.

Karn, J.F. (2001) Phosphorus nutrition of grazing cattle: a review. *Animal Feed Science Technology* 89, 133–153.

Kenny, D., Cambre, R.C., Lewandowski, A., Pelto, J.A., Irlbeck, N.A., Wilson, H., Mierau, G.W., Sill, F.G. and Alberto Pasas Garcia, M.V.Z. (1993) Suspected vitamin D_3 toxicity in pacas (*Cuniculus paca*) and agoutis (*Dasyprocta aguti*). *Journal of Zoo and Wildlife Medicine* 24, 129–139.

Ledwaba, M.F. and Roberson, K.D. (2003) Effectiveness of twenty-five-hydroxycholecalciferol in the prevention of fibial dyschondroplasia in Ross cockerels depends on dietary calcium level. *Poultry Science* 82, 1769–1777.

McKenzie, R.A., Gartner, R.J.W., Blaney, B.J. and Glanville, R.J. (1981) Control of nutritional secondary hyperparathyroidism in grazing horses with calcium and phosphorus supplementation. *Australian Veterinary Journal* 57, 554–557.

McKenzie, R.A., Bell, A.M., Storie, G.J., Keenan, F.J., Cornack, K.M. and Grant, S.G. (1988) Acute oxalate poisoning of sheep by buffel grass (*Cenchrus ciliaris*). *Australian Veterinary Journal* 65, 26.

Nagy, K.A., Shoemaker, V.H. and Costa, W.R. (1976) Water, electrolyte and nitrogen budgets of jackrabbits (*Lepus californicus*) in the Mojave Desert. *Physiological Zoology* 49, 351–363.

Nijboer, J., van Brug, H., Tryfonidou, M.A. and van Leeuwen, J.P.T.M. (2003) UV-B and vitamin D_3 metabolism in juvenile Komodo dragons (*Varanus komodoensis*). In: Fidgett, A., Clauss, M., Ganslosser, U., Hatt, J.-M. and Nijboer, J. (eds) *Zoo Animal Nutrition*, Vol II. Filander Verlag, Fürth, Germany, pp. 233–246.

Ott, E.A. and Asquith, R.L. (1995) Trace mineral supplementation of yearling horses. *Journal of Animal Science* 73, 466–471.

Pehrson, A. (1983) Digestibility and retention of food components in caged mountain hares (*Lepus timidus*) during the winter. *Holarctic Ecology* 6, 395–403.

Pitcher, T. and Buffenstein, R. (1994) Passive uptake in the small intestine and active uptake in the hindgut contribute to the highly efficient mineral metabolism of the common mole-rat, *Cryptomys hottentotus*. *British Journal of Nutrition* 71, 573–582.

Pitcher, T. and Buffenstein, R. (1995) Intestinal calcium transport in mole-rats (*Cryptomys camarensis* and *Heterocephalus glaber*) is independent of both genomic and non-genomic vitamin D mediation. *Experimental Physiology* 80, 597–608.

Pitcher, T., Buffenstein, R., Keegan, J.D., Moodley, G.P. and Yahav, S. (1992) Dietary calcium content, calcium balance and mode of uptake in a subterranean mammal, the Damara mole-rat. *Journal of Nutrition* 122, 108–114.

Pitcher, T., Sergeev, I.N. and Buffenstein, R. (1994) Vitamin D metabolism in the Damara mole-rat is altered by exposure to sunlight yet mineral metabolism is unaffected. *Journal of Endocrinology* 143, 367–374.

Rennie, J.S. and Whitehead, C.C. (1996) Effectiveness of dietary 25- and 1-hydroxycholecalciferol in combating tibial dyschondroplasia in broiler chickens. *British Poultry Science* 37, 413–421.

Rennie, J.S., Fleming, R.H., McCormack, H.A., McCorquodale, C.C. and Whitehead, C.C. (1997) Studies on effects of nutritional factors on bone structure and osteoporosis in laying hens. *British Poultry Science* 38, 417–424.

Savage, C.J., McCarty, R.N. and Jeffcott, L.B. (1993) Effects of dietary energy and protein on induction of dyschondroplasia in foals. *Equine Veterinary Journal* Suppl. 16, 74–79.

Schmidt-Nielsen, K. (1964) *Desert Animals. Physiological Problems of Heat and Water.* Oxford University Press, London.

Schryver, H.F., Meakim, D.W., Lowe, J.E., Williams, J., Soderholm, L.V. and Hintz, H.F. (1987) Growth and calcium metabolism in horses fed varying levels of protein. *Equine Veterinary Journal* 19, 280–287.

Smith, B.S.W. and Wright, H. (1984) Relative contributions of diet and sunshine to the overall vitamin D status of the grazing ewe. *The Veterinary Record* 115, 537–538.

Thompson, K.N., Baker, J.P. and Jackson, S.G. (1988a) The influence of supplemental feed on growth and bone development of nursing foals. *Journal of Animal Science* 66, 1692–1696.

Thompson, K.N., Jackson, S.G. and Baker, J.P. (1988b) The influence of high planes of nutrition on skeletal growth and development of weanling horses. *Journal of Animal Science* 66, 2459–2467.

Ullrey, D.E. and Bernard, J.B. (1989) Meat diets for performing exotic cats. *Journal of Zoo and Wildlife Medicine* 20, 20–25.

Van Rensburg, I.B.J. and Lowry, M.H. (1988) Nutritional secondary hyperparathyroidism in a lion cub. *Journal of the South African Veterinary Association* 59, 83–86.

Van Saun, R.J., Smith, B.B. and Watrous, B.J. (1996) Evaluation of vitamin D status of llamas and alpacas with hypophoshatemic rickets. *Journal of the American Veterinary Medical Association* 209, 1128–1133.

Wu, W., Nelson, P.E., Cook, M.E. and Smalley, E.B. (1990) Fusarochromanone production by *Fusarium* isolates. *Applied Environmental Microbiology* 56, 2989–2993.

Yarger, J.G., Quarles, C.L., Hollis, B.W. and Gray, R.W. (1995) Safety of 25-hydroxycholecalciferol in poultry rations. *Poultry Science* 74, 1437–1446.

19 The Integument, Pigmentation, Membranes and Extracellular Matrix

Hair Growth

Production of hair is important in certain farmed carnivorous species such as mink and foxes. It is also important in sheep and goats; wool, mohair and cashmere are types of hair. The quality of the hair is also important in most livestock species and companion animals, in which a sleek, glossy hair coat is considered desirable. Hair growth is also very important in wild species; the insulatory properties of hair provide a first line of defence against extremes in environmental temperature.

Nutrients important in hair growth include protein, energy-providing nutrients, specific minerals such as iron and copper, vitamins including biotin and pantothenic acid, and essential fatty acids. These nutrients will be discussed following a general consideration of hair growth.

Hair **follicles** develop as extensions of the outer layer of the skin. At birth, an animal has its full complement of primary hair follicles; subsequent development of the hair coat depends mainly on nutritional and environmental factors. At the base of the follicle is a highly vascular layer called the **papilla**, which provides the developing hair with nutrients. The growth of the hair occurs from the matrix plate directly above the papilla. The hair cells become cornified shortly after their formation, so the hair fibre, as it emerges from the skin, consists of dead cornified cells.

There are two main types of hair follicles, the primary and the secondary follicles. The **primary follicles** produce the longest type of hair, the **guard hair**, and the shorter, intermediate guard hairs grow from lateral primary follicles, while the underfur grows from secondary follicles. The primary follicles are arranged as a triad, with a central follicle and two laterals. The primary follicles have an arrector pili muscle, which allows erection of the guard hair during fright or anger and, under cold conditions, increases insulatory properties by trapping air in the coat. The **secondary follicles**

lack the arrector muscle. The primary follicles have a sebaceous gland that secretes lipid, giving the fur its glossy appearance and providing water-shedding properties. Hairs in fur animals are grouped into bundles containing a guard hair and several underfur hairs. Hairs in a bundle emerge from a common opening to the skin surface. In some bundles, the guard hair is so tiny that the difference in structure from underfur hairs is not visible to the naked eye. In mink winter fur, there are about 15 underfur hairs per bundle, whereas the winter fur of the blue fox contains about 40 underfur hairs per bundle (Valtonen *et al.*, 1995; Blomstedt, 1998). The dense winter coat is a result of an increase in the number of secondary follicles that can branch to form new follicles. These derived follicles are temporary structures. The development of the winter coat is due to the action of **melatonin**, a hormone produced by the pineal gland. Melatonin production and secretion are regulated by day length (photoperiod). The metabolic effects of melatonin on hair growth are mediated by its effects on prolactin synthesis and secretion (Rose *et al.*, 1984; Worthy *et al.*, 1986).

The hair coat undergoes a growth cyle (Fig. 19.1). At one stage in the cycle, it reaches a state referred to as the **prime** condition. The pelt of fur animals must be harvested when the fur is prime. If the pelt is not prime, the garment manufactured from it will shed hair and be unattractive. A hair undergoes three distinct growth phases in which periods of active growth alternate with resting periods. These periods are: (i) the anagen phase; (ii) the catagen phase; and (iii) the telogen phase. During the **anagen phase**, the hair shaft undergoes rapid growth. The follicle is embedded deep in the skin. Pigments are actively synthesized in this phase and move up the hair shaft as it grows. The hair pigment cells, called **melanocytes**, can be seen as dark-coloured areas on the leather side of an unprimed pelt (Fig. 19.2). As the growth cycle proceeds, the hair follicle shortens until its base is located just below the sebaceous gland in the upper layer of the skin and the papilla atrophies. These processes occur in the **catagen phase**. During the **telogen phase**, the hair is in a resting state, and the pigment cells have been drawn up into the hair shaft. At this stage, the pelt is prime. The leather side of the prime pelt is creamy white because the pigmented cells are in the hair shaft, and the last grown part of the hair does not contain any colour (Fig. 19.2). Following the telogen phase, a new cycle begins with a new hair beginning growth in the same follicle, forcing out the old hair and causing it to be shed (moulting). The length of the hair growth cycle is characteristic of the species. For example, the anagen phase is approximately 3 months in the mink winter fur, 21–26 days in the rat, 2–8 years in the human scalp and 7 years in the Merino sheep. In most mammals, the cycle of hair growth is seasonal and is related to day length and hormonal activity, resulting in regular periods of shedding or moulting (Ben-Ari, 2000).

In the manufacture of fur garments from pelts of mink or other fur animals, the leather side of the pelts may be shaved (i.e. like planing wood) to make them of uniform thickness. If the pelt is not completely in prime condition (see Fig. 19.1c), the shaving process may cut off the bottom of the hair follicles, causing the hair to fall out (see Fig. 19.1a). The skin of male animals is thicker than the skin of females (which accounts for gender differences in susceptibility to skin wrinkling in humans), so pelts from male animals require removal of more skin.

Hair is composed of **keratin**, a protein with a high cystine content. Keratin is a chain of amino acids in a helical coil, where cysteine forms sulfhydryl bonds between the coils giving the hair elasticity. Hairs consist of a central core of cells, the medulla, surrounded by the cortex. The cortex is covered with an outer layer of cells called the cuticle; the cuticle cells give water-repellent properties by overlapping like shingles. The medulla contains air spaces. The hair colour is determined by its structure and the pigments **melanin** (brown, black) and **pheomelanin** (yellow, red). These pigments are synthesized from the amino acid tyrosine. The conversion of tyrosine to melanin involves an enzyme, **tyrosinase**, which requires copper and iron as

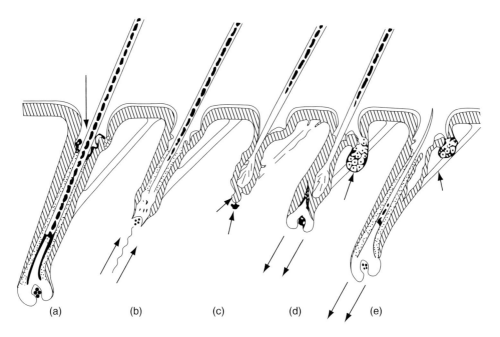

(a) (b) (c) (d) (e)

Fig. 19.1. The hair growth cycle. The growth of a new hair or anagen phase (a), is followed by the catagen phase (b), during which the lower part of the follicle atrophies. Melanin pigments move up the hair fibre from the dermis to the epidermal area. When this occurs, the underside of the pelt changes from dark to white (see Fig. 19.2) indicating that the hair is prime (c and d). In the telogen phase (d), a new hair follicle is formed and a new hair begins growth (e), which causes the previous hair to be shed.

(a)

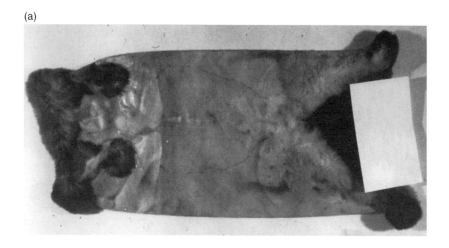

(b)

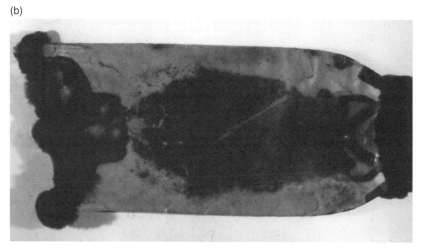

Fig. 19.2. Examples of prime (a) and non-prime (b) pelts turned inside out. The dark areas on the skin of the non-prime pelt correspond to (a) or (b) in Fig. 19.1 and consist of the melanin pigment granules that have not yet moved up the hair shaft (courtesy of N.P. Johnston, Brigham Young University, Utah, USA).

cofactors. White hair results both from a lack of pigment and reflection of light off the intercellular air spaces. Other factors affecting **hair colour** include cuticle structure (rough or smooth) and the degree of glossiness produced by sebaceous gland secretions. Feeding sources of unsaturated fats, such as vegetable oils, increases sebaceous gland secretion and produces a glossy hair coat (sheen, bloom).

Detailed consideration of the chemistry, biosynthesis and functions of melanin pigments is provided by Jimbow *et al.* (1986) and Pawelek and Korner (1982). In brief, tyrosinase oxidizes tyrosine in two steps. An hydroxyl group is added,

which then is further oxidized to dihydroxyphenylalanine (DOPA) and then to DOPA-quinone (Fig. 19.3). The DOPA-quinone rearranges to form an indole group; melanin arises from the condensation of several indole molecules (Fig. 19.3). In the production of pheomelanin, reaction with cysteine is involved (Fig. 19.3). Pheomelanin makes up a large portion of the skin pigment of red-haired people. Pheomelanin is unstable in the presence of UV light, accounting for sunlight-induced freckles and increased susceptibility to skin cancer in 'red-heads' (Jimbow *et al.*, 1986). Melanin in human skin is both constitutive and inducible. Ethnic and racial differences in skin colour are a result of the amount of constitutive melanin produced, while inducible skin colour (sun tan) is elicited by exposure of the skin to UV light (Jimbow *et al.*, 1986).

Numerous dietary factors influence **feather pigmentation** of avian species (Grau *et al.*, 1989), with considerable species differences in responses. A characteristic sign of lysine deficiency in bronze turkeys, chickens and Japanese quail is absence of melanin synthesis, producing white wing feathers (Fig. 19.4). Dietary deficiencies of phenylalanine, tyrosine, pantothenic acid, folic acid, iron and copper reduce melanin deposition in feathers (Grau *et al.*, 1989). In contrast, deficiencies of vitamin D and calcium increase pigmentation of chicken feathers (Grau *et al.*, 1989). The roles of carotenoids in feather pigmentation are discussed later in this chapter.

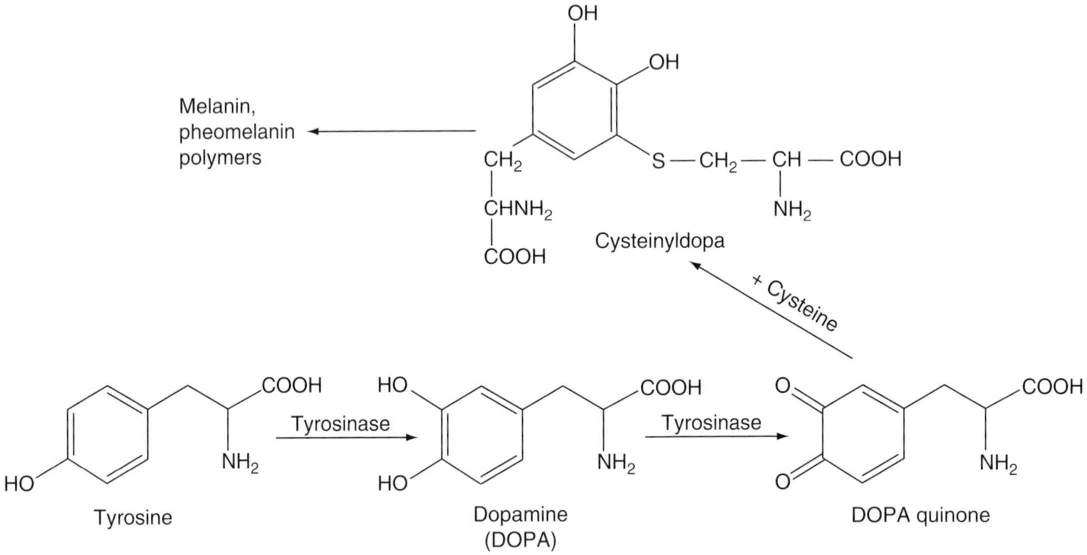

Fig. 19.3. Synthesis pathway of melanin and pheomelanin polymers.

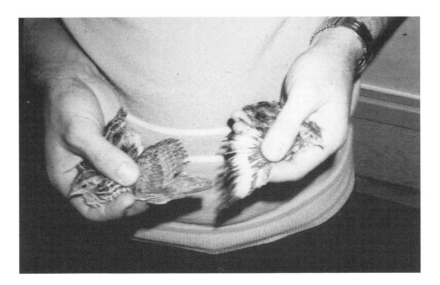

Fig. 19.4. White wing band characteristic of lysine deficiency in quail.

Because hair is composed almost entirely of protein, it is not surprising that dietary protein is one of the main nutritional factors affecting hair growth. Methionine is commonly the first-limiting amino acid for fur growth in mink and foxes (Dahlman *et al.*, 2003). A high methionine requirement during periods of rapid hair growth is related to the high content of sulfur-containing amino acids, especially cystine, in hair.

Nutritional status affects the wool growth of sheep. Although wool is essentially pure protein, the daily protein requirement for wool growth is only a small component of the total protein requirement. However, microbial protein does not contain an adequate amino acid balance to support maximal wool growth. Australian researchers demonstrated that post-ruminal administration of sources of methionine or high quality proteins to sheep markedly stimulated wool production (Colebrook and Reis, 1969). Utilization of sulfur-amino-acid-rich sources of non-degradable protein in sheep feeding might be a feasible way of increasing wool production. Similarly, supplementation of musk oxen with rumen-protected methionine increased wool production (Robertson *et al.*, 1998). Usually, the main nutritional factor limiting wool growth is energy intake (Ryder and Stephenson, 1968). Limitations to feed intake or increased energy requirements for productive functions (e.g. lactation) reduce the rate of wool growth. Severe stress, such as a short period of starvation, may cause cessation of wool growth and a break in the fibre after wool growth resumes. This results in fleece shedding.

Achromatrichia is the production of hair lacking pigmentation. Achromatrichial nutrients, which cause loss of hair pigmentation when deficient, include iron, copper, biotin and pantothenic acid. Iron and copper are cofactors of the enzyme tyrosinase which converts tyrosine to melanin. Generally there is a greying of dark hair in copper-deficient animals. Copper-deficient Hereford cattle develop yellow instead of red hair, while the normally black hair of Holstein cattle may be red. Pantothenic acid deficiency in rats causes dark fur to turn grey, but there is no indication that this occurs in other species. Grey hair in humans is characteristic of the ageing process. In the telogen phase of hair growth, a new hair follicle is made. Keratinocytes (epidermal cells) synthesize a new hair from the bottom up, stacking atop one another and eventually dying, leaving behind a hair shaft of keratin. As the keratinocytes build the hair fibre, melanocytes synthesize the melanin pigments. The keratinocytes and melanocytes are formed from stem cells at the base of the follicle. For unknown reasons, melanocyte stem cells have a much shorter longevity than keratinocyte stem cells, leading to the lack of pigment formation and grey or white hair.

Induced iron deficiency in mink occurs with diets containing substantial amounts of raw fish of the cod family, including Pacific hake, Atlantic whiting and coalfish (Table 19.1). Marine fish contain high contents of **trimethylamine oxide (TMAO)** in their tissues. The TMAO in marine fish may have osmotic roles, such as lowering the freezing point in the body fluids of polar species (Seibel and Walsh, 2002). TMAO binds iron by forming insoluble iron oxide hydroxides in the digestive tract, preventing its absorption and inducing severe iron deficiency. The TMAO is enzymatically converted to **formaldehyde** during cold storage in fish species of the cod family. This process is an unusual enzymatic reaction in which the enzyme is activated by freezing. The formaldehyde produced may add to the iron deficiency problem by impairing iron absorption due to reactions with protein in the intestinal mucosa. Both formaldehyde and TMAO may bind iron in the digestive tract, preventing its absorption and inducing severe iron deficiency. Mink that are fed raw fish of these species become severely anaemic and fur pigmentation is disturbed (Stout *et al.*, 1960; Costley, 1970). The underfur developed during severe iron deficiency anaemia is white or grey, causing the pelt to be almost worthless (Fig. 19.5). Mink ranchers have termed this the **cotton fur syndrome**. Heat treatment of the fish and supplementation with suitable iron sources prevent the condition. Iron deficiency impairs the enzymatic conversion of tyrosine to melanin in the hair follicle. Copper is a cofactor also. Aulerich *et al.* (1982) observed that use of copper sulfate at feed additive concentrations in mink diets (100–200 ppm Cu) resulted in darker fur, presumably from increased melanin synthesis.

The trimethylamine in gadid fish (e.g. pollock, cod) may have implications in the nutrition of Steller **sea lions**, which are declining drastically in number in the North Pacific. Signs of iron deficiency, such as anaemia, reduced growth and weight loss have been observed in sea lions feeding on pollock (Rosen and Trites, 2000; Trites and Donnelly, 2003). Other factors, such as low gross energy content of these fish, due to their low fat

Table 19.1. Iron absorption by rats and mink fed raw or cooked Pacific hake (adapted from Costley, 1970).

| | Mean iron absorption (% of administered dose) | | | |
| | Rats | | Mink | |
Form of iron	Raw hake diet	Cooked hake diet	Raw hake diet	Cooked hake diet
[59]Ferric chloride	6.2[*b]	15.2[†]	3.4[*]	8.9[†]
[59]Ferrous sulfate[a]	7.1[*]	8.4[*]	1.3[*]	9.3[†]

[a]Ferrous citrate for the mink.
[b]Values marked with [*]are different from those marked with [†]($P < 0.05$) within a species.

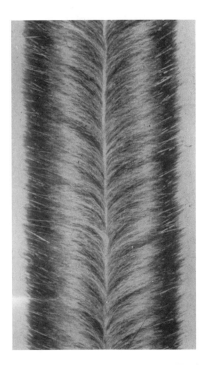

Fig. 19.5. A 'cotton fur' pelt of a dark mink. The fur is white because of a diet-induced iron deficiency. Iron deficiency impairs the enzymatic conversion of tyrosine to melanin in the hair follicle. Iron is a cofactor for the enzyme involved.

content, may also be involved (Donnelly *et al.*, 2003).

Biotin deficiency in mink and other animals can be induced by an inhibitor in raw avian egg white and avian oviducts. Raw eggs contain **avidin**, a glycoprotein that binds biotin and prevents its absorption. Feeding raw eggs, spray-dried eggs or poultry viscera containing eggs to mink may cause biotin-deficiency symptoms, including grey underfur, 'spectacle eyes'

(loss of hair around the eyes), foot pad dermatitis, poor growth and reproductive failure. Turkey eggs have a very high avidin content; the condition was often noted when turkey viscera were fed to mink, leading to the term '**turkey waste greying**' for the syndrome. Heat treatment inactivates avidin (Wehr *et al.*, 1980).

Tall fescue toxicosis is another factor that affects hair pigmentation of cattle. The black hair of Angus cattle may turn brown or bronze (Lipham *et al.*, 1989), probably due to the effects of melatonin via reduced prolactin concentrations (Porter *et al.*, 1994). Fescue toxicosis causes drastic decreases in prolactin secretion.

Essential fatty acids are components of cell membranes. Because skin cells are rapidly growing and the skin undergoes continuous turnover, dietary essential-fatty-acid deficiency is reflected in abnormal skin cells and flaky dermatitis. Essential fatty acids are also exuded from the hair follicles, causing the hair to be sleek and glossy (Fig. 19.6).

Antler Growth

Nutritional requirements for **antler growth** in deer have received considerable study (Kay and Staines, 1981), mainly because deer are farmed for antler production. Antler growth requires a high intake of energy, protein and minerals, especially calcium. The organic matrix of antlers is entirely protein and the hardened antler contains about 40% organic matter, so there is a **high protein requirement** for antler formation (Asleson *et al.*, 1996). **Copper deficiency** results in malformed antlers (Gogan *et al.*, 1988). Usually antler growth does not represent a nutritional problem for the wild animal, because it takes place during the summer when feed availability and intake are high. The maturation of antlers, shedding of the velvet and

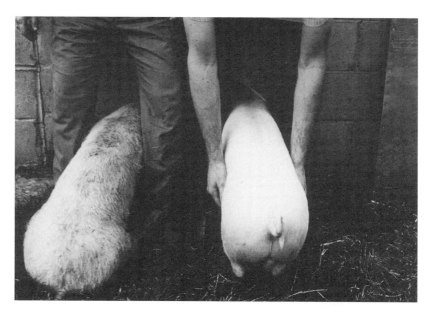

Fig. 19.6. The maize-fed pig on the right shows the favourable effects of the maize oil on the skin. The pig on the left was fed a diet deficient in essential fatty acids.

maintenance of the antlers in the hard, functional condition are dependent on testosterone concentrations, which vary seasonally (West and Nordan, 1976). In New Zealand, deer have been domesticated for production of antlers, which are exported to China to be used for medicinal purposes. Deer farming for meat production has begun in the USA (Buckmaster, 1988) using fallow deer. An advantage of fallow deer is that they resemble the bulk and roughage eaters (grazers) more than the concentrate selectors (see Chapter 3). Thus, fallow deer thrive on grass and are not susceptible to omasal impaction when fed hay. Nutritional requirements of red deer for meat production have been reviewed by Kay *et al.* (1984) and Barry and Wilson (1994).

Hooves and Feet

Foot health

A number of nutrients affect foot health. The B-complex vitamin **biotin** is often implicated in maintaining hoof and foot health. Biotin is widely distributed in common feedstuffs but has a low bioavailability in some grains (e.g. wheat, barley, sorghum, oats). Biotin deficiency in poultry fed wheat-based diets has been a common problem.

Biotin deficiency in non-ruminants causes dermatitis and cracks in the feet (**foot-pad dermatitis**). Biotin supplementation can increase fingernail thickness in humans (Mock, 1996). The metabolic role of biotin in these effects is not clear. One possible explanation is that biotin has a role in maintaining cell division or mitosis (Zempleni, 2001). Fast-growing tissues would be most affected by impaired cell division. The major metabolic role of biotin is participation in carboxylation reactions. It is unclear if these reactions play a role in the effects of biotin on foot health.

Supplementary biotin is often used to improve hoof health in dairy cattle (Fitzgerald *et al.*, 2000) and horses (Linden, 2001). Biotin supplementation of these animals often reduces hoof cracks and lesions. Ruminal biotin synthesis may be compromised in dairy cows fed high-energy grain-based diets (Fitzgerald *et al.*, 2000).

Laminitis

Laminitis, or founder, is inflammation of the laminae in the hoof and general hoof inflammation. The laminae are leaf-like structures that support the coffin bone (Fig. 19.7). When they become inflamed and swollen, blood flow in the hoof is impaired. Elevated blood pressure

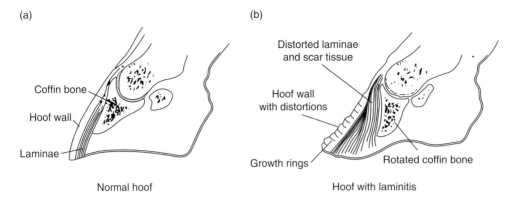

(a)

Coffin bone

Hoof wall

Laminae

Normal hoof

(b)

Distorted laminae
and scar tissue

Hoof wall
with distortions

Growth rings

Rotated coffin bone

Hoof with laminitis

Fig. 19.7. (a) In the normal hoof, the hoof wall and the laminae are parallel. (b) In laminitis, the laminae are distorted, causing rotation of the coffin bone. Pain, distorted hoof structure and lameness result.

(hypertension) precedes development of the symptoms. Blood is shunted through a circulatory bypass away from the arterioles in the hoof, through dilated (enlarged) **arteriovenous anastomoses** (**AVAs**) (a vessel that directly interconnects an artery and a vein, acting as a shunt to bypass a capillary bed). Absorbed toxins, including histamine, lactic acid and bacterial endotoxins produced in the gut, can cause AVA dilation, reduced blood supply to the hoof and inflammation of laminae.

Laminitis is particularly important in horses and cattle. The etiology in each case will be considered.

Equine laminitis

Laminitis in horses is a serious problem, because virtually all uses of the horse require that it have sound hooves and legs. Laminitis is often a sequel to other disorders, such as grain or lush pasture overload, other gastrointestinal disturbances, infections, retained placenta, insulin resistance (Chapter 16) and plant-induced toxicosis (e.g. black walnut poisoning). Garner *et al.* (1975) developed a technique for inducing laminitis for research purposes, by dosing with starch to cause carbohydrate overload of the hindgut. Excessive carbohydrate in the hindgut results in rapid proliferation of microbes and production of large quantities of lactic acid and bacterial endotoxins. Absorbed lactic acid and endotoxin cause venoconstriction in the hoof, resulting in the expansion of AVA shunts at the level of the coronary band (Moore *et al.*, 1989). Rowe *et al.* (1994) found that oral administration of the antibiotic virginiamycin to horses prevented

laminitis induced by grain feeding, by inhibiting the Gram-positive bacteria which produce lactic acid.

The initial event in laminitis is venoconstriction, impeding blood flow in the laminar capillaries (Moore and Allen, 1996), with the increase in capillary pressure causing fluid to move into the interstitial space. This event is accompanied by development of thrombosis (clotting) in the affected blood vessels in the hoof, probably due to activation of platelets by endotoxins or other products of hindgut fermentation (Weiss *et al.*, 1994, 1995, 1996). The reduced laminar blood flow is accompanied by shunting of blood away from the affected area by the AVA bypass.

Many horses and especially ponies (Fig. 19.8) are susceptible to development of laminitis when grazing lush, succulent pasture with high protein and soluble carbohydrate contents. Overloading the

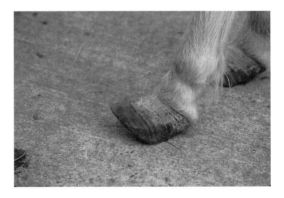

Fig. 19.8. Hoof of a foundered pony, showing abnormal growth rings and placement of the weight on the heel, to minimize pain.

hindgut with readily fermentable nutrients in low fibre forages results in excessive lactic acid and bacterial endotoxin production. Grasses often contain significant quantities of fructans, which may play a role in equine laminitis. **Fructans** (polymers of fructose) are not digested in the small intestine and undergo fermentation in the large intestine, thus contributing to lactic acid and endotoxin production (Longland *et al.*, 1999). Diurnal variation in fructan contents are seen, with maximum levels at midday, suggesting that it might be advisable to avoid access of horses to pasture during the midday period (Longland *et al.*, 1999). In cool season (temperate) C3 grasses, the stems contain the highest concentrations of fructans (Longland and Byrd, 2006). Thus grasses which have headed out (established stems and seed heads) may be a greater risk for inducing laminitis. Van Eps and Pollitt (2006) confirmed that dosing horses with fructan (inulin) induced clinical and histological laminitis. Similar results were also obtained with oligofructose-induced laminitis in cattle (Thoefner *et al.*, 2004). Harris *et al.* (2006) and Elliott and Bailey (2006) have provided excellent reviews of the etiology of equine laminitis. **Carbohydrate overload of the hindgut** (with starch and fructans) results in a proliferation of Gram-positive bacteria, notably *Streptococcus bovis* and lactic acid-producing lactobacilli and streptococci. These microbes produce a number of metabolites which can have inflammatory activity in the hooves. These include D-lactic acid, various amines and bacterial endotoxins. A number of **vasoactive amines** are produced in the equine hindgut, including phenylethylamine and isoamylamine (Bailey *et al.*, 2002) and tryptamine (Elliott and Bailey, 2006). Ergot alkaloids (e.g. ergotamine) contained in endophyte-infected tall fescue may also play a role in digital vasoconstriction by activating 5-hydroxytryptamine receptors (Harris *et al.*, 2006). A summary of the etiology of equine laminitis is given in Fig. 19.9.

The high susceptibility of ponies to laminitis may reflect their evolutionary heritage. 'Survival of species evolving in nutritionally sparse environments, including hunter-gatherer humans and rugged pony breeds, was probably facilitated by thrifty genes and insulin resistance,' according to Treiber *et al.* (2006a). Ponies with recurrent laminitis have been observed to be insulin resistant (Bailey *et al.*, 2007). Dietary fructans enhance insulin resistance in these ponies (Bailey *et al.*, 2007). Insulin-resistant equines are commonly viewed as 'easy keepers'.

The enzyme **matrix metalloproteinase** (**MMP**) breaks down the basement membrane bonding the dermal to the epidermal lamellae in the hoof (Harris *et al.*, 2006). A number of the metabolites of Gram-positive bacteria are activators of MMP, such as **thermolysin** produced by *S. bovis* (Mungall and Pollitt, 2002). Oxidative damage may play a role in laminitis. Increased **free radical** formation may occur as a result of changes in glucose/insulin metabolism and the development of insulin resistance (Treiber *et al.*, 2006b).

Consumption of **black walnut** (*Juglans nigra*) wood shavings by horses causes laminitis. True *et al.* (1978) reported that racehorses bedded down with chips or sawdust developed laminitis. MacDaniels (1983) discussed the toxic effect on herds of racehorses in Wisconsin and Michigan where severe allergenic reactions to the shedding of walnut pollen occurred as well as to the shedding of leaves in the autumn. In these instances, the problems were sufficiently serious that all the walnut trees were cut down, the stumps bulldozed and the soil removed from the paddocks and stables. Ralston and Rich (1983) reported an incident in Colorado involving horse stalls bedded with pine shavings containing 20% black walnut shavings as a contaminant. Within 12 h of exposure, the horses exhibited signs of toxicosis, including reluctance to move, early acute laminitis, slight oedema of the limbs and depression. Uhlinger (1989) reported an outbreak of black walnut toxicosis in horses bedded with black walnut shavings, with signs of severe abdominal pain and laminitis.

Water extracts of black walnut wood cause laminitis when administered to horses (Galey *et al.*, 1990, 1991). Galey *et al.* (1991) suggested that this procedure provides a good model for induction of laminitis for research purposes, without the complications of electrolyte imbalance, shock and colic that may occur when carbohydrate overload is used to induce the condition. The active laminitis-inducing principle of black walnut has not been identified. Black walnuts and other members of the walnut family (Persian or English walnuts, butternuts, hickories and pecans) contain **juglone** (5-hydroxy-1,4-naphthoquinone), a phenolic derivative of naphthoquinone. Juglone is an allelopathic substance which inhibits the growth of other plants. Tomatoes, potatoes and other vegetables, as well as many other trees and shrubs, are inhibited in their growth by juglone released into the soil from black walnut roots As a result, competition to

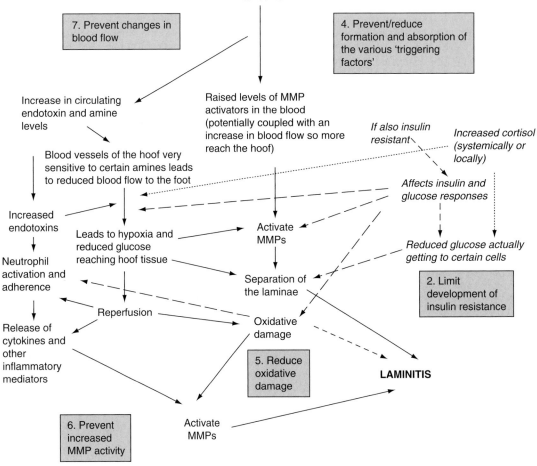

Ingestion of an
'excessive' amount of rapidly fermentable carbohydrate
e.g. an 'overload' of starch from cereal grains or sugar and/or fructan and/or starch from pasture

1. Identify animals predisposed to laminitis

3. Avoid high intakes of rapidly fermentable material

❖ Too much reaches hindgut – rapidly fermented
❖ Produces lactic acid – pH decreases – increases mucosal permeability
❖ Some bacteria die releasing endotoxin and other unwanted factors
❖ Other bacteria change internal metabolism in response to the pH decrease – produce for example certain amines
❖ Increased concentration of various substances including exotoxins (bacterial proteases) in particular matrix metalloproteinase (MMP) activating factors, as well as amines within the gastrointestinal tract
❖ With change in permeability increased risk that certain factors cross into the blood in increased amounts

7. Prevent changes in blood flow

4. Prevent/reduce formation and absorption of the various 'triggering factors'

Increase in circulating endotoxin and amine levels

Raised levels of MMP activators in the blood (potentially coupled with an increase in blood flow so more reach the hoof)

If also insulin resistant

Increased cortisol (systemically or locally)

Blood vessels of the hoof very sensitive to certain amines leads to reduced blood flow to the foot

Affects insulin and glucose responses

Increased endotoxins

Leads to hypoxia and reduced glucose reaching hoof tissue

Activate MMPs

Reduced glucose actually getting to certain cells

Neutrophil activation and adherence

Separation of the laminae

2. Limit development of insulin resistance

Reperfusion

Oxidative damage

Release of cytokines and other inflammatory mediators

5. Reduce oxidative damage

LAMINITIS

6. Prevent increased MMP activity

Activate MMPs

Fig. 19.9. Events leading to the onset of equine laminitis. Seven countermeasures are indicated in shaded boxes (courtesy of the *Journal of Nutrition* and P. Harris, Royal Veterinary College, London).

walnuts from other plants is reduced. True and Lowe (1980) found that large oral doses of juglone given to horses induced mild clinical signs of laminitis, but the naturally occurring condition could not be duplicated. Precursors of juglone may be involved in black walnut toxicosis (MacDaniels, 1983). Black walnut toxicosis in other animals besides horses does not seem to occur. It is recommended that walnut trees, particularly black walnuts, are not planted in horse pastures and that black walnut chips and sawdust are not used for bedding.

Bovine laminitis

Laminitis in beef and dairy cattle is an important problem for economic and animal welfare reasons. Laminitis is probably the major cause of bovine lameness (Vermunt and Greenough, 1994). Typically, laminitis is associated with high concentrate diets or with lush, succulent pasture high in protein and soluble carbohydrates.

High concentrate diets support a high rate of ruminal fermentation, with abundant production of VFAs, including lactic acid. **Lactic acid** is a stronger acid than the other VFAs, and contributes to a drop in rumen pH. The lowered rumen pH is accompanied by changes in the rumen microbes from Gram-negative to Gram-positive bacteria such as *S. bovis* and *Lactobacillus* spp. **Endotoxins** are released from the cell walls of lysed Gram-negative bacteria. Absorbed endotoxin may cause allergenic reactions in the arterioles of the hoof, impairing blood supply to the tissue. Lactic acid and histamine absorbed from the rumen contribute to the circulatory dysfunction (Vermunt and Greenough, 1994). Dilated AVAs in the corium of the hoof shunt blood away from the hoof tissue. Histamine stimulates AVA dilation. Dietary administration of the antibiotic virginiamycin, which inhibits Gram-positive bacteria, is effective in reducing lactic acid production in the rumen (Godfrey *et al.*, 1992). Ruminal administration of a lactate-utilizing microbe, *Megasphaera elsdenii*, also has shown potential in reducing rumen lactate concentrations (Kung and Hession, 1995).

Nutrition is a major factor in the development of laminitis in cattle. As in the equine founder syndrome, carbohydrate overload of the gut resulting in excessive microbial growth is the principal contributing factor. In ruminants, carbohydrate overload of the rumen produces changes in the microflora, high rates of production of VFAs and lactic acid, lowered rumen pH and increased microbial toxin production (endotoxins, histamine). High-producing dairy cows, with high feed intakes of high-energy, low-roughage diets, are particularly likely to develop laminitis.

Cattle on heavily fertilized pastures are also susceptible to laminitis. Vermunt (1992) speculated that elevated pasture nitrate levels could be involved. Nitrate is converted to nitrite in the rumen. Absorbed nitrite can produce pronounced vasodilation (Vermunt, 1992), which by promoting the AVA shunt in the hoof could contribute to laminitis. High protein intakes have been implicated in laminitis (Vemunt, 1992). The mechanism of action of protein in this effect has not been elucidated. The laminitis-inducing effects of lush, heavily fertilized pastures may be a consequence of both the high protein and the high soluble carbohydrate contents.

Block (1994) suggested that because laminitis in dairy cattle is related to blood acid–base balance, the dietary cation–anion balance could play a role in the disorder. Further research is needed to validate this suggestion.

Cell Membranes

Various types of membranes occur in animal tissue. The **plasma membrane** separates cells from the extracellular fluid. Other membranes enclose internal organelles such as mitochondria, endoplasmic reticulum, Golgi complexes, secretory granules, lysosomes and the nucleus. Cell membranes provide a means of keeping body fluids compartmentalized. Water makes up about 60% of the lean body mass of humans and many animals. It is distributed between **intracellular and extracellular fluids**, with about two-thirds being intracellular. These compartments differ substantially in composition. The intracellular fluid is enriched in the cations K^+ and Mg^{++}, with phosphate as the major anion. Extracellular fluid is high in Na^+ and Ca^{++}, with chloride as the major anion.

Membranes are composed largely of protein and lipid. The major lipids are phospholipids, glycosphingolipids and cholesterol. The two major types of phospholipids are the phosphoglycerides and sphingomyelin. **Phosphoglycerides** (Fig. 19.10) consist of glycerol with two esterified fatty acids in positions 1 and 2, and a phosphate on position 3. The fatty acids are usually C16 and C18, both saturated and unsaturated. **Sphingomyelin** contains a sphingosine backbone rather than glycerol (Fig. 19.10). The **glycosphingolipids** contain monosaccharides such as galactose and glucose bound to ceramide (Fig. 19.10). They are found mainly in the plasma membranes. The most common sterol in cell membranes is cholesterol. **Cholesterol** occurs in association with the phospholipids, with its

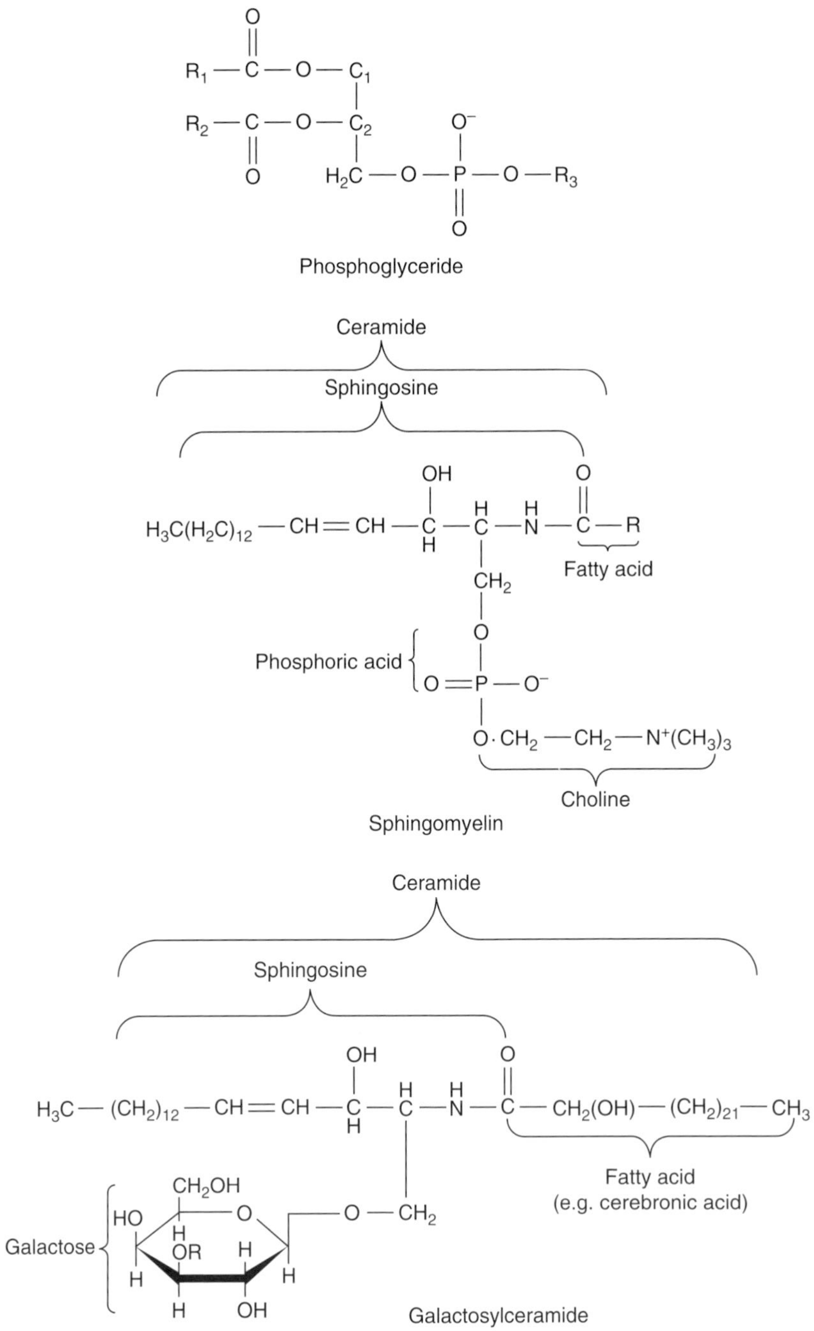

Fig. 19.10. Structures of phosphoglycerides and sphingolipids that function in membrane structure.

hydroxyl group at the aqueous interface. Vitamin E is another lipid in cell membranes, providing protection against auto-oxidation.

The lipids in cell membranes are amphipathic; that is, they have both hydrophobic (non-polar) and hydrophilic (polar) regions. They form **lipid bilayers**, which exist as sheets with the hydrophilic region exposed to the cellular fluids and the hydrophobic region constituting the core of the membrane. The bilayer is impermeable to most water-soluble molecules, because they are insoluble in the hydrophobic core. Non-lipid molecules can pass through channels in the membrane. **Channels** are formed by proteins in the membrane that allow the movement of ions, small molecules and transport proteins that carry larger molecules. There are specific ion channels for Na^+, K^+, Ca^{++} and Cl^-. Some bacteria synthesize small organic molecules, **ionophores**, that shuttle ions across membranes. Ionophores are used as feed additives for cattle (e.g. Rumensin®) and poultry (e.g. monensin). In ruminants, ionophores disrupt membrane function in Gram-positive bacteria such as *S. bovis*, while in poultry they disrupt membrane function in the protozoa (*Eimeria* spp.) which cause coccidiosis.

Hormones can affect membrane structure. For example, insulin increases glucose transport across membranes in adipose tissue and muscle. Membranes also have **active transport** mechanisms, such as ATPase, which are energy requiring. The Na^+-K^+ ATPase system is also called the sodium-potassium pump, and serves to maintain the high concentration gradients of these elements between extracellular and intracellular fluids.

Muscle Tissue and the Extracellular Matrix

Muscle constitutes the largest single tissue in the body. The three major types of muscle are: (i) skeletal; (ii) cardiac; and (iii) smooth. Skeletal and cardiac muscles are striated; smooth muscle is non-striated. The two major proteins in muscle tissue are actin and myosin. Skeletal muscle protein is the major non-fat source of stored energy in the body; during starvation, there is a very large loss of muscle tissue (wasting), such as in the condition of marasmus in humans (see Chapter 6). During intracellular breakdown of actin and myosin, 3-methylhistidine is formed and excreted in the urine. The urinary output of this methylated amino

acid can be used as a measure of protein degradation. Calcium plays an important role in muscle contraction, entering muscle cells through calcium channels. Abnormal accumulation of calcium occurs in degenerating muscle tissue, such as in white muscle disease, a degeneration of skeletal and cardiac tissue caused by selenium deficiency (see Chapter 13).

Muscle tissue secretes a network of macromolecules called the **extracellular matrix** (ECM) often referred to as **connective tissue**. The ECM contains three major classes of molecules: (i) the structural proteins collagen, elastin and fibrillin; (ii) certain specialized proteins such as fibrillin, fibronectin and laminin; and (iii) proteoglycans. There are at least 19 different vertebrate collagens (Velleman, 2002). **Collagens** are the most abundant protein in animal tissue, constituting about 25% of the body protein. The major collagens of skin, bone and cartilage are collagens I and II. All collagens have a triple helix structure, with three polypeptide chains coiled together in a right-handed helix. A major characteristic of collagen is the occurrence of glycine at every third position of the triple helical portion of the polypeptide units. Other characteristic amino acids are hydroxyproline and hydroxylysine, which are formed post-translationally by hydroxylases. Cofactors are ascorbic acid (vitamin C) for hydroxyproline and copper for hydroxylysine. Collagen fibres are stabilized by covalent cross-links involving hydroxylysine between the helical units. Collagen is relatively stable, but can be degraded during starvation and inflammatory states.

Proteoglycans are proteins that contain glycosaminoglycans, which include hyaluronic acid, chrondroitin sulfate, keratans, heparin and heparin sulfate. **Glycosaminoglycans** contain repeating units of disaccharides, one of which is always an amino sugar, either D-glucosamine or D-galactosamine. The other component of the disaccharide is a uronic acid, such as L-glucuronic acid. Except for hyaluronic acid, all the glycosaminoglycans are sulfated.

Proteoglycans are widely distributed in all tissues as major components of the ECM. Type I collagen is the organic matrix of bone. Type II collagen is the principal protein in cartilage. In osteoarthritis, disrupted formation and occurrence of proteoglycans involving chondroitin sulfate and hyaluronic acid occurs. Changes also occur in the ECM of the skin during ageing.

The Skin

Skin growth

Skin is one of the most actively growing tissues of the body, undergoing continuous formation. Thus nutritional deficiencies are often first observed in the skin.

Zinc is a constituent (metalloenzyme) or cofactor of a variety of enzymes in the body, including a number involved in nucleic acid and protein metabolism. Examples include thymidine kinase and DNA and RNA polymerases. Cell differentiation and cell replication are impaired in zinc deficiency. Therefore, the most rapidly growing tissues are the first to show signs of zinc deficiency. These include the skin, gastrointestinal tract, wound-repair tissue and the reproductive tract.

Zinc deficiency in pigs and poultry causes **parakeratosis**, or severe dermatitis with dry, scaly, cracked skin, and poor feathering in poultry. Diets containing soybean meal increase zinc requirements, because of the high phytic acid content of this product. Supplementary zinc is often provided in a chelated form, such as zinc methionine.

Essential fatty acids (linoleic, α-linolenic) and arachidonic acids are structural lipids occurring in cell membranes. Essential-fatty-acid deficiency results in rough, scaly skin (dermatitis). These symptoms occur prominently because the skin tissue has a rapid turnover time. Addition of vegetable oils to animal diets improves the appearance of the skin (Fig. 19.6). Unsaturated fatty acids such as EPA and DHA (Chapter 10) are also precursors of eicosanoids (e.g. prostaglandins, leukotrienes) which inhibit inflammatory responses in the skin.

Pigmentation of the skin and feathers

Melanin and pheomelanin are major skin pigments. They have been discussed previously under 'Hair growth' (this chapter).

The major **pigmenting agents** with a dietary origin are the carotenoid pigments. **Carotenoids** are plant pigments with a range of yellow to red coloration. Over 600 specific carotenoid structures have been identified. Some carotenoids function in photosynthesis, while others provide coloration of leaves, flowers and fruits. Carotenoids are divided into two groups: (i) **carotenes**; and (ii) **xanthophylls** (Fig. 19.11). They may be non-cyclic (e.g. lycopene) or contain five- or six-membered rings at one or both ends of the hydrocarbon chain (e.g. β-carotene, lutein). Xanthophylls are oxycarotenoids, with alcohol, keto or ester groups on the terminal rings. The position and type of these groups determine the colour of xanthophylls, and complexing of xanthophylls with proteins may shift the colour or give irridescence in birds (Klasing, 1998).

Carotenoids are of interest in the human diet because of their **antioxidant activity**. Each carotenoid molecule has at least nine double bonds in the side chain, capable of interacting with ROS, accounting for their antioxidant activity (Garcia-Casal, 2006).

Carotenoids are important in the coloration of wild birds, reptiles, domestic poultry and fish. In chickens, pigmentation of the egg yolks and skin is commercially important. There are differences in consumer preferences for pigmentation; in some areas, consumers prefer highly pigmented egg yolks and broiler skin, whereas in other areas poultry products with little pigmentation are preferred. Sources of xanthophyll pigments for poultry include green plants such as lucerne, yellow maize and a variety of yellow or red plant materials (Table 19.2). The richest commercial source of natural xanthophylls is marigold petal meal. It contains 6000–10,000 mg xanthophylls/kg; in comparison, dehydrated lucerne meal contains approximately 200 mg/kg and maize contains 20 mg/kg. The major xanthophyll in lucerne is **lutein**, which is yellow, whereas in maize and maize gluten meal the major pigment is **zeaxanthin**, which imparts an orange-red colour. Xanthophylls have no known nutritional value except as a source of pigment. In some cases, they have antioxidant activity, particularly those which have one or more exposed hydroxyl group. Synthetic carotenoids (e.g. canthaxanthin) have been developed and are increasingly used in the poultry industry in place of lucerne meal or marigold meal.

Dried marine algae are good sources of both carotenoid pigments and ω-3 fatty acids, and can be used as feed additives to enhance both ω-3 fatty acid and carotenoid contents of poultry products. Marine microalgae are the original source of ω-3 fatty acids in fish. **Astaxanthin** and **canthaxanthin** are two synthetic xanthophylls used to provide the pink skin coloration of salmon and trout. Shrimp, crabs, krill and herbivorous fish accumulate phytoplankton carotenoids, mainly astaxanthin and are used as pigmenting agents in diets for farmed salmon and trout (contrary to what may be popular

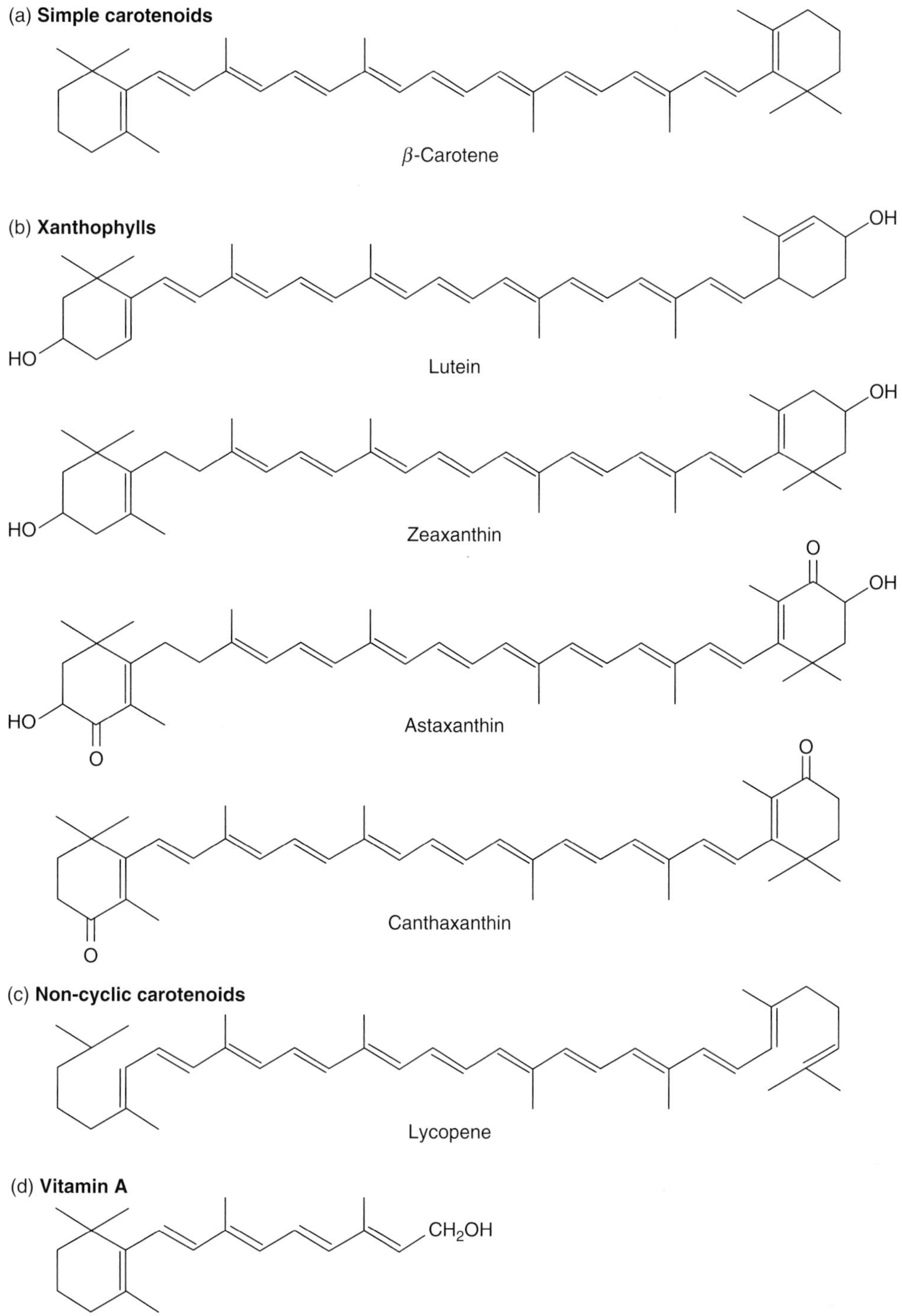

(a) **Simple carotenoids**

β-Carotene

(b) **Xanthophylls**

Lutein

Zeaxanthin

Astaxanthin

Canthaxanthin

(c) **Non-cyclic carotenoids**

Lycopene

(d) **Vitamin A**

CH₂OH

Fig. 19.11. Structure of common carotenoids and xanthophylls involved in skin and feather pigmentation.

The Integument, Pigmentation, Membranes and Extracellular Matrix

Table 19.2. Carotenoid pigment contents of some common pigment sources (from Klasing, 1998).

Pigment source	Carotenoid	Amount (mg/kg[a])
Krill	Astaxanthin	22–77
Copepod	Astaxanthin	39–84
Shrimp	Astaxanthin	100
Salmon	Astaxanthin	5
Algae (*Spirulina*)	Cryptoxanthin	389
	Zeaxanthin	80
Tomatoes	Total carotenoids	51
Red peppers	Total carotenoids	127–248
Lucerne meal	Total xanthophylls	220–330
Paprika	Total xanthophylls	275
Chilli peppers (dry)	Total xanthophylls	185
Carrots (dry)	Total xanthophylls	65
Yellow maize	Total xanthophylls	20–25
Marigold petals	Total xanthophylls	8000

[a]Wet weight basis.

belief, farmed salmon are not injected with dyes to colour their flesh!).

The unique colours of wild birds are largely due to carotenoid pigments (Table 19.3). Complete reviews of this subject are provided by Brush (1990) and Stradi (1998). Browns, blacks and greys are provided by melanin pigments synthesized in melanocytes in the developing feather. Structural colours are those produced by the surface or internal organization of the keratin proteins in the feather. White feathers are caused by light scattering from an unpigmented structure. The feather structure is such that it appears white from all viewing angles. Blue coloration is visually a structural feature. Structural blue of feathers is the result of light scattering. The external feather surface is blue while the back is black (Brush, 1990). The integrity of the colour can be destroyed mechanically (e.g. by a hammer blow). Iridescence is produced by intermixed layers of keratin and melanin (e.g. peacock tail feathers). Plants contain blue and purple anthocyanin pigments, which are absorbed in animals (Talavera *et al.*, 2004), but they are not involved in blue feather pigmentation. Although anthocyanins are not involved in animal pigmentation, they are potent antioxidants. Schaefer *et al.* (2008) observed that birds can actively select fruits based on anthocyanin content; fruits rich in anthocyanins are black or UV reflecting. On the other hand, birds cannot use colour to determine the carotenoid contents of fruits (Schaefer *et al.*, 2008).

Carotenoids provide the distinct coloration of many species exhibited in zoos. Many of the birds with brilliant plumage, such as the flamingo and scarlet ibis, as well as reptiles and amphibians with brightly coloured skin, require dietary carotenoids for this pigmentation. Canthaxanthin is included in flamingo diets for this purpose; β-carotene can also be used because it can be catabolized to canthaxanthin. Different species have different abilities to metabolize carotenoids; the carmine bee-eater, for example, does not metabolize canthaxanthin and instead appears to use lutein for its feather pigmentation (Dierenfeld and Sheppard, 1996). Simple chemical changes can cause biologically significant changes in plumage of wild birds. For example, only a single chemical change is responsible for the seasonal change from red (canthaxanthin) to yellow (isozeaxanthin) in the male scarlet tanager (Brush, 1990). The chemical change is simply the

Table 19.3. Distribution of carotenoids in birds (adapted from Klasing, 1998).

Species	Colour	Carotenoids
Flamingo	Pink	Astaxanthin, canthaxanthin
Canary	Yellow	Lutein
Canary	Golden-yellow	Zeaxanthin, lutein
Cedar waxwing	Red	Astaxanthin
Northern cardinal	Red	Canthaxanthin
Orange dove	Orange	Rhodoxanthin
Resplendent quetzal	Red	Canthaxanthin
Roseate spoonbill	Pink	Canthaxanthin, astaxanthin
Scarlet ibis	Pink-red	Canthaxanthin, astaxanthin
Toco toucan	Yellow, orange feathers and beak	Lutein, rhodoxanthin, zeaxanthin
Chicken	Golden yellow egg	Lutein, zeaxanthin
	Yellow skin, beak	Lutein

conversion of a keto group to an hydroxyl group. Another common change is to alter the number or position of double bonds in carotenoids. Pigmentation within a species of wild birds can vary depending upon the available diet. For example, a rapid change in some populations of cedar waxwings from a yellow to red tail band was associated with dietary differences of the populations (Brush, 1990).

Vultures have highly pigmented heads. Rotten flesh and bones, the typical diet of vultures, are low in carotenoids. Negro et al. (2002) observed that the colourful head pigmentation of the Egyptian vulture is derived from carotenoid pigments in cattle dung, which the birds regularly consume. Lutein was the dominant carotenoid in cattle dung. Consumption of excrement is common among several vulture species and is probably the primary means of acquiring carotenoids.

In many species of free-living birds, carotenoids are required for breeding success, as poorly coloured birds are less likely to mate. Thus carotenoids can be considered as dietary essentials for free-living birds for communication of reproductive fitness (Klasing, 1998), including mating displays and for advertising dominant status. The highest concentrations of carotenoids in bird tissue have been reported for the throat pouches of male frigate birds (Jucola et al., 2008). The main carotenoid responsible for this coloration is astaxanthin, acquired through consumption of fish, crustaceans and squid.

Lycopene is a non-cyclic carotenoid with 11 linearly arranged conjugated double bonds (Fig. 19.11). It is the characteristic red pigment of tomatoes. A diet rich in lycopene has been associated with reduced incidence of prostate and gastrointestinal cancers in humans (Clinton, 1998; Giovannucci, 1999). Lycopene is stable in cooked products and the bioavailability is even increased by cooking (Castenmiller and West, 1998). Representative lycopene contents of various food products are shown in Table 19.4.

Although carotenoids are a major source of pigmentation of birds, there are other pigment classes, including melanins, porphyrins, psittacofulvins and iron oxides (McGraw et al., 2007). Parrots display a spectrum of red-to-yellow hues in their feathers, but do not use carotenoids to generate these colours (McGraw and Nogare, 2004). Parrots use a novel class of red, orange and yellow pigments called **psittacofulvins**. These compounds are

Table 19.4. Approximate lycopene content of various foods (adapted from Clinton, 1998).

Food	Lycopene content (mg/100 g[a])
Tomatoes	
Fresh	0.88–4.20
Very red strains	5
Yellow	0.5
Tomato	
Sauce	6.20
Paste	5.40–150.0
Soup	8.0
Juice	5.0–11.6
Ketchup	9.9–13.4
Dried apricot	0.86
Pink grapefruit	3.36
Fresh watermelon	2.3–7.2
Fresh papaya	2.0–5.3

[a]Wet weight basis.

not derived from the diet but are synthesized in the follicles of growing feathers. Their synthesis is influenced by environmental conditions such as nutritional stress (Masello et al., 2008). Although parrots do not use carotenoids in feather pigmentation, they do have high blood concentrations of both dietary (lutein, zeaxanthin, β-cryptoxanthin) and metabolically derived (anhydrolutein, dehydrolutein) carotenoids (McGraw and Nogare, 2004).

McGraw et al. (2007) identified unique fluorescent yellow pigments in penguin feathers, which appear to be pterin pigments. Pterins are common yellow pigments in insects and the skin of fish, amphibians and reptiles. According to McGraw et al. (2007), these pigments have never before been identified in bird feathers. In the case of penguins, they may have a dietary origin (pterin-containing fish). Other colourful structures in penguins, such as orange beaks in king and emperer penguins, do contain carotenoid pigments.

Except for β-carotene which has provitamin A activity, carotenoids are considered to be non-nutritive. There is some evidence that β-carotene may have specific reproductive effects in dairy cattle (see Chapter 22). Carotenoids (β-carotene, lycopene, lutein, zeaxanthin) have also been demonstrated to improve iron absorption in humans (Garcia-Casal, 2006).

The **β-carotene** molecule consists of two vitamin A molecules joined together. Enzymes in the intestinal mucosa convert β-carotene to vitamin A by splitting it. The efficiency of this conversion varies among species. In humans, cattle and horses, significant amounts of carotene may be absorbed. This accounts for the yellow coloration of milk and body fat of Jersey and Guernsey cattle and the yellow skin pigmentation of vegetarians consuming large amounts of carrots and other carotene-rich vegetables. The fat of grass-fed cattle is often very yellow, because of the accumulation of carotenoid pigments. Sheep rarely have yellow fat, because of their efficient metabolism of carotenoids (Yang *et al.*, 1992).

Metabolic Roles of Vitamin A

Vitamin A is the only carotenoid that is an essential nutrient. Vitamin A is required for diverse metabolic functions, including roles in growth and differentiation of epithelial tissues, formation of visual pigments, reproduction (Chapter 22) and bone growth (Chapter 18). The vitamin A molecule can exist as an alcohol (retinol), an aldehyde (retinal or retinaldehyde) and an acid (retinoic acid) (Fig. 19.12). Retinoic acid is not able to fulfil the functions of retinol in vision or reproduction, but can sustain normal growth.

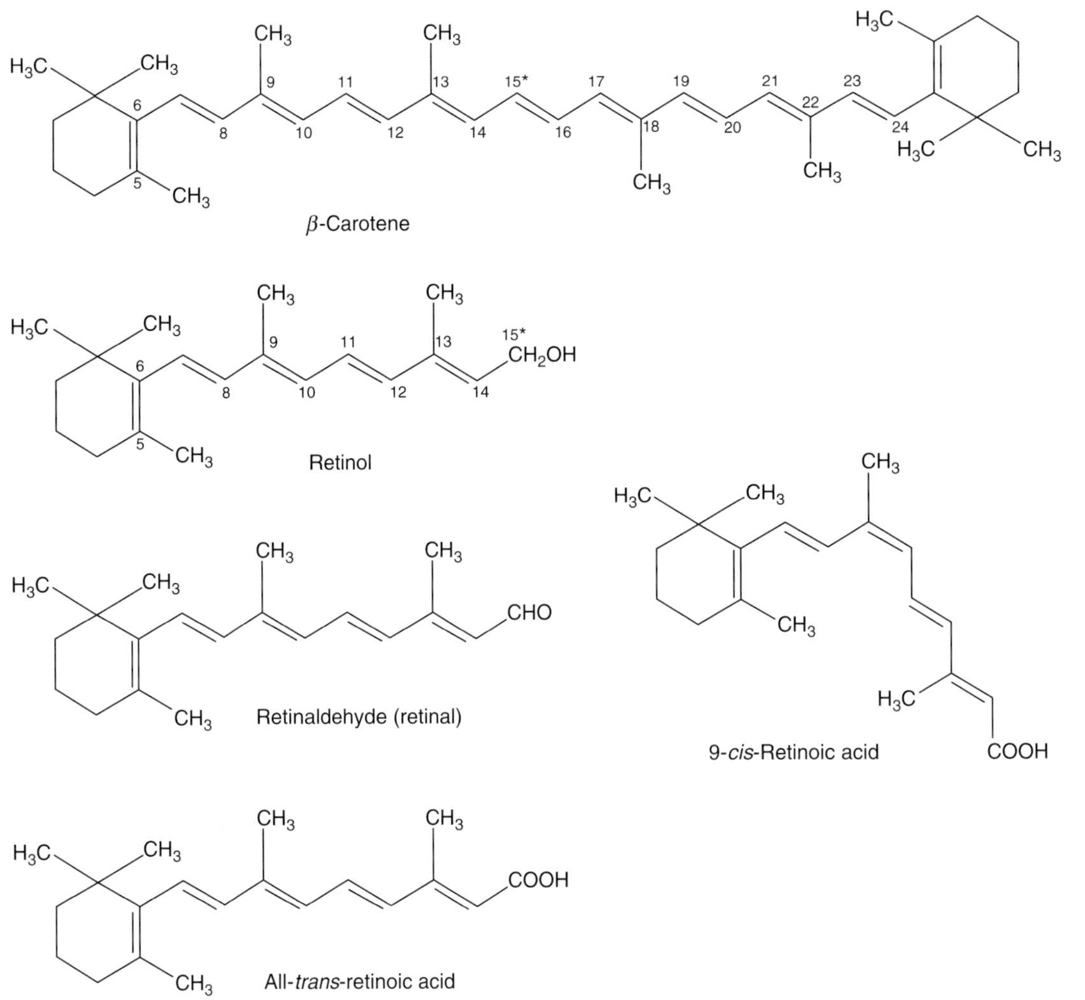

Fig. 19.12. Various chemical forms of vitamin A. The asterisk on carbon-15 indicates the site of cleavage of β-carotene into two retinols.

Vitamin A deficiency signs reflect these metabolic actions. In **vitamin A deficiency**, the normal epithelial tissues of the skin and mucous membranes are replaced by keratinized epithelium. Mucous-secreting cells fail to differentiate. This results in intestinal dysfunction and increased susceptibility of mucous membranes of the alimentary, genital, reproductive, urinary and respiratory tracts to infection. An example of the effect of keratinization of epithelial tissue in vitamin A deficiency is the condition of **xerophthalmia** (dry eye), characterized by a dry condition of the cornea and conjunctiva, cloudiness and ulceration. Vitamin A plays a role in the synthesis of glycoproteins that form mucopolysaccharides such as chondroitin sulfate.

Absorption and transport of vitamin A

The main dietary sources with vitamin A activity are provitamin A carotenoids (mainly β-carotene) and **retinol esters** such as retinyl palmitate. Intestinal mucosal tissue converts β-carotene to vitamin A by the action of two enzymes: (i) a cleavage enzyme which cleaves the central double bond to yield two molecules of retinaldehyde; and (ii) a reductase which reduces retinaldehyde to retinol. There is considerable species variability in the extent to which β-carotene is converted to retinol. Absorbed carotene is deposited in the liver and fatty tissues as a yellow pigment.

Vitamin A esters are hydrolysed in the intestine by pancreatic retinyl ester hydrolase. Vitamin A is then absorbed as free retinol, which is re-esterified to palmitate in chylomicrons. Retinol is transported in the blood in association with a plasma protein, **retinol-binding protein** (**RBP**). Newly absorbed retinyl esters are taken up by hepatocytes. Liver storage of vitamin A is in the hepatocytes and in fat-storage stellate (Ito) cells, and is in the form of retinyl ester. When liver vitamin A is mobilized, the retinyl ester is hydrolysed and free retinol released, bound to RBP. Blood concentrations of retinol are not a reliable indicator of vitamin A status, because a normal blood concentration is maintained until liver stores are exhausted. A more reliable measure of vitamin A status is the liver concentration. In livestock, use of liver biopsy is a common research technique for obtaining a liver sample for vitamin A analysis.

Role of vitamin A in vision

Vitamin A has several essential roles in the visual process. The retina contains two types of cells, rods and cones. In the retina, retinal (retinaldehyde) functions as the prosthetic group in light-sensitive opsin proteins, forming **rhodopsin** (in rods) and **iodopsin** (in cones). A particular cone cell contains only one type of opsin and is sensitive to only one colour. In the retina's pigment epithelium, all-*trans*-retinal is isomerized to 11-*cis*-retinol and oxidized to 11-*cis*-retinal. 11-*cis*-Retinal reacts with a lysine in opsin, forming rhodopsin (Fig. 19.13). The absorption of light by rhodopsin causes isomerization of the retinal from 11-*cis* to all-*trans*, and a series of conformational changes in opsin (photorhodopsin, lumi-rhodopsin, meta-rhodopsin – see Fig. 19.13). This causes release of retinal from the protein and initiation of a nerve impulse in the optic nerve. The all-*trans*-retinol is converted back to 11-*cis*-retinal, so that vitamin A is continually recycled in the visual process. In vitamin A deficiency, this recycling is inadequate, so that the time taken to adapt to darkness and the ability to see in low light are impaired (**night blindness**). These processes (Fig. 19.14) were elucidated by George Wald (1968), who received the Nobel Prize in Medicine for this achievement.

Vitamin A toxicity

Vitamin A toxicity (hypervitaminosis A) occurs when the ability of the liver to store retinol is exceeded, causing the blood retinol concentration to increase. Signs of toxicity reflect central nervous system effects, with headache, nausea, ataxia and anorexia, all associated with elevated cerebrospinal fluid pressure. Other effects include liver damage, hypercalcaemia, bone deformities and skin damage (excessive dryness, desquamation and alopecia). Vitamin A toxicity also causes reproductive disorders (see Chapter 22). The livers of certain Arctic animals often contain high concentrations of vitamin A. **Polar bears** store extremely high amounts of vitamin A in the liver, in specialized perisinusoidal cells known as **Ito** or **stellate** cells (Leighton *et al.*, 1988). This ability to sequester vitamin A is important because of the extremely high vitamin A intake from consumption of seals, which are rich in the vitamin. The build-up of vitamin A in the Arctic food chain begins with the consumption of

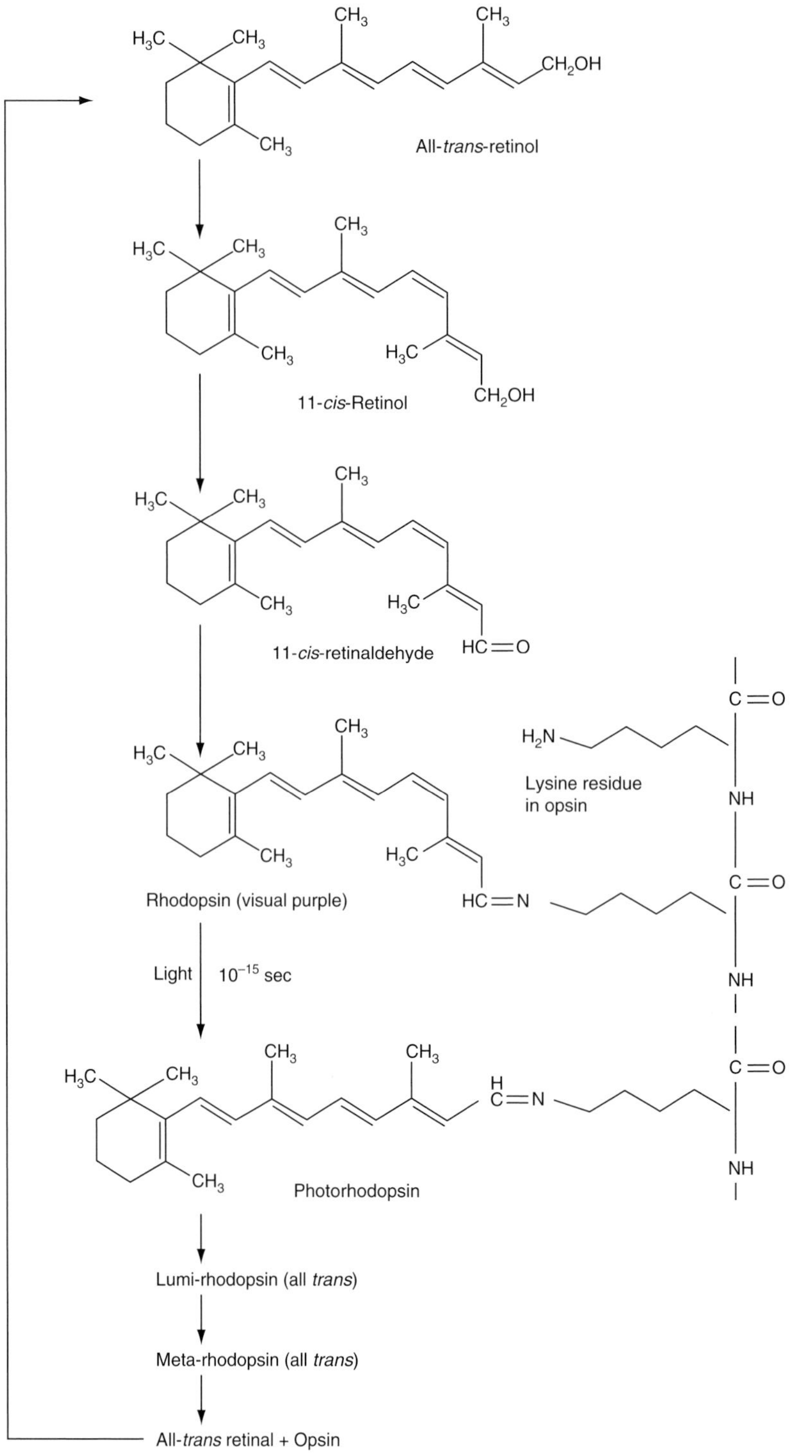

Fig. 19.13. Conversions of vitamin A during the reception of light in the visual process.

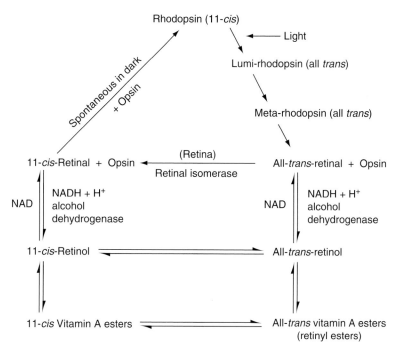

Fig. 19.14. Metabolism of vitamin A in vision.

carotene-rich plankton by fish. Although the polar bear is resistant to hypervitaminosis A, care to prevent overdosing with the vitamin should be taken with other species.

Dogs and other **carnivores** in the Canidae (canine) and Mustelidae (weasel) families have been reported with very high blood concentrations of **vitamin A**, up to 10–50 times higher than for other species (Schweigert *et al.*, 1990; Slifka *et al.*, 1999). The majority of the blood vitamin A in canines and mustelids occurs in the form of **retinyl esters**, primarily as retinyl stearate, bound to lipoproteins. In contrast to other species, the blood vitamin A concentrations are readily influenced by dietary vitamin A intake (Schweigert *et al.*, 1990). In most species, blood vitamin A exists as retinol bound to RBP. Only traces of retinyl esters occur and blood concentrations do not reflect intake. In other species, the occurrence of retinyl esters is a sign of severe vitamin A toxicosis. Another difference between canines and other species is that vitamin A is excreted in the urine of canines (Schweigert *et al.*, 1991), mostly as retinyl palmitate/oleate. Schweigert *et al.* (1990, 1991) speculate that these phenomena allow canines to cope with large amounts of dietary vitamin A in prey –

perhaps ecologically on a seasonal basis – without developing **vitamin A intoxication**. Anecdotal accounts of vitamin A toxicity have been reported in zoo carnivores – primarily snakes – fed whole rodents that have been shown to contain excessive concentrations of preformed vitamin A (Douglas *et al.*, 1994). Vitamin A concentrations measured in free-ranging rodents are about one-tenth the amounts reported in whole prey raised on commercial laboratory rodent diets. Because insects as a whole are known to contain low amounts of vitamin A (Barker *et al.*, 1998), it is possible that insectivorous species may be more sensitive to dietary excesses, but this has not been investigated systematically.

Vitamin A toxicity with fatalities has occurred with numerous Arctic and Antarctic explorers, in the early days of polar exploration. Explorers were sometimes forced to kill their sled dogs and eat them, including the livers which contain extremely high contents of vitamin A. Polar bear and seal livers are also toxic.

Consumption of high concentrations of β-carotene does not cause vitamin A toxicity. The conversion of carotene to vitamin A is suppressed when tissue saturation with vitamin A has occurred.

Questions and Study Guide

1. Name the nutrients which cause achromatrichia, and explain how they function in hair pigmentation.
2. What is the role of trimethylamine oxide in causing cotton fur syndrome in mink?
3. Biotin is extensively used, especially with horses, as a dietary aid in maintaining healthy hooves. How does biotin function in this role?
4. What is the postulated role of fructans in causing laminitis in horses?
5. Why are ponies especially susceptible to laminitis?
6. What are some differences in concentrations of minerals in intracellular and extracellular fluids?
7. Why does meat contain cholesterol? What is its function in meat tissue?
8. What is the extracellular matrix?
9. What is the most abundant protein in the animal body?
10. What is the difference between a proteoglycan and a glycosaminoglycan?
11. What tissues are rich in either Type I or Type II collagen?
12. What is the difference between carotenes and xanthophylls?
13. Why do wild salmon have pink flesh?
14. Some birds (e.g. bluebirds, blue jays) are blue in colour. What is responsible for the blue coloration of their feathers?
15. Why do vultures have colourful heads?
16. What foods are rich in lycopene? Why might lycopene be important in the human diet? Which is a better source of lycopene: fresh tomatoes or ketchup?
17. Grass-fed cattle may have yellow body fat. Why?
18. What is the difference between retinol and retinal?
19. What is rhodopsin?
20. Why does vitamin A deficiency cause night blindness?
21. Polar bear and dog liver cause vitamin A intoxication in humans (e.g. Arctic explorers). Why?

References

Asleson, M.A., Hellgren, E.C. and Varner, L.W. (1996) Nitrogen requirements for antler growth and maintenance in white-tailed deer. *Journal of Wildlife Management* 60, 744–752.

Aulerich, R.J., Ringer, R.K., Bleavins, M.R. and Napolitano, A. (1982) Effects of supplemental dietary copper on growth, reproductive performance and kit survival of standard dark mink and the acute toxicity of copper to mink. *Journal of Animal Science* 55, 337–343.

Bailey, S.R., Rycroft, A. and Elliott, J. (2002) Production of amines in equine cecal contents in an *in vitro* model of carbohydrate overload. *Journal of Animal Science* 80, 2656–2662.

Bailey, S.R., Menzies-Gow, N.J., Harris, P.A., Habershon-Butcher, J.L., Crawford, C., Berhane, Y., Boston, R.C. and Elliott, J. (2007) Effect of dietary fructans and dexamethasone administration on the insulin response of ponies predisposed to laminitis. *Journal of the American Veterinary Medical Association* 231, 1365–1373.

Barker, D., Fitzpatrick, M.P. and Dierenfeld, E.S. (1998) Nutrient composition of selected whole invertebrates. *Zoo Biology* 17, 123–134.

Barry, T.N. and Wilson, P.R. (1994) Venison production from farmed deer. *Journal of Agricultural Science* 123, 159–165.

Ben-Ari, E.T. (2000) Hair today. Untangling the biology of the hair follicle. *BioScience* 50, 303–308.

Block, E. (1994) Manipulation of dietary cation–anion difference on nutritionally related production diseases, productivity, and metabolic responses of dairy cows. *Journal of Dairy Science* 77, 1437–1450.

Blomstedt, L. (1998) Pelage cycle in blue-fox (*Alopex lagopus*): a comparison between animals born early and late in the season. *Acta Agriculturae Scandinavica Section A, Animal Science* 48, 122–128.

Brush, A.H. (1990) Metabolism of carotenoid pigments in birds. *FASEB Journal* 4, 2969–2977.

Buckmaster, R. (1988) Deer farming: a new veterinary frontier. *Large Animal Veterinarian* 43, 20–24.

Castenmiller, J.J.M. and West, C.E. (1998) Bioavailability and bioconversion of carotenoids. *Annual Review of Nutrition* 18, 19–38.

Clinton, S.K. (1998) Lycopene: chemistry, biology and implications for human health and disease. *Nutrition Reviews* 56, 35–51.

Colebrook, W.F. and Reis, P.J. (1969) Relative value for wool growth and nitrogen retention of several proteins administered as abomasal supplements to sheep. *Australian Journal of Biological Science* 22, 1507–1516.

Costley, G.E. (1970) Involvement of formaldehyde in depressed iron absorption in mink and rats fed Pacific hake (*Merluceius productus*). PhD thesis, Oregon State University, Oregon.

Dahlman, T., Valaja, J., Jalava, T. and Skrede, A. (2003) Growth and fur characteristics of blue foxes (*Alopex lagopus*) fed diets with different protein levels and with or without DL-methionine supplementation in the growing-furring period. *Canadian Journal of Animal Science* 83, 239–245.

Dierenfeld, E.S. and Sheppard, C.D. (1996) Canthaxanthin pigment does not maintain color in carmine bee-eaters. *Zoo Biology* 15, 183–185.

Donnelly, C.P., Trites, A.W. and Kitts, D.D. (2003) Possible effects of pollock and herring on the growth and reproductive success of Steller sea lions (*Eumetopias jubatus*): insights from feeding experiments using an alternative animal model, *Rattus norvegicus. British Journal of Nutrition* 89, 71–82.

Douglas, T.C., Pennino, M. and Dierenfeld, E.S. (1994) Vitamins E and A, and proximate composition of whole mice and rats used as feed. *Comparative Biochemistry and Physiology* 107A, 419–424.

Elliott, J. and Bailey, S.R. (2006) Gastrointestinal derived factors are potential triggers for the development of acute equine laminitis. *Journal of Nutrition* 136, 2103S–2107S.

Fitzgerald, T., Norton, B.W., Elliott, R., Podlich, H. and Svendsen, O.L. (2000) The influence of long-term supplementation with biotin on the prevention of lameness in pasture fed dairy cows. *Journal of Dairy Science* 83, 338–344.

Galey, F.D., Beasley, V.R., Schaeffer, D. and Davis, L.E. (1990) Effect of an aqueous extract of black walnut (*Juglans nigra*) on isolated equine digital vessels. *American Journal of Veterinary Research* 51, 83–88.

Galey, F.D., Whiteley, H.E., Goetz, T.E., Kuenstler, A.R., Davis, C.A. and Beasley, V.R. (1991) Black walnut (*Juglans nigra*) toxicosis: a model for equine laminitis. *Journal of Comparative Pathology* 104, 313–326.

Garcia-Casal, M.N. (2006) Carotenoids increase iron absorption from cereal-based food in the human. *Nutrition Research* 26, 340–344.

Garner, H.E., Coffman, J.R., Hahn, A.W., Hutcheson, D.P. and Tumbleson, M.E. (1975) Equine laminitis of alimentary origin: an experimental model. *American Journal of Veterinary Research* 36, 441–444.

Giovannucci, E. (1999) Tomatoes, tomato-based products, lycopene, and cancer: review of the epidemiologic literature. *Journal of the National Cancer Institute* 91, 317.

Godfrey, S.I., Boyce, M.D. and Rowe, J.B. (1992) Changes within the digestive tract of sheep following engorgement with barley. *Australian Journal of Agricultural Research* 44, 1093–1101.

Gogan, P.J.P., Jessup, D.A. and Barrett, R.H. (1988) Antler anomalies in tule elk. *Journal of Wildlife Diseases* 24, 656–662.

Grau, C.R., Roudybush, T.E., Vohra, P., Kratzer, E.H., Yang, M. and Nearenberg, D. (1989) Obscure relations of feather melanization and avian nutrition. *World's Poultry Science Journal* 45, 241–246.

Harris, P., Bailey, S.R., Elliott, J. and Longland, A. (2006) Countermeasures for pasture-associated laminitis in ponies and horses. *Journal of Nutrition* 136, 2114S–2121S.

Jimbow, K., Fitzpatrick, T.B. and Quevedo, W.C., Jr (1986) Formation, chemical composition and function of melanin pigments. In: Bereiter-Hahn, J., Matoltsy, A.G. and Richards, K.S. (eds) *Biology of the Integument*, Vol. 2 *Invertebrates*. Springer-Verlag, Berlin, pp. 278–291.

Jucola, F.A., McGraw, K. and Dearborn, D.C. (2008) Carotenoids and throat pouch coloration in the great frigatebird (*Fregata minor*). *Comparative Biochemistry and Physiology Part B* 149, 370–377.

Kay, R.N.B. and Staines, B.W. (1981) The nutrition of the red deer (*Cervus elaphus*). *Nutrition Abstracts and Reviews* 51(B), 601–622.

Kay, R.N.B., Milne, J.A. and Hamilton, W.J. (1984) Nutrition of red deer for meat production. *Proceedings of the Royal Society of Edinburgh (Biology)* 82, 231–242.

Klasing, K.C. (1998) *Comparative Avian Nutrition*. CAB International, Wallingford, Oxon, UK.

Kung, L., Jr and Hession, A.O. (1995) Preventing *in vitro* lactate accumulation in ruminal fermentations by inoculation with *Megasphaera elsdenii*. *Journal of Animal Science* 73, 250–256.

Leighton, F.A., Cattet, M., Norstrom, R. and Trudeau, S. (1988) A cellular basis for high levels of vitamin A in livers of polar bears (*Ursus maritimus*): the Ito cell. *Canadian Journal of Zoology* 66, 480–482.

Linden, J.E. (2001) *The Role of Biotin in Improving the Hoof Condition of Horses*. Hoffman-LaRoche, Basel, Switzerland.

Lipham, L.B., Thompson, F.N., Stuedemann, J.A. and Sartin, J.L. (1989) Effects of metoclopramide on steers grazing endophyte-infected fescue. *Journal of Animal Science* 67, 1090–1097.

Longland, A.C. and Byrd, B.M. (2006) Pasture nonstructural carbohydrates and equine laminitis. *Journal of Nutrition* 136, 2099S–2102S.

Longland, A.C., Cairns, A.J. and Humphreys, M.O. (1999) Seasonal and diurnal changes in fructan concentration in *Lolium perenne*: implications for the grazing management of equines pre-disposed to laminitis. In: *Proceedings of the 16th Equine Nutrition and Physiology Symposium*, North Carolina State University, Raleigh, North Carolina, 2–5 June 1999, pp. 258–259.

MacDaniels, L.H. (1983) Perspective on the black walnut toxicity problem – apparent allergies to man and horse. *Cornell Vet* 73, 204–207.

Masello, J.F., Lubjuhn, T. and Quillfeldt, P. (2008) Is the structural and psittacofulvin-based coloration of wild burrowing parrots *Cyanoliseus patagonus* condition dependent? *Journal of Avian Biology* 39, 653–662.

McGraw, K.J. and Nogare, M.C. (2004) Carotenoid pigments and the selectivity of psittacofulvin-based coloration systems in parrots. *Comparative Biochemistry and Physiology* 138B, 229–233.

McGraw, K.J., Toomey, M.B., Nolan, P.M., Morehouse, N.I., Massaro, M. and Jouventin, P. (2007) A description of unique fluorescent yellow pigments in penguin feathers. *Pigment Cell Research* 20, 301–304.

Mock, D.M. (1996) Biotin. In: Ziegler, E.E. and Filer, L.J., Jr (eds) *Present Knowledge in Nutrition*, 7th edn. ILSI Press, Washington, DC, pp. 220–235.

Moore, J.N. and Allen, D., Jr (1996) The pathophysiology of acute laminitis. *Veterinary Medicine* 91, 936–393.

Moore, J.N., Allen, D., Jr and Clark, E.S. (1989) Pathophysiology of acute laminitis. *Veterinary Clinics of North America: Equine Practice* 5, 67–72.

Mungall, B.A. and Pollitt, C.C. (2002) Thermolysin activates equine lamellar hoof matrix metalloproteinases. *Journal of Comparative Pathology* 126, 9–16.

Negro, J.J., Grande, J.M., Tella, J.L., Garrido, J., Hornero, D., Donazar, J.A., Sanchez-Zapata, J.A., Benitez, J.R. and Barcell, M. (2002) Coprophagy: an unusual source of essential carotenoids. *Nature* 416, 807–808.

Pawelek, J.M. and Korner, A.M. (1982) The biosynthesis of mammalian melanin. *American Scientist* 70, 136–145.

Porter, J.K., Stuedemann, J.A., Thompson, F.N., Buchanan, B.A. and Tucker, H.A. (1994) Melatonin and pineal neurochemicals in steers grazed on endophyte-infected tall fescue: effects of metoclopramide. *Journal of Animal Science* 71, 1526–1531.

Ralston, S.L. and Rich, V.A. (1983) Black walnut toxicosis in horses. *Journal of the American Veterinary Medical Association* 183, 1095.

Robertson, M.A., Rowell, J. and White, R.G. (1998) Effect of rumen-protected methionine on wool production and protein turnover in muskoxen (*Ovibos moschatus*). In: *Proceedings of the 2nd Comparative Nutrition Society Conference*, Banff, Canada, pp. 179–181.

Rose, J., Stormshak, F., Oldfield, J. and Adair, J. (1984) Induction of winter fur growth in mink (*Mustela vison*) with melatonin. *Journal of Animal Science* 58, 57–61.

Rosen, D.A.S. and Trites, A.W. (2000) Pollock and the decline of Steller sea lions: testing the junk-food hypothesis. *Canadian Journal of Zoology* 78, 1243–1250.

Rowe, J.B., Lees, M.J. and Pethick, D.W. (1994) Prevention of acidosis and laminitis associated with grain feeding in horses. *Journal of Nutrition* 124, 2742S–2744S.

Ryder, M.L. and Stephenson, S.K. (1968) *Wool Growth*. Academic Press, New York.

Schaefer, H.M., McGraw, K. and Catoni, C. (2008) Birds use fruit colour as honest signal of dietary antioxidant rewards. *Functional Ecology* 22, 303–310.

Schweigert, F.J., Ryder, O.A., Rambeck, W.A. and Zucker, H. (1990) The majority of vitamin A is transported as retinyl esters in the blood of most carnivores. *Comparative Biochemistry and Physiology* 95A, 573–578.

Schweigert, F.J., Thomann, E. and Zucker, H. (1991) Vitamin A in the urine of carnivores. *International Journal for Vitamin and Nutrition Research* 61, 110–113.

Seibel, B.A. and Walsh, P.J. (2002) Trimethylamine oxide accumulation in marine animals: relationship to acylglycerol storage. *Journal of Experimental Biology* 295, 297–306.

Slifka, K.A., Bowen, P.E., Stacewicz-Sapuntikis, M. and Crissey, S.D. (1999) A survey of serum and dietary carotenoids in captive wild animals. *Journal of Nutrition* 129, 380–390.

Stout, F.M., Oldfield, J.E. and Adair, J. (1960) Aberrant iron metabolism and the cotton fur abnormality in mink. *Journal of Nutrition* 72, 46–52.

Stradi, R. (1998) *The Color of Flight*. Solei Gruppo Editoriale Informatico, Milan, Italy.

Talavera, S., Felgines, C., Texier, O., Besson, C., Manach, C., Lamaison, J.-L. and Remesy, C. (2004) Anthocyanins are efficiently absorbed from the small intestine in rats. *Journal of Nutrition* 134, 2275–2279.

Thoefner, M.B., Pollitt, C.C., van Eps, A.W., Milinovich, G.J., Trott, D.J., Wattle, O. and Andersen, P.H. (2004) Acute bovine laminitis: a new induction model using alimentary oligofructose overload. *Journal of Dairy Science* 87, 2932–2940.

Treiber, K.H., Kronfeld, D.S. and Geor, R.J. (2006a) Insulin resistance in equids: possible role in laminitis. *Journal of Nutrition* 136, 2094S–2098S.

Treiber, K.H., Kronfeld, D.S., Hess, T.M., Byrd, B.M., Splan, R.K. and Staniar, W.B. (2006b) Evaluation of genetic and metabolic predispositions and nutritional risk factors for pasture-associated laminitis in ponies. *Journal of the American Veterinary Medical Association* 228, 1538–1545.

Trites, A.W. and Donnelly, C.P. (2003) The decline of Steller sea lions *Eumetopias jubatus* in Alaska: a review of the nutritional stress hypothesis. *Mammal Review* 33, 3–28.

True, R.G. and Lowe, J.E. (1980) Induced jugalone toxicosis in ponies and horses. *American Journal of Veterinary Research* 41, 944–945.

True, R.G., Lowe, J.E., Heissen, J.E. and Bradley, W. (1978) Black walnut shavings as a cause of acute laminitis. *Proceedings of the American Association of Equine Practitioners* 24, 511–515.

Uhlinger, C. (1989) Black walnut toxicosis in ten horses. *Journal of the American Veterinary Medical Association* 195, 343–344.

Valtonen, M., Vakkuri, O. and Blomstedt, L. (1995) Autumnal timing of photoperiodic manipulation critical via melatonin to winter pelage development in the mink. *Animal Science* 61, 589–596.

Van Eps, A.W. and Pollitt, C.C. (2006) Equine laminitis induced with oligofructose. *Equine Veterinary Journal* 38, 203–208.

Velleman, S.G. (2002) Role of the extracellular matrix in muscle growth and development. *Journal of Animal Science* 80(E. Suppl. 2), E8–E13.

Chapter 19

Vermunt, J.J. (1992) 'Subclinical' laminitis in dairy cattle. *New Zealand Veterinary Journal* 40, 133–138.

Vermunt, J.J. and Greenough, P.R. (1994) Predisposing factors of laminitis in cattle. *British Veterinary Journal* 150, 151–164.

Wald, G. (1968) Molecular basis of visual excitation. *Science* 162, 230–239.

Wehr, N.B., Adair, J. and Oldfield, J.E. (1980) Biotin deficiency in mink fed spray-dried eggs. *Journal of Animal Science* 50, 877–885.

Weiss, D.J., Geor, R.J., Johnston, G. and Trent, A.M. (1994) Microvascular thrombosis associated with the onset of acute laminitis in ponies. *American Journal of Veterinary Research* 55, 606–612.

Weiss, D.J., Trent, A.M. and Johnston, G. (1995) Prothrombotic events associated with the prodromal stages of acute laminitis. *American Journal of Veterinary Research* 56, 986–991.

Weiss, D.J., Monreal, L., Angles, A.M. and Monasterio, J. (1996) Evaluation of thrombin-antithrombin complexes and fibrin fragment D in carbohydrate-induced acute laminitis. *Research in Veterinary Science* 61, 157–159.

West, N.O. and Nordan, H.C. (1976) Hormonal regulation of reproduction and the antler cycle in the male Columbian black-tailed deer (*Odocoileushemionus hemionus columbianus*). Part I. Seasonal changes in the histology of the reproductive organs, serum testosterone, sperm production, and the antler cycle. *Canadian Journal of Zoology* 54, 1617–1636.

Worthy, G.A., Rose, J. and Stormshak, F. (1986) Anatomy and physiology of fur growth: the pelage priming process. In: Novak, M., Baker, J.A., Obbard M.E. and Mallock, B. (eds) *Wild Furbearer Management and Conservation in North America*. Ministry of Natural Resources, Toronto, pp. 827–841.

Yang, A., Larsen, T.W. and Tume, R.K. (1992) Carotenoid and retinol concentrations in serum, adipose tissue and liver and carotenoid transport in sheep, goats and cattle. *Australian Journal of Agricultural Research* 43, 1809–1817.

Zempleni, J. (2001) Biotin. In: Bowman, B.A. and Russell, R.M. (eds) *Present Knowledge in Nutrition*, 8th edn. ILSI Press, Washington, DC, pp. 241–252.

PART VII
Water and Body Fluids

This part is intended to discuss water utilization by animals and fluid compartments of the body.

Part Objectives

1. To discuss differences among animals in their requirements and utilization of water.
2. To discuss water conservation strategies of desert and arid-land animals.
3. To discuss blood components related to nutrition, such as blood proteins, haemoglobin and the nutrients involved in its synthesis, and electrolytes, including dietary electrolyte balance.

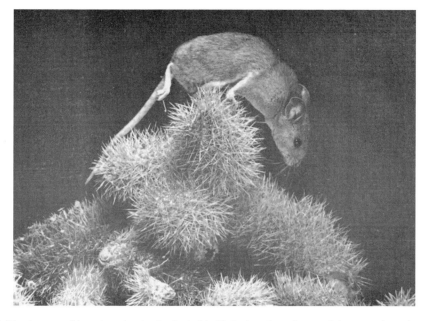

The pack rat (*Neotoma* spp.) is a desert animal adapted to life in American deserts. It has an adapted water metabolism strategy for survival in arid environments. (Courtesy of Oxford University Press, London).

20 Water

Water is the fluid matrix of the animal body in which are embedded the living cells with their contained protoplasm and the intercellular substance giving form and structure to the body and protection from environmental stress. The high solvent power of water permits the formation of a large variety of solutions, true and colloidal, within which the reactions of metabolism occur. Most, but not all, enzymes are soluble in water. The high dielectric constant of water promotes ionization of organic, and especially inorganic, solutes, thus facilitating the initiation and velocity of metabolic reactions. Water enters into many metabolic reactions (hydrolyses) and is produced in many others.... The low thermal conductivity of water and its high specific heat narrow the amplitude of variation in body temperature induced by warming or cooling of its environment.... The high heat of vaporization of water accounts in part for the high proportion of the body heat dissipated in the production of water vapor on the external surfaces of the body.

H.H. Mitchell (1962)

Water is required in greater quantity than any other orally ingested substance. Sources of water include drinking water, water occurring in feedstuffs and metabolic water arising from nutrient metabolism. Examples of **metabolic water** include that produced when lipids, carbohydrates and amino acids are catabolized to carbon dioxide and water. In some desert animals, metabolic water may make up the major or sole source of water. The **kangaroo rat**, for example, never drinks (Schmidt-Nielsen, 1964). It has a very low rate of water loss, achieved by having no sweat glands, excreting a highly concentrated urine, and having a low evaporation rate from the expired air because of a countercurrent cooling mechanism in the nasal passages. Kangaroo rats eat a diet of dry seeds and plant material, with very little green or succulent matter, although more recently, Tracy and Walsberg (2002) reported that insects and succulent vegetation do constitute a part of the diet of the kangaroo rat and may make a significant contribution to their water economy. In contrast, another desert rodent, the **pack rat**, has a very high water requirement, which it meets by consuming succulent vegetation such as cactus. The behavioural and physiological adaptations of desert animals to a dry environment have been discussed in detail by Schmidt-Nielsen (1964).

Marine mammals (e.g. sea lions, seals, walrus, whales) and most marine fish never drink, but obtain their water from their food. Diets for most **marine mammals** in zoos (e.g. seals, sea lions, porpoises) are based on fish. Frozen fish should be thawed in a refrigerator rather than air thawed. Air thawing may result in a loss of 10–15% of the moisture.

One of the factors influencing species differences in water requirements is the nature of the nitrogenous end products of protein metabolism excreted in the urine. Most mammals excrete urea, which is toxic to the tissues unless in dilute solution. Thus large amounts of water are required to dilute it. Birds have a lower water requirement than mammals because they excrete uric acid in a nearly solid form. Fish excrete ammonia directly from the gills, and many have such low water requirements that they never drink. With mammals, high protein diets increase the amount of water required for dilution of urinary urea. The nature of the digestive tract and feeding strategy also influence water requirements. Ruminants require large quantities of water to form a suspension of ingesta in the rumen and, therefore, have higher water requirements than non-ruminant species. Feedstuffs with high water-absorbing characteristics, such as wheat bran and dried forage (e.g. lucerne hay), increase the water requirements. Average water requirement figures for livestock are given in Table 20.1. Water requirements are increased in cold weather because feed intake is increased. Mature beef cattle and sheep can rely solely on snow as a water source, but more productive animals, such as feedlot cattle and dairy animals, must have free access to drinking water (Degen and Young, 1990).

Table 20.1. Expected water consumption of various classes of adult livestock in a temperate climate (adapted from National Research Council, 1974).

Species	Water (l/day)
Beef cattle	26–66
Dairy cattle	38–110
Horses	30–45
Pigs	11–19
Sheep and goats	4–15
Chickens	0.2–0.4
Turkeys	0.4–0.6

Toxins in Water

The concentration of minerals in water is normally not of sufficient magnitude to be nutritionally significant. More commonly, water can be a source of mineral toxicity. Highly **saline water** may contain sufficient calcium, magnesium, sodium, bicarbonate, chloride and sulfate ions to exert toxic effects. Sulfates are more injurious than chlorides; hydroxides are more harmful than carbonates, which are more harmful than bicarbonates. The National

Research Council (1974) recommendations concerning saline water are given in Table 20.2.

One of the most common toxic substances in water is the **nitrate** ion. Contamination of water sources with nitrate is common in areas with a high concentration of animals (e.g. feedlots), with heavy fertilization of fields with manure or nitrogenous fertilizers, or with contamination from septic tanks. Concentrations of 200 ppm nitrate in water are potentially hazardous; concentrations above 1500 ppm may cause acute toxicity. Nitrate is converted to nitrite ion in the rumen; nitrite combines with the haemoglobin molecule to prevent it from transporting oxygen. Death is thus from anoxia. The blood of affected animals is chocolate in colour due to the colour of **methaemoglobin**, formed when nitrite reacts with haemoglobin.

Iron salts in groundwater sometimes cause problems with water quality. Iron in oxygen-free ground water is normally in the soluble, reduced state (Fe^{2+}). When exposed to oxygen or chlorine, it is oxidized to the reddish, less soluble Fe^{3+} form (rust), which produces iron deposits in pipes, tanks and fixtures. Wells may become contaminated with

Table 20.2. A guide to the use of saline waters for livestock and poultry (adapted from National Research Council, 1974).

Total soluble salts content of waters (mg/l)	Comment
Less than 1,000	These waters have a relatively low level of salinity and should present no serious burden to any class of livestock or poultry
1,000–2,999	These waters should be satisfactory for all classes of livestock and poultry. They may cause temporary and mild diarrhoea in livestock not accustomed to them or watery droppings in poultry (especially at the higher levels) but should not affect their health or performance
3,000–4,999	These waters should be satisfactory for livestock, although they might very possibly cause temporary diarrhoea or be refused at first by animals not accustomed to them. They are poor waters for poultry, often causing watery faeces and (at the higher levels of salinity) increased mortality and decreased growth, especially in turkeys
5,000–6,999	These waters can be used with reasonable safety for dairy and beef cattle, sheep, pigs and horses. It may be well to avoid the use of those approaching the higher levels for pregnant or lactating animals. They are not acceptable waters for poultry, almost always causing some type of problem, especially near the upper limit, where reduced growth and production, or increased mortality, will probably occur
7,000–10,000	These waters are unfit for poultry and probably for pigs. Considerable risk may exist in using them for pregnant or lactating cows, horses, sheep, the young of these species or for any animals subjected to heavy heat stress or water loss. In general, their use should be avoided, although older ruminants, horses, and even poultry and pigs may subsist on them for long periods of time under conditions of low stress
More than 10,000	The risks with these highly saline waters are so great that they cannot be recommended for use under any conditions

iron-utilizing bacteria; these cause foul odours and plug water lines. Treatment of the water system and well with bleach may control bacteria.

Pesticides and other agricultural chemicals may enter water supplies from agricultural runoff, accidental spills or faulty waste-disposal systems. The organophosphates, such as malathion, are the most toxic. Insecticides of plant origin, such as pyrethrins and rotenones, are not considered a hazard.

Lakes and stock-watering ponds may have a heavy 'bloom' of toxic **blue-green algae** (cyanobacteria). Many species of algae produce extremely potent toxins (Beasley *et al.*, 1989). Signs of blue-green algae toxicosis in pigs include vomiting, frothing at the mouth, coughing, muscle tremors, rapid breathing and bloody diarrhoea (Chengappa *et al.*, 1989). Severe liver damage occurs. In dairy cattle, clinical signs include anorexia, reluctance to move, dementia and ruminal atony. Serum enzymes characteristic of liver damage are elevated (Galey *et al.*, 1987) and death is due to massive liver damage.

Blue-green algae in farm ponds can be controlled by dragging a porous bag containing copper sulfate through the pond. However, this sometimes leads to proliferation of copper-tolerant green algae. Though these algae are normally controlled by zooplankton, which feed on them, high concentrations of copper kill the zooplankton, allowing the green algae to proliferate. The green algae are not usually toxic, but they can cause severe water quality problems, leading to turbid, odiferous, bad-tasting water.

Water quality can influence development of **polioencephalomalacia** (**PEM**) in feedlot cattle. PEM, also known as cerebrocortical necrosis, is a non-infectious disease of ruminants (*polio*: Greek for grey; *encephalo*: Greek for brain; *malacia*: Greek for softness; thus softening of the grey matter of the brain). Clinical signs of the disorder include aimless wandering, disorientation, blindness, recumbancy and opisthotonus (stargazing posture). The brain is oedematous, with yellowish discoloration of the cerebral cortex. Affected animals often respond dramatically to administration of thiamin. Water high in sulfates promotes PEM, apparently via a complex interaction involving copper, sulfur and thiamin. Gooteratne *et al.* (1989) and Cummings *et al.* (1995) reviewed these interrelationships. When water is a major source of dietary sulfate, risk of PEM may increase in hot weather because of increased water consumption (McAllister *et al.*, 1997).

Water Economy of Desert Herbivores

Humans and livestock are potentially competitive for several types of resources, including land, cereal grains and water. In arid regions, including much of the western USA, rapidly expanding human populations are creating an ever-increasing demand on water resources. The use of large amounts of water for livestock, and especially cattle, is of concern (Tamminga, 1996; Van Horn *et al.*, 1996). Besides the water actually used by animals, the amount of water excreted is also important as a potential source of groundwater contamination. Cattle, in fact, are poor utilizers of water and in semi-arid regions, other kinds of animals might be better choices. Maloiy *et al.* (1979) classified large herbivores into three main physiological ecotypes:

1. Wet tropical and wet temperate. Herbivores with high rates of water and energy use and poor urine concentrating ability, for example, buffalo, cattle, pig, eland, waterbuck, elephant, horse, moose and reindeer.
2. Warm, dry savannah, semi-arid. Herbivores with intermediate rates of water and energy use and good renal concentrating ability, for example, sheep, wildebeest and donkey.
3. Arid zone animals with low rates of energy and water turnover and medium to high urine-concentrating ability, for example, camel (Fig. 20.1), goat, oryx, gazelle and ostrich.

Thus cattle are relatively unadapted to semi-arid conditions. Zebu breeds are only slightly superior to European breeds in water utilization. Sheep are considerably more efficient in water utilization than cattle and, under temperate conditions, can often meet their water needs from forage alone. Cattle, however, virtually always require access to drinking water. Adaptations of sheep include a good urine-concentrating ability, the excretion of relatively dry faecal pellets, and the insulatory properties of the fleece, reducing the need for evaporative cooling (Silanikove, 1992). Of the common domestic ruminants, goats are clearly the best adapted to arid conditions, especially the **Bedouin goat**, raised by Bedouin nomads on the deserts of the Middle Eastern countries. These animals can lose as much as 40% of their body weight through dehydration and still continue to feed normally (Silanikove, 1992, 1994). When provided access to water, they can replenish this loss within 2 min (Fig. 20.2). In these goats, the rumen acts as an osmotic barrier,

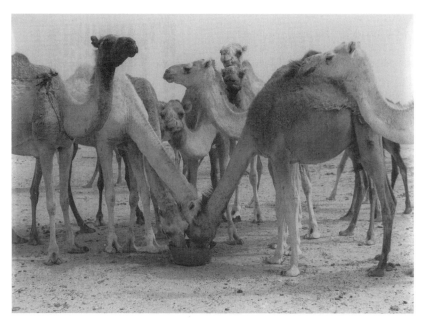

Fig. 20.1. Livestock differ greatly in their efficiency of water utilization. Animals adapted to arid conditions have various mechanisms to conserve body water and survive dehydration. Camels have lower water requirements than other domestic animals.

preventing osmotic shock to the tissues after rapid rehydration (Shkolnik *et al.*, 1980; Louw, 1984). Because the Bedouin goats need drink only once every 2–4 days, they can utilize forage resources

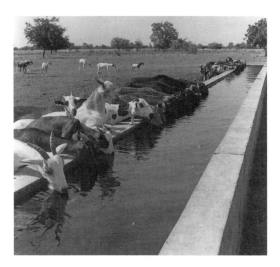

Fig. 20.2. Desert goats need drink only once every 2–4 days. Thus they can use forage resources that are far removed from water supplies more effectively than most other domestic animals.

that are far removed from water. In cattle rehydrated after water deprivation, about 20% of ingested water bypasses the rumen to the intestine (Cafe and Poppi, 1994). Other herbivores well adapted to desert conditions include the oryx, gazelle (e.g. springbok), ostrich and camel. In terms of conversion of the meagre desert forage into meat or milk, the oryx and goat seem to have the most potential (Louw, 1984).

Animals adapted to arid conditions have physiological adaptations to minimize water loss. Besides urinary excretion, as already discussed, there is also the potential for large faecal water losses. Clauss *et al.* (2004) measured the faecal dry matter content of 81 species of captive ruminants with a variety of feeding strategies: frugivores (n = 5), browsers (n = 16), intermediate feeders (n = 35) and grazers (n = 25). There were no clear-cut differences in faecal dry matter contents among the various feeding types, although grazing ruminants produced both the driest and the wettest faeces. Unfortunately, domestic ruminants were not included. The lowest dry matter contents were for species resembling cattle in their rumen anatomy – wild cattle (banteng, gaur, bison and buffalo). Clauss *et al.* (2004) attribute these differences to the length of the colon descendens (distal colon), where most water absorption occurs. Thus desert animals have elongated colons. For example, the **oryx** has an especially long colon (Hofmann, 1989). Clauss *et al.* (2003) speculate that the competition for space within the abdominal cavity in grazers led to the evolutionary decrease in the capacity of the hindgut, and the consequent higher faecal water losses in large grazing ruminants poses an intrinsic body size limitation.

The rumen plays an important role in the adaptation of ruminants to arid environments. The digestive tract can constitute as much as 25% of a ruminant animal's body weight (Silanikove, 1994). The rumen functions as a reservoir of stored water which is used during dehydration, and also accommodates a large volume of water upon rehydration. Desert goats are the most efficient ruminants with regard to their ability to withstand dehydration, and can lose as much as 40% of their body weight during dehydration. Camels can also undergo long periods (up to 15 days) of water deprivation, by utilizing gut stores of water. Desert ruminants are characterized by the ability to regain water equilibrium by rapidly drinking an amount equal to the water lost during dehydration. Rapid rehydration in many species causes **water toxicity**, characterized

by hypo-osmotic effects in the blood, with consequent red blood cell haemolysis. In desert ruminants, a high rate of sodium secretion into the rumen via saliva serves to buffer the water of rehydration, preventing water toxicity (Silanikove, 1994).

In non-ruminant herbivores such as the horse, the hindgut plays a role in water homeostasis analogous to the role of the rumen in ruminants (Sneddon and Argenzio, 1998). In horses, the hindgut constitutes 75% of total gut volume. The greatest volume by far is in the proximal (ascending) colon. According to Sneddon and Argenzio (1998), 'Donkeys appear to be in a league of their own in that both dry matter intake per unit body mass and digestive efficiency on high fibre diets are superior to that of other equids, under dry grazing conditions.'

The **oryx** (*Oryx gazelle*) (Fig. 20.3a) is a grazing ruminant native to East Africa that is adapted to extremely arid conditions without surface water. Efforts to domesticate the oryx are in progress (Stanley-Price, 1985a, b). Oryx can be quickly tamed and moved as a closely packed herd and are highly adapted to desert conditions. The oryx has an extremely low rate of evaporative water loss (Stanley-Price, 1985a) and a low metabolic rate. It ruminates at night when the heat of fermentation is

(a)

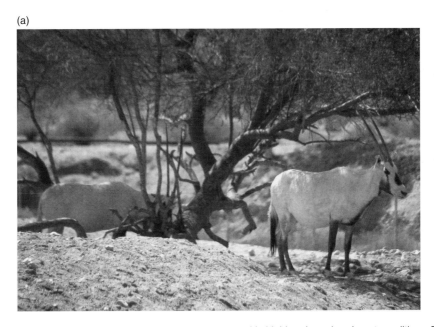

Fig. 20.3. (a) The oryx has extremely low water requirements and is highly adapted to desert conditions. Efforts to domesticate the oryx are in progress.

Continued

(b)

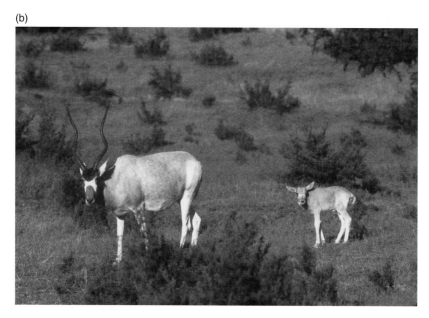

Fig. 20.3. Continued. (b) The addax, like the oryx, is well adapted to arid environments (photographs courtesy of E. Spevak, St Louis Zoo, Missouri, USA).

least burdensome and this eliminates the need for increased thermogenesis at night, when temperatures are often quite cold in the desert. Another grazer, the addax (*Addax nasomaculatus*) (Fig. 20.3b), is native to the Sahara Desert, has a low water turnover and a capacious water-storing rumen (Hummel *et al.*, 2008).

Thus the efficiency of conversion of forage and water to useful products in many arid and semi-arid regions of the world might be enhanced by utilizing animals with superior biochemical and behavioural adaptations to an arid environment. These animals might not be the traditional domesticated ruminants but perhaps newly domesticated species like the oryx.

Questions and Study Guide

1. What is metabolic water?
2. The kangaroo rat and the pack rat are desert rodents. Compare their strategies for coping in an environment that lacks drinking water.
3. How do seals and whales meet their water needs?
4. Why does dietary protein concentration affect water requirements of many animals?
5. Why do cattle excrete 'cow pies' whereas most desert ruminants excrete pelleted faeces?
6. What are some adaptations of oryx to desert conditions?

References

Beasley, V.R., Cook, W.O., Dahlem, A.M., Hoover, S.B., Lovell, R.A. and Valentine, W.M. (1989) Algae intoxication in livestock and waterfowl. *Veterinary Clinics of North America: Food Animal Practice* 5, 345–361.

Cafe, L.M. and Poppi, D.P. (1994) The fate and behavior of imbibed water in the rumen of cattle. *Journal of Agricultural Science* 122, 139–144.

Chengappa, M.M., Pace, L.W. and McLaughlin, B.G. (1989) Blue-green algae (*Anabaena spiroides*) toxicosis in pigs. *Journal of the American Veterinary Medical Association* 194, 1724–1725.

Clauss, M., Frey, R., Kiefer, B., Lechner-Doll, M., Lochlein, W., Polster, C., Rossner, G.E. and Streich, W.J. (2003) The maximum attainable body size of herbivorous mammals: morphophysiological constraints on foregut, and adaptations of hindgut fermenters. *Oecologia* 136, 14–27.

Clauss, M., Lechner-Doll, M. and Streich, W.J. (2004) Differences in the range of faecal dry matter content between feeding types of captive wild ruminants. *Acta Theriologica* 49, 259–267.

Cummings, B.A., Gould, D.H., Caldwell, D.R. and Hamas, D.W. (1995) Ruminal microbial alterations associated with sulfide generation in steers with dietary sulfate-induced polioencephalomalacia. *American Journal of Veterinary Research* 56, 1390–1395.

Degen, A.A. and Young, B.A. (1990) The performance of pregnant cows relying on snow as a water source. *Canadian Journal of Animal Science* 70, 507–515.

Galey, F.D., Beasley, V.R., Carmichael, W.W., Kleppe, G., Hooser, S.B. and Haschek, W.M. (1987) Blue-green algae (*Microcystis aeruginosa*) hepatotoxicosis in dairy cows. *American Journal of Veterinary Research* 48, 1415–1420.

Gooteratne, S.R., Buckley, W.T. and Christensen, D.A. (1989) Review of copper deficiency and metabolism in ruminants. *Canadian Journal of Animal Science* 69, 819–845.

Hofmann, R.R. (1989) Evolutionary steps of ecophysiological adaptation and diversification of ruminants: a comparative view of their digestive system. *Oecologia* 78, 443–457.

Hummel, J., Steuer, P., Sudekum, K.-H., Hammer, S., Hammer, C., Streich, W.J. and Clauss, M. (2008) Fluid and particle retention in the digestive tract of the addax antelope (*Addax nasomaculatus*) – adaptations of a grazing desert ruminant. *Comparative Biochemistry and Physiology* 149, 142–149.

Louw, G.N. (1984) Water deprivation in herbivores under arid conditions. In: Gilchrist, F.M.C. and Mackie, R.I. (eds) *Herbivore Nutrition in the Subtropics and Tropics*. The Science Press, Craighall, Republic of South Africa, pp. 106–126.

Maloiy, G.M.O., Macfarlane, W.V. and Shkolnik, A. (1979) Mammalian herbivores. In: Maloiy, G.M.O. (ed.) *Comparative Physiology of Osmoregulation in Animals*, Vol. 11. Academic Press, London, pp. 185–209.

McAllister, M.M., Gould, D.H., Raisbeck, M.F., Cummings, B.A. and Loneragan, G.H. (1997) Evaluation of ruminal sulfide concentrations and seasonal outbreaks of polioencephalomalacia in beef cattle in a feedlot.

Journal of the American Veterinary Medical Association 211, 1275–1279.

Mitchell, H.H. (1962) *Comparative Nutrition of Man and Domestic Animals*. Academic Press, New York.

National Research Council (1974) *Nutrients and Toxic Substances in Water for Livestock and Poultry*. National Academy Press, Washington, DC.

Schmidt-Nielsen, K. (1964) *Desert Animals. Physiological Problems of Heat and Water*. Oxford University Press, London.

Shkolnik, A., Maltz, E. and Choshniak, I. (1980) The role of the ruminant's digestive tract as a water reservoir. In: Ruckebusch, Y. and Thivend, P. (eds) *Digestive Physiology and Metabolism in Ruminants*. AVI Publishing Co., Westport, Connecticut, pp. 731–742.

Silanikove, N. (1992) Effects of water scarcity and hot environment on appetite and digestion in ruminants: a review. *Livestock Production Science* 30, 175–194.

Silanikove, N. (1994) The struggle to maintain hydration and osmoregulation in animals experiencing severe dehydration and rapid rehydration: the story of ruminants. *Experimental Physiology* 79, 281–300.

Sneddon, J.C. and Argenzio, R.A. (1998) Feeding strategy and water homeostasis in equids: the role of the hind gut. *Journal of Arid Environments* 38, 493–509.

Stanley-Price, M.R. (1985a) Game domestication for animal production in Kenya: feeding trials with oryx, zebu cattle and sheep under controlled conditions. *Journal of Agricultural Science* 104, 367–374.

Stanley-Price, M.R. (1985b) Game domestication for animal production in Kenya: the nutritional ecology of oryx, zebu cattle and sheep under free-range conditions. *Journal of Agricultural Science* 104, 375–382.

Tamminga, S. (1996) A review on environmental impacts of nutritional strategies in ruminants. *Journal of Animal Science* 74, 3112–3124.

Tracy, R.L. and Walsberg, G.E. (2002) Kangaroo rats revisited: re-evaluating a classic case of desert survival. *Oecologia* 133, 449–457.

Van Horn, H.H., Newton, G.L. and Kunkle, W.E. (1996) Ruminant nutrition from an environmental perspective: factors affecting whole-farm nutrient balance. *Journal of Animal Science* 74, 3082–3102.

21 Blood, Electrolytes, Fluid Balance and Diet-induced Anaemias

A number of nutrients function in regulating blood composition and fluid balance. These include protein (for synthesis of blood proteins), electrolytes (sodium, potassium, chlorine), iron, copper, folic acid and vitamin B_{12} (for formation of haemoglobin) and vitamin K (for blood clotting). The specific roles of these nutrients will be discussed.

Blood Proteins

The proteins of blood plasma can be separated into three main groups: (i) fibrinogen; (ii) albumin; and (iii) globulins. Most plasma proteins are synthesized by the liver. Most are glycoproteins, with either N- or O-linked oligosaccharide chains. An exception is albumin, which contains no carbohydrate.

Albumin is the major protein in plasma, constituting about 60% of the total plasma protein. In humans, the liver produces about 12 g of albumin/day, representing about 25% of total hepatic protein synthesis. In liver disease, the synthesis of albumin decreases markedly, with a decrease in the albumin:globulin ratio. Accompanying **liver disease** (or protein malnutrition) is **oedema** (accumulation of fluid in the tissues) and **ascites** (accumulation of fluid in the abdominal cavity). Albumin is responsible for most of the osmotic pressure of plasma. Reduced serum albumin in liver disease accounts for the oedema and ascites, caused by a disturbance in the **osmotic balance** between plasma and the tissue fluids. Albumin is a solute (dissolved substance) that, along with amino acids, sugars and minerals contributes to osmotic pressure of body fluids. Another role of albumin is the transport of copper in the blood (see section on 'Copper' in this chapter). Albumin also transports long-chain fatty acids.

In inflammatory conditions, the concentrations of **acute phase proteins**, such as C-reactive protein, increase in the plasma. These proteins play a role in the body's response to inflammation. **Nuclear factor kappa-B** (**NFκB**) is a transcription factor involved in the stimulation of the synthesis of acute phase proteins. NFκB binds to a number of gene promoters in the nucleus and activates transcription of genes involved in the inflammatory response.

Blood Clotting and Vitamin K

A number of plasma proteins are involved in **blood clotting**. These include fibrinogen, prothrombin and a number of factors from Factor 1 (fibrinogen) to Factor XIII (fibrin-stabilizing factor). Blood clotting initially involves the formation of a loose and temporary platelet aggregation at the site of injury. Platelet activation involves a change in shape of the platelets, facilitating aggregation. Platelet aggregation initiates release of factors (**thromboplastin**) which start a cascade of events leading to formation of a clot. Thromboplastin activates **prothrombin** to an enzyme, thrombin. This activation involves the action of vitamin K and calcium binding, described below. **Thrombin** acts as an enzyme to split one or more peptides from fibrinogen, altering its solubility and causing it to precipitate as a clot (Fig. 21.1).

Prothrombin is activated by the addition of a carboxyl group to glutamic acid residues in the molecule. The added carboxyl group provides a calcium-binding site for ionic bonding of a calcium ion between two carboxyl groups (Fig. 21.2). The addition of calcium activates prothrombin to the active enzyme thrombin. The carboxylase reaction for the addition of the carboxyl group to glutamic acid residues in prothrombin is **vitamin K-dependent**. The hydroquinone (reduced) form of vitamin K is required, and an epoxide-containing quinone is produced in the reaction. This is regenerated to the hydroquinone form by the vitamin K cycle in the liver (Fig. 21.3). **Dicumarol**, contained in mouldy sweet clover hay, is an inhibitor of

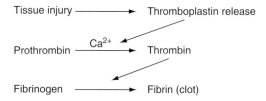

Fig. 21.1. The events involved in blood clotting. Vitamin K is involved in the conversion of prothrombin to thrombin.

2,3-expoxide reductase, which converts the epoxide to the quinone. **Sweet clover poisoning** causes bleeding and haemorrhage. **Warfarin** has the same effect and is used as a rodenticide for this reason. The structures of compounds with vitamin K activity are shown in Fig. 21.4.

Haemoglobin Formation: Iron, Copper, Folic Acid, Vitamin B$_{12}$

Iron

Iron is a constitutent of several metalloenzymes, including the respiratory pigments such as haemoglobin, cytochromes and myoglobin, and various enzymes such as peroxidase and catalase. Quantitatively, the major metabolic requirement for iron is synthesis of haemoglobin and other respiratory pigments. Thus the classic sign of iron deficiency is microcytic, hypochromic **anaemia,** characterized by smaller than normal erythrocytes.

Haemoglobin is a complex protein consisting of a haem group (porphyrin) containing ferrous (Fe^{2+}) iron and a protein (globin). The protein portion consists of four peptide chains coiled in a helix, with haem in a cavity within the helix structure. The unique function of haemoglobin is its ability to maintain iron in the ferrous state, with the ability to form a stable complex with oxygen.

Iron absorption is regulated according to need, by control at the level of the intestinal mucosa. Dietary iron occurs either as ionic iron (ferric and ferrous iron) or as a component of haem. **Non-haem iron** is absorbed primarily in the ferrous (Fe^{2+}) state. Ferric iron is reduced (addition of an electron) to ferrous iron in the intestine. Reducing agents such as ascorbic acid increase iron absorption by reducing ferric iron. Iron in meat (**haem iron**) is absorbed more efficiently than non-haem (ionic) iron, because the iron in haem is in the ferrous state. In the enterocyte haem is split into ferrous iron and bilirubin by haem oxygenase. The consumption of meat or other animal tissue enhances the absorption of non-haem iron. There is evidence that low-molecular-weight carbohydrates in muscle tissue are responsible for increasing the uptake of non-haem iron from meat (Huh *et al.*, 2004). Polymers of fructose, such as inulin and fructooligosaccharides (FOS), are fermented in the hindgut, producing short chain VFAs. These apparently increase iron solubility in the colon. In a study with young pigs, Yasuda *et al.* (2006) found that dietary inulin significantly increased iron absorption from maize-soy diets.

Inhibitors of iron absorption include phytates and polyphenols (tannins). The effects of tannins on iron status are discussed in Chapter 13, and may account for anaemia in browsers such as the black rhinoceros. Trimethylamine oxide (TMAO) and formaldehyde in fish also impair iron absorption (see Chapter 19).

Iron is absorbed at the level of duodenum enterocytes. Incoming iron in the Fe^{3+} state is reduced by ferrireductase present on the enterocyte surface.

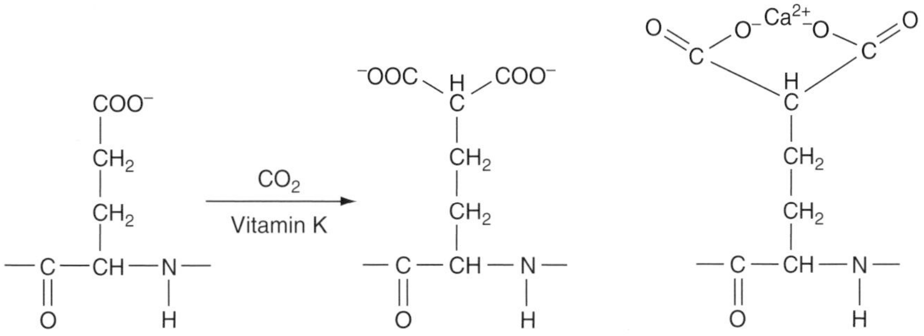

Fig. 21.2. Vitamin K functions in the addition of carboxyl groups to prothrombin to create calcium-binding sites.

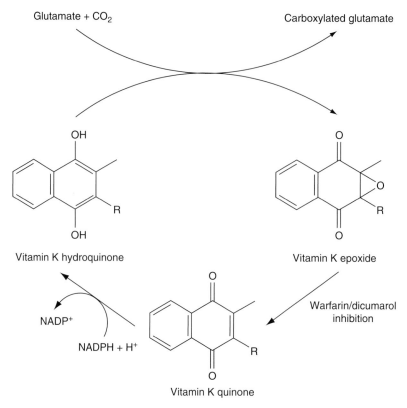

Glutamate + CO$_2$ Carboxylated glutamate

Vitamin K hydroquinone

Vitamin K epoxide

NADP$^+$

NADPH + H$^+$

Warfarin/dicumarol inhibition

Vitamin K quinone

Fig. 21.3. Dicumarol and warfarin create a vitamin K deficiency by inhibiting the vitamin K cycle for the regeneration of the metabolically active form of vitamin K.

Once inside the enterocyte, iron can be stored as **ferritin** (an iron-containing protein) or transferred across the basolateral membrane into the plasma. Iron transported across the basolateral membrane (absorbed iron) binds to **transferrin**, the plasma protein which transports iron in the blood. Regulation of iron absorption occurs at the level of the enterocyte, where further iron absorption is blocked (mucosal block) by the action of a plasma peptide called **hepcidin**.

Red blood cells (rbc) are continuously being replaced by newly synthesized rbc, with old rbc being processed in the reticuloendothelial system (liver, spleen, bone marrow). When haemoglobin is degraded, globin is converted to its constituent amino acids. The porphyrin portion of the molecule is also degraded. The iron enters the body's iron pool, and the iron-free porphyrin is converted to biliverdin and bilirubin. These are excreted in the bile as bile pigments. Excess iron is stored in the liver, bone marrow and spleen, either as ferritin or **haemosiderin**, another iron-containing protein.

Copper

Studies in the early days of nutrition research demonstrated that feeding rats a diet consisting only of milk produced anaemia, and that in addition to iron, copper was required to cure the anaemia. This established the existence of a role of copper in haemoglobin formation. The mode of action appears to be that a copper-containing blood protein, **ceruloplasmin** (also known as ferroxidase), functions in the oxidation of ferrous (Fe^{2+}) to ferric (Fe^{3+}) iron in transferrin. This is necessary for the mobilization of stored iron.

Like iron, copper is absorbed according to need. **Metallothionein**, a cysteine-rich protein in the enterocytes, is involved in copper absorption. About 90% of the copper in plasma is associated with ceruloplasmin and the remainder with albumin. Ceruloplasmin binds copper tightly, so the albumin-bound copper is more available to tissues.

In ruminants, there is an important interaction between copper, molybdenum and inorganic sulfate.

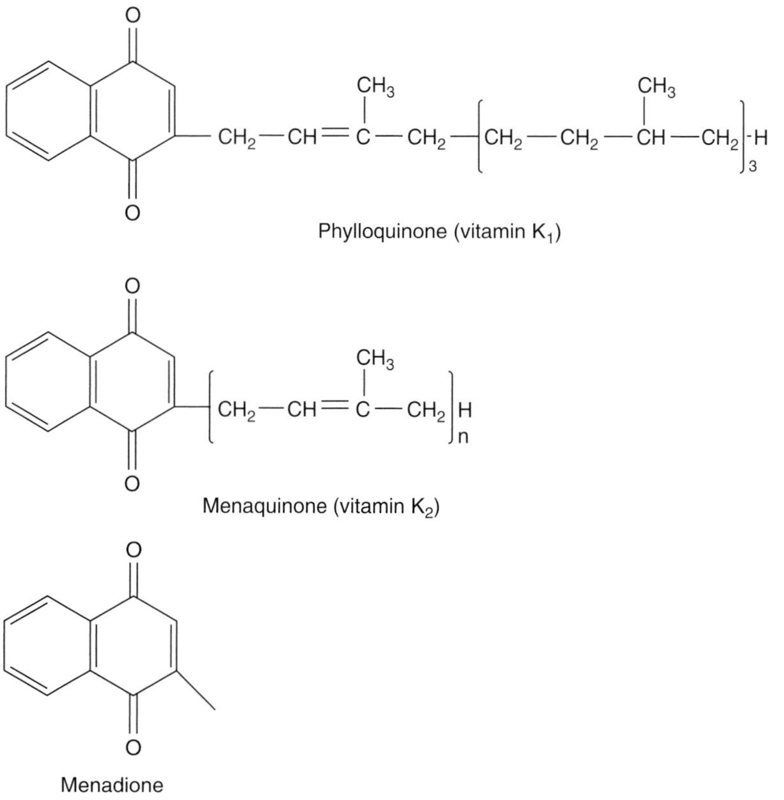

Phylloquinone (vitamin K₁)

Menaquinone (vitamin K₂)

Menadione

Fig. 21.4. Structures of compounds with vitamin K activity.

High dietary **molybdenum** intensifies copper deficiency or may induce a copper deficiency even though forage copper concentrations may be normal. The mechanism of action is that sulfide produced from sulfates or sulfur amino acids in the rumen reacts with molybdate ions to produce **thiomolybdates**, including trithiomolybdates ($MoSO_3^{2-}$) and tetrathiomolybdates ($MoSO_4^{2-}$) (Price *et al.*, 1987). The thiomolybdates react with copper ions to form products in which the copper is physiologically unavailable. The interactions between copper, molybdenum and sulfur in ruminant nutrition have been reviewed in depth by Suttle (1991).

Besides anaemia, other signs of copper deficiency include hair depigmentation (Chapter 19), skeletal deformity, aortic rupture, ataxia, infertility and severe diarrhoea. **Aortic rupture and skeletal deformity** are a reflection of the role of copper in the synthesis of collagen and other connective tissues. Copper is an activator of **lysyloxidase**, an enzyme involved in the cross-linking of collagen and elastin

fibres. **Ataxia** in copper-deficient animals is caused by a deficiency of cytochrome oxidase activity in the motor neurons of the central nervous system. Copper is a constituent of cytochromes. **Infertility** due to copper deficiency is a result of impaired ovarian steroid hormone synthesis (Kendall *et al.*, 2006). In cattle, severe **diarrhoea** may occur in copper deficiency. This is a malabsorption syndrome, caused by atrophy of villi and diminished cytochrome oxidase activity in mucosal cells.

Folic Acid and Vitamin B₁₂

The B-complex vitamins folic acid (folacin, folate) and vitamin B_{12} (cyanocobalamin) have interrelated functions in preventing anaemia.

Folacin consists of a pteridine bicyclic ring, p-aminobenzoic acid and one or more glutamic acid residues (Fig. 21.5). The active form of folic acid is **tetrahydrofolate** (THF). Dietary folates may have several glutamic acid groups, which are

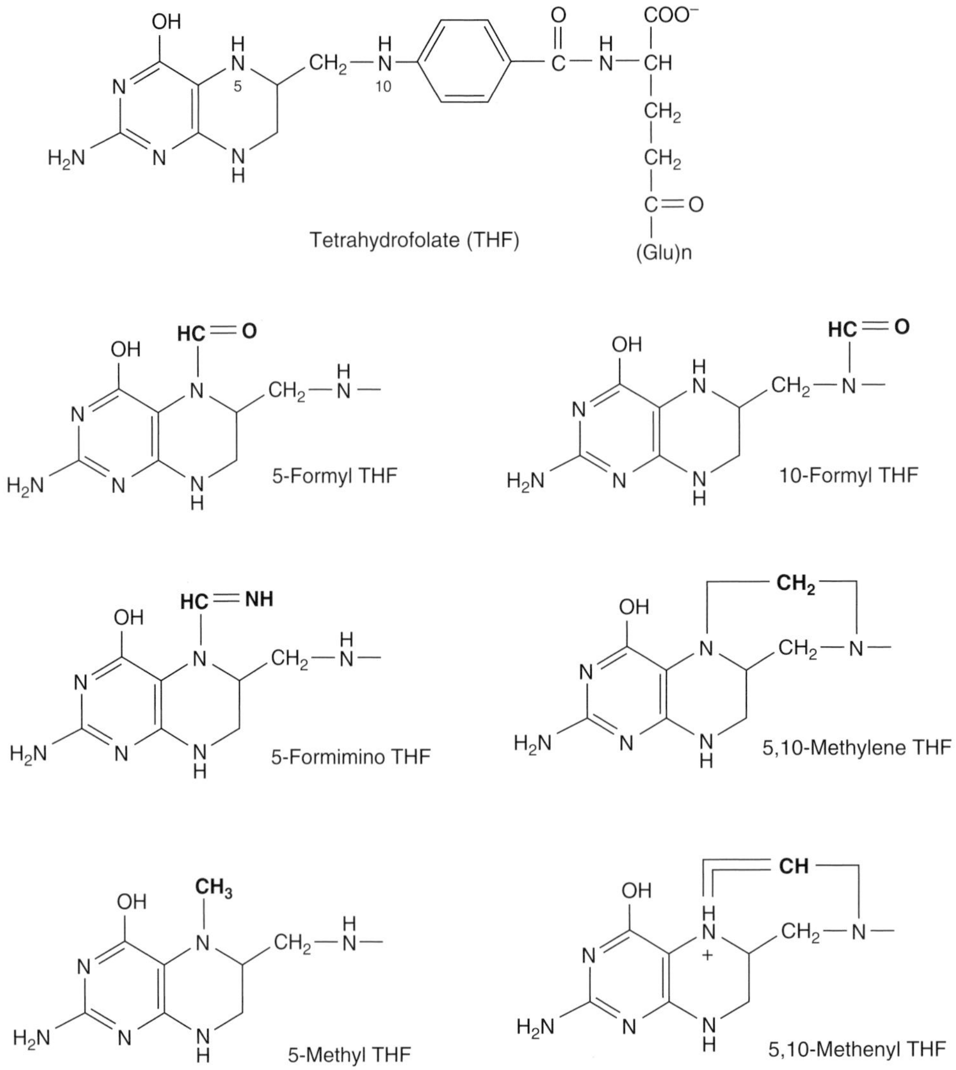

Fig. 21.5. Tetrahydrofolic acid and the one-carbon substituted folates.

cleaved off in the intestine by a γ-glutamate carboxy peptidase in the brush border.

THF is a carrier of one-carbon (1-C) fragments, attached to N-5, N-10 or the N-5, N-10 bridge (Fig. 21.5). Folate-requiring reactions include amino acid metabolism, purine and pyrimidine synthesis (Fig. 21.6) and the formation of the primary methylating agent, S-adenosyl methionine (SAM) (Fig. 21.7). When acting as a **methyl donor,** SAM forms homocysteine, which can be remethylated by 5-methyl THF, catalysed by methionine synthase to form methionine (Fig. 21.8). Methionine synthase is a vitamin B_{12}-containing enzyme. Impairment of methionine synthase in vitamin B_{12} deficiency causes the accumulation of 5-methyl THF, inducing a deficiency of folate. Deficiency of either folate or vitamin B_{12} affects rapidly dividing cells because they have a large requirement for thymidine for DNA synthesis. Thymidine synthesis requires a one-carbon fragment in association with THF. This affects the synthesis of rbc in bone marrow, causing the rbc to remain in an immature state. Immature rbc are large (macrocytic) and contain organelles such as nuclei that are not found in

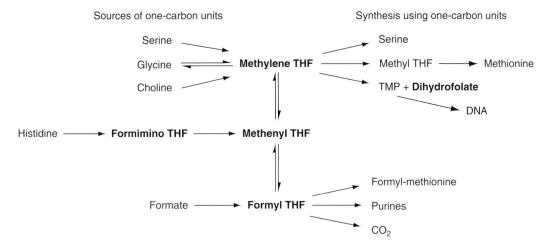

Fig. 21.6. Sources and utilization of one-carbon-substituted folates.

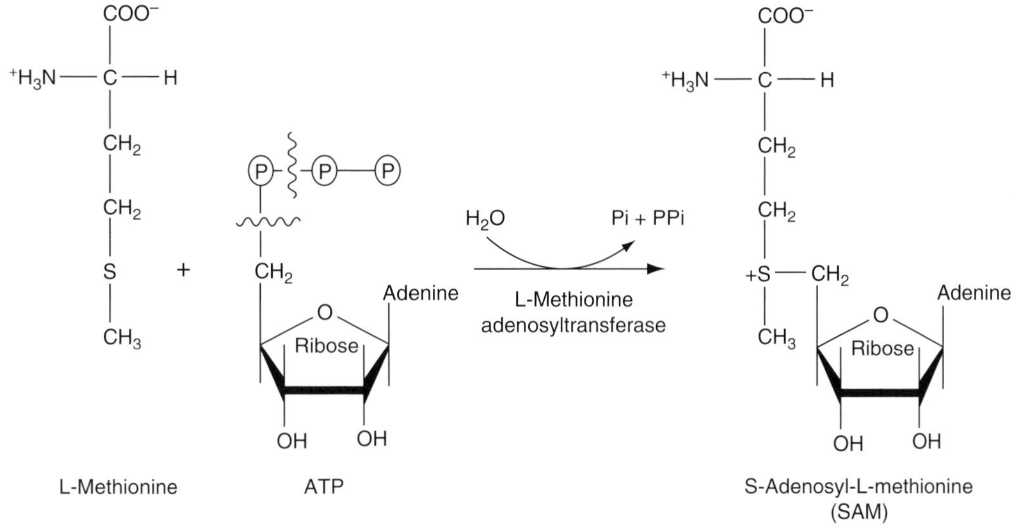

Fig. 21.7. S-adenosyl methionine (SAM) is the metabolically active form of methionine (active methionine) involved in methylation reactions.

mature erythrocytes. Thus either folate or vitamin B_{12} deficiency results in **macrocytic (megaloblastic) anaemia**.

Vitamin B_{12} (cobalamin) is a complex molecule containing a cobalt ion (see Fig. 9.8 in Chapter 9). Vitamin B_{12} is synthesized exclusively by microbes, so is found only in foods of animal origin (arising from microbial synthesis in the gut). Vitamin B_{12} is absorbed bound to a small glycoprotein secreted by the gastric mucosa, called the **intrinsic factor**.

In individuals lacking secretion of the intrinsic factor, **pernicious anaemia** (macrocytic anaemia) occurs.

Fumonisins are mycotoxins produced by a common fungal contaminant of maize, *Fusarium verticilliodes*. Fumonisins inhibit an enzyme, ceramide synthase, involved in the acylation of sphinganine, reducing the formation of sphingomyelin, a sphingolipid involved in formation of neural tissue and some membrane proteins, including the folic-acid-binding transporter (Marasas *et al.*, 2004).

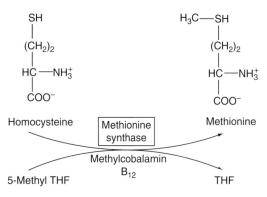

Fig. 21.8. The folate trap. A deficiency of vitamin B_{12} causes the accumulation of 5-methyl THF, inducing a deficiency of folate.

Fumonisins cause embryonic neural tube and craniofacial defects that are prevented by supplementary folic acid. High incidences of **neural tube defects** occur in some regions of the world (Guatemala, South Africa, China, South Texas) where substantial intake of fumonisins in contaminated maize has been documented (Marasas *et al.*, 2004). In Texas, for example, there is a significant association between neural tube defects and tortilla consumption.

Chronic **arsenic poisoning** affects as many as 100 million people in India, Bangladesh, Vietnam, Cambodia and Nepal, because of high arsenic concentrations in well water. Excretion of arsenic involves folate-dependent methylation of inorganic arsenic to methylated arsenic acids. Supplementation of arsenic-exposed individuals with folic acid increases urinary arsenic elimination and decreases blood arsenic concentrations (Gamble *et al.*, 2007) and may be a feasible means of treating widespread arsenic poisoning in Asia.

Diet-induced Anaemias

Besides the nutrients involved in iron metabolism and haemoglobin synthesis (described above), a number of dietary conditions can cause haemolytic anaemia, involving destruction of the rbc membrane.

A classic sign of vitamin E deficiency is the susceptibility of rbc to *in vitro* haemolysis. **Vitamin E** is a component of cell membranes, where it functions as an antioxidant. Several powerful oxidants are produced during metabolism of the **rbc**. These include superoxide (O_2^-), hydrogen peroxide

(H_2O_2), peroxyl radical (ROO^-) and hydroxyl radicals (OH^-), which collectively are referred to as **reactive oxygen species (ROS)**. A deficiency of vitamin E reduces the resistance of the rbc to ROS, causing the membrane to break, allowing the haemoglobin to escape. Thus vitamin E deficiency causes rbc haemolysis. Increased susceptibility of rbc from rats fed a hepatotoxic agent (pyrrolizidine alkaloid) to *in vitro* erythrocyte haemolysis (see Fig. 13.4 in Chapter 13) has been observed (Cheeke, 1989). Liver damage results in impaired hepatic synthesis of vitamin-E-transporting plasma proteins and lowered plasma and liver vitamin E concentrations (Lulay *et al.*, 2007).

After the discovery of **selenium** as an essential nutrient, there was an intensive search for its mode of action. It was observed that dietary selenium sometimes, but not always, prevented *in vitro* haemolysis of rat rbc. Serendipitously, it was discovered that dietary selenium was effective if the *in vitro* medium contained added glucose (Rotruck *et al.*, 1973). Examination of the role of added glucose led to the discovery that glucose metabolism by the pentose phosphate pathway maintained a supply of reduced glutathione (GSH) in the rbc. The GSH reduced ROS such as hydrogen peroxide:

$$2GSH + H_2O_2 \xrightarrow{\text{Glutathione peroxidase}} G\text{-}S\text{-}S\text{-}G + 2H_2O$$

Subsequent work demonstrated that the enzyme **glutathione peroxidase** contained selenium (Rotruck *et al.*, 1973). At least five selenium-containing glutathione peroxidases have been identified (Sunde, 2006). There are also several non-selenium-containing glutathione peroxidases. The generation of hydrogen for maintaining cellular GSH begins with the metabolism of glucose to phosphogluconic acid, and the production of NADPH + H⁺. The hydrogen of NADPH + H⁺ is transferred to oxidized glutathione (G-S-S-G) to produce GSH. The role of selenium, as part of glutathione peroxidase, is to then transfer the hydrogen to ROS (Fig. 13.2).

Several human and animal anaemias result from impairment of the above enzyme system. In some regions of the world, especially the Mediterranean region, haemolytic anaemia occurs in people who consume fava beans (*Vicia faba*). The disorder is known as **favism**. Individuals susceptible to favism have low rbc activity of **glucose-6-phosphate dehydrogenase (G6PD)**, the enzyme of the pentose phosphate cycle which metabolizes glucose to produce reducing equivalents (NADPH) in the rbc. Fava beans contain oxidants which attack the rbc membrane. At least 100 million people of Mediterranean and African ancestry have low rbc activities of G6PD. Low activity of G6PD is linked to resistance to malaria. **Malaria** is caused by a protozoan parasite that invades the rbc. ROS oxidize the protozoal cell membrane, which is more susceptible to haemolysis than the rbc. Thus in areas where malaria is endemic, there has been natural selection for individuals with low G6PD, because a slight surplus of ROS favours antiprotozoal activity. Anti-malarial drugs such as quinine and primaquine are oxidants and act by oxidizing the malarial protozoan cell membrane. Thus favism-susceptible individuals with low G6PD are more sensitive to excessive doses of anti-malarial drugs than people with higher G6PD levels.

A number of plants contain haemolytic agents which cause haemolysis in livestock and other domestic animals. Plants in the genus *Brassica*, such as kale, rape, cabbage, cauliflower and turnips, are important livestock feeds. Ruminants fed a diet of *Brassica* may develop severe haemolytic anaemia after 3–4 weeks. The first sign of clinical disease is the appearance of stainable granules within the rbc. These are called Heinz-Ehrlich bodies or Heinz bodies (Fig. 21.9). They are composed of haemichrome, an oxidized form of haemoglobin which is unstable and rapidly precipitates. The formation of haemichrome is the first sign of oxidative damage to haemoglobin. **Brassica anaemia** results from the rumen metabolism of **S-methylcysteine sulfoxide** (SMCO) an amino acid in *Brassica* spp. SMCO is metabolized in the rumen to produce dimethyl disulfide, a haemolytic agent (Fig. 21.10). It is an oxidant that attacks the rbc membrane. It is inactivated by reduction with GSH and glutathione peroxidase to produce CH_3SH (methylmercaptan).

Onions are toxic to many animals. Onions contain a number of sulfur-containing compounds which are converted to thiosulfinates when onions are macerated. A major one is dipropyl disulfide, an oxidant. Signs of **onion poisoning** are rbc Heinz bodies and haemolytic anaemia. Dogs are very sensitive to onion toxicity because of a lack of rbc GSH-G6PD protection against oxidative damage.

The consumption of wilted or dried leaves and bark of the red maple (*Acer rubrum*) can cause haemolytic anaemia and Heinz body formation in horses. Methaemoglobin is also produced in **red maple poisoning**. Methaemoglobin is formed by oxidant activity; it is detoxified by methaemoglobin reductase, which requires NADH as a cofactor. Horses have a low activity of this enzyme.

Saponins are surfactants occurring in many plant species. They are potent haemolytic agents when injected intravenously. Dietary saponins do not cause haemolysis because they are not absorbed.

Favism, brassica anaemia, onion poisoning, red maple poisoning and saponins are discussed in more detail by Cheeke (1998).

Copper toxicity causes rbc haemolysis with a severe haemolytic crisis. Copper accumulates in the liver until the liver cells are saturated with the element, causing oxidative damage to the liver. Copper catalyses the conversion of hydrogen peroxide to the hydroxyl radical, causing lipid peroxidation of cell membranes (Haywood *et al.*, 2005). The breakdown of liver cells releases large amount of copper into the blood, where the rbc are damaged by the same oxidative mechanism. Haemolysis of rbc occurs, causing anaemia, jaundice and red urine due to excretion of haemoglobin pigments.

Sheep are especially susceptible to copper toxicity, due to a low ability to excrete copper in the bile (Haywood *et al.*, 2005). At a liver copper concentration of greater than 1000 µg/g hepatic necrosis may result in a haemolytic crisis with profound jaundice (the yellows) which is generally fatal. Sheep breeds vary in susceptibility to copper. The Merino is the most tolerant, while a primitive breed, the North Ronaldsay, is the most susceptible. This breed lives on the beach of a barren island off the coast of Scotland and subsists on seaweed washed up on the beach. Seaweed has a very low (2 ppm) copper content. The North Ronaldsay

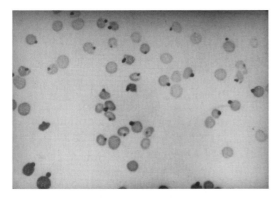

Fig. 21.9. Erythrocytes showing Heinz bodies, which are clumps of denatured haemoglobin.

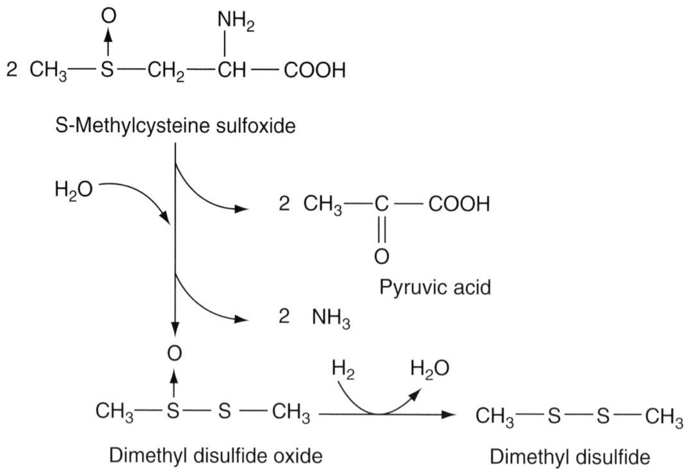

$$2\ CH_3-\overset{\displaystyle O}{\overset{\displaystyle \uparrow}{S}}-CH_2-\underset{\displaystyle NH_2}{\overset{\displaystyle |}{CH}}-COOH$$

S-Methylcysteine sulfoxide

H_2O

$$2\ CH_3-\underset{\displaystyle O}{\overset{\displaystyle ||}{C}}-COOH$$

Pyruvic acid

$2\ NH_3$

$$CH_3-\overset{\displaystyle O}{\overset{\displaystyle \uparrow}{S}}-S-CH_3$$

Dimethyl disulfide oxide

H_2 H_2O

$$CH_3-S-S-CH_3$$

Dimethyl disulfide

Fig. 21.10. Rumen metabolism of S-methylcysteine sulfoxide (SMCO), a haemolytic amino acid in *Brassica* spp.

breed has adapted to a low copper diet by efficient copper uptake and retention, but as a consequence is very susceptible to copper toxicity. Efforts to preserve flocks of this breed in other locations have been impeded by virtual inability of the animals to consume normal vegetation without developing copper toxicity (MacLachlan and Johnston, 1982). The liver mitochondria of North Ronaldsay sheep have increased susceptibility to copper-induced oxidative stress (Haywood *et al.*, 2005).

Pyrrolizidine alkaloids, found in a number of poisonous plants such as *Senecio* spp., cause accumulation of copper in the liver (Cheeke, 1998). In Australia, chronic copper toxicity in sheep occurs in animals consuming pyrrolizidine-alkaloid-containing plants. The pyrrolizidine alkaloids cause liver damage which decreases the ability to secrete bile, a major excretory route for excess copper. A severe haemolytic crisis follows (Howell *et al.*, 1991a,b).

The Electrolytes

Sodium, potassium and chlorine

Sodium, potassium and chlorine are considered together because they are closely interrelated in their metabolism. **Common salt** (NaCl) is routinely added to animal feeds and provided as a free choice to grazing animals. In North America and Europe, provision of salt to livestock is almost universal. One of the principal reasons for this is that ani-

mals, particularly ruminants, have an innate desire to consume salt, which has often been interpreted as reflecting a physiological and nutritional need. However, as Morris (1980) points out, animals (particularly herbivores) have a salt appetite and consume much more salt than required for optimal health. In contrast, the salt appetite in humans is acquired primarily as a result of social and dietary customs. In humans, excessive salt consumption has been linked with hypertension, but in livestock, there is no evidence that 'luxury consumption' of salt has harmful effects so long as adequate water is available. If water availability is limited, salt toxicity can occur. Diets of herbivores tend to be high in potassium; the sodium-to-potassium imbalance may be a contributing factor in the salt appetite of these animals.

Ruminants have a pronounced ability to conserve **sodium**. The rumen acts as a sodium storehouse. When sodium-deficient diets are consumed, rumen sodium is drawn upon to counteract blood sodium depletion, and potassium, which is abundant in grass, replaces sodium in saliva. These mechanisms allow ruminants to adapt to the large sodium-deficient areas of the world, which include most non-coastal land areas. Northern ruminants, such as moose, eat large amounts of sodium-containing aquatic plants during a 3-month season and draw on the rumen sodium pool during the rest of the year (Botkin *et al.*, 1973).

Under range conditions, strategic placement of salt can be used to control the distribution of livestock. Salt is often used as a vehicle for providing trace elements, worming agents and antibloat compounds. Iodized salt and trace-mineralized salt are the forms normally used. For supplementing range cattle with protein, protein supplements can be mixed with salt to limit consumption. A mixture containing 40% salt will usually result in adequate but not excessive intake. Supplements containing salt can also be used to increase water intake of cattle to aid in preventing urinary calculi. A supplement containing 15% salt is adequate for this purpose (Bailey, 1981). For pig and poultry diets, the addition of 0.25–0.5% salt is a standard practice. Usually the salt also contains trace minerals. Many **trace-mineralized salt preparations** are available commercially.

Potassium deficiency is not commonly encountered in livestock production, but it can occur under certain circumstances. Most feedstuffs contain adequate **potassium**, with grains tending to be lower than good quality roughages. Mature, weathered, poor quality roughages may lack adequate amounts. Feedlot cattle fed high concentrate diets sometimes respond positively to dietary potassium supplementation. There has been interest in the effect of stress on potassium. Stress conditions, such as in transporting and marketing feeder cattle and pigs, may stimulate adrenal cortex activity and increase potassium excretion. Dehydration and diarrhoea increase loss of the element. Hutcheson and Cole (1986) reported that supplementation of receiving diets for feedlot calves with potassium to provide a total daily intake of 26 g potassium/100 kg body weight was necessary for optimal weight gains. In contrast, Brumm and Schricker (1989) found no beneficial effects from supplementation of transport-stressed feeder pigs with potassium chloride and concluded that maize-soy diets contain sufficient potassium for pigs experiencing stress in marketing and transport. Further work is necessary to conclusively demonstrate a role for potassium supplementation under practical conditions.

Because lucerne and grains have a fairly high potassium content, forage crops grown in association with dairy farms may have a high potassium content. As the dairy industry intensifies, there is a trend towards large numbers of cows being kept in confinement, with the manure being disposed of on surrounding crop land, which is often used for forage (e.g. maize silage) production. Forage potassium contents in excess of 5% are being encountered (Fisher *et al.*, 1994). When these **high-potassium forages** are fed to dairy cattle, there is an increase in water consumption and urine volume, creating management problems. High potassium intakes interfere with magnesium and calcium absorption and may promote hypomagnesaemia and milk fever in dairy cattle. The high potassium intake may adversely affect cation–anion balance (see next section).

Dietary electrolyte balance

Sodium, potassium and chlorine are interrelated in regulating **electrolyte balance** of animal tissues. **Electrolytes** are electrically charged dissolved substances. The animal body is electrically neutral; acid–base balance is determined as the difference between total cation and anion intake and excretion. **Dietary fixed ions** are bioavailable ions that are not metabolized (e.g. Ca^{2+}, Cl^-), whereas the term **dietary undetermined anion** refers to ions, such as bicarbonate, that balance the dietary fixed cations:

$$\text{Dietary undetermined anion} = (Na^+ + K^+ + Ca^{2+} + Mg^{2+}) - (Cl^- + S^{2-} + P^{2-})$$

Dietary cations are usually present in excess of dietary anions; therefore, to maintain electrical neutrality, they are balanced by the dietary undetermined anions.

The **dietary electrolyte balance** can be calculated as the sum of cations minus the sum of non-metabolizable anions:

$$\text{Macromineral balance (meq/kg)} = (Na^+ + K^+ + Ca^{2+} + Mg^{2+}) - (Cl^- + P^{2-} + S^{2-})$$

The ions are expressed as milliequivalents because electrolyte balance deals with the equivalence of electrical charges.

The acidogenicity or alkalinogenicity of the diet is largely determined by the relative deficit or excess, respectively, of **metabolizable anions**, such as acetate and citrate (Patience *et al.*, 1987; Patience and Chaplin, 1997). Under most circumstances, the dietary mineral balance is adequately expressed as $Na + K - Cl$ (meq/kg). For poultry, the optimal electrolyte balance is about 250 meq/kg (Mongin, 1981; Johnson and Karunajeewa, 1985; Hulan *et al.*, 1987); electrolyte imbalance results in reduced growth and induces leg abnormalities such as tibial dyschondroplasia (slipped tendon). For pigs, the $Na + K - Cl$ (meq/kg) should be in the 100–200 range for optimal performance.

The number of milliequivalents per kilogram of diet can be calculated as follows.

Na: meq/kg diet = mg Na/kg ÷ 23.0

K: meq/kg diet = mg K/kg ÷ 39.1

Cl: meq/kg diet = mg Cl/kg ÷ 35.5

Ca: meq/kg diet = mg Ca/kg ÷ 20.0

Mg: meq/kg diet = mg Mg/kg ÷ 12.15

P: meq/kg diet = mg P/kg ÷ 10.3

S: meq/kg diet = mg S/kg ÷ 16.0

The electrolyte balance is influenced by the form in which minerals are provided, that is, inorganic (e.g. NaCl) or organic (e.g. Na citrate) salts. Organic salts contain a metabolizable anion (e.g. citrate is converted to carbon dioxide and water); thus diets high in metabolizable anions will have an excess of cations relative to anions, giving an alkalinogenic diet.

Amino acid status can influence electrolyte balance, particularly in poultry. In birds, certain amino acids are degraded in the kidney; these include arginine, lysine, histidine, isoleucine and tyrosine. The enzyme involved is kidney arginase. An excess of dietary lysine causes marked elevation of kidney arginase, resulting in excessive degradation of arginine and arginine deficiency. This lysine-arginine antagonism is influenced by electrolyte status (Austic and Calvert, 1981). The effect of excess lysine is magnified by an excess of chloride. Conversely, responses to dietary supplements of sodium or potassium bicarbonate in pigs and poultry fed lysine-deficient diets have been reported (Patience *et al.*, 1987). When the dietary electrolyte balance decreases below about 175 meq/kg, blood pH and bicarbonate drop, indicating a metabolic acidosis. Thus, there is a complex interrelationship among dietary electrolytes, amino acids and acid–base balance. Typical maize-soy pig diets have an electrolyte balance of approximately 175 meq/kg. The trend to replacement of part of the soybean meal with synthetic lysine (lysine-HCl), thus reducing potassium and increasing chloride, could lead to increased concerns with acid–base balance (Patience *et al.*, 1987).

Electrolyte balance in ruminants is complicated by a number of factors, which are reviewed by Fredeen *et al.* (1988). Diets containing maize silage and grains have cation deficits and are acidogenic, whereas lucerne has a cation excess and is alkalinogenic.

Ruminant diets are often supplemented with sodium and potassium-containing buffers, calcium carbonate and magnesium oxide. Prepartum alkalosis may increase the incidence of parturient paresis (milk fever), whereas acidosis may help prevent it (Fredeen *et al.*, 1988; Leclerce and Block, 1989). Diets that are acidic (excess anions) have greater calcium absorption. Those with excess cations may have reduced calcium availability. High cation prepartum diets, especially those high in potassium and sodium, can cause milk fever in cows because they induce a metabolic alkalosis that reduces the ability of the cow to maintain calcium homeostasis at the onset of lactation (Goff *et al.*, 2004). Cows fed diets high in cations have a reduced ability to mobilize bone calcium and a reduced ability to produce 1,25-dihydroxyvitamin D. Thus, in ruminants, the complete macromineral balance equation, which includes calcium, magnesium, phosphorus and sulfur, in addition to sodium, potassium and chloride, probably should be used in calculating electrolyte balance.

There is increasing recognition of the importance of electrolyte balance in the feeding of all types of livestock and poultry. Acid–base balance can influence growth and appetite, leg disorders in poultry, response to thermal stress, incidence of milk fever in dairy cattle, and the metabolism of various amino acids, minerals and vitamins (Patience, 1990).

Downer Cow Syndrome

Downer cow syndrome mainly refers to dairy cows that have become non-ambulatory for a variety of reasons. Because of animal welfare considerations, they have become a major concern in the livestock industry. Of particular concern is the appearance of downer cows at slaughter facilities. In the USA, non-ambulatory livestock are by law not to be slaughtered, to be kept out of the human food chain. One reason is because there is an increased risk of bovine spongiform encephalitis (BSE; mad cow disease) in animals that are unable to stand or walk.

Some of the major causes of downer cow syndrome are milk fever, grass tetany, low blood phosphorus, low blood potassium, ketosis, coliform mastitis, trauma (e.g. caused by cows in heat being mounted, slipping on slick floors) and energy/protein wasting (metabolic exhaustion).

For periparturient cows, milk fever (hypocalcaemia) is the major cause of down cows (Goff, 2006). The transition from non-lactating to lactation at calving presents a tremendous challenge to serum calcium homeostasis. Hypocalcaemia results when bone calcium mobilization and intestinal calcium absorption are unable to keep up with the needs of lactation. Often suboptimal blood concentrations of magnesium, phosphorus and potassium are also involved. Hypomagnesaemia affects calcium metabolism by reducing parathyroid hormone (PTH) secretion in response to hypocalcaemia, and reducing tissue sensitivity to PTH (Goff, 2006). In addition, magnesium functions at neuromuscular junctions in the transmission of nerve impulses to muscle tissue. This is another way that hypomagnesaemia is involved in the downer cow syndrome. Metabolic alkalosis predisposes cows to milk fever and reduces response to

PTH. For this reason, dietary cation–anion balance is important. Urine pH provides an inexpensive assessment of blood pH. For optimal control of subclinical hypocalcaemia, the average pH of the urine of Holstein cows should be between 6.2 and 6.8, while in Jerseys it should be between 5.8 and 6.3 (Goff, 2006). Limiting dietary cations has only a slight effect on blood pH; to substantially lower urine pH, the addition of anions to the diet is required.

Cows laying on one side for 6 h or more can develop nerve and muscle damage, and may never be able to stand even if successfully treated for milk fever. Thus prevention and very early treatment of affected animals are of paramount importance.

Questions and Study Guide

1. What is the major protein in blood? What is its major function?
2. How does vitamin K function in blood clotting? What is the role of calcium in blood clotting?
3. Why is the iron in meat absorbed efficiently in humans?
4. How does vitamin C affect iron absorption?
5. Compare the functions of ferritin, transferrin and haemosiderin.
6. What is the metabolic role of ceruloplasmin?
7. What is the relationship among copper, molybdenum and inorganic sulfate in ruminant nutrition?
8. Copper deficiency can cause anaemia, ataxia, achromatrichia, skeletal deformity, infertility and diarrhoea. Explain the metabolic causes in each case.
9. What causes pernicious anaemia?
10. Why does folic acid supplementation reduce arsenic toxicity in humans?
11. Why does vitamin E deficiency cause erythrocyte haemolysis?
12. Dietary selenium will prevent *in vitro* haemolysis of red blood cells from vitamin-E-deficient rats, if the blood is supplemented with glucose. What is the role of glucose in this process?
13. What are some plants that can induce red blood cell haemolysis in livestock?
14. What is unusual about the North Ronaldsay breed of sheep?
15. Why do domestic and wild animals often show a craving for salt?
16. How does dietary electrolyte balance affect calcium metabolism in dairy cows?
17. How does hypomagnesaemia contribute to development of downer cow syndrome?

References

Austic, R.E. and Calvert, C.C. (1981) Nutritional interrelationships of electrolytes and amino acids. *Federation Proceedings* 40, 63–67.

Bailey, C.B. (1981) Silica metabolism and silica urolithiasis: a review. *Canadian Journal of Animal Science* 61, 219–235.

Botkin, D.B., Jordan, P.A., Dominski, A.S., Lowendorf, H.S. and Hutchinson, G.E. (1973) Sodium dynamics in a northern ecosystem. *Proceedings of the National Academy of Sciences USA* 70, 2745–2748.

Brumm, M.C. and Schricker, B.R. (1989) Effect of dietary potassium chloride on feeder pig performance, marker shrink, carcass traits and selected blood parameters. *Journal of Animal Science* 67, 1411–1417.

Cheeke, P.R. (1989) Pyrrolizidine alkaloid toxicity and metabolism in laboratory animals and livestock. In: Cheeke, P.R. (ed.) *Toxicants of Plant Origin*, Vol. 1. CRC Press, Boca Raton, Florida, pp. 1–22.

Cheeke, P.R. (1998) *Natural Toxicants in Feeds, Forages, and Poisonous Plants*. Prentice Hall, Upper Saddle River, New Jersey.

Fisher, L.J., Dinn, N., Tait, R.M. and Shelford, J.A. (1994) Effect of level of dietary potassium on the absorption and excretion of calcium and magnesium by lactating cows. *Journal of Animal Science* 74, 503–509.

Fredeen, A.H., DePeters, E.J. and Baldwin, R.L. (1988) Effects of acid–base disturbance caused by differences in dietary fixed ion balance on kinetics of calcium metabolism in ruminants with high calcium demand. *Journal of Animal Science* 66, 174–184.

Gamble, M.V., Liu, X., Slavkovich, V., Pilsner, J.R., Ilievski, V., Factor-Litvak, P., Levy, D., Alam, S., Islam, M., Parvez, F., Ahsan, H. and Graziano, J.H. (2007) Folic acid supplementation lowers blood arsenic. *American Journal of Clinical Nutrition* 86, 1202–1209.

Goff, J.P. (2006) Macromineral physiology and application to the feeding of the dairy cow for prevention of milk fever and other periparturient mineral disorders. *Animal Feed Science and Technology* 126, 237–257.

Goff, J.P., Ruiz, R. and Horst, R.L (2004) Relative acidifying activity of anionic salts commonly used to prevent milk fever. *Journal of Dairy Science* 87, 1245–1255.

Haywood, S., Simpson, D.M., Ross, G. and Beynon, R.J. (2005) The greater susceptibility of North Ronaldsay sheep compared with Cambridge sheep to copper-induced oxidative stress, mitochondrial damage and hepatic stellate cell activation. *Journal of Comparative Pathology* 133, 114–127.

Howell, J.McC., Deol, H.S. and Dorling, P.R. (1991a) Experimental copper and *Heliotropium europaeum* intoxication in sheep: clinical syndromes and trace element concentrations. *Australian Journal of Agricultural Research* 42, 979–992.

Howell, J.McC., Deol, H.S., Dorling, P.R. and Thomas, J.B. (1991b) Experimental copper and heliotrope intoxication in sheep: morphological changes. *Journal of Comparative Pathology* 105, 49–74.

Huh, E.C., Hotchkiss, A., Brouillette, J. and Glahn, R.P. (2004) Carbohydrate fractions from cooked fish promote iron uptake by Caco-2 cells. *Journal of Nutrition* 134, 1681–1689.

Hulan, H.W., Simons, P.C.M., Van Schagen, P.J.W., McRae, K.B. and Proudfoot, F.G. (1987) Effect of cation–anion imbalance and calcium content on general performance and incidence of leg abnormalities of broiler chickens. *Canadian Journal of Animal Science* 67, 165–177.

Hutcheson, D.P. and Cole, N.A. (1986) Management of transit-stress syndrome in cattle: nutritional and environmental effects. *Journal of Animal Science* 62, 555–560.

Johnson, R.J. and Karunajeewa, H. (1985) The effects of dietary minerals and electrolytes on the growth and physiology of the young chick. *Journal of Nutrition* 115, 1680–1690.

Kendall, N.R., Marsters, P., Guo, L., Scaramuzzi, R.J. and Campbell, B.K. (2006) Effect of copper and thiomolybdates on bovine theca cell differentiation *in vitro*. *Journal of Endocrinology* 189, 455–463.

Leclere, H. and Block, E. (1989) Effects of reducing dietary cation–anion balance for prepartum dairy cows with specific reference to hypocalcemic parturient paresis. *Canadian Journal of Animal Science* 69, 411–423.

Lulay, A.L., Leonard, S.W., Traber, M.G., Keller, M.R. and Cheeke, P.R. (2007) Effects of dietary pyrrolizidine

(*Senecio*) alkaloids on plasma and liver vitamin E distribution in broiler chickens. In: Panter, K.E., Wierenga, T.L. and Pfister, J.A. (eds) *Poisonous Plants. Global Research and Solutions*. CAB International, Wallingford, Oxon, UK, pp. 77–81.

MacLachlan, G.K. and Johnston, W.S. (1982) Copper poisoning in sheep from North Ronaldsay maintained on a diet of terrestrial herbage. *Veterinary Record* 111(13), 299–301.

Marasas, W.F.O., Riley, R.T., Hendricks, K.A., Stevens, V.L., Sadler, T.W., van Waes, J.G., Missmer, S.A., Cabrera, J., Torres, O., Gelderblom, W.C.A., Allegood, J., Martinez, C., Maddox, J., Miller, J.D., Starr, L., Sullards, M.C., Roman, A.V., Voss, K.A., Wang, E. and Merrill, A.H., Jr (2004) Fumonisins disrupt sphingolipid metabolism, folate transport, and neural tube development in embryo culture and *in vivo*: a potential risk factor for human neural tube defects among populations consuming fumonisin-contaminated maize. *Journal of Nutrition* 134, 711–716.

Mongin, P.J. (1981) Recent advances in dietary anion–cation balance. Applications in poultry. *Proceedings of the Nutrition Society* 40, 285–294.

Morris, J.G. (1980) Assessment of sodium requirements of grazing beef cattle: a review. *Journal of Animal Science* 50, 145–152.

Patience, J.F. (1990) A review of the role of acid–base balance in amino acid nutrition. *Journal of Animal Science* 68, 398–408.

Patience, J.F. and Chaplin, R.K. (1997) The relationship among dietary undetermined anion, acid–base balance, and nutrient metabolism in swine. *Journal of Animal Science* 75, 2445–2452.

Patience, J.F., Austic, R.E. and Boyd, R.D. (1987) Effect of dietary electrolyte balance on growth and acid–base status in swine. *Journal of Animal Science* 64, 457–466.

Price, J., Will, A.M., Paschaleris, G. and Chesters, J.K. (1987) Identification of thiomolybdates in digesta and plasma from sheep after administration of [99]Mo-labelled compounds into the rumen. *British Journal of Nutrition* 58, 127–138.

Rotruck, J.T., Pope, A.L., Ganther, H.E., Swanson, A.B., Hafeman, D.G. and Hoekstra, W.G. (1973) Selenium: biochemical role as a component of glutathione peroxidase. *Science* 179, 588–590.

Sunde, R.A. (2006) Selenium. In: Brown, B.A. and Russell, R.M. (eds) *Present Knowledge in Nutrition*, Vol. I, 9th edn. International Life Sciences Institute (ILSI), Washington, DC, pp. 480–497.

Suttle, N.F. (1991) The interactions between copper, molybdenum, and sulphur in ruminant nutrition. *Annual Review of Nutrition* 111, 121–140.

Yasuda, K., Roneker, K.R., Miller, D.D., Welch, R.M. and Lei, X.G. (2006) Supplemental dietary inulin affects the bioavailability of iron in corn and soybean meal to young pigs. *Journal of Nutrition* 136, 3033–3038.

PART VIII
Reproduction and the Immune System

This part is intended to discuss the most important nutritional effects on reproduction in animals and on the immune system.

Part Objectives

1. To discuss the effects of energy status and nutrients that affect energy metabolism (e.g. phosphorus) on reproduction.
2. To review evidence that compounds in plants may provide dietary cues for reproduction in small rodents (e.g. meadow voles).
3. To discuss the roles of vitamin A, β-carotene and vitamin E in reproduction.
4. To discuss other dietary factors (gossypol, ergot alkaloids, phyto-oestrogens, environmental pollutants) related to reproduction.
5. To discuss nutritional effects on the immune system in ruminants.
6. To discuss the relationship between nutrition and inflammation.

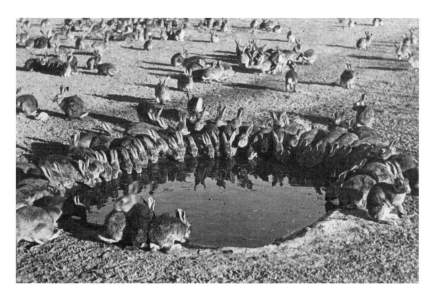

Many animals have the ability to suspend reproduction during times of nutritional stress. The cue for this stress is usually inadequate energy intake. Some animals, such as these wild rabbits in Australia, resorb their fetuses when feed availability is low, as during a drought.

22 Nutrition and Reproduction

Nutrition plays important roles in reproductive success. Growth of the fetus and placental tissues have a high priority for nutrients, especially those relating to energy and protein requirements. The ultimate role of all organisms is the successful completion of reproduction.

Energy Metabolism and Reproduction

On an evolutionary basis, animals developed physiological mechanisms which inform them metabolically as to whether undertaking reproduction at a particular time is wise. For example, it would not be an evolutionarily sound strategy for wild ungulates in northern regions to give birth in mid-winter. Various environmental cues aid in focusing reproductive efforts to periods when success is likely. If a severe drought is imminent, it would be wise to delay reproduction. A developing drought would result in reduced feed availability and thus reduced availability of energy-providing nutrients. Reduced energy intake could provide a cue to alter hormonal status to inhibit reproduction. In general, low energy intakes and poor body condition will tend to impair reproduction. Nutrients that are involved in energy metabolism, such as enzyme cofactors, will if deficient impair reproduction. For example, **phosphorus** has a role in phosphorylation of sugars in carbohydrate metabolism and is a component of ATP. Dietary phosphorus deficiency thus provides a cue that energy metabolism is impaired. **Phosphorus deficiency** of livestock is relatively common in various parts of the world where soil contents of the mineral are low. Such conditions are prevalent in parts of South America (e.g. the savannahs of Colombia, Venezuela and Brazil) where the soils are acid and infertile. Phosphorus-deficient grazing animals often have a depraved appetite (**pica**) and consume wood, bones and so on. Calving intervals under these conditions are very long (several years) or reproduction may cease entirely. Deficiencies this severe rarely occur in the USA. Less obvious phosphorus inadequacy may nevertheless impair reproductive performance; cattle may not have normal oestrous cycles and may not experience oestrus or heat periods. Thus, conception rates are low and calving intervals are extended. In parts of the tropics, cows may not produce a calf more often than once every 2 or 3 years or may not even come into oestrus because of severe phosphorus deficiency. Phosphorus nutrition of grazing cattle has been reviewed by Karn (2001).

Another example of a possible dietary cue for reproduction is the presence of substances in plants that may function in regulating reproduction in small herbivorous mammals, such as the meadow vole and the lemming, by providing dietary cues as to when food supplies (energy) are adequate for reproduction. Berger *et al.* (1977) found that cinnamic acids and their related vinyl phenols inhibited reproductive function in the meadow vole (*Microtus montanus*). When fed these compounds, the animals exhibited decreased uterine weight, inhibition of follicular development and a cessation of breeding activity. The compounds were at highest concentration in native plants at the end of the vegetative growing season, possibly providing a dietary cue to turn off reproduction. Later studies by these workers (Berger *et al.*, 1981; Sanders *et al.*, 1981) demonstrated that a plant-derived cyclic carbamate, **6-methoxybenzoxazolinone (6-MBOA)**, stimulates reproductive activity in meadow voles. They suggest that 6-MBOA may trigger reproductive activity in the spring when food supplies are abundant. The significance, if any, of these compounds in livestock production is not known. However, if late-season forage contains phenolics that inhibit reproductive processes and spring forage has reproduction-stimulating compounds, there would be potential implications for livestock production. 6-MBOA has a structural resemblance to melatonin (Fig. 22.1), a hormone

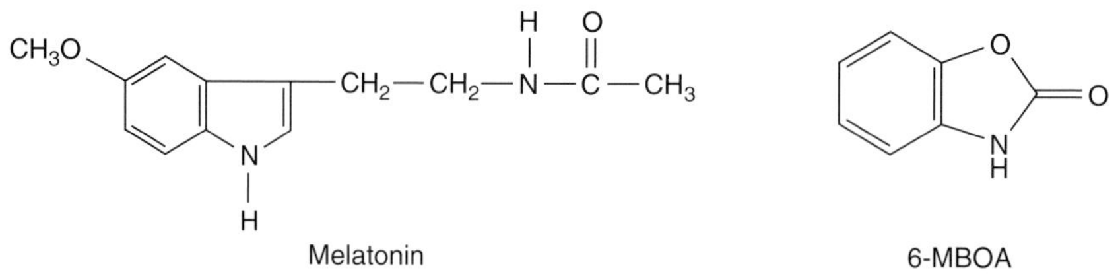

Fig. 22.1. Structures of melatonin and 6-methoxybenzoxazolinone (6-MBOA), illustrating structural similarity.

whose activity is related to light exposure and pro-lactin secretion. Melatonin is produced in the pineal gland and may have a role in the regulation of seasonal breeding. Thus, 6-MBOA may exert its effects through an interaction with melatonin.

Vitamin and Mineral Roles in Reproduction

Vitamin E was in the past sometimes called the 'fertility vitamin' or 'antisterility factor'. This designation was an accident of history. In the early days of vitamin research, what had been called 'fat-soluble vitamin A' was fractionated into what we now know as vitamin A and vitamin D. Rats fed with these two vitamins along with all other nutrients known at that time did not reproduce normally. Supplementation of the rats with various foods restored fertility. Wheat germ oil was especially effective. The active component was isolated and named vitamin E. When the chemical structure was elucidated, it was named 'tocopherol' from the Greek words for childbirth and 'to bear'. However, despite this early association with reproduction, vitamin E functions primarily as an antioxidant (Chapter 13). Its reproductive effects are actually due to the maintenance of tissue structural integrity by antioxidant activity.

Vitamin A is essential for reproductive function in both males and females, and for fetal development (Chew, 1993). Vitamin A deficiency results in weak, dead or malformed offspring. Chew (1993) cites evidence that vitamin A functions in steroidogenesis (synthesis of steroid hormones) such as progesterone. Vitamin A may also have a direct effect on the uterine environment, including formation of normal uterine epithelial tissue. Vitamin A also affects embryo development by regulating cell differentiation and proliferation. In the male, vitamin A is required for spermatogenesis. Hypervitaminosis A can also cause reproductive problems, including abortion, fetal resorption, birth defects and low neonatal viability. Interestingly, both deficiency and excess of vitamin A cause similar problems. For example, fetal **hydrocephalus** (Fig. 22.2) occurs with both deficient and toxic vitamin A states.

There is evidence that β-carotene may play a role in reproduction (Weiss, 1998). The corpus luteum of cows contains high concentrations of β-carotene, an observation which has stimulated research on its effects on dairy cow reproduction. There is a tendency of lowered incidence of retained placenta in cows receiving β-carotene. Arechiga *et al.* (1998) found that in a hot climate (Florida), the characteristic decline in dairy cow fertility in the hot months was reduced with β-carotene supplementation, and milk yield was increased. They attributed these responses to an antioxidant effect. Heat stress is accompanied by increased tissue free radical formation. Arechiga *et al.* (1998) suggest that β-carotene increases embryonic survival under heat stress conditions by counteracting free radical formation in the embryo.

As discussed in Chapter 21, **copper deficiency** causes infertility as a result of impaired ovarian steroid hormone synthesis.

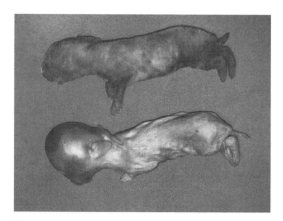

Fig. 22.2. Hydrocephalus (fluid on the brain) in a newborn rabbit from a female rabbit fed a vitamin A-deficient diet (bottom) compared to a normal kit (top).

Other Dietary Factors and Reproduction

Gossypol is a toxin found in cottonseed and cottonseed meal. Gossypol has some interesting effects on reproduction. Much of the interest stems from observations on humans in China and the possible development of a male birth control pill. A Chinese scientist reported that in a 10-year period, not a single child had been born in Wang village in Jiangsu (Hron *et al.*, 1987). It was discovered that a crude, homemade cottonseed oil preparation had been used for cooking in this village. Women lacked menstrual cycles and men were sterile. Subsequent investigation linked these conditions to the consumption of gossypol. Large-scale testing in China of gossypol as a male contraceptive was begun in the 1970s and terminated in 1998 (Waites *et al.*, 1998) because of concerns that the infertility was irreversible and that an abnormally high rate of hypoalkaemia (low blood potassium) was observed. Studies continue in Brazil (Coutinho, 2002). Coutinho (2002) suggests that the lack of reversibility could be an advantage; gossypol could be used as a non-surgical alternative to vasectomy.

Randel *et al.* (1992) reviewed the effects of cottonseed products and gossypol on reproduction. Gossypol causes males to be infertile because of non-motile sperm and depressed sperm counts. Specific lesions occur in the spermatozoa and in the germinal epithelium. Randel *et al.* (1992) concluded: 'Extensive damage to the germinal epithelium has been shown in both rams and bulls fed diets containing gossypol and is of major concern.' These authors recommend that sources of free gossypol should be avoided in the diets of breeding male ruminants. Testosterone concentrations in growing bulls are not affected by gossypol consumption, but testicular morphology changes occur (Chase *et al.*, 1994). Cusack and Perry (1995) found no effect on fertility of bulls fed whole cottonseed to provide calculated daily intakes of 7.6–19.8 g free gossypol. However, they speculated that a high mineral level in the water may have resulted in binding of minerals with free gossypol in the rumen, inactivating it. Thus the mineral intakes via feed and water can be important determinants of the toxic concentration of gossypol. In non-ruminants, the direct toxic effects of gossypol are such that they mask the more chronic antifertility effects.

In females, gossypol disrupts oestrous cycles, pregnancy and early embryo development (Randel *et al.*, 1992), particularly in non-ruminants. The ruminant female is somewhat insensitive to the antifertility effects of gossypol (Randel *et al.*, 1992; Gray *et al.*, 1993).

Tall fescue grass infected with microscopic fungi called endophytes contains endophyte-produced ergot alkaloids. Pronounced impairment of reproduction occurs in livestock consuming endophyte-infected tall fescue (Porter and Thompson, 1992). Horses are the only livestock whose reactions to the toxic tall fescue are almost exclusively related to poor reproduction (Cross *et al.*, 1995). Mares on toxic tall fescue pasture may experience prolonged gestation, dystocia, agalactia (lack of lactation), thickened, oedematous placentas and have large, weak foals with elongated hooves (McCann *et al.*, 1992). Foal survival is very low (Putnam *et al.*, 1991). Abortion may also occur. Clinically, affected mares have low serum prolactin and progesterone (McCann *et al.*, 1992) and decreased triiodothyronine (T3) concentrations (Boosinger *et al.*, 1995). Low prolactin causes agalactia while suppression of progesterone may be a contributing factor to prolonged gestation. The fescue effects are manifested when the mares are consuming toxic fescue from day 300 of pregnancy. Removal of mares from toxic fescue by day 300 results in a normal parturition (Putnam *et al.*, 1990). Pregnant mares on toxic fescue exhibit no direct signs of toxicity except for intermittent diarrhoea and excessive sweating, presumably in response to hyperthermia (Putnam *et al.*, 1991).

The reproductive effects in horses are caused by the ergopeptine alkaloids in endophyte-infected tall fescue. Similar signs occur in horses consuming the ergot bodies of *Claviceps purpurea* (Riet-Correa *et al.*, 1988). Mechanisms involved include reduced serum prolactin, reduced placental blood flow because of vasoconstrictive effects, and ergot-stimulated contraction of uterine muscle causing abortion. Administration of bromocriptine, a synthetic ergot alkaloid, to pregnant mares produces the same adverse reproductive effects as endophyte-infected tall fescue (Ireland *et al.*, 1991). Domperidone, a D2 dopamine receptor antagonist, prevents the inhibitory effects of ergovaline on prolactin release, and may offer potential as a treatment for fescue toxicosis in horses (Redmond *et al.*, 1994; Cross *et al.*, 1995).

Impaired reproduction of cattle on endophyte-infected tall fescue occurs (Paterson *et al.*, 1995). Reduced calving rates may be due to altered luteal function and reduced levels of circulating progesterone (Porter and Thompson, 1992). Lowered milk production may occur. General reproductive efficiency is impaired, without the pronounced effects on the fetus and parturition events that occur in horses. Impaired reproduction may be in part a consequence of general unthriftiness and weight loss of cattle on toxic tall fescue (Paterson *et al.*, 1995).

Relatively little information is available on the effects of tall fescue and ergot alkaloids on male reproduction. Bromocriptine-induced hypoprolactaemia in rams reduces expression of sexual behaviour such as libido (Regisford and Katz, 1994). The absence of much data suggests that effects of toxic tall fescue on male reproduction are probably minor.

A number of other mycotoxins, such as zearalenone, have oestrogenic activity and can adversely affect reproduction of livestock (Cheeke, 1998).

Subterranean clover (*Trifolium subterraneum*) has been widely sown for sheep pasture in many parts of Australia. It is also extensively grown on hill pasturelands in the US Pacific Northwest. It is a winter annual, sprouting with the autumn rains and providing forage during the winter and spring. In late spring, it produces seeds in burs that are pushed into the ground at maturity, so the plant reseeds itself. This characteristic provides the origin of its name. Sub clover, as it is commonly known, has greatly increased pasture productivity in regions where it is well adapted. In the early 1940s, as sub clover became an important pasture species in Western Australia, a dramatic decrease in the fertility of sheep to a level of about 30% fertility was noted. The infertility was expressed as a failure to conceive and was accompanied by a cystic glandular hyperplasia of the cervix and uterus. Lactation in non-pregnant ewes and wethers suggested that a plant oestrogen was involved in the so-called 'clover disease'. Australian researchers in the early 1950s extracted nearly 5 t of fresh clover, from which they were able to isolate and identify two isoflavones, genistein and formononetin, that had oestrogenic activity. These and other plant oestrogens are referred to as **phyto-oestrogens**. Since that time, a great deal of Australian research has helped to identify the modes of action of phyto-oestrogens (Adams, 1989, 1995).

Pasture species that cause livestock problems because of their phyto-oestrogen content include sub clover, red clover (*Trifolium pratense*), and lucerne (*Medicago sativa*). The oestrogens in clovers are usually **isoflavones**, while lucerne contains **coumestans**. Structures of some common phyto-oestrogens are shown in Fig. 22.3. Their resemblance to estradiol is apparent. The phyto-oestrogens occur in plant tissue as water-soluble glycosides. The isoflavones are synthesized by plants from phenylalanine, while the coumestans are synthesized from cinnamic acid.

The mouse uterine weight bioassay has been extensively used in studies of phyto-oestrogens. Plant extracts or the isolated oestrogens are injected into immature female mice and 24 h later the uterine weight is measured. Oestrogens cause an increase in uterine weight (Fig. 22.4). Examples of some typical dose responses are shown in Table 22.1.

The equivalent potencies at a dosage required to produce a 25 mg uterus were: estrone, 6900; coumestrol, 35; genistein, 1; daidzein, 0.75; biochanin A, 0.46; and formononetin, 0.26. These results show that the phyto-oestrogens have an exceedingly low potency as compared to estrone. However, they can produce significant biological effects through an additive action with endogenous oestrogen, and they may occur in plants at very high levels. The isoflavone content of sub clover may reach 5% of the dry weight.

A puzzling observation was that the oestrogenic activity of sub clover pastures, as assessed by teat length of wethers, was correlated with the **formononetin** content of the pasture. Formononetin has a very low oestrogenic activity in the uterine weight bioassay (Table 22.1). The explanation resides in rumen metabolism. In the sheep rumen, biochanin A and genistein are degraded to p-ethylphenol and a phenolic acid, whereas formononetin is demethylated to daidzein and then metabolized to equol (Fig. 22.5). Equol is oestrogenic. Hence, formononetin is bioactivated by sheep rumen microorganisms to a more potent oestrogen (Davies and Hill, 1989). There is also evidence that formononetin is directly oestrogenic in sheep (Wang *et al.*, 1994). The same metabolism of formononetin to equol occurs in the rumen of cows (Dickinson *et al.*, 1988); the absorbed equol is excreted more rapidly in cattle, so they are less susceptible than sheep to the oestrogenic effects of clover isoflavones. Diets that are rapidly fermented promote a more rapid ruminal metabolism of formononetin than those lacking readily fermentable carbohydrate (Davies and Hill, 1989). Lundh (1990, 1995) and Lundh *et al.* (1990) demonstrated

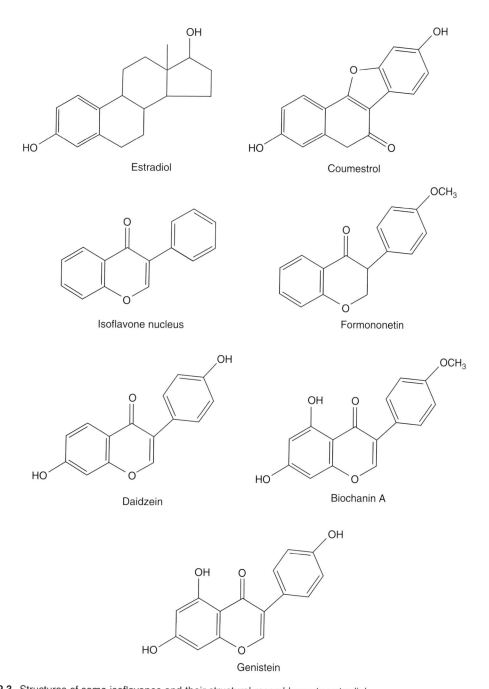

Fig. 22.3. Structures of some isoflavones and their structural resemblance to estradiol.

differences between sheep and cattle in glucuronide conjugation of phyto-oestrogens, but concluded that the most likely explanation for the greater sensitivity of sheep to phyto-oestrogens is species differences in oestrogen receptor activity.

After sheep have grazed oestrogenic pasture for several years, the fertility of the flock becomes depressed. A typical example from Australia is shown in Table 22.2, indicating that with a high-oestrogen cultivar of sub clover, fertility of the flock

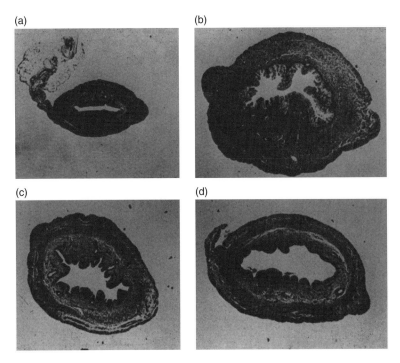

Fig. 22.4. Photomicrographs of cross-sections of uteri from rats receiving phyto-oestrogens. Pre-pubertal (a) and pubertal (b) normal intact rats. (c) Pre-pubertal rat administered a red clover (*T. pratense*) extract. (d) Pre-pubertal rat administered coumestrol acetate, a phyto-oestrogen from lucerne. Note the great enlargement of the uterus in the animals given phyto-oestrogens (courtesy of W.D. Kitts, University of British Columbia, British Columbia, Canada).

eventually declined to zero. This condition of permanent infertility is known as **clover disease**. The main cause of the infertility is a failure of fertilization associated with poor sperm penetration to the oviduct. The **cervical mucus** has an altered consistency which impairs sperm storage in the cervix. Sperm are stored in the cervix after mating; in clover-affected ewes, the number of sperm present after 24 h is less than 5% of that expected. Adams (1990) suggests that the change in mucus consistency is due to an altered responsiveness to stimulation with oestrogen. Therefore, the cervix and vagina of ewes with clover disease fail to respond normally to endogenous oestrogen stimulation to 'prime' the cervix during the breeding season.

In ewes affected by clover disease, the cervix shows structural and functional changes. The cervical tissue changes in morphology to look more like uterine tissue than a cervix. The normal cervix has folds; in clover disease, the folds of the cervix fuse together, trapping epithelial tissue to make it look like glands. Permanent infertility develops with prolonged exposure to the phyto-oestrogens.

Table 22.1. Dose response with phyto-oestrogens using mouse uterine weight bioassay (adapted from Livingston, 1978).

Compound	µg/mouse	Uterine weight (mg)
Control	0	9.6
Estrone	0.5	14.7
	1	23.8
	2	45.3
Coumestrol	100	13.8
	200	24.2
	400	40.7
Genistein	5,000	19.4
	8,000	27.0
	12,000	32.4
Daidzein	5,000	17.3
	10,000	24.8
	15,000	31.2
Biochanin A	10,000	20.3
	20,000	27.9
	40,000	45.5
Formononetin	15,000	16.8
	25,000	23.2
	40,000	26.1

Chapter 22

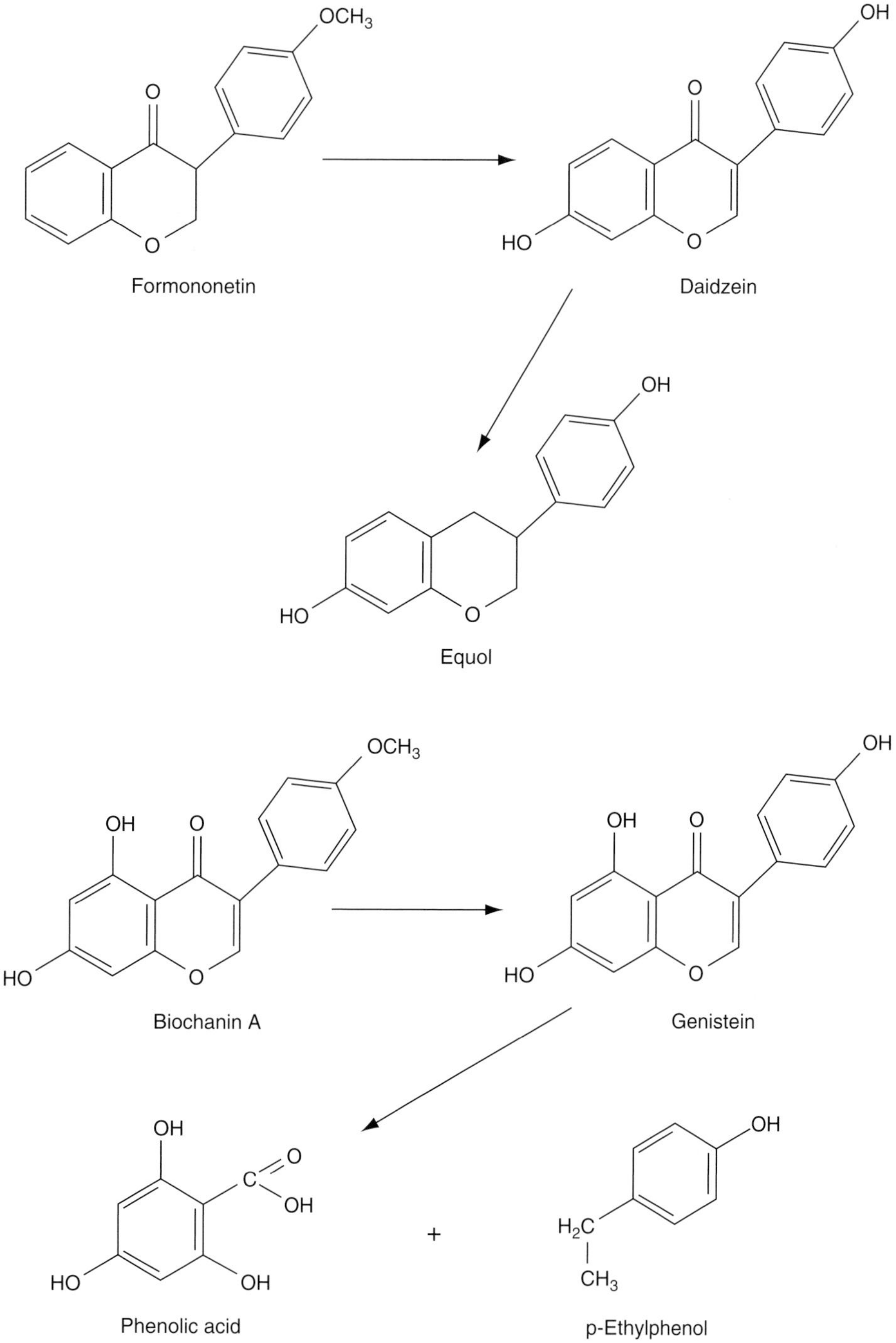

Fig. 22.5. Metabolism of subterranean clover isoflavones in the sheep rumen.

Table 22.2. Effect of formononetin content of subterranean clover on percentage of ewes lambing (from Neil *et al.*, 1974).

Year	Pasture type (% formononetin)				
	Non-oestrogenic control (0%)	Woogenellup (0.15%)	Geraldton (0.79%)	Dinninup (1.19%)	Dwalaganup (1.30%)
1	91	76	87	78	89
2	73	84	78	72	56
3	86	69	56	53	30
4	59	41	42	35	6
5	84	63	53	41	8
6	85	67	52	38	0

If sheep are bred while grazing oestrogenic pasture, fertility depression can occur. The infertility does not persist if they are subsequently maintained on non-oestrogenic pastures. This temporary infertility is especially pertinent to the coumestans. Problems in breeding have occurred with dairy cattle fed lucerne. These included decreased fertility because of cystic ovaries and irregular oestrous cycles, as well as precocious mammary and genital development in heifers. Coumestans suppress oestrus and inhibit ovulation, probably by lowering ovarian oestrogen secretion. Sheep grazing oestrogenic clover do not show the normal seasonal changes in serum luteinizing hormone (Chamley *et al.*, 1981).

The fertility and sperm production of rams does not seem to be affected by their grazing on oestrogenic pastures. Wethers may develop enlarged teats and begin lactating. Teat enlargement of wethers has been used as a sensitivity index of the potency of pastures.

An interesting situation is that phyto-oestrogens may be involved in the regulation of reproduction of California quail. Leopold *et al.* (1976) reported that during dry years, stunted desert plants produced high contents of oestrogenic isoflavones that inhibited quail reproduction. In normal or wet years, the plants grow abundantly and the levels of phyto-oestrogens are low, resulting in higher reproduction rates in the quail. Hughes (1988) has proposed an evolutionary role of phyto-oestrogens as defensive chemicals to modulate the fertility of vertebrate herbivores to limit herbivory.

Phyto-oestrogens may act as 'anti-oestrogens'. A high blood concentration of phyto-oestrogens may inhibit the release of gonadotropic hormones from the pituitary and may compete with endogenous oestrogens for receptor sites in target tissues such as the uterus and cervix.

Problems associated with phyto-oestrogens and ewe fertility in Australia are much less than they once were. A major reason has been the development of low-formononetin cultivars of sub clover. Also, animal management to limit oestrogenic exposure is practised. However, moderate depression of fertility is still observed and it has been estimated that about 4 million ewes fail to lamb each year in Australia because of phyto-oestrogen exposure (Adams, 1995). The problem will persist for many years because of the difficulty of eliminating the high-oestrogen cultivars from existing pastures. Sub clover has a high percentage of hard seeds which resist germination and therefore a reservoir of seeds of the original cultivars persists in pastures that have been newly seeded to the low-formononetin types. There is genetic variability among sheep in their susceptibility to clover-induced infertility and selection of ewes for resistance to clover disease shows promise (Croker *et al.*, 1989). Little (1996) developed a strategic grazing plan in which phyto-oestrogen levels in sub clover are monitored, with the least oestrogenic pasture reserved for young ewes, to reduce likelihood of permanent infertility.

Setchell *et al.* (1987) found that the poor reproduction of captive cheetahs in zoological parks in North America may be due in part to the effects of **phyto-oestrogens** in soybean meal used in a commercial zoo feline diet. Setchell *et al.* (1987) suggested that because cats have a low activity of liver enzymes involved in metabolism and excretion of toxins, they may be more sensitive than livestock are to plant oestrogens. Carnivores would be expected, on an evolutionary basis, to have a lower ability to detoxify plant toxins than have herbivores, which have coevolved with plants heavily defended with toxic chemicals. Thus, the inclusion of plant products such as soybean meal in diets for carnivores may have unanticipated detrimental effects.

The presence of phyto-oestrogens in diets for laboratory rodents is a common but often unrecognized problem. Diets containing soybean meal will contain isoflavones (mainly daidzein and genistein) while lucerne contains coumestrol. Many commercial rodent diets used in research contain soybean meal and/or lucerne meal. The presence of phyto-oestrogens in the control diet can compromise studies of endocrine disruptors such as environmental oestrogens (Thigpen *et al.*, 2004).

Lucerne tablets have become a common dietary supplement for humans, available in health food stores. Elakiovich and Hampton (1983) analysed three brands of commercial lucerne tablets for their phyto-oestrogen content, which ranged from 20 to 190 ppm. They warned that this level of intake, in conjunction with other extraneous oestrogen sources such as birth control pills and oestrogen replacement therapy, could be potentially harmful. The benefits, if any, of consuming lucerne tablets are unclear.

Adlercreutz (1990a,b) has proposed that the high fat, low fibre Western diet promotes a high incidence of hormone-dependent cancers, including breast, prostate and colon cancer. A Western-type diet results in elevated plasma levels of sex hormones and decreases the **steroid hormone-binding globulin (SHBG)** fraction of the blood, thus increasing the plasma concentration of free steroids (Adlercreutz *et al.*, 1987). Phyto-oestrogens in soybean products and other plant-based foods stimulate hepatic synthesis of SHBG, reducing the concentration of free steroid hormones in the blood. They may also interfere with the uptake of oestrogens at the tissue level by binding with oestrogen receptors. Thus dietary sources of phyto-oestrogens may have protective effects against oestrogen-dependent cancers (Adlercreutz *et al.*, 1991). Oestrogens have two opposing effects on cancer, depending on dosage. Large doses inhibit breast cancer tumour development and suppress growth of tumours already present, but small doses promote tumour development (Kaldas and Hughes, 1989).

Nutrition and Reproduction in Livestock

Energy intake of **beef cows** is a major determinant of reproductive efficiency. It is of particular concern in relation to oestrous cycles and initiation of pregnancy. After calving, beef cows should be rebred within 60–90 days to maintain a once-per-year calving interval. This postpartum period is one of high energy requirements to support lactation. If a cow is not able to consume sufficient feed to maintain a positive energy balance, initiation of oestrous cycling may not occur, resulting in a **prolonged calving interval**. Grazing cattle may not be able to consume a sufficient amount of forage to maintain a positive energy balance and may have a prolonged **postpartum anoestrus** period. Cows with high milk production are particularly susceptible. Short and Adams (1988) reviewed the effects of nutrition on beef-cow reproduction. The effects of energy intake appear to be mediated by blood glucose concentration, which in turn influences the release of gonadotropins that control the oestrous cycle (Richards *et al.*, 1989).

Nutrition has an effect on **dystocia** (difficult calving), although the effects are not always consistent and predictable. Very high and very low planes of nutrition for cows in late gestation are undesirable. High energy intakes cause obesity and deposition of fat in the birth canal, reducing the pelvic opening and causing dystocia. Low planes of nutrition do not necessarily reduce dystocia incidence and result in weak, less active calves and in impairment of subsequent reproduction potential of the cow.

Dairy cattle (in developed countries) are fed high energy diets, so reproduction is not normally influenced by energy intake. **Retained placenta** is a common reproductive problem in dairy cows. Deficiencies in trace nutrients have been shown to increase the incidence of retained fetal membranes in dairy cattle (LeBlanc *et al.*, 2002). Specifically, deficiencies in vitamin E and selenium have been linked to retained placenta.

Feeding fat to dairy cows results in improved reproductive performance. One mode of action is simply the provision of extra energy to prevent negative energy balance. There is a specific advantageous effect of polyunsaturated fatty acids on dairy cow reproduction, causing changes in plasma estradiol, progesterone and prostaglandins, with stimulation of ovarian follicular growth (Thomas *et al.*, 1997).

Ewes respond well to **flushing** or an improvement in nutritional status just prior to breeding. Flushing provides a dietary cue that it is a good time to reproduce because feed is abundant. Although ewe response to flushing is variable, producers can expect to improve lambing rates by 10–20% from flushing. About 2 weeks before the rams are turned in, the ewes should be put on lush grass pasture or other good quality feed, or fed about 228–454 g of grain/ewe for 2 weeks before and 2–3 weeks after breeding begins. Legume pastures, such as red clover, should not be used for flushing ewes because of the potential for **phyto-oestrogen-induced infertility**.

After breeding, ewes in the early stages of pregnancy are fed just above maintenance conditions for approximately 3.5 months on good pasture or hay. Ewe lambs bred to lamb at 12–13 months in age need to be fed at higher levels to allow for continued growth as well as fetal development. For the last third of pregnancy, the rapidly increasing size of the fetus(es) and the decreased rumen volume (Forbes, 1970) necessitate that the nutrient density of the diet be increased. During the last trimester of pregnancy, ewes are quite susceptible to ketosis, which may result in pregnancy disease (pregnancy paralysis or twin-lamb disease). **Ketosis** is caused by a metabolic shortage of glucose and excessive reliance on mobilized body lipid to meet energy requirements. These events reflect the increased metabolic requirements of the fetuses for glucose and the inability of a roughage diet to supply sufficient gluconeogenic precursor (propionate). Mobilization of body lipid produces ketogenic long-chain fatty acids coincident with impaired glucose biosynthesis. Symptoms of ketosis, such as coma, are due to inadequate blood glucose to support brain metabolism, while excess acetate from fatty acid catabolism is converted to ketones (e.g. β-hydroxybutyrate). Metabolic events associated with ketosis are discussed in Chapter 16.

Fetal growth in late pregnancy is met largely by placental transfer of maternal glucose and amino acids (Bell, 1995). These increased maternal demands are met partly by increased feed intake and partly by an array of metabolic adaptations, including increased hepatic gluconeogenesis from endogenous substances, decreased peripheral glucose utilization, increased fatty acid mobilization from adipose tissue, and increased amino acid mobilization from muscle (Bell, 1995).

There is some indication that mild feed restriction in mid-pregnancy might be desirable because overfat ewes are susceptible to feed intake reduction in late pregnancy, making them more likely to experience ketosis (Wilkinson and Chestnutt, 1988). For the last trimester of pregnancy, nutrient restrictions should be avoided since inadequate levels at this time will result in lighter lambs at birth, unequal birth weights in twins, increased perinatal lamb losses, reduced mothering instincts and lowered milk production.

With **horses**, broodmares should be in adequate body condition before breeding, as conception rate is influenced by the condition of the mare. A useful **condition-scoring** system (Henneke *et al.*, 1984) quantifies palpable fat cover over the ribs, vertebrae, pelvis, neck and shoulder to evaluate horses. The system ranks horses with a score of 1 to 9, where 1 is emaciated and 9 is obese. Broodmares should be maintained between 5 and 7, or in moderate to fleshy condition. The ribs should not be visually discernible but should be able to be felt, the back should be level to having a slight crease, and the neck and withers should blend smoothly. As with other livestock, a flushing response may be seen with animals gaining weight at the time of breeding. A good-quality roughage diet is adequate for the non-working mare during the first two trimesters. During the last trimester and during lactation, a concentrate supplement should be provided. Each horse's diet should be adjusted according to its individual needs, as assessed by body condition. Obesity in horses caused by overfeeding should be avoided. When Gill *et al.* (1985) restricted mares to 70% of protein requirements during pregnancy and lactation, birth weights were not affected, but growth rate of the foal to 90 days was reduced in the restricted group compared to mares fed at National Research Council requirements.

Reproduction in **rabbits** is influenced by nutrition. Inadequate energy intake may result in resorption of the fetuses or small, weak litters at birth. Excessively fat does will similarly have small, weak litters and poor milking ability. One of the major causes of poor reproduction during the winter is inadequate energy intake of does, often a result of limit-feeding the same amount of feed as provided in the summer. In cold-climate areas, feed intake must be increased during the winter to meet the animals' higher energy requirements. Another common source of reproductive problems is **vitamin A malnutrition**. Deficient (less than 5000 IU/kg of diet) or toxic (more than 70,000 IU/kg) amounts of vitamin A can result in fetal resorption, abortion, fetal hydrocephalus (Fig. 22.2) and small, weak, non-viable litters. Maintenance of adequate vitamin A status is complicated by variability in quality of lucerne meal, which is usually the main ingredient of rabbit diets. Green lucerne meal usually contains adequate vitamin A activity (as β-carotene) while brown or bleached lucerne is generally deficient (Cheeke, 1987). Fetal resorption or abortion in wild rabbits is an evolutionary adaptation to aid in survival of the female if feed supply becomes severely limiting. It is a superior evolutionary strategy to halt reproduction instead of putting both the female and the litter in jeopardy.

Environmental Pollutants and Reproduction

A variety of environmental pollutants have adverse effects on reproduction in wildlife (Tyler *et al.*, 1998). They primarily exert their effects through modulating or disrupting the endocrine system. Many mimic endogenous hormones in chemical structure. Synthetic (man-made) chemicals that act as hormone mimics include organochlorine pesticides (DDT and its metabolites, endosulfan, toxaphene, dieldrin), polychlorinated biphenyls (PCBs), dioxins and a further variety of industrial chemicals (Tyler *et al.*, 1998). Many of these **endocrine-disrupting chemicals** affect oestrogen and androgen metabolism. There is some evidence of declining sperm counts in humans that may be linked to environmental pollutants (Sharpe and Skakkebaek, 1993; Safe, 1995).

The reproductive effects of **DDT** and its metabolites have been extensively studied. Of particular concern have been the effects on raptors (e.g. bald eagles) at the top of the food chain and waterfowl (e.g. gulls). The primary effect is eggshell thinning and cracking, preventing successful embryo development (Colborn *et al.*, 1993). DDT induces cytochrome P_{450} activity in the liver, modifying steroid metabolism. Calcium metabolism in birds is regulated by two steroids, estradiol and vitamin D. Increased vitamin D metabolism induced by dietary DDT may modify calcium absorption with adverse effects on eggshell thickness. The adverse effects of DDT are not seen in all species of birds because of hepatic differences in cytochrome P_{450} enzymes.

Effluents from sewage treatment plants contain estradiol and estrone at concentrations sufficient to adversely affect fish reproduction (Tyler *et al.*, 1998). The primary source of these oestrogens is women, both from endogenous excretion and from contraceptive pills.

Questions and Study Guide

1. Why does phosphorus deficiency of cattle adversely affect reproduction?
2. What is the postulated role of 6-MBOA in regulating reproduction in herbivorous rodents?
3. What is the metabolic effect of vitamin E on reproduction?
4. What are the effects of vitamin A and β-carotene on reproduction?
5. Does endophyte-free tall fescue pasture adversely affect reproduction in pregnant mares? Explain.
6. What types of common feedstuffs for livestock contain phyto-oestrogens?
7. The insecticide DDT adversely affects reproduction in bald eagles and herring gulls, but when fed to chickens or quail, has no adverse effects. Explain.

References

Adams, N.R. (1989) Phytoestrogens. In: Cheeke, P.R. (ed.) *Toxicants of Plant Origin*, Vol. IV. CRC Press, Boca Raton, Florida, pp. 23–51.

Adams, N.R. (1990) Permanent infertility in ewes exposed to plant oestrogens. *Australian Veterinary Journal* 67, 197–201.

Adams, N.R. (1995) Detection of the effects of phytoestrogens on sheep and cattle. *Journal of Animal Science* 73, 1509–1515.

Adlercreutz, H., Hockerstedt, K., Bannwart, C., Bloigu, S., Hamalainen, E., Fotsis, T. and Ollus, A. (1987) Effect of dietary components, including lignans and phytoestrogens, on enterohepatic circulation and liver metabolism of estrogens and on sex hormone binding globulin (SHBG). *Journal of Steroid Biochemistry and Molecular Biology* 27, 1135–1144.

Adlercreutz, H. (1990a) Diet, breast cancer, and sex hormone metabolism. *Annals of the New York Academy of Sciences* 595, 281–290.

Adlercreutz, H. (1990b) Western diet and Western diseases: some hormonal and biochemical mechanisms and associations. *Scandanavian Journal of Clinical Laboratory Investigation* 50, 3–23.

Adlercreutz, H., Honjo, H., Higashi, A., Fotsis, T., Hamalainen, E., Hasegawa, T. and Okada, H. (1991) Urinary excretion of lignans and isoflavonoid phytoestrogens in Japanese men and women consuming a traditional Japanese diet. *American Journal of Clinical Nutrition* 54, 1093–1100.

Arechiga, C.F., Staples, C.R., McDowell, L.R. and Hansen, P.J. (1998) Effects of timed insemination and supplemental β-carotene on reproduction and milk yield of dairy cows under heat stress. *Journal of Dairy Science* 81, 390–402.

Bell, A.W. (1995) Regulation of organic nutrient metabolism during transition from late pregnancy to early lactation. *Journal of Animal Science* 73, 2804–2819.

Berger, P.J., Sanders, E.H., Gardner, P.D. and Negus, N.C. (1977) Phenolic plant compounds functioning as reproductive inhibitors in *Microtus montanus*. *Science* 195, 575–577.

Berger, P.J., Negus, N.C., Sanders, E.H. and Gardner, P.D. (1981) Chemical triggering of reproduction in *Microtus montanus*. *Science* 214, 69–70.

Boosinger, T.R., Brendemuehl, J.P., Bransby, D.L., Wright, J.C., Kemppainen, R.J. and Kee, D.D. (1995) Prolonged gestation, decreased triiodothyronine concentration, and thyroid gland histomorphologic features in newborn foals of mares grazing *Acremonion coenophialum*-infected fescue. *American Journal of Veterinary Research* 56, 66–69.

Chamley, W.A., Adams, N.R., Hooley, R.D. and Carson, R. (1981) Hypothalamic-pituitary function in normal ewes and ewes which grazed oestrogenic subterranean clover for several years. *Australian Journal of Biological Sciences* 34, 239–244.

Chase, C.C., Jr, Bastidas, P., Rutle, J.L., Long, C.R. and Randel, R.D. (1994) Growth and reproductive development in Brahman bulls fed diets containing gossypol. *Journal of Animal Science* 72, 445–452.

Cheeke, P.R. (1987) *Rabbit Feeding and Nutrition*. Academic Press, San Diego.

Cheeke, P.R. (1998) *Natural Toxicants in Feeds, Forages, and Poisonous Plants*. Prentice Hall, Upper Saddle River, New Jersey.

Chew, B.P. (1993) Effects of supplemental β-carotene and vitamin A on reproduction in swine. *Journal of Animal Science* 71, 247–252.

Colborn, T., vom Saal, F.S. and Soto, A.M. (1993) Developmental effects of endocrine-disrupting chemicals in wildlife and humans. *Environmental Health Perspectives* 101, 378–384.

Coutinho, E. (2002) Gossypol: a contraceptive for men. *Contraception* 59, 259–263.

Croker, K.P., Lightfoot, R.J., Johnson, T.J., Adams, N.R. and Carrick, M.J. (1989) The effects of selection for resistance to clover infertility on the reproductive performances of Merino ewes grazed on oestrogenic pastures. *Australian Journal of Agricultural Research* 40, 165–176.

Cross, D.L., Redmond, L.M. and Strickland, J.R. (1995) Equine fescue toxicosis: signs and solutions. *Journal of Animal Science* 73, 899–908.

Cusack, P.M.V. and Perry, V. (1995) The effect of feeding whole cottonseed on the fertility of bulls. *Australian Veterinary Journal* 72, 463–466.

Davies, H.L. and Hill, J.L. (1989) The effect of diet on the metabolism in sheep of the tritiated isoflavones formononetin and biochanin A. *Australian Journal of Agricultural Research* 40, 157–163.

Dickinson, J.M., Smith, G.R., Randel, R.D. and Pemberton, I.J. (1988) *In vitro* metabolism of for-

mononetin and biochanin A in bovine rumen fluid. *Journal of Animal Science* 66, 1969–1973.

Elakiovich, S.D. and Hampton, J.M. (1983) Analysis of coumestrol, a phytoestrogen, in alfalfa tablets sold for human consumption. *Journal of Agricultural and Food Chemistry* 32, 173–175.

Forbes, J.M. (1970) Voluntary food intake of pregnant ewes. *Journal of Animal Science* 31, 1222–1227.

Gill, R.J., Potter, G.D., Kreider, J.L., Schelling, G.T., Jenkins, W.L. and Hines, K.K. (1985) Nitrogen status and postpartum pH levels of mares fed varying levels of protein. *Proceedings of Equine Nutrition and Physiology Society Symposium* 9, 84–86.

Gray, M.L., Greene, L.W. and Williams, G.L. (1993) Effects of dietary gossypol consumption on metabolic homeostasis and reproductive endocrine function in beef heifers and cows. *Journal of Animal Science* 71, 3052–3059.

Henneke, D.R., Potter, G.D. and Kreider, J.L. (1984) Body condition during pregnancy and lactation and reproductive efficiency of mares. *Theriogenology* 21, 897–900.

Hron, R.J., Koltun, S.P., Pominski, J. and Abraham, G. (1987) The potential commercial aspects of gossypol. *Journal of the American Oil Chemists' Society* 64, 1315–1319.

Hughes, C.L., Jr (1988) Phytochemical mimicry of reproductive hormones and modulation of herbivore fertility by phytoestrogens. *Environmental Health Perspectives* 78, 171–175.

Ireland, F.A., Loch, W.E., Worthy, K. and Anthony, R.V. (1991) Effects of bromocriptine and perphenazine on prolactin and progesterone concentrations in pregnant pony mares during late gestation. *Journal of Reproduction and Fertility* 92, 179–186.

Jimbow, K., Fitzpatrick, T.B. and Quevedo, W.C., Jr (1986) Formation, chemical composition and function of melanin pigments. In: Bereiter-Hahn, J., Matoltsy, A.G. and Richards, K.S. (eds) *Biology of the Integument*, Vol. 2, *Invertebrates*. Springer-Verlag, Berlin, pp. 278–291.

Kaldas, R.S. and Hughes, C.L., Jr (1989) Reproductive and general metabolic effects of phytoestrogens in mammals. *Reproductive Toxicology* 3, 81–89.

Karn, J.F. (2001) Phosphorus nutrition of grazing cattle: a review. *Animal Feed Science and Technology* 89, 133–153.

LeBlanc, S.J., Duffield, T.F., Leslie, K.E., Bateman, K.G., TenHag, J., Walton, J.S. and Johnson, W.H. (2002) The effect of prepartum injection of vitamin E on health in transition dairy cows. *Journal of Dairy Science* 85, 1416–1426.

Leopold, A.S., Erwin, M., Oh, J. and Browning, B. (1976) Phytoestrogens. Adverse effects on reproduction in California quail. *Science* 191, 98–99.

Little, D.L. (1996) Reducing the effects of clover disease by strategic grazing of pastures. *Australian Veterinary Journal* 73, 192–193.

Livingston, L. (1978) Forage plant estrogens. *Journal of Toxicology and Environmental Health* 4, 301–324.

Lundh, T.J.-O. (1990) Conjugation of the plant estrogens formononetin and daidzein and their metabolite equol by gastrointestinal epithelium from cattle and sheep. *Journal of Agricultural and Food Chemistry* 38, 1012–1016.

Lundh, T. (1995) Metabolism of estrogenic isoflavones in domestic animals. *Proceedings of the Society for Experimental Biology and Medicine* 208, 33–39.

Lundh, T.J.-O., Pettersson, H.I. and Martinsson, K.A. (1990) Comparative levels of free and conjugated plant estrogens in blood plasma of sheep and cattle fed estrogenic silage. *Journal of Agricultural and Food Chemistry* 38, 1530–1534.

McCann, J.S., Caudle, A.B., Thompson, F.N., Stuedemann, J.A., Heusner, G.L. and Thompson, D.L., Jr (1992) Influence of endophyte-infected tall fescue on serum prolactin and progesterone in gravid mares. *Journal of Animal Science* 70, 217–223.

Neil, H.G., Lightfoot, R.J. and Fels, H.E. (1974) Effect of legume species on ewe fertility in South Western Australia. *Proceedings of the Australian Society of Animal Production* 10, 136.

Paterson, J., Forcherio, C., Larson, B., Samford, M. and Kerley, M. (1995) The effects of fescue toxicosis on beef cattle productivity. *Journal of Animal Science* 73, 889–898.

Porter, J.K. and Thompson, F.N., Jr (1992) Effects of fescue toxicosis on reproduction in livestock. *Journal of Animal Science* 70, 1594–1603.

Putnam, M.R., Brendemuehl, J.P., Boosinger, T.R., Bransby, D.I., Kee, D.D., Schumacher, J. and Shelby, R.A. (1990) The effect of short term exposure to and removal from the fescue endophyte *Acremonium coenophialum* on pregnant mares and foal viability. In: Quisenberry, S.S. and Joost, R.E. (eds) *Proceedings of the International Symposium on Acremonium/ Grass Interactions*. Louisiana Agricultural Experiment Station, Baton Rouge, Louisiana, pp. 255–258.

Putnam, M.R., Bransby, D.I., Schumacher, J., Boosinger, T.R., Bush, L., Shelby, R.A., Vaughan, J.T., Ball, D. and Brendemuehl, J.P. (1991) Effects of the fungal endophyte *Acremonium coenophialum* in fescue on pregnant mares and foal viability. *American Journal of Veterinary Research* 52, 2071–2074.

Randel, R.D., Chase, C.C., Jr and Wyse, S.J. (1992) Effects of gossypol and cottonseed products on reproduction of mammals. *Journal of Animal Science* 70, 1628–1638.

Redmond, L.M., Cross, D.L., Strickland, J.R. and Kennedy, S.W. (1994) Efficacy of domperiodone and sulpiride as treatments for fescue toxicosis in horses. *American Journal of Veterinary Research* 55, 722–729.

Regisford, E.G.C. and Katz, L.S. (1994) Effects of bromocriptine treatment on the expression of sexual behavior in male sheep (*Ovis aries*). *Journal of Animal Science* 72, 591–597.

Richards, M.W., Wettemann, R.P. and Schoenemann, H.M. (1989) Nutritional anestrus in beef cows: concentrations of glucose and nonesterified fatty acids in plasma and insulin in serum. *Journal of Animal Science* 67, 2354–2362.

Riet-Correa, F., Mendez, M.C., Schild, A.L., Bergamo, P.N. and Flores, W.N. (1988) Agalactica, reproductive problems and neonatal mortality in horses associated with the ingestion of *Claviceps purpurea*. *Australian Veterinary Journal* 65, 192–193.

Safe, S.H. (1995) Environmental and dietary estrogens and human health: is there a problem? *Environmental Health Perspectives* 103, 346–351.

Sanders, E.H., Gardner, P.D., Berger, P.J. and Negus, N.C. (1981) 6-methoxybenzox-azolinone: a plant derivative that stimulates reproduction in *Microtus montanus*. *Science* 214, 67–69.

Setchell, K.D.R., Gosselin, S.J., Welsh, M.B., Johnston, J.O., Balistreri, W.F., Kramer, L.W., Dresser, B.L. and Tarr, M.J. (1987) Dietary estrogens: a probable cause of infertility and liver disease in captive cheetahs. *Gastroenterology* 93, 225–233.

Sharpe, R.P. and Skakkebaek, N.E. (1993) Are oestrogens involved in falling sperm counts and disorders of the male reproductive tract? *Lancet* 341, 1392–1395.

Short, R.E. and Adams, D.C. (1988) Nutritional and hormonal interrelationships in beef cattle reproduction. *Canadian Journal of Animal Science* 68, 29–39.

Thigpen, J.E., Setchell, K.D.R., Saunders, H.E., Haseman, J.K., Grant, M.G. and Forsythe, D.B. (2004) Selecting the appropriate rodent diet for endocrine disruptor research and testing studies. *International League of Associations for Rheumatology Journal* 45, 401–416.

Thomas, M.G., Bao, B. and Williams, G.L. (1997) Dietary fats varying in their fatty acid composition differentially influence follicular growth in cows fed isoenergetic diets. *Journal of Animal Science* 75, 2512–2519.

Tyler, C.R., Jobling, S. and Sumpter, J.P. (1998) Endocrine disruption in wildlife: a critical review of the evidence. *Critical Reviews in Toxicology* 28, 319–361.

Waites, G.M.H., Wang, C. and Griffin, P.D. (1998) Gossypol: reasons for its failure to be accepted as a safe, reversible male antifertility drug. *International Journal of Andrology* 21, 8–12.

Wang, W., Tanaka, Y., Han, Z. and Cheng, J. (1994) Radioimmunoassay for quantitative analysis of formononetin in blood plasma and rumen fluid of wethers fed red clover. *Journal of Agricultural and Food Chemistry* 42, 1584–1587.

Weiss, W.P. (1998) Requirements of fat-soluble vitamins for dairy cows: a review. *Journal of Dairy Science* 81, 2493–2501.

Wilkinson, S.C. and Chestnutt, D.M.B. (1988) Effect of level of food intake in mid and late pregnancy on the performance of breeding ewes. *Animal Production* 47, 411–419.

23 Nutrition and Immunity in Ruminants

NEIL E. FORSBERG,[1] YONGQIANG WANG,[1]
STEVEN B. PUNTENNEY[1] AND JEFFERY A. CARROLL[2]

[1]OmniGen Research, Corvallis, Oregon, USA; [2]USDA-ARS, Livestock Issues
Research Unit, Lubbock, Texas, USA

Introduction

Nutrition has an impact on every physiological process in the body. Hence, it should not be surprising that nutrition also has important implications on immunity and incidence of disease. While scientists have known for many years that nutrition influences immunity, only in recent years have specific mechanisms by which nutrients affect immunity become apparent. The purpose of this chapter will be to acquaint readers with some general concepts of immunology and to review what is now known about how specific nutrients benefit the immune system of ruminant livestock.

General Concepts of Immunology

The immune system can be generally separated into three broad components: (i) natural immunity; (ii) innate immunity; and (iii) acquired immunity. All of these must be fully developed and functioning properly to provide adequate immunological protection. Natural and innate immunity are typically grouped together under the category of innate immunity. Therefore, for this chapter, the immune system will be presented as two distinct 'arms' which work in tandem to prevent infections. These are the 'innate' immune system and the 'acquired' immune system (Janeway et al., 2005). The innate immune system, as its name implies, consists of readily available mechanisms that 'fight' the first stages of infection. This system essentially provides the first line of defence against pathogens, whether bacterial, viral, protozoal or fungal. By providing this front-line barrier, the innate system provides the time required by the acquired system to develop an antibody response against a specific pathogen.

Developing the antibodies against specific pathogens requires several days to several weeks.

Innate immunity

The innate immune system is an evolutionarily ancient mechanism to fight disease and represents the antigen-non-specific defence mechanisms of the immune system that is elicited immediately or within several hours (0–4 h) after exposure to an antigen. It consists of several anatomic, physiologic and cellular components. Anatomic aspects include the epithelial barriers to infection provided by the skin, lung, mammary and gastrointestinal tract. Secretion of hydrochloric acid and digestive enzymes by the gastrointestinal tract also aids in preventing entry of pathogens into the body. Complement is also considered a component of innate immunity. But, in addition to these, animals possess a cellular component of innate immunity. The cellular component consists of phagocytic cells (e.g. neutrophils and macrophages) that are activated at sites of infection and then attack and kill pathogens before pathogens have the opportunity to proliferate and cause a significant infection.

The term 'innate immunity' implies that it is stable or unwavering. But, this is not the case. Innate immunity, although always present to some degree, is regulated and may be 'strengthened' or 'weakened' by a number of factors including wounds, dehydration, nutritional status, genetics and even stress.

Innate immunity is a non-selective immune system. It does not modify itself depending upon the type of pathogen challenge. Instead, it prevents infection by targeting general properties of pathogens. For example, few pathogens can withstand the low pH of the stomach (abomasum) and most should be digested by the digestive enzymes of the gastrointestinal tract. In fact, the majority of organisms encountered by an animal on a daily basis do not cause disease under normal circumstances as they are readily detected and eliminated by the innate immune system.

The cellular component of innate immunity identifies pathogens by their presentation of distinct 'pathogen-associated molecular patterns' (PAMPs; Janeway *et al.*, 2005). Specifically, pathogens contain molecules not typically found in mammalian cells and via this strategy cells of the innate system are able to recognize invading pathogens. Examples of molecules associated with pathogens which are recognized by innate cells include lipotechoic acid, double-stranded RNA, CpG DNA sequences and unusual sugar residues (e.g. mannans) among others. Binding of PAMPs to Toll-like receptors initiates killing mechanisms by the neutrophils and macrophages. In all, it is estimated that the innate immune system recognizes approximately 10^3 molecular patterns.

Acquired (adaptive) immunity

The second arm of the immune system is termed the 'adaptive system' and is characterized by the production of antibodies which are directed against specific antigens (Janeway *et al.*, 2005). The use of vaccines to protect animals from various pathogens is an example of acquired immunity. Acquired immunity can be classified as either cell-mediated or humoral immunity. Cell-mediated immunity represents the immunological response associated with immune cells which act directly against pathogen-infected cells. Humoral immunity on the other hand involves the generation of specific antibodies that are directed against the invading pathogens. Acquired immunity requires the involvement of specialized white blood cells (T and B cells), various cytokines and antibodies to provide long-term immunological protection. The T cells, which develop in the thymus, provide cell-mediated immunity and are divided into two groups: (i) the T-helper (T_H) cells; and (ii) cytotoxic T-lymphocytes (CTLs). The T_H cells produce cytokines to help the other T and B cells to grow and divide, and grow and divide themselves to produce more cells to fight future infections. The CTLs are responsible for destroying pathogen-infected cells. Pathogens can be phagocytosed and digested by antigen-presenting cells

(e.g. macrophages, B lymphocytes and dendritic cells). Digested pieces of pathogens are presented on the surface of the antigen-presenting cell to T_H cells. The T_H cells may then stimulate clonal expansion of a B-cell lineage which then secretes antibodies. Alternatively, the T_H cell, in response to a cytokine termed 'interleukin-2 (IL-2)', will develop into a CTL. CTLs express antibodies (T receptors) tethered to their cell surface and can mediate destruction of cells infected with a pathogen.

Antibodies may take on a variety of forms and are referred to as immunoglobulins (Ig). The most common Ig are IgM and IgG. IgMs are the first antibodies to be produced by the immune system in response to an infection. Although they 'arrive on the scene' as the first antibody type following an infection, they possess relatively low affinity against antigen. The more-specific IgG isotypes (IgG1, IgG2, IgG3 and IgG4) require additional time for their development.

Relationship of the innate and acquired immune system

Discussion of innate and acquired arms of the immune system separately implies that these systems function independently. However, we now know that the two arms communicate with one another and, to some extent, rely upon similar communication molecules. Up-regulation of the innate system provides an important feed-forward system for antibody production. For example, activation of neutrophils by an invading pathogen causes neutrophils to release IL-1β which, in turn, stimulates the acquired system.

Nutrition and Immunology

Methodology

A challenge facing those with interest in the interface between nutrition and immunity is: what are the best predictors of immune status? 'Immunity' is an extremely broad concept and there are literally dozens of methods available for assessing immune function. No one laboratory is capable of completing all assays of immunity and, as a result, it is often difficult to make comparisons from one study to the next. The general strategies which have been used to assess impact of a treatment or nutrient on immune function have included the following (Chew and Park, 2004).

Immunoglobulin production

One may assess total IgM and IgG concentrations in blood as indexes of immunity. These do not provide very definitive information on immunity, however, because the total IgM or IgG fraction represents the combined titre against all antigens to which an organism has been exposed. Nutritionists should be wary of studies which examine total IgG or IgM responses. More useful information is derivable from titre.

Titre

Titre provides specific insight into concentrations of antibodies (whether IgM or IgG) directed towards a specific antigen.

Immune cell proliferation

T and B cells can be induced to proliferate by the addition of specific chemicals (mitogens) to their environment. The rate of cell division induced by a mitogen provides an index of the ability of the humoral immune system to 'ramp-up' following an infection. Typical mitogens added to stimulate T- and B-cell division include poke weed mitogen and lipopolysaccharide.

Killing activity of lymphocytes (lymphocyte cytotoxic assay)

This assay determines the ability of T cells to kill target cells.

Cytokine production

Communication among cells which mediate immunity is carried out by a large number of hormones called 'cytokines'. Common signalling cytokines include IL-1, IL-2, IL-4, IL-5, IL-6, IL-10, **tumour necrosis factor-alpha (TNF-α)** and **interferon-gamma (IFN-γ)**. Measuring concentrations of cytokines in biological samples can provide useful information on activities of specific aspects of the immune system.

Delayed-type hypersensitivity (DTH) assay

A standard means of assessing a cell-mediated immune response is to perform a DTH test, which is done by injecting an antigen of interest intradermally and then determining if there is a delayed induration (swelling reaction at the site). The degree of DTH reactivity is determined in humans and guinea pigs by the diameter of induration 48 h after antigen injection or in mice by the amount of ear or footpad swelling 24 h after antigen injection (Nichols et al., 2002).

Molecular diagnostics

Availability of genomic sequences for pathogens and new molecular screening techniques have given rise to methods which assess specific components of immunity.

Nutrition and immunity

Calder and Kew (2002) published a review on nutrients with known effects on immunity. In non-ruminants, essential amino acids, linoleic acid, vitamin A, folic acid, vitamin B_6, vitamin B_{12}, vitamin C, vitamin E, zinc, copper, iron and selenium affect one or more indexes of immunity (Calder and Kew, 2002). Tam et al. (2003) have also published a review on potential roles of magnesium in support of the immune system. Vitamin E and zinc have received the most attention as immunostimulatory nutrients (Calder and Kew, 2002).

The most recent essential nutrient with reported benefit to the immune system is vitamin D. Liu et al. (2006) recently reported a link between Toll-like receptors and vitamin D-mediated innate immunity and suggested that differences in ability of human populations to produce vitamin D may contribute to susceptibility to microbial infection. Since this original report, dozens of studies on the relationship of vitamin D and immunity have now been completed. A Pubmed search using the keywords of 'vitamin D and immunity' in early 2010 yielded 601 peer-reviewed articles; 187 since 2006.

Less is known about the nutritional regulation of immunity in ruminant livestock. But, it may safely be assumed that nutrients, at the tissue level, will have similar effects on immunity in ruminants as in non-ruminants. Perhaps dietary sources of the immunostimulatory B-vitamins (B_6, B_{12}, folic acid), vitamin C and the essential amino acids are less important in ruminants as these are either endogenously synthesized (i.e. vitamin C) or provided by a healthy microbial population (i.e. essential amino acids, B-vitamins). Spears (2000) reported that selenium, vitamin E, chromium, cobalt, copper and vitamin A have immune regulatory properties in cattle.

Energy usage and immune responses

While activation of physiological processes within the animal in response to an immunological challenge is necessary for survival, there is an associated energy cost which reduces the overall productivity potential. Indeed, creating and maintaining a febrile response alone is very energy intensive. It has been estimated that there is approximately a 10–15% increase in energy usage for every degree of body temperature increase associated with an immune response. Additional energy, above and beyond that necessary for the febrile response, is required for processes such as increased production of inflammatory cytokines, acute phase proteins and antibody formation. Information of the precise energetic requirements of immunity in ruminant animals is lacking. However, an older study in humans (Shizgal and Martin, 1988) reported that sepsis in humans resulted in a 44% increase in energy requirement. Based on this, one would expect that severe infections in ruminants (e.g. mastitis, metritis) would be similarly calorically expensive. In an effort to compensate for these direct energy requirements, animals will display various behavioural responses such as increased sleep, decreased social activity, decreased sexual behaviour and decreased foraging in an effort to conserve energy. Additionally, there are various metabolic changes which occur relative to glucocorticoid and norepinephrine activity which take place in an effort to liberate energy in response to illness. While these behavioural and metabolic responses aid in the animal's effort to conserve energy, they have an overall negative impact on productivity. Utilizing energy resources to mount an adequate immunological response limits the energy that could otherwise be used for other economically important biological functions such as growth, reproduction and lactation. However, the reality is that activation of the immune system is necessary to prevent disease within the animal, and without diverting nutrients to support immunological functions, there would be significant economic losses associated with death loss, decreased feed efficiency and reduced average daily gain.

How do specific nutrients affect immunity in dairy cattle?

A general mechanism by which nutrients support the immune system is via provision of antioxidants. Immune cells are characterized by high levels of reactive oxygen species (ROS) which are used, in part, to kill ingested pathogens. In addition to high ROS generation, immune cell membranes are rich in the poly-unsaturated fatty acids which are susceptible to ROS-mediated damage (Chew and Park, 2004). Nutrients with antioxidant properties (carotenes, vitamin E, vitamin C, zinc and selenium), therefore, support immunity. A brief summary of how individual nutrients affect immune function in ruminants is given below.

Carotenoids

Carotenoids are plant pigments and antioxidants that include β-carotene, lutein, canthaxanthin, lycopene and astaxanthin (Chew and Park, 2004). Carotenoids (i.e. β-carotene) have traditionally been viewed as a source of vitamin A via the cleavage of β-carotene precursor into active forms of vitamin A. However, carotenoids have immunostimulatory properties independent of their roles as precursors of vitamin A. Bendich and Shapiro (1986) were the first to document immunostimulatory properties of carotenoids. Specifically, they reported that canthaxanthin increased mitogenstimulated lymphocyte proliferation in rats. Since then, many additional projects have documented mechanisms by which carotenoids, independent of vitamin A, benefit immunity. In dairy cattle, for example, supplementation with β-carotene at dryoff reduced mammary gland infections (Chew, 1987). β-Carotene increased lymphocyte blastogenesis (Daniel et al., 1990) and increased neutrophil killing activity (Tjoelker et al., 1988; Michal et al., 1994).

Vitamin E and selenium

Vitamin E and selenium play overlapping and essential roles in support of the immune system in ruminant animals. A large portion of the benefits of these nutrients is related to their functions as antioxidants. Feeding supplementary selenium to ruminant animals reduces incidence of diseases (including intra-mammary infections: e.g. Smith et al., 1984) and several studies have identified potential mechanisms. For example, Hogan et al. (1990) reported that selenium enhanced neutrophil killing activity. Maddox et al. (1999) have reported that selenium deficiency increases neutrophil adherence, and Spears (2000) has speculated that altered adherence could affect ability of neutrophils to attack and sequester pathogen. Politas et al. (1995) reported that vitamin E prevented the peripartum reduction in neutrophil superoxide anion production and impaired IL-1 production by monocytes. Two studies have reported that vitamin E supplementation increases lymphocyte proliferation (Reddy et al., 1986; Garber et al., 1996) and Cao et al. (1992) reported that selenium and vitamin E increased antibody responses of dairy cattle. Parnousis et al. (2001) reported that injection of selenium either alone or in combination with vitamin E significantly improved the production of specific antibodies against E. coli, and that the production of specific antibodies was greater after the administration of selenium alone. These two nutrients have shown the most consistent effects on the ruminant immune system.

Omega-3 (ω-3) and -6 (ω-6) fatty acids

Dietary fatty acids can affect immunity through the production of the cytokines (Lessard et al., 2003). A mechanism by which fatty acids affect immunity is through production of eicosenoids (e.g. prostaglandins) and leukotrienes. Diets rich in the ω-6 fatty acids, such as linoleic acid (C18:2), lead to the formation of **arachidonic acid** whereas diets rich in the ω-3 fatty acids (such as linolenic acid, C18:3, flaxseed and fish oils) lead to the formation of, for example, **eicosapentaenoic acid (EPA)**. Eicosenoids synthesized from arachidonic acid tend to have strong inflammatory potential whereas those synthesized from EPA have lesser potential. Hence, feeding fatty acid mixtures which are enriched in the ω-3 fatty acids reduces inflammatory reactions and reduces production of pro-inflammatory cytokines including IL-1, IL-6 and TNF-α.

Several studies have examined the value of feeding flaxseed, a source of ω-3 fatty acids, on dairy immune function. Petit and Trawiramungu (2002) reported that flaxseed modified **prostaglandin (PG)** production and reproduction. Another study (Lessard et al., 2003) reported that flaxseed increased progesterone and PGE_4 concentrations but did not have consistent effects on other indexes of immunity (proliferation responses of lymphocytes, titre to ovalbumin immunization, IFN-γ or PGE_2). In the third study Lessard et al. (2004) re-investigated effects of flaxseed on markers of immune function during the periparturient period. They documented that transition was associated with reduced lymphocyte proliferation in response to mitogen stimulation. Furthermore, transition was associated with reduced IFN-γ and increased TNF-α and **nitric oxide (NO)**. Modulation of the dietary ω-3:ω-6 ratio with flaxseed had limited effects on these parameters and the authors concluded that more work was needed to fully explore the potential for use of fatty acids to regulate immunity in dairy cattle.

Diets enriched in the ω-3 fatty acids have been introduced into the pet food market as a strategy to reduce inflammation and a product with bypass of high ω-3:ω-6 ratios is available for improving reproduction in dairy cattle. However, there is not yet enough information on the value of modifying fatty acids in ruminants as a strategy to benefit immunity.

Chromium

Spears (2000) has reviewed studies on the value of adding chromium to livestock diets vis-à-vis immune health. Individual studies have yielded conflicting results which Spears (2000) attributed to variations in chromium status, supplementation protocol and to physiological states of animals.

Several studies have indicated that supplementation of chromium to dairy cattle, in a biologically available form (e.g. chromium–amino acid complex or chromium-yeast), benefits immunity. For example, Burton et al. (1993) reported increased concanavalin A-induced blastogenesis in chromium-supplemented periparturient cattle. Chang et al. (1994) reported increased blastogenesis in lymphocytes recovered from sick calves. However, this effect was not detected in lymphocytes taken from healthy calves. Burton et al. (1993) reported that chromium increased development of titre to ovalbumin immunization and in 1994 reported increased titre in chromium-supplemented cows following immunization with infectious bovine rhinotracheitis virus (IBRV) antigen (but not parainfluenza virus Type 3). More recently, Fladyna et al. (2003) reported that chromium, fed as a chelate, increased IgG2 antibody response to tetanus toxoid.

Many studies have reported that chromium supplementation did not affect immune parameters (as cited in Spears, 2000). A common theme among studies which *have* detected a benefit to chromium supplementation may be the presence of a stressor (shipping, parturition, weaning). It is possible that stress and consequent immunosuppression are required for clear benefits of chromium supplementation to be detected.

Copper

Natural copper deficiency increases susceptibility of ruminant animals to disease (Spears, 2000). However, experimental models of copper deficiency often fail to increase incidence of disease. Several studies have investigated effects of copper on immunity in ruminant animals. It should not be surprising that copper supports immunity as it is associated with many proteins. However, specific studies have yielded equivocal results (Spears, 2000). Some studies have shown that supplementation of copper-deficient diets augments markers of immune function whereas others do not. Mechanisms by which copper specifically supports immune function have not been described in ruminants.

Jones and Suttle (1981) published one of the first studies with ruminant animals which indicated that copper supports immunity. Specifically, copper increased neutrophil killing activity of a common mould: *Candida albicans*. Low copper status reduced mitogen-stimulated blastogenesis following weaning and IBRV challenge (Wright *et al.*, 2000). Ward *et al.* (1997) reported that copper enhanced cell-mediated immunity (DTH-response) and Salyer *et al.* (2004) reported that neither supplemental copper nor zinc affected performance or morbidity of lightweight, newly received heifers; however, the source of both copper and zinc affected the humoral immune response to ovalbumin immunization. Beyond these studies, there are few which directly implicate copper in immune function and many which have produced equivocal results (Spears, 2000).

Zinc

In a recent review, Rink and Gabriel (2000) summarized the known effects of zinc on immunity in non-ruminants. Specific roles that zinc plays in support of immunity are plentiful, well established and too numerous to report in this brief review. However, it should not be surprising that zinc plays an essential role as an 'immunonutrient' as it is associated with over 300 proteins. Clearly, a zinc deficiency has opportunity to impact a large number of cellular events which might compromise immunity.

As one example, zinc plays an important role in transcriptional control through its action as a zinc-finger motif. Cells deficient in zinc have reduced ability to proliferate. The immune response requires rapid proliferation of cells (e.g. T and B lymphocytes) in response to specific antigens and, therefore, zinc deficiency prevents this aspect of immunity from developing.

Spears (2000) reported that, in contrast to studies with humans and laboratory animals, marginal zinc deficiency has little effect on immune function in ruminant animals but that zinc supplementation may be beneficial. For example, Salyer *et al.* (2004) reported increased antibody response to a bioavailable zinc supplement when fed to beef heifers and Galyean *et al.* (1995) reported that morbidity from respiratory diseases was reduced by addition of zinc to weaned calf diets.

Novel Nutritional Strategies to Augment Immunity

In addition to providing adequate amounts of all essential vitamins and minerals, other opportunities may exist for augmentation of immune function. Provision of microbiological fractions (cell wall fractions) and probiotics (live microorganisms) in the diet have potential to support the immune system. Although it is not fully clear how this form of nutritional supplementation benefits the immune system, it is possible it includes Toll-like receptor signalling in the gastrointestinal tract (Harris *et al.*, 2006). Wang *et al.* (2007, 2009) have hypothesized that these products increase gastrointestinal signalling via Toll-like receptor signalling that feeds forward and increases immune function. **Toll-like receptors** are membrane receptors that recognize molecules derived from microbes after they have breached physical barriers such as the skin or gut mucosa. They have a key role in the innate immune system. Their name derives from their similarity to the Toll gene first identified in *Drosophila*.

Little research has been completed on biochemical mechanisms by which novel feed supplements may benefit the ruminant immune system. A series of studies on how one product (OmniGen-AF) alters innate immunity in ruminant livestock has been completed (Wang *et al.*, 2007, 2009) and has demonstrated that neutrophil function is enhanced by the provision of the additive. Specifically, molecular markers of neutrophil function (L-selectin, interleukin-1β, interleukin converting enzyme and interleukin-8 receptor) are all up-regulated on neutrophils as a result of feeding this product. Microarray analysis confirmed the increased expression of neutrophil genes involved in signal transduction and in apoptosis in animals fed this product (Wang *et al.*, 2009).

Conclusion

The 20th century focused on discovery of the nutrients and identification of their roles in biology. In the past two decades, the field of immunology has emerged as a dominant field in animal health and it is now clear that the traditional nutrients play key roles in supporting the immune system. As we learn more about signalling and control of immune function, it is likely that additional nutritional strategies will be utilized to maintain and support immune function and health of livestock species.

Questions and Study Guide

1. What is the difference between innate immunity and acquired immunity?
2. How do cells of the innate immune system recognize invading pathogens?
3. What are the limitations of IgM and IgG as measures of immune status?
4. Why does the febrile response (fever) increase energy requirements?
5. Why is the metabolic requirement for antioxidants increased when the immune system is activated? What are the nutrients with antioxidant activity?
6. How might the favourable immune responses with supplementary chromium be explained by the metabolic roles of chromium?

References

Bendich, A. and Shapiro, S.S. (1986) Effect of β-carotene and canthaxanthin on the immune response of the rat. *Journal of Nutrition* 116, 2254–2262.

Burton, J.L., Mallard, B.A. and Mowat, D.N. (1993) Effects of supplemental chromium on immune responses of periparturient and early lactation dairy cows. *Journal of Animal Science* 71, 1532–1539.

Burton, J.L., Mallard, B.A. and Mowat, D.N. (1994) Effects of supplemental chromium on antibody responses of newly weaned feedlot calves to immunization with infectious bovine rhinotracheitis and parainfluenza 3 virus. *Canadian Journal of Animal Science* 58, 148–151.

Calder, P.C. and Kew, S. (2002) The immune system: a target for functional foods? *British Journal of Nutrition* 88(Supplement 2), S165–S177.

Cao, Y., Maddox, J.F., Mastro, A.M., Scholz, R.W., Hildenbrandt, G. and Reddy, C.C. (1992) Selenium deficiency alters the lipoxygenase pathway and mitogenic response of bovine lymphocytes. *Journal of Nutrition* 122, 2121–2127.

Chang, X., Mallard, B.A. and Mowat, D.N. (1994) Proliferation of peripheral blood lymphocytes of feeder calves in response to chromium. *Nutrition Research* 14, 851–864.

Chew, B.P. (1987) Vitamin A and carotene on host defense. *Journal of Animal Science* 70, 2732–2743.

Chew, B.P. and Park, J.S. (2004) Carotenoid action on the immune response. *Journal of Nutrition* 134, 257S–261S.

Daniel, L.R., Chew, B., Tanaka, T.S. and Tjoelker, L.W. (1990) β-Carotene and vitamin A effects on bovine phagocyte function during the periparturient period. *Journal of Dairy Science* 74, 124–133.

Faldyna, M., Pechova, A. and Krejci, J. (2003) Chromium supplementation enhances antibody response to vaccination with tetanus toxoid in cattle. *Journal of Veterinary Medicine B, Infectious Diseases and Veterinary Public Health* 7, 326–331.

Galyean, M.L., Malcolm-Callis, K.J., Gunter, S.A. and Berrie, R.A. (1995) Effect of zinc source and level and added copper lysine in the receiving diet on performance by growing and finishing steers. *Professional Animal Scientist* 11, 139–148.

Garber, M.J., Roeder, R.A., Davidson, P.M., Pumfey, W.M. and Schelling, G.T. (1996) Dose-response effects of vitamin E supplementation on growth performance and meat characteristics on beef and dairy steers. *Canadian Journal of Animal Science* 76, 63–72.

Harris, P., Bailey, S.R., Elliott, J. and Longland, A. (2006) Countermeasures for pasture-associated laminitis

---

in ponies and horses. *Journal of Nutrition* 136, 2114S–2121S.

Hogan, J.S., Smith, K.L., Weiss, W.P., Todhunter, D.A. and Schockley, W.L. (1990) Relationships among vitamin E, selenium and bovine blood neutrophils. *Journal of Dairy Science* 73, 2372–2378.

Janeway, C.A., Travers, P., Walport, M. and Shlomchik, M.J. (2005) *Immunobiology: the Immune System in Health and Disease.* Garland Publishing, New York.

Jones, D.G. and Suttle, N.F. (1981) Some effects of copper deficiency on leukocyte function in sheep and cattle. *Research in Veterinary Sciences* 31, 151–156.

Lessard, M., Gagnon, N. and Petit, H.V. (2003) Immune responses of postpartum dairy cows fed flaxseed. *Journal of Dairy Science* 86, 2647–2657.

Lessard, M., Gagnon, N., Godson, D.L. and Petit, H.V. (2004) Influence of parturition and diets enriched in *n*-3 or *n*-6 polyunsaturated fatty acids on immune response of dairy cows during the transition period. *Journal of Dairy Science* 87, 2197–2210.

Liu, P.T., Stenger, S., Li, H., Wenzel, L., Tan, B.H., Krutzik, S.R., Ochoa, M.T., Schauber, J., Wu, K., Meinken, C., Kamen, D.L., Wagner, M., Bals, R., Steinmeyer, A., Zügel, U., Gallo, R.L., Eisenberg, D., Hewison, M., Hollis, B.W., Adams, J.S., Bloom, B.R. and Modlin, R.L. (2006) Toll-like receptor triggering of a vitamin D-mediated human antimicrobial response. *Science* 311(5768), 1770–1773.

Maddox, J.F., Aherne, K.M., Reddy, C.C. and Sordillo, L.M. (1999) Increased neutrophil adherence and adhesion molecule mRNA expression in endothelial cells during selenium deficiency. *Journal of Leukocyte Biology* 65, 658–664.

Michal, J.J., Chew, B., Wong, T.S., Heirman, L.R. and Standaert, F.E. (1994) Modulatory effects of dietary β-carotene on blood and mammary leukocyte function in peripartum dairy cows. *Journal of Dairy Science* 77, 1408–1422.

Nichols, K.L., Bauman, S.K., Schafer, F.B. and Murphy, J.W. (2002) Differences in components at delayed-type hypersensitivity reaction sites in mice immunized with either a protective or a nonprotective immunogen of *Cryptococcus neoformans. Infection and Immunity* 70, 591–600.

Parnousis, N., Roubies, N., Karatzias, H., Frydas, S. and Papasteriadis, A. (2001) Effect of selenium and vitamin E on antibody production by dairy cows vaccinated against *E. coli. Veterinary Record* 149, 643–646.

Petit, H.V. and Trawiramungu, H. (2002) Reproduction of dairy cows fed flaxseed, Megalac or micronized soybeans. *Journal of Animal Science* 80, 312.

Politas, I., Hidiroglow, M., Batra, T.R., Gilmore, J.A., Gorewit, R.C. and Scherf, H. (1995) Effects of vitamin E on immune function. *American Journal of Veterinary Research* 56, 179–184.

Reddy, P.G., Morrill, J.L., Minocha, H.C., Morrill, M.B., Dayton, A.D. and Frey, R.A. (1986) Effect of supplemental vitamin E on the immune system of calves. *Journal of Dairy Science* 69, 164–171.

Rink, L. and Gabriel, P. (2000) Zinc and the immune system. *Proceedings of the Nutrition Society* 59, 541–552.

Salyer, G.B., Galyean, M.L., Defoor, P.J., Nunnery, G.A., Parsons, C.H. and Rivera, J.D. (2004) Effects of copper and zinc on performance and humoral immune response of newly received, lightweight beef heifers. *Journal of Animal Science* 82, 2467–2473.

Shizgal, H.M. and Martin, M.F. (1988) Caloric requirement of the critically ill septic patient. *Critical Care Medicine* 16(4), 312–317.

Smith, L.K., Harrison, J.H., Hancock, D.D., Todhunter, D.A. and Conrad, H.R. (1984) Effects of vitamin E and selenium supplementation on incidence of clinical mastitis and duration of clinical symptoms. *Journal of Dairy Science* 67, 1293–1300.

Spears, J.W. (2000) Micronutrients and immune function in cattle. *Proceedings of the Nutrition Society* 59, 587–594.

Tam, M., Gomez., S., Gonzalez-Cross, M. and Marcos, A. (2003) Possible roles of magnesium on the immune system. *European Journal of Clinical Nutrition* 57, 1193–1197.

Tjoelker, L.W., Chew, B., Tanaka, T.S. and Daniel, L.R. (1988) Bovine vitamin A and β-carotene intake and lactational status. 1. Responsiveness of peripheral blood polymorphonuclear cells to vitamin A and β-carotene challenge *in vitro. Journal of Dairy Science* 71, 3112–3119.

Wang, Y.Q., Puntenney, S.B., Burton, J. and Forsberg, N.E. (2007) Ability of a commercial feed additive to modulate expression of innate immunity in sheep immunosuppressed with Dexamethasone. *Animal* 1, 945–951.

Wang, Y.Q., Puntenney, S.B., Burton, J. and Forsberg, N.E. (2009) Use of gene profiling to evaluate the effects of a feed additive on immune function in periparturient dairy cattle. *Journal of Animal Physiology and Animal Nutrition* 93, 66–75.

Ward, J.D., Gengelbach, G.P. and Spears, J.W. (1997) The effects of copper deficiency with or without high dietary iron or molybdenum on immune function of cattle. *Journal of Animal Science* 75, 1400–1408.

Wright, C.L., Spears, J.W., Brown, T.T., Lloyd, K.E. and Tiffany, M.W. (2000) Effects of chromium and copper on performance and immune function in stressed steers. *Journal of Animal Science* 78, 1.

24 Nutrition and the Inflammatory Response

Two major categories of the immune system are the innate and acquired immune systems. The **innate immune system** is the first line of defence against pathogenic invasion of the body. A major component of the innate immune system is the **inflammatory response**, which is the result of the production of **pro-inflammatory cytokines** such as interleukin-1 (IL-1), tumour necrosis factor-α (TNF-α), interleukin-6 (IL-6), interleukin-8 (IL-8) and interferon-α (INF-α). Other inflammatory chemicals include those from damaged cells such as histamine and kinins (e.g. bradykinin). Plasma proteins such as **acute phase proteins** and C-reactive protein are also involved. These latter substances are mediators of cytokines that through feedback loops regulate the production of pro-inflammatory cytokines. The plasma concentrations of these proteins are elevated during chronic inflammatory states.

Cytokines are composed of small water-soluble proteins and glycoproteins. They are produced in a wide variety of cell types, including blood cells. They function in cell signalling, such as signalling immune cells (e.g. T cells, macrophages) to move to sites of infection. Each cytokine binds to a specific cell-surface receptor. Subsequent cascades of intracellular signalling then alter cell functions, including up-regulation and/or down-regulation of genes or transcription factors.

The production of cytokines initiates events that assist the body in warding off a bacterial or viral invasion. In particular, nutrients are repartitioned away from normal metabolic processes to pathways that bolster defence against pathogens. For example, there is increased muscle protein degradation to provide amino acids for energy metabolism to increase body temperature and metabolic rate. Cytokines can influence the endocrine system, by modifying the release of hormones, affecting hormone receptors or secondary messenger pathways. For example, TNF-α results in a decrease

in responsiveness to growth hormone releasing hormone (GHRH) and thyrotropin releasing hormone (TRH) (Elasser *et al.*, 1997). GHRH functions in release of growth hormone and prolactin from the pituitary, whereas TRH stimulates the release of thyrotropin stimulating hormone (TSH), thus regulating metabolic rate, growth, and all thyroid functions.

Another inflammatory chemical is **nitric oxide (NO)**, which is synthesized from L-arginine by **nitric oxide synthase (NOS)**. There are constitutive forms of NOS and an inducible form (**iNOS**). iNOS is induced by pro-inflammatory agents such as bacterial endotoxins (e.g. bacterial lipopolysaccharide, LPS) and the cytokines. Enhanced formation of NO following induction of iNOS is a component of inflammation. Cytokine stimulation of iNOS involves stimulated production of **nuclear transcription factor kappa B (NFκB)**. NFκB is a transcription factor (transcription is transfer of genetic code from DNA to produce RNA) that is involved in the stimulation of synthesis of acute phase proteins. NFκB is also involved in the expression of cytokines and other factors involved in immunologic expression. It exists in an inactive form in the cytosol but is activated and translocated to the nucleus via cytokines such as IL-1 produced in inflammatory events.

During disease challenges, the first immune response of the animal involves generation of free radicals by macrophages and neutrophils to kill bacteria. An example of an important free radical in inflammatory responses is **superoxide anion**, produced by a one-electron reduction of molecular oxygen. In acute and chronic inflammation, the production of superoxide is increased such that it overwhelms the capacity of **superoxide dismutase (SOD)** to remove it. Superoxide has beneficial effects in fighting pathogenic invasion, but also reacts with NO to produce **peroxynitrite** which has pro-inflammatory activity. These reactive oxygen species (ROS) are effective in destroying invading pathogens but also cause host cell damage. Host pathology is an inevitable consequence of disease fighting by the immune system.

An invariable effect of pro-inflammatory activity in fighting disease is a reduction in feed intake. About 70% of the decrease in growth rate that accompanies an inflammatory response is due to **reduced feed intake**, while 30% is due to inefficiencies in nutrient absorption and metabolism. Dantzer (2001) coined the term 'cytokine-induced sickness behaviour' (**sickness behaviour**)[1] to describe the non-specific symptoms of infection and inflammation that include weakness, malaise, listlessness, inability to concentrate, depression, lethargy and anorexia. IL-1 is an important cytokine for the induction of sickness behaviour. In animals with subclinical infection, the changes may be subtle, but there can be a reduction in feed intake and a shift in the partitioning of dietary nutrients away from skeletal muscle accretion to metabolic responses that support the immune system (Johnson, 1997).

The PG_2 series and TX_2 series of **eicosanoids** (see Chapter 10) are inflammatory agents produced in response to immunostimulation. They are synthesized by the **cyclooxygenase** (**COX**) pathway. There are two major COX isoenzymes, COX1 and COX2. Aspirin and other non-steroidal anti-inflammatory drugs (NSAID) inhibit COX enzyme activity. *Yucca schidigera* products, which are used as feed additives, inhibit NO formation and have anti-inflammatory activity (Marzocco *et al.*, 2004) and inhibit COX activity (Wenzig *et al.*, 2008). Yucca contains **resveratrol**, a polyphenolic anti-inflammatory agent (Oleszek *et al.*, 2001). Resveratrol, also abundant in grape skins and red wine, inhibits COX enzymes and NO formation.

Omega-3 fatty acids have anti-inflammatory properties when provided in optimal proportions with omega-6 fatty acids. Both ω-3 and ω-6 fatty acids are precursors of eicosanoids, including prostaglandins, thromboxanes and leukotrienes. The ω-6 fatty acids produce eicosanoids that have inflammatory properties, while the eicosanoids synthesized from the ω-3 series of fatty acids (EPA, DHA) have anti-inflammatory properties (Simopoulos, 2002). The inflammatory properties of ω-6 fatty acids are attributed to arachidonic acid. EPA competitively inhibits the production of inflammatory prostaglandins and leukotrienes by

competing as a substrate for COX enzymes and 5-lipoxygenase (Simopoulos, 2002). In dogs, ω-3 fatty acids are used as dietary supplements to control inflammatory responses (Wander *et al.*, 1997; Kearns *et al.*, 1999). Dietary supplements of cod liver oil, a source of ω-3 fatty acids, reduce the severity of rheumatoid arthritis in humans (Galarraga *et al.*, 2008).

Immune Stimulation and Animal Performance

Although seemingly counter-intuitive, stimulation of the immune system can be a negative in livestock and poultry production. In essence, when the immune system is activated, nutrients are diverted from growth to formation of immuno-components such as cytokines, acute phase proteins and antibody proteins. If the immune system is responding to a mild or slight pathogenic threat, the result is a negative effect on growth. The main factor responsible for growth inhibition, as mentioned earlier, is a depression in feed intake associated with an inflammatory response (Klasing, 1988, 1998). The **segregated early weaning** (**SEW**) system of pig production was developed to avoid the growth-depressing effects of an immune response. The SEW system is based on weaning the pigs while maternal antibody protection is at its peak, and then moving the pigs to an isolated housing building to prevent disease exposure and activation of the immune system. For the first 2–3 weeks of life, the baby pig has passive immunity obtained via maternal antibodies in the mother's colostrum. However, this immunity is limited only to the antigens to which the mother was exposed prior to farrowing. In the SEW system, pigs are weaned at about 14–17 days of age and moved to isolated, clean facilities without exposure to any other pigs. This weaning method has been adopted as a standard practice by most of the pig industry, combined with the **all-in and all-out facility management concept**. This means the buildings are completely emptied to allow clean up, sanitizing and (preferably) 1 day of vacancy prior to refilling the building with same-source and same-age pigs. This SEW system minimizes the young pigs' exposure to diseases (antigens), which also minimizes the activation of their immune system. **Activation of the immune system** by exposure to antigens reduces growth performance of the pig, because nutrients are diverted from growth to the synthesis of **cytokines** and other components of the immune system (Dritz *et al.*, 1996; Williams *et al.*, 1997a, b, c). Thus, preventing the activation of a pig's immune system by minimizing its exposure to antigens results in more efficient nutrient utilization for growth. Pigs raised in the SEW system have higher amino acid requirements than conventionally reared pigs (Williams *et al.*, 1997a,b) and the diets should contain protein sources with highly digestible amino acids (Bergstrom *et al.*, 1997). The advantages of the SEW system are maintained throughout the entire growth period (Williams *et al*, 1997c) with increased growth rate, feed conversion efficiency and carcass leanness. Therefore, the pigs' level of chronic immune system activation will affect nutrient requirements at all stages of growth.

Johnson (1997), Johnson *et al.* (1997) and Klasing (1988) summarized the nutritional effects of cytokine production (Table 24.1) and the mechanisms by which pro-inflammatory cytokines inhibit growth. Energy, protein, lipid, carbohydrate and mineral metabolism are all negatively impacted. The repartitioning of nutrients may be a defence mechanism against invading pathogens. For example, a pathogen challenge causes a shift in **iron** from transferrin in the extracellular fluids to intracellular ferritin. Decreased plasma iron lowers the proliferation and virulence of pathogens. Lactoferrin is a glycoprotein in milk that has antimicrobial and anti-inflammatory properties (Wu *et al.*, 2007) by virtue of its ability to scavenge free iron, thus depriving microbes of this nutrient. In poultry, **biotin** is sequestered bound to avidin during an inflammatory response, preventing bacteria from acquiring biotin. Providing extra water-soluble vitamins to poultry undergoing disease challenge may actually be providing nutrients to the pathogens rather than to the host. Genetic selection of livestock and poultry for maximal productivity has reduced their ability to respond to an immune challenge because of a change in the partition of nutrients between tissue growth and the immune system. This, according to these authors, has increased the susceptibility of modern strains of livestock and poultry to infectious diseases.

The **endocrine system** is involved in the metabolic shift away from growth-related processes to immune function during disease stress (Elasser *et al.*, 1997; Johnson *et al.*, 1997; Spurlock, 1997). Various endocrine hormones and cytokine signals participate in redirecting nutrient use during disease stress (Elasser *et al.*, 1997). According to Elasser *et al.* (1997), 'In an intricate interplay, hormones and cytokines regulate, modify, and modulate each other's production and tissue interactions to alter metabolic priorities.' Dietary protein and energy intakes affect blood patterns of hormones and cytokines after disease challenge. Growth hormone has a regulatory role on cytokine production during disease stress (Elasser *et al.*, 1997).

The mucosal membranes of the gut are the largest interface of an animal with its environment and are the major sites of entry of foreign antigens (Bar-Shira and Friedman, 2005). Thus the gut has the body's major immunologic defences, the **gut-associated lymphoid tissue (GALT)**. GALT is

Table 24.1. Partial list of effects of immune system activation on nutrient metabolism (adapted from Klasing, 1988; Johnson, 1997; Johnson *et al.*, 1997).

Metabolic target	Effect[a]
Central nervous system	Fever
	Anorexia
	Hypothalamic-pituitary axis
Protein metabolism	Breakdown of skeletal muscle
	Increased hepatic amino acid uptake
	Acute-phase protein synthesis
Lipid metabolism	Lipolysis
	De novo fatty acid synthesis
	Inhibition of lipoprotein lipase activity
	Decreased uptake of blood TAGs
	Increased hepatic VLDL secretion
	Hypertriglyceridaemia
Mineral metabolism	Hypozincaemia
	Hypoferraemia
	Hypercupraemia
	Hypercalcaemia
Carbohydrate metabolism (biphasic response)	Phase I Hyperglycaemia
	Gluconeogenesis
	Glycogenolysis
	Phase II Hypoglycaemia
	Decreased PEPCK activity
	Increased glucose oxidation

[a]Abbreviations: PEPCK, Phosphoenolpyruvate carboxykinase (an enzyme used in the metabolic pathway of gluconeogenesis); TAGs, triacylglycerols; VLDL, very low density lipoprotein.

composed of cells interspaced between epithelial cells and in organized lymphatic tissue, including various structures such as **Peyer's patches** of lymphoid tissue at the ileocaecal junction, and the **Bursa of Fabricius** in chickens. The functional development of the hindgut lymphoid tissue precedes that of the small intestine, because the hindgut is heavily populated with bacteria which provide immunologic challenges. The GALT is the largest immune organ of the body. It produces large quantities of immunoglobulin A (IgA), which is the only class of antibody that is efficiently secreted into the gastrointestinal tract.

Infections of the mammary gland (mastitis) and uterus (metritis) are common sources of inflammation in lactating dairy cows, particularly near the periparturient period (Waldron *et al.*, 2006). There may be associations between immunologic disorders and metabolic problems such as ketosis and milk fever. To investigate this possibility, Waldron *et al.* (2006) produced experimental mastitis by administering *E. coli* LPS into the mammary tissue of early-lactation cows. Acute mastitis did not induce ketosis, but rather increased glucose synthesis by the liver and decreased plasma non-esterified fatty acids (NEFA) and ketone bodies. However, acute mastitis induced by LPS markedly depressed plasma calcium (Waldron *et al.*, 2003) suggesting a possible association of milk fever with mastitis.

Anti-inflammatory Effects of Growth Promoter Antibiotics

Antibiotics have been used as **antimicrobial growth promoters** (AGP) for many years, but despite their widespread use, their mode of action in promoting growth has not been conclusively identified. Klasing (1988) proposed that antibiotics may alter intestinal microflora to reduce the production of **immunogens** that provoke an immune response. Diversion of nutrients away from growth to cytokine synthesis to respond to immunogens could reduce growth. Antibiotics may thus act by reducing the microbial burden of the animal, providing greater nutrient availability for growth. It is well known that the antibiotic growth response is greater in a dirty environment than a clean one, supporting the hypothesis that microbial burden is involved.

Niewold (2007) has proposed a new explanation for the antibiotic growth response, based on anti-inflammatory activity. At least four major mechanisms have been proposed to explain AGP-mediated growth enhancement:

1. AGP inhibit intestinal microbes that produce immunogens (substances that elicit an immune response), thus reducing the metabolic costs of the innate immune system (Klasing, 1988).
2. AGP reduce growth-depressing metabolites such as ammonia and bile acid degradation products produced by microbes.
3. AGP reduce microbial use of nutrients.
4. AGP enhance the uptake and utilization of nutrients by causing a thinning of the intestinal mucosa.

Niewold (2007) refutes these proposed mechanisms, all of which share the common hypothesis that the intestinal microflora depress growth. The AGP are fed at sub-therapeutic concentrations, below the minimum inhibitory concentration for pathogens. Chronic feeding of antibiotics induces antibiotic resistance in enteric microbes, but the growth promoting activity remains. AGP have similar effects in animals (e.g. poultry and pigs) that differ greatly in the composition of intestinal microbes. Antibiotics are of numerous different chemical types and different antimicrobial spectra (e.g. Gram-positive versus Gram-negative) but give similar growth promoting effects. Not all antibiotics have growth-promoting activity, whereas they all inhibit microbes. Based on these and other considerations, Niewold (2007) proposed that AGP have a target that is not the intestinal microflora. He suggests that AGP accumulate in inflammatory cells in the intestine (macrophages, polymorphonucleocytes). Antibiotics have been demonstrated to inhibit inflammatory activity, such as production of pro-inflammatory cytokines and ROS. **Intestinal inflammation** leads to an accumulation of inflammatory cells in the mucosa, leading to a thicker intestinal wall. The thinner intestinal wall when AGP are fed is consistent with reduced inflammation. Thus Niewold (2007) concludes that AGP inhibit intestinal inflammation, reducing the acute phase response and obviating a shift in nutrients away from growth. Phagocytic inflammatory cells can accumulate high concentrations of antibiotics, which could attenuate the ability of these cells to destroy microbes, further reducing the likelihood of an inflammatory response.

Note

[1] Spire (2010) provides an excellent review of sickness behaviour in livestock, particularly in feedlot cattle.

References

Bar-Shira, E. and Friedman, A. (2005) Ontogeny of gut associated immune competence in the chick. *Israel Journal of Veterinary Medicine* 60(2), 42–50.

Bergstrom, J.R., Nelssen, J.L., Tokach, M.D., Goodband, R.D., Dritz, S.S., Owen, K.Q. and Nessmith, W.B., Jr (1997) Evaluation of spray-dried animal plasma and select menhaden fish meal in transition diets of pigs weaned at 12 to 14 days of age and reared in different production systems. *Journal of Animal Science* 75, 3004–3009.

Dantzer, R. (2001) Cytokine-induced sickness behavior: mechanisms and implications. *Annals of the New York Academy of Sciences* 933, 222–234.

Dritz, S.S., Owen, K.Q., Goodband, R.D., Nelssen, J.L., Tokach, M.D., Chengappa, M.M. and Blecha, F. (1996) Influence of lipopolysaccharide-induced immune challenge and diet complexity on growth performance and acute-phase protein production in segregated early-weaned pigs. *Journal of Animal Science* 74, 1620–1628.

Elasser, T.H., Kahl, S., Steele, N.C. and Rumsey, T.S. (1997) Nutritional modulation of somatotropic axis-cytokine relationships in cattle: a brief review. *Comparative Biochemistry and Physiology* 116A(3), 209–221.

Galarraga, B., Ho, M., Youssef, H.M., Hill, A., McMahon, H., Hall, C., Ogston, S., Nuki G. and Belch, J.J.F. (2008) Cod liver oil (*n*-3 fatty acids) as a non-steroidal anti-inflammatory drug sparing agent in rheumatoid arthritis. *Rheumatology*. Available at: rheumatology.oxfordjournals.org/cgi/content/abstract/ken024v1

doi:10.1093/rheumatology/ken024 (accessed 2 February 2010).

Johnson, R.W. (1997) Inhibition of growth by pro-inflammatory cytokines: an integrated view. *Journal of Animal Science* 75, 1244–1255.

Johnson, R.W., Arkins, S., Dantzer, R. and Kelley, K.W. (1997) Hormones, lymphohemopoietic cytokines and the neuroimmune axis. *Comparative Biochemistry and Physiology* 116A, 183–201.

Kearns, R.J., Hayek, M.G., Turek, J.J., Meydani, M., Burr, J.R., Greene, R.J., Marshall, C.A., Adams, S.M., Borgert, R.C. and Reinhart, G.A. (1999) Effect of age, breed and dietary omega-6 (*n*-6):omega-3 (*n*-3) fatty acid ratio on immune function, eicosanoid production, and lipid peroxidation in young and aged dogs. *Veterinary Immunology and Immunopathology* 69, 165–183.

Klasing, K.C. (1988) Nutritional aspects of leukocytic cytokines. *Journal of Nutrition* 118, 1436–1446.

Klasing, K.C. (1998) Nutritional modulation of resistance to infectious diseases. *Poultry Science* 77, 1119–1125.

Marzocco, S., Piacente, S., Pizza, C., Oeszek, W., Stochmal, A., Pinto, A., Sorrentino, R. and Autore, G. (2004) Inhibition of inducible nitric oxide synthase expression by yuccaol C from *Yucca schidigera* Roezl. *Life Sciences* 75, 1491–1501.

Niewold, T.A. (2007) The nonantibiotic anti-inflammatory effect of antimicrobial growth promoters, the real mode of action? A hypothesis. *Poultry Science* 86, 605–609.

Oleszek, W., Sitek, M., Stochmal, A., Piacente, S., Pizza, C. and Cheeke, P. (2001) Resveratrol and other phenolics from the bark of *Yucca schidigera* Roezl. *Journal of Agricultural and Food Chemistry* 49, 747–752.

Simopoulos, A.P. (2002) Omega-3 fatty acids in inflammation and autoimmune diseases. *Journal of the American College of Nutrition* 21, 495–505.

Spire, M.F. (2010) Cattle sickness behaviour complex. *Feedstuffs* 82 (16), 13–16.

Spurlock, M.E. (1997) Regulation of metabolism and growth during immune challenge: an overview of cytokine function. *Journal of Animal Science* 75, 1773–1783.

Waldron, M.R., Nonnecke, B.J., Nishida, T., Horst, R.L. and Overton, T.R. (2003) Effect of lipopolysaccharide infusion on serum macromineral and vitamin D concentrations in dairy cows. *Journal of Dairy Science* 86, 3440–3446.

Waldron, M.R., Kulick, A.E., Bell, A.W. and Overton, T.R. (2006) Acute experimental mastitis is not causal toward the development of energy-related metabolic disorders in early postpartum dairy cows. *Journal of Dairy Science* 89, 596–610.

Wander, R.C., Hall, J.A., Gradin, J.L., Du, S.H. and Jewell, D.E. (1997) The ratio of dietary (*n*-6) to (*n*-3) fatty acids influence immune system function, eicosanoid metabolism, lipid peroxidation and vitamin E status in aged dogs. *Journal of Nutrition* 127, 1198–1205.

Wenzig, E.M., Oleszek, W., Stochmal, A., Kunert, O. and Bauer, R. (2008) Influence of phenolic constituents from *Yucca schidigera* bark on arachidonate metabolism *in vitro*. *Journal of Agricultural and Food Chemistry* 56, 8885–8890.

Williams, N.H., Stahly, T.S. and Zimmerman, D.R. (1997a) Effect of chronic immune system activation on the rate, efficiency, and composition of growth and lysine needs of pigs fed from 6 to 27 kg. *Journal of Animal Science* 75, 2463–2471.

Williams, N.H., Stahly, T.S. and Zimmerman, D.R. (1997b) Effect of chronic immune system activation on body nitrogen retention, partial efficiency of lysine utilization, and lysine needs of pigs. *Journal of Animal Science* 75, 2472–2480.

Williams, N.H., Stahly, T.S. and Zimmerman, D.R. (1997c) Effect of level of chronic immune system activation on the growth and dietary lysine needs of pigs fed from 6 to 112 kg. *Journal of Animal Science* 75, 2481–2496.

Wu, S.-C., Chen, H.-L., Yen, C.-C., Kuo, M.-F., Yang, T.-S., Wang, S.-R., Weng, C.-N., Chen, C.-M. and Cheng, W.T.K. (2007) Recombinant porcine lactoferrin expressed in the milk of transgenic mice enhances offspring growth performance. *Journal of Agricultural and Food Chemistry* 55, 4670–4677.

Appendix:
Answers to Study Guide Questions

Chapter 1

1. Dietetics is the formulation and preparation of diets to meet the needs of humans. School lunch programmes, meals for seniors, cafeteria meals, etc., are examples. Dieticians are nutrition professionals who help people make dietary changes and healthy food choices. Animal scientists who formulate diets and feeding programmes for animals are called diet formulators or nutrition consultants.

2. A nutrient is a dietary essential for one or more species of animal. Water is a dietary essential in animals that meet their water needs from food that they eat. Marine mammals, for instance, don't drink salt water but obtain water from their diet, such as fish tissue. In zoos, fish used for marine mammal food are usually stored frozen and may become dehydrated. This may lead to water deprivation in fish-eating species that don't consume water directly.

3. Organic compounds consist of substances based on carbon. Proteins, carbohydrates, lipids and vitamins are organic compounds. Mineral elements are inorganic and contain no carbon (mineral salts, such as calcium carbonate, may contain carbon).

4. (a) Amino acids are the basic building blocks (basic units) of protein structure. (b) The simple sugars (monosaccharides) are the basic units of carbohydrate structure. For example, cellulose and starch are large molecules consisting entirely of glucose molecules joined together.

5. Carbohydrates contain carbon, and hydrogen and oxygen in the proportions found in water, so carbohydrates are 'hydrates of carbon' $(CH_2O)_n$.

6. The Kjeldahl procedure involves digesting feed or tissue samples with concentrated acid, and then measuring the nitrogen content of the digest. It is assumed, validly, that virtually all the nitrogen was derived from amino acids.

7. It would be very difficult and expensive to measure all the individual proteins in a feed. Instead, the Kjeldahl procedure is used to measure the nitrogen content. Crude protein is then calculated as $N \times 6.25$.

8. Maize is a C4 plant, having a tropical origin. C4 plants are metabolically more efficient than C3 plants (e.g. barley) in use of solar energy to synthesize carbohydrate.

9. Saturated fatty acids contain all the hydrogen that they are chemically capable of containing; that is, they are saturated with hydrogen. Unsaturated fatty acids contain one or more double bonds, so they can take up hydrogen. This is what happens when maize (corn) oil is converted to margarine, for example.

10. The main chemical difference between animal fats and vegetable oils is that animal fats have a higher content of saturated fatty acids.

11. Vitamins are organic substances other than proteins, carbohydrates and lipids that have specific roles in metabolism and are required in the diet in very small amounts. Some vitamins can be obtained in a non-dietary manner, such as niacin which can be synthesized by animals from the amino acid tryptophan. Vitamin D can be synthesized in the skin with exposure to sunlight. The last vitamin to be discovered was vitamin B_{12}, in 1948.

12. Nutraceuticals are dietary supplements other than known nutrients that are perceived as having some other type of beneficial property, such as anti-inflammatory activity. In many cases, their efficacy has not been established by scientific evidence. They are particularly promoted in the equine industry.

13. In a double-blind study, neither the experimental subject nor the investigator knows which treatment is which. This procedure is followed to reduce bias and to avoid the placebo effect.

14. Enzymes are biological catalysts which accelerate or facilitate biochemical reactions. A catalyst is not used up in a chemical reaction and can be re-used. Cofactors and coenzymes are minerals and vitamins that are required to activate enzymes.

For example, many enzymes require the presence of a mineral element such as copper or zinc (metal-activated enzymes). Several B vitamins function as constituents of coenzymes, which are organic cofactors. The best known is probably coenzyme A (CoA), containing the vitamin pantothenic acid. CoA is vital for many reactions of cellular metabolism.

15. Homeostasis refers to 'constancy of the internal environment'. The body attempts to maintain a constant blood concentration of certain constituents, such as glucose and calcium. Any deviation from normal results in the action of homeostatic hormones, such as insulin, to return the constituent to its normal concentration.

16. Hormones are produced in a gland and transported to target tissues via the circulatory system. Their secretion is subject to feedback regulation. Examples include the thyroid hormones (thyroxine, calcitonin), pancreatic hormones (insulin, glucagon), and numerous others. Although classified as a nutrient, vitamin D actually functions as a steroid hormone.

17. Metabolism is the summation of catabolism and anabolism. Catabolism is breaking down while anabolism is building up. Thus the oxidation of glucose to yield ATP is catabolism, while the synthesis of tissue proteins from amino acids is anabolism. Many people are familiar with the term 'anabolic steroids'. These are derivatives of testosterone which stimulate build-up of muscle tissue.

18. Biochemical individuality refers to the fact that each individual has a unique internal chemistry. The term was coined many years ago, and has been given new life by the emerging field of metabolomics. In the future, it may be possible to customize nutritional or drug-treatment regimes according to the unique biochemistry of an individual.

Chapter 2

1. Probably the best example of a specialist feeder is the koala (which is not a bear!). It feeds only on a few species of eucalyptus trees. The pygmy rabbit feeds almost exclusively on sagebrush. The giant panda consumes mainly bamboo, but will consume other vegetation and even small animals.

2. The giant panda is taxonomically in the order Carnivora. It has the dental and digestive tract characteristics of a true carnivore (flesh eater) but in fact consumes a primarily vegetarian diet. Thus, paradoxically, it is a vegetarian carnivore.

3. Autoenzymatic digestion involves digestive enzymes secreted by the animal itself, while allo-enzymatic digestion involves an exogenous source of enzymes from the gut microbes.

4. All animals have only one stomach, so are monogastric (mono = one; gastric = stomach). Ruminants such as cattle and deer do not have four stomachs. They have one stomach divided into four compartments.

5. Hydrochloric acid in the stomach causes the pH of the stomach to be highly acidic. Most ingested bacteria, including pathogens, are killed by the acid. In addition, the low pH has some digestive effects, causing some hydrolysis of proteins and polysaccharides, and denaturation of proteins. The hydrochloric acid also causes activation of pepsinogen to the active enzyme pepsin.

6. (a) A major cause of stomach ulcers in humans is infection by the bacterium *Helicobacter pylori*, which weakens or degrades the mucous coating of the stomach, allowing invasion of the stomach lining by other bacteria. (b) In pigs, gastric ulcers are associated with high energy, low fibre diets, leading to fermentation and acid production in the oesophageal region of the stomach.

7. Digestion is the preparation of ingested food for absorption of nutrients, or, simply put, digestion is preparation for absorption. Proteins, carbohydrates and lipids are large molecules which must be digested. Minerals and vitamins do not require digestion, although in some cases vitamins occur in plants in a bound form that must be degraded to facilitate absorption. Mineral sources may require digestion of phytates by phytases to release the bound minerals.

8. Villi are projections of the intestinal mucosa, and are lined by a single layer of cells called enterocytes. Each enterocyte has an outer layer of projections called microvilli. The villi and microvilli greatly increase the intestinal surface area.

9. Goblet cells produce and secrete mucus, which protects the intestinal lining from digestive enzymes and also provides lubrication to facilitate movement of digesta through the gut.

10. The glycocalyx is a filamentous web attached to the microvilli. This web-like structure helps retard the rate of passage at the lining of the intestine, increasing the time available for digestion and absorption. The glycocalyx 'traps' particles so that digestion in the brush border can be completed.

11. The term 'unstirred water layer' refers to the contents of the intestine that are in contact with the

brush border (intestinal mucosa). The rate of movement is slower than in the lumen of the intestine. An analogy is a water pipe. Water moves fastest in the interior (lumen) of the pipe, and is slowed down by friction against the wall of the pipe.

12. Peristalsis refers to muscular contractions which propel digesta through the digestive tract. Anti-peristalsis refers to muscular contractions which move gut contents 'backwards', from the colon to the caecum for example.

13. Birds have a segmented stomach with a true gastric stomach (the proventriculus) and the gizzard. They also have two caeca, whereas mammals have one caecum.

14. Birds have embryonic but non-functional teeth. The grinding functions of teeth in mammals are accomplished by the gizzard of birds.

Chapter 3

1. Fermentation is defined as anaerobic respiration, and applies mainly to the anaerobic catabolism of carbohydrates. Because oxidation is not complete under anaerobic conditions, end products of fermentation include non-oxidized carbon fragments such as volatile fatty acids (VFAs) in bacterial fermentation in the rumen and ethanol in wine and beer fermentation by yeasts.

2. The four compartments of the ruminant stomach are the rumen, reticulum, omasum and abomasum. The rumen and reticulum are the major sites of fermentation, the reticulum also traps foreign particles, the omasum acts as a sieve to retain large particles in the rumen, and the abomasum is the gastric stomach where hydrochloric acid is secreted.

3. Hofmann classified ruminants into groups based on feeding strategy: (i) concentrate selectors; (ii) bulk and roughage feeders (grazers); and (iii) intermediate feeders. As discussed in the chapter, these categories are controversial but in general are valid.

4. Very small ruminants such as mouse deer are extremely susceptible to omasal impaction. In the wild, they feed on very succulent, low fibre substances such as fruit.

5. Moose and giraffes are concentrate selectors, and like the small ruminants in Question 4, they are very susceptible to omasal impaction. They are subject to 'wasting disease' because of gut impactions. Moose are especially difficult to raise in captivity.

6. The ventricular groove is a temporary muscular tube that functions to transport liquids (milk) directly from the oesophagous to the omasum, thus bypassing rumen fermentation. It is desirable in suckling animals that milk does not enter the rumen. The young animal is intolerant of the stomach acids produced by fermentation, and is susceptible to bloating from the gases produced.

7. Cattle are well adapted as grazing animals. They have strong chewing muscles, that aid in the grazing of grass. Cattle have a large rumen capable of holding a large quantity of roughage. The rumen is muscular, allowing thorough mixing of the contents. They have a high capacity for rumination, facilitating the physical maceration of forage into smaller particles. They have a well-developed omasum, which aids in the retention of ingested forage in the rumen. They produce large quantities of saliva. Thus the stomach of cattle is well adapted to the grazing of grass and utilization of coarse forage. Despite these attributes, cattle in North America, such as feedlot and dairy cattle, are commonly fed low roughage, high grain diets. This development arose with the availability of large amounts of inexpensive feed maize. Increasing use of maize as a feedstock for fuel (ethanol) production may result in a 'backing off' from high grain diets for ruminants in the future.

8. In wild ruminants, and domestic ruminants raised on forage, protein and energy are obtained as a result of rumen fermentation. Microbial protein is a major source of protein to the ruminant animal, while much of their energy is obtained from the catabolism of absorbed VFAs.

9. Rumination involves the regurgitation from the rumen of ingested feed, to be re-chewed and degraded into smaller particle sizes. Eructation is the process by which the fermentation gases are expelled from the rumen.

10. Major types of rumen microbes are bacteria, protozoa and fungi. Rumen bacteria and protozoa can be subdivided into further categories, such as amylolytic and cellulolytic bacteria, and holotrich and entodiniomorph protozoa.

11. An example of an avian arboreal folivore (a tree-dwelling leaf-eating bird) is the hoatzin. The koala is a mammalian arboreal folivore, which lives in eucalyptus trees and feeds upon the tree leaves.

12. Phytobezoars are similar in principle to hair balls (trichobezoars). Phytobezoars are ball-like masses of undigested plant fibre that obstruct the digestive tract. They are mainly a problem in foregut fermenters fed highly lignified and poorly digested tree leaves.

13. Hoatzins are birds native to the tropics of Central and South America. They are the only known avian foregut fermenter. They have numerous adaptations for a tree-leaf-based diet. They are poor flyers, but the ability to fly at all gives them a competitive advantage over other arboreal feeders. They have functional wing claws that aid in climbing trees and holding on to branches. They have an enlarged foregut with microbial fermentation, and are selective feeders, selecting only high quality, readily digested leaves with low concentrations of secondary compounds (toxins).

14. The rabbit is not a good model for horse nutrition studies. The hindgut of the rabbit functions to selectively sort out and excrete fibre, while the hindgut of the horse is adapted for fibre retention and digestion. As a result, digestibility coefficients for forages are very different between the horse and the rabbit, with fibre digestibilities much higher in horses.

15. Coprophagy is the consumption of faeces. Caecotrophy refers to a specific hindgut adaptation by which caecal contents are formed into boluses which are consumed directly from the anus. For example, the rabbit engages in caecotrophy, while dogs often practise coprophagy and horses sometimes do also.

16. Very small animals are not usually ruminants. Relative to body weight, small animals have very high metabolic rates. It is difficult to sustain a high rate of metabolism from fermentation of forage. Small herbivores must consume high quality and readily digestible diets to be able to satisfy their energy requirements. On the other hand, very large animals would not be able to ingest and transport huge quantities of forage – there is an upper limit to the weight of digestive tract contents that an animal could consume and still be able to move.

17. The large size of the rumen in the grazer (cattle) takes up most of the space in the abdominal cavity, thus decreasing the space available for the colon. Therefore, a smaller colon size reduces the capacity for water reabsorption. Sheep, on the other hand, have a less voluminous rumen and a greater colonic capacity for water reabsorption.

18. Equids (zebra) and ruminants (antelope) have different digestive strategies for dealing with forages. Ruminants have an omasum which functions to retain fibrous material in the rumen until it has been digested. With very poor quality, highly fibrous forages, this retention of fibre 'plugs up' the digestive tract. In contrast, equids can pass very large quantities of forage through the gut, and even if it is very low in nutritional value, they can survive by deriving nutrients from a very large volume of forage.

19. Production of maize in the USA is subsidized, resulting in it being quite inexpensive. Maize production is not subject to the classic economic control of supply and demand. This situation has prevailed since the end of World War II. As a result, maize has been the least expensive energy source for feeding livestock and poultry. Because maize has a high digestible energy value, animals perform very well on maize-based diets. A large feedlot industry for fattening beef cattle has developed, using maize as the major feed ingredient, because it is the least expensive way to feed cattle. Even though cattle evolved as grazers, they are reasonably tolerant of high grain diets, although there are various problems associated with lactic acidosis. The era of cheap maize for feed in the USA may be nearly over as increasing amounts are being used to produce biofuel (ethanol).

Chapter 4

1. There are about (depends on species) 20 amino acids that are metabolic requirements for tissue protein synthesis. In the plant kingdom, there are hundreds of known amino acids. According to one author (Wink, see Chapter 1), the number may be as high as 900 amino acids.

2. Proline is not really an amino acid; it is an imino acid, because its amino group occurs within a ring structure.

3. An α-carbon is the first carbon atom in a carbon chain that is attached to a functional group. In the case of α-amino acids, the amino and carboxyl groups are the functional groups attached to the α-carbon.

4. Glycine does not exist as D- and L-isomers because it lacks an asymmetric carbon atom.

5. Polar amino acids contain ionized groups, such as the ionized carboxyl group (COO^-). Non-polar amino acids lack charged (ionized) groups. The presence or absence of charged groups is a function of the pH of the medium, as well as the composition of the side chain.

6. The essential amino acids are: arginine, histidine, isoleucine, leucine, tryptophan, lysine, methionine, phenylalanine, threonine and valine.

7. The term 'essential' is a bit confusing as it is applied to amino acids. All the amino acids are metabolically essential. Those that are called 'essential amino acids' are those which must be provided in the diet. The so-called non-essential amino acids are essential to protein synthesis, but can be formed in the liver and other tissues by interconversions so do not need to be present as such in the diet. Thus the term 'essential' is with specific reference to being required as such in the diet.

8. There are two peptide bonds in a tripeptide (there are three amino acids but only two bonds are needed to connect them together).

9. (a) The amino acid cysteine contains a sulfhydryl group. (b) When two cysteine molecules are joined to form cystine, a disulfide bond is formed.

10.

Note that lysine has an extra amino group in its side chain, while glutamic acid has a carboxyl group. Neither of these participate in peptide bond formation; it is the amino and carboxyl groups attached to α-carbons that form peptide bonds.

11. Keratin and carotene may sound alike, but they are totally different substances. Keratin is a type of protein found in hooves and hair, while carotene is a plant pigment and source of vitamin A (vitamin A is synthesized from β-carotene).

12. The crimp of a wool fibre is caused by intramolecular bonding of non-adjacent cysteines to form cystine. The disulfide bonds in cystine hold the protein of the wool fibre (keratin) in its secondary structure.

13. When proteins are denatured, by heat for example, the secondary structure is disrupted.

14. (a) Albumin is a blood protein. (b) Albumen is a protein in eggs (remember the 'e' form of albumen occurs in 'e'ggs).

15. Gelatin is produced by boiling a source of collagen in water or dilute acid or base.

Chapter 5

1. (a) Endopeptidases hydrolyse peptide bonds within the primary structure of a protein, splitting it into smaller fragments, the polypeptides. Trypsin is an example of an endopeptidase. Exopeptidases cleave amino acids off the terminal ends of a protein molecule. (b) Aminopeptidases and carboxypeptidases are types of exopeptidases, acting on the end with a free carboxyl group (carboxypeptidases) or free amino group (amino peptidases).

2. Pepsin and rennin function in the stomach.

3. The pancreas gland is the source of these enzymes, which were named prior to the time that a standard convention for naming enzymes with an 'ase' ending was established.

4. Soybeans are well known for containing trypsin inhibitors. Soybeans and soybean meal to be fed to non-ruminants must be heated to destroy trypsin inhibitors. Legume seeds in general (beans, peas) contain trypsin inhibitors.

5. Ptomaines are toxic amines produced when the carboxyl group is removed from amino acids by intestinal bacteria.

6. Skatole (3-methyl indole) is produced by bacterial catabolism of tryptophan. Skatole is one of the main constituents of faecal odour. Absorbed skatole is responsible for the 'boar taint' of the meat of male pigs.

7. Undigested dietary protein is fermented by bacteria in the hindgut. Several amino acids when fermented produce unpleasant smelling compounds such as amines, phenols and skatole. Ammonia and hydrogen sulfide are also products of intestinal fermentation of amino acids.

8. Excess dietary urea is poisonous to ruminants. Urea is converted to ammonia in the rumen by bacterial urease. The ammonia is utilized by the rumen bacteria to synthesize bacterial protein. If the amount of ammonia in the rumen exceeds the amount needed for microbial protein synthesis, the excess is absorbed. At high levels, it exceeds the capacity of the liver to remove it and convert it back into urea. Then ammonia escapes detoxification (by conversion to urea) and enters the general blood supply (the general circulation). Ammonia is extremely toxic to cells, especially those of the brain. Detoxification of ammonia in the brain depletes the organ of carbohydrate (α-ketoglutaric acid) needed for energy metabolism.

9. Diets high in readily fermentable carbohydrates promote efficient utilization of urea, by supporting a high rate of bacterial growth in the rumen to 'sop up' the ammonia. The high rate of fermentation results in a high production rate of VFA, which lowers the rumen pH. Ammonia is absorbed more

slowly under acidic conditions, helping to prevent ammonia toxicity.

10. Urea recycling refers to the secretion of blood urea back into the rumen, via the saliva and directly across the rumen wall.

11. Bypass protein is protein that is not fermented in the rumen, but 'bypasses' rumen fermentation to be digested by the animal in the small intestine. This process is beneficial with high quality proteins. Microbial protein is of moderate quality (content and balance of essential amino acids) so it is desirable to avoid the conversion of high quality dietary protein to lower quality microbial protein in the rumen.

12. Replace the amino group of methionine with an hydroxyl group.

13. Soybeans don't synthesize trypsin inhibitors to inhibit the growth of poultry and pigs! Trypsin inhibitors are part of the chemical defence system of the plant. Some plant-feeding insects secrete proteolytic enzymes to digest leaf and seed proteins. Inhibition of these insect proteases is the driving force behind the evolution of trypsin inhibitors in plants.

Chapter 6

1. The reaction is illustrated in Fig. 6.3 in the chapter.

2. A Schiff base is formed when the B vitamin pyridoxine (vitamin B_6) reacts with the amino group of an amino acid, to transfer it to a keto acid from carbohydrate metabolism, to form a new amino acid. This process is called transamination.

3. An ideal protein is defined as one which meets an animal's amino acid requirements precisely. Its determination involves use of ileal cannulas to measure absorbed amino acids.

4. It is well documented that it is possible to meet the protein requirements of humans with a totally plant-based diet. A common question asked of vegetarians is 'where do you get your protein?'. The protein requirements for maintenance of an adult human are actually quite low and are not difficult to meet.

5. (a) Lysosomes are subcellular organelles which act as the cell's garbage disposal unit. They contain proteases such as cathepsins which break down 'worn out' cellular proteins to amino acids which can be reused. (b) Ubiquitins are small proteins which function in disposal of defective proteins and non-functional enzymes.

6. The Dalmation dog excretes uric acid in its urine, in addition to urea. The uric acid is derived from the catabolism of nucleic acids. In other dog breeds, uric acid is converted to a more water-soluble product, allantoin, for urinary excretion.

7. Ornithine and citrulline are two non-protein amino acids which function as components of the urea cycle. The urea cycle enzymes function in converting ammonia to urea in the liver.

8. Chickens (and other birds) do not have a functioning urea cycle system. As a result, they cannot synthesize arginine, so they have a higher dietary requirement than mammals for this amino acid. Instead of converting ammonia to urea, birds convert it to uric acid, which requires glycine and methionine for its synthesis. Therefore chickens have higher requirements than pigs for arginine, methionine and glycine.

9. The white substance in the excreta (faeces plus urine) of birds is uric acid crystals.

10. Although ammonia is alkaline in reaction, it can contribute to acid rain by reacting with atmospheric sulfuric acid to form ammonium sulfate, which can be oxidized in soil to produce nitric and sulfuric acids.

11. In fish, ammonia is excreted through the gills and sometimes through the skin. Urea is also excreted by some fish.

12. There are numerous examples of nutrients which have a sparing effect on other nutrients. For example, cysteine in the diet reduces (spares) the amount of methionine needed. As will be discussed in Chapter 13, vitamin E and selenium have a sparing effect on their respective requirements. Niacin has a sparing effect on the tryptophan requirement.

13. Choline, as a constituent of lecithin, aids in mobilizing lipid from the liver, preventing fatty liver syndrome.

14. Creatine is a source for muscle contraction. Creatinine is produced by its metabolism, and is excreted in the urine.

15. Kwashiorkor is a severe protein deficiency in children. Marasmus is a severe deficiency of both protein and energy.

16. Taurine is not an amino acid, because it does not have an α-carbon with amine and carboxyl groups attached. It is a derivative of sulfur amino acids, and is a dietary requirement of cats and large breeds of dogs.

17. Male cats synthesize several sulfur-containing amino acids such as isovalthine and felinine, which function in territorial marking.

18. An indole has a five-membered carbon ring containing a nitrogen. The amino acid tryptophan contains an indole group. A tryptophan derivative, serotonin, is a neurotransmitter in the brain. Skatole (3-methyl indole) is produced by bacteria from fermentation of tryptophan. Skatole produced in the rumen can be absorbed and causes lung lesions. Skatole produced in the hindgut contributes to faecal odour, and is responsible for the 'boar taint' in the meat of male pigs. Certain grasses such as reed canary grass contain alkaloids with an indole structure. These tryptamine alkaloids are structurally similar to serotonin and cause neurological disturbances as a result.

19. Boar taint is caused by accumulation of skatole in the muscle tissue of intact male pigs. The male hormone androstenone inhibits the liver enzymes that convert skatole to metabolites to be excreted in the urine.

20. In the conversion of tryptophan to niacin, there are species differences in enzyme activities. Cats synthesize picolinic acid instead of niacin, and therefore have a dietary requirement for niacin.

21. A number of hormones are synthesized from the amino acid tyrosine. These include the thyroid hormones, and the adrenal hormones adrenalin and noradrenalin. Tyrosine is also the precursor of melanin, the black-brown pigment of hair.

22. Glutathione is a tripeptide containing cysteine. The sulfhydryl group of cysteine in this structure is very reactive, and also readily undergoes oxidation-reduction. Glutathione has important roles in detoxifying toxic substances, either by conjugation with them to facilitate excretion, or by reducing them by providing hydrogen. Glutathione has a role in preventing red blood cell haemolysis, by adding hydrogen to oxidizing agents such as hydrogen peroxide. This is discussed in more detail in Chapter 13.

23. Grouse and ptarmigan are birds which excrete conjugates of ornithine. These are called ornithurates.

24. Two drugs that are used to influence NO activity are nitroglycerin and Viagra.

25. The Maillard (browning) reaction is stimulated by heat. In this reaction, reducing sugars (see Chapter 7) react with free amino groups (e.g. epsilon amino groups of lysine) to produce indigestible brown pigments.

26. Red clover has high polyphenol oxidase activity. This enzyme causes the oxidation of phenols, which can then participate in browning reactions.

Rained-on red clover hay quickly turns black because of this reaction.

27. Because it has a free amino group at the end of its side chain, lysine is the amino acid most affected by the browning reaction.

28. There is evidence that nucleotides may stimulate growth of baby pigs, suggesting that they might be considered nutrients.

29. Gout is caused by crystals of insoluble uric acid precipitating in joints. Pigs don't get gout because they convert uric acid to water-soluble allantoin.

Chapter 7

1. The basic units of carbohydrate structure are the monosaccharides (simple sugars).

2. Starch and cellulose are both made up entirely of glucose molecules. Starch is a polymer of maltose and cellulose is a polymer of cellobiose (a polymer is a large molecule made up of a large number of identical units). In the case of maltose and starch, the bond joining the glucoses in the carbohydrate chain is an α-1,6 bond, while in cellulose it is a β-1,6 bond. It is remarkable that because of this seemingly small difference, starch (e.g. a potato) and cellulose (wood) have completely different physical properties.

3. Table sugar (sucrose) is not a reducing sugar because it does not have a free aldehyde group to react with copper in the Benedict's and Fehling's tests.

4. Oligosaccharides are believed to act as growth factors for beneficial gut bacteria. They also stimulate the intestinal immune system.

5. Amylopectin differs from amylase by having a branched structure while amylase is a straight chain of glucose molecules.

6. A polymer is a large molecule composed of multiples of a specific repeating unit. In starch the repeating unit is maltose; in cellulose it is cellobiose. In proteins and polypeptides, there are no repeating units. They are composed of chains of different amino acids, without any specific repeating group.

7. Two carbohydrates of animal origin are glycogen and lactose.

8. Fructans are a constituent of the nitrogen-free extract (NFE) fraction of the proximate analysis scheme.

9. The difference between ADF and NDF is that the NDF includes the hemicellulose fraction.

10. Forage will have a low sugar content early in the morning, because the plant cellular respiration will have been utilizing sugars all night. A cold night will reduce the rate of respiration so the following morning the forage should have a higher sugar content than normal. By the afternoon, photosynthesis should have produced a lot of sugars, particularly on a sunny day.

Chapter 8

1. There is evidence that humans have adapted to the presence of dietary starch from grains by having higher amylase secretion than populations of hunter-gatherers who do not have a starch-based diet. People whose ancestors had a dairying culture tend to have higher lactase secretion rates than people from non-dairying cultures, who are more likely to exhibit lactose intolerance.

2. Barley contains non-starch polysaccharides such as β-glucans. These are viscous, poorly water-soluble gums that tend to clog up the intestinal mucosa and interfere with fat absorption. They are also hydroscopic, and draw water into the gut, causing wet litter in poultry houses.

3. The two major types of feed enzymes used commercially are phytases and enzymes (β-glucanases, pentosanases) that digest non-starch polysaccharides (NSP) in wheat and barley. Phytases improve mineral availability, and the glucanases and pentosanases improve the digestion of NSP, thus increasing the metabolizable energy values of wheat and barley for poultry.

4. Cheese or pizza consumption should not affect people with lactose intolerance. Cheese is made by separating the milk protein and fat from the lactose. The protein and fat become cheese, and the water-soluble lactose is the whey. There is virtually no lactose in cheese.

5. The major VFAs produced in rumen fermentation are acetic, propionic and butyric acids. Smaller amounts of other VFAs such as lactic acid, valeric acid and isovaleric and isobutyric acids are also produced.

6. Baby animals do not secrete sucrase, so are unable to digest sugar (sucrose). Undigested sucrose causes osmotic diarrhoea.

7. Rumen fungi are believed to solubilize lignin and improve the digestibility of fibre in ruminants.

8. Holotrichs are ciliated over the entire body while in entodiniomorphs the cilia are restricted to the mouth region.

9. Various chemicals, such as detergents and copper sulfate, kill rumen protozoa, thus acting as defaunating agents.

10. The acrylate pathway is one of the pathways leading to the formation of propionic acid in rumen fermentation.

11. Ionophores stimulate the production of propionate and reduce methane production.

12. Ionophores stimulate production of propionate, which yields more energy when metabolized by the animal than acetate and butyrate.

13. *Streptococcus bovis* proliferates rapidly when cattle are switched abruptly to a high starch (high grain) diet. *S. bovis* produces D-lactic acid, a strong acid which causes lactic acidosis.

14. Parakeratosis in cattle is damage to the rumen papillae. In pigs, parakeratosis refers to skin lesions, such as those caused by zinc deficiency.

15. Propionate is one of the VFAs produced in rumen fermentation, so, as in other ruminants, bighorn sheep would absorb propionate, which in the blood exists as sodium and calcium salts. Propionic acid and propionate salts have antifungal activity. An interesting and apparently unstudied question is whether or not rumen propionate inhibits rumen fungi. This could be an explanation as to why rumen fungi occur only when high roughage diets (which produce low propionate as percentage of total VFA) are fed.

Chapter 9

1. The two major pathways are: (i) glycolysis; and (ii) the citric acid cycle (Krebs cycle, tricarboxylic acid cycle or TCA cycle).

2. Hydrogen is released during glycolysis and citric acid cycle reactions, and transferred to hydrogen receptors such as NAD. When the NADH is oxidized in the electron transport reactions, hydrogen reacts with oxygen to produce water, and the energy released in that reaction is used to synthesize ATP.

3. Thiamin is a coenzyme for decarboxylation reactions (the removal of carbon to form carbon dioxide). Thiamin functions in this way in the conversion of pyruvate (3C) to acetyl CoA (2C) and, in the citric acid cycle, in the conversion of α-ketoglutarate to succinyl CoA.

4. The four vitamins are thiamin, pantothenic acid, niacin and riboflavin. Thiamin functions in decarboxylation of α-ketoglutarate, pantothenic acid is a constituent of coenzyme A, niacin is a component of NAD and NADP, and riboflavin is a component of FAD.

5. Chastek's paralysis is caused by thiamin deficiency, induced by thiaminase in raw fish such as carp.

6. Glucose can be metabolized in the pentose phosphate pathway, in the red blood cells, in which two hydrogens are transferred to NADP. These hydrogens are further transferred to glutathione, from which they can be transferred to oxidizing agents (e.g. hydrogen peroxide) to reduce them to nontoxic products (e.g. water). If not reduced, the oxidizing agents attack the red blood cell membrane.

7. Absorbed acetate is converted to acetyl CoA and enters the citric acid cycle. Butyrate is converted to two acetyl CoAs. Propionate is converted in several steps to succinyl CoA, an intermediate in the citric acid cycle.

8. Cobalt is a constituent of vitamin B_{12}, which is synthesized by bacteria in the rumen. In a cobalt deficiency, vitamin B_{12} cannot be synthesized, creating a vitamin B_{12} deficiency in the animal. Vitamin B_{12} is necessary for propionate metabolism, and the synthesis of haemoglobin. Inability to metabolize propionate causes emaciation and impairment of haemoglobin synthesis causes anaemia.

9. When propionate is produced, there is less hydrogen released to form methane than when acetate is produced. Therefore a high ratio of acetate to propionate (A:P ratio) will result in higher methane production.

Chapter 10

1. Unsaturated fatty acids have one or more double bonds.

2. 18:3 ω6 and 18:3Δ6,9,12 are the same fatty acid (see chemical structure at bottom of page).

Fish oils are a rich source of omega-3 (ω-3) fatty acids. Their beneficial effects on human health were first noted when it was observed that Greenland Eskimos consuming their traditional diet experienced virtually no 'diseases of civilization' such as cardiovascular disease, even though they consumed a diet very high in fat such as seal, walrus and whale blubber. The fat of these marine animals has a high content of ω-3 fatty acids. The reason for this is that phytoplankton in the ocean synthesize these fatty acids, which then accumulate in the food chain. Small herbivorous fish eat phytoplankton, larger carnivorous fish eat the herbivorous fish, marine mammals eat the carnivorous fish, and the Eskimos eat the marine mammals. Each species in this trophic pyramid has body fat enriched in ω-3 fatty acids.

3. Oleic acid is of the *cis* configuration and elaidic acid is *trans*.

4. Methylene interrupted double bonds: –CH=CH–CH$_2$–CH=CH–; Conjugated double bonds: –CH=CH–CH=CH–

5. Fats have a high proportion of saturated fatty acids, while oils have a high content of unsaturated fatty acids. An exception is the tropical oils (coconut and palm oils) which are highly saturated but liquid at room temperature.

6. Most people associate the word 'steroids' with anabolic steroids, which are illicit (banned) drugs. Most steroids are essential in metabolism, such as cholesterol, bile acids, vitamin D, androgens, oestrogens, progestins, etc.

7. Eicosanoids are substances such as prostaglandins, prostacyclins, thromboxanes and leuketrienes, which are derived from C20 and C22 fatty acids. DHA and EPA are two fatty acids in fish oils, from which eicosanoids are synthesized.

8. The main essential fatty acids are linoleic and α-linolenic acids. Some authorities also include arachidonic acid as a dietary essential.

Chapter 11

1. Primary bile acids are synthesized in the liver and secreted in the bile. Secondary bile acids are produced by bacterial metabolism of primary bile acids in the hindgut.

Chapter 10, question 2.

18 : 3 ω 6

CH$_3$—CH$_2$—CH$_2$—CH$_2$—CH$_2$—CH=CH—CH$_2$—CH=CH—CH$_2$—CH=CH—CH$_2$—CH$_2$—CH$_2$—C$\lessgtr$ $^O_{OH}$

18 : 3 Δ 6, 9, 12

CH$_3$—CH$_2$—CH$_2$—CH$_2$—CH$_2$—CH=CH—CH$_2$—CH=CH—CH$_2$—CH=CH—CH$_2$—CH$_2$—CH$_2$—C$\lessgtr$ $^O_{OH}$

2. Micelles disperse non-polar products of fat digestion in the aqueous medium of the intestine. The bile acids which form the structure of micelles are amphipathic, meaning that they have both water and lipid solubility properties.

3. Bile pigments such as biliverdin are metabolized in the gut by bacteria to produce urobilinogens. Urobilinogens are oxidized to brown pigments when faeces are exposed to air.

4. Dietary lipids are digested somewhat poorly by ruminants. There is no emulsifying agent such as bile secreted into the rumen. Rumen microbes are not efficient in fat digestion, and in fact are inhibited by unsaturated fatty acids. The rumen is a reducing (high hydrogen) environment. Under reducing conditions, unsaturated fatty acids are partially or completely hydrogenated. In the rumen, this produces a cascade of unsaturated fatty acids, including a number of forms of conjugated linoleic acid (CLA). Several unique fatty acids are produced, including vaccenic and rumenic acids.

5. The odour of lamb and mutton is in part caused by medium-length branched-chain fatty acids. They are formed from methylmalonate, an intermediate in propionate metabolism. Because propionate production is highest on concentrate diets, the odour is more pronounced with grain-fed sheep than those grazing on grass.

Chapter 12

1. 'Good cholesterol' is the high density (HDL) cholesterol. This designation refers to the density of the blood lipoprotein to which the cholesterol is attached. Proteins in solution have a high density (they sink in water); lipids have low density (they float on water). HDL has a high protein content (see Table 12.1). HDL cholesterol is considered good because that is the form in which cholesterol is transported from the tissues to the liver. The LDL-bound cholesterol is considered bad, because it is the form in which cholesterol is transported to the tissues such as artery walls. The cholesterol molecule is the same in each case; it is just bound to different lipoproteins.

2. As discussed in Question 1 above, a lipoprotein has a high density when it contains a high content of protein, and a low density when it has a high lipid content.

3. Chylomicrons are almost pure lipid, so of course they have a low density.

4. The liver has important roles in fat metabolism. It produces bile, which is necessary for the emulsification of fats in the digestive tract. The liver synthesizes the lipoproteins which transport lipids in the blood. The liver is also an important site for catabolism of fatty acids and the synthesis of triacylglycerols (TAGs).

5. Statin drugs inhibit the synthesis of cholesterol in the liver. The specific reaction they inhibit is the rate-limiting step in cholesterol biosynthesis, catalysed by the enzyme HMG-CoA reductase.

6. Enterohepatic circulation refers to the secretion of substances into the digestive tract, and then subsequent reabsorption farther down the tract. For example, bile acids are secreted into the gut, where they participate in micelle formation and then are reabsorbed.

7. Most fatty acids are synthesized by the sequential addition of a two-carbon unit, beginning from acetyl CoA. So fatty acid elongation will proceed C2, C4, C6, C8 … C16. Fatty acids with an odd number of carbons (e.g. C17) are quite uncommon.

8. Glucose can be converted to acetyl CoA, which can then be synthesized into fatty acids. However, this is not reversible, so when fatty acids are oxidized to acetyl CoA, the acetyl CoA cannot be used to synthesize glucose. By 'no net synthesis' is meant that although carbon atoms from acetyl CoA, if radioactive, might be found in glucose, there can be no increase in the amount of glucose from acetyl CoA derived from fat metabolism.

9. Eicosanoids are substances derived from the eicosa (C20) polyunsaturated fatty acids (mainly from fish oils). Examples of eicosanoids include prostaglandins, prostacyclins, thromboxanes, leukotrienes and lypoxins. These have hormone-like activity.

10. *Trans*-fatty acids are unsaturated fatty acids with the *trans* configuration about the double bond(s). They are produced industrially from the partial hydrogenation of vegetable oils to produce margarine and other solid fats. *Trans*-fatty acids are also produced by biohydrogenation of unsaturated fatty acids in the rumen. The possible negative effects of ruminant *trans*-fatty acids on human health are offset by the beneficial effects of the CLA that are produced during biohydrogenation.

11. Beef fat may contain odd-chain (odd number of carbons) and branched-chain fatty acids because of microbial metabolism of lipids in the rumen. One reason is because in the rumen microbial fatty acid synthesis can begin with odd-chain and branched-chain VFAs such as propionic, valeric and isobutyric acids.

12. Milk fat depression is considered undesirable because in many cases dairy farmers are paid more for milk with a higher fat content. The fat is important if the milk will be used for manufacturing cheese and butter.

13. The basis of the 'biohydrogenation theory' of milk fat depression is that certain intermediates of fatty acid biohydrogenation are absorbed and inhibit the expression of lipogenic enzymes in the mammary gland, causing a reduction in milk fat synthesis. Examples of absorbed fatty acids which have this effect are *trans*-10, *cis*-12 CLA, *trans*-9, *cis*-11 CLA and *cis*10, *trans*-12 CLA.

14. Cats are unable to convert linoleic acid to arachidonic acid because they lack Δ6 desaturase, and therefore they require a dietary source of arachidonic acid. They normally acquire this fatty acid from consumption of prey.

15. The citrate cleavage enzyme in non-ruminants functions in converting citrate into acetyl CoA and oxaloacetate in the cytosol. This is a means of transporting acetyl CoA from the mitochondria to the cytosol, where fatty acid synthesis occurs. Acetyl CoA is unable to directly pass across the mitochondrial membrane. In ruminants, the citrate cleavage enzyme is involved in producing NADPH for fatty acid synthesis. See Figs. 12.6 and 12.7.

16. Rumenic and vaccenic acids are intermediates in CLA formation. They are unsaturated. They differ in isomerization from linoleic acid, and differ from stearic acid which is fully saturated.

Chapter 13

1. Rancidity is the process by which unsaturated fatty acids react with oxygen to produce peroxides.

2. Antioxidants prevent auto-oxidation by providing hydrogen (reduction) to oxidizing agents such as free radicals and peroxides.

3. There is a widespread perception that preservatives are harmful to human health. On the contrary, they improve human health by preventing growth of moulds on foods (antifungal agents) and prevent rancidity (antioxidants). They may also have beneficial antioxidant activity in the tissues following their absorption.

4. Vitamin C is an antioxidant because it can provide hydrogen to oxidants. It also functions in the recycling of vitamin E, increasing its effectiveness as an antioxidant.

5. Canola oil and especially olive oil are high in monounsaturated fatty acids. These have cholesterol lowering properties, but are less susceptible than polyunsaturated fatty acids to auto-oxidation and production of peroxides.

6. Vitamin E is not a single, discrete substance. Numerous chemical structures have vitamin E activity. These include the tocopherols and tocotrienols, both of which exist as numerous isomeric forms.

7. Natural vitamin E (RRR-α-tocopherol) is more potent than synthetic (all-rac-α-tocopherol acetate or succinate).

8. A quinone is a structure containing a six-carbon ring with two oxygens attached by double bonds.

9. Increasing the vitamin E content of meat reduces the oxidation of lipids in the tissue, delaying the discoloration of the product with exposure to air.

10. Rhinos in zoos are not fed diets that exactly mimic what they would consume in the wild. Vitamin E concentrations in browse plants consumed by wild rhinos are much higher than in grasses and pelleted diets typically fed to zoo animals. Also, the nature of the fatty acids in the diets of wild and captive rhinos differs. Ingestion of seeds and kernels favours linoleic acid intake, while ingestion of native browse leaves favours linolenic acid. Rapid degradation of stored feed occurs, while no loss would occur with browsed feed in the wild. These factors could increase the vitamin E requirements of captive rhinos.

11. The main metabolic function of selenium is as a component of the enzyme glutathione peroxidase. This enzyme transfers hydrogen from reduced glutathione (GSH) to oxidants such as hydrogen peroxide.

12. Humans, other primates and a few other animals lack the enzyme L-gulonolactone oxidase, which is required for the synthesis of ascorbic acid.

13. Vitamin C stimulates iron absorption by reducing Fe^{3+} to Fe^{2+}. Iron is absorbed most efficiently when in the Fe^{2+} state (see Chapter 21). Iron absorption is lowered in vitamin-C-deficient individuals.

14. Resveratrol is a phenolic antioxidant in grape skins, and is believed to be the substance responsible for the healthful effects of red wine, which include beneficial effects against cardiovascular disease.

15. DDT is an organic compound which is metabolized by the cytochrome P_{450} enzymes in the liver, making it more water soluble and easier to excrete. Non-polar substances that require detoxification in the liver stimulate the activity of the enzymes that detoxify them. They induce enzyme activity, so are said to be inducing agents. The detoxification defence system of the body is under normal conditions 'idling', and when there is a need to increase detoxification abilities it is 'kicked into gear'.

16. Cytochrome P_{450} is part of an enzyme system, the mixed-function oxidase (MFO) system, which is responsible for detoxification of toxins by increasing their water solubility, facilitating their excretion in the urine.

Chapter 14

1. The respiratory quotient (RQ) is determined by measuring gaseous exchange: oxygen consumption and carbon dioxide elimination. The RQ is CO_2/O_2. It is mainly used in research on energy metabolism. It is useful in the determination of the nature of the metabolic fuel being used. For example, the RQ of a hibernating bear could be determined to find out if hibernating animals use fat or protein (muscle) as their major fuel source.

2. A calorie is the amount of heat required to raise the temperature of 1 g of water by 1°C. Calories are determined in an instrument called a bomb calorimeter. The heat produced by the burning of a given amount of feed is determined by measuring the increase in temperature of a known quantity of water.

3. The comparative slaughter technique has been extensively used to measure the net energy contents of feedstuffs used in feeding cattle, especially those in feedlots. It measures the amount of energy gain by an animal fed a specific amount of feed.

4. White adipose tissue is normal body fat. Brown adipose tissue is a special type of stored fat that has a high content of mitochondria, which are responsible for its brown colour (see Chapter 15). The mitochondrial metabolism produces a lot of heat, which helps maintain the body temperature of a hibernating animal. Fat-storing hibernators rely on both white and brown adipose tissue as their major metabolic fuel during hibernation.

5. Amino acids are deaminated in the liver. Deamination is the removal of their amino group. The remaining carbon structure then enters the basic metabolic pathways of the animal: glycolysis and the citric acid (TCA) cycle. The point at which they enter these pathways depends upon their specific structure.

6. The carbon skeletons of some amino acids can be converted to oxaloacetic acid (OAA), which can then by the reversal of glycolysis produce glucose. Fatty acids are catabolized to acetyl CoA, which cannot be used to synthesize glucose. Every acetyl CoA catabolized in the citric acid cycle reacts with an OAA, and in the functioning of the citric acid cycle one OAA is produced. Thus one OAA is used up and another one created, so there is no net increase in OAA to be drawn off for gluconeogenesis.

Chapter 15

1. Glycogenolysis is the process of catabolism of glycogen. Gluconeogenesis is the reversal of glycolysis to synthesize glucose. 'Neogenesis' refers to the formation of glucose from new sources (neo = new); in other words, from non-carbohydrate sources such as amino acids.

2. Brown adipose tissue or brown fat has a large number of mitochondria which are responsible for the brown colour.

3. Lipotropes are substances that promote mobilization of fat from the liver, thus preventing fatty liver syndrome. Examples of lipotropes are choline, betaine, vitamin B_{12} and methionine.

4. The fat of wild ruminants has a higher proportion of ω-6 and ω-3 unsaturated fatty acids than the body fat of maize-fed cattle. Wild ruminants also have higher phospholipid contents of their fat.

5. The domestication of cereal grains has increased the food supply for humans, and fostered the development of civilization. However, the consumption of grain-based diets has led to various nutritional problems such as vitamin and mineral deficiencies that were not experienced by hunter-gatherers.

6. Nutritional distortion refers to the selective removal of certain components of foods and then consuming them in excess of amounts that could normally be obtained from foods. For example, modern humans process foods to isolate oils and sugar, and then consume these products in large quantities. We have distorted foods by selectively removing those fractions which we have an innate desire for, such as sugar and lipid, and consuming them out of context of how they occur in nature.

7. Diseases of Western civilization are maladies such as heart disease, cancer, diabetes and obesity. While these diseases do occur in virtually all cultures, they are especially prevalent in modern societies. Excessive consumption of sugar and fat, and lack of fibre may be major contributory factors, especially when the sugar and fat are consumed in processed foods such as fast food, chips, doughnuts and other pastries, etc.

8. Marbled beef can be considered an example of nutritional distortion. The meat of feedlot cattle has been distorted by the excessive feeding of calories from grain, at levels far greater than the level cattle would consume on their natural diet of grass.

9. The ratio of ω-6 to ω-3 fatty acids has changed from about 1:1 in pre-agricultural times to about 10–20:1 today, mainly because of our excessive consumption of vegetable oils (mainly ω-6) and grain-fed meat animals with carcass fat that is high in saturated and ω-6 fatty acids. In the USA, maize (corn) oil is the main contributory factor to both vegetable oil and marbled meat consumption.

Chapter 16

1. There is no net synthesis of glucose from acetyl CoA. In the ruminant, sodium acetate is converted to acetyl CoA. Therefore, it would not be an effective treatment to increase glucose synthesis in ketotic cows.

2. Ketosis involves a metabolic shortage of glucose. By decreasing their production of milk, dairy cows can reduce their metabolic demand for glucose needed for synthesis of lactose in milk. Sheep, however, are unable to reduce the glucose demands of developing fetuses (except by aborting them).

3. A cold-adapted pregnant ewe would probably reduce its feed intake when penned up in a warm barn. This could result in the mobilization of body fat for energy, increasing acetyl CoA and inducing ketosis.

4. The glycaemic index is a measure of the blood glucose-raising potential of foods. The concept was developed for humans, but might have application to horses. Feeds with a high glycaemic index would be detrimental to horses with equine metabolic syndrome, and could provoke the condition in previously healthy animals.

5. The 'thrifty gene hypothesis' relates to indigenous peoples who have adapted to the 'feast or famine' of adverse environmental conditions. Their metabolism is oriented towards storing energy when food is abundant for its utilization during lean times. People adapted to 'feast or famine' conditions are not adapted to a constant 'feast' condition of processed foods and fast foods that are very high in calories. Obesity and diabetes are the inevitable result.

6. A glucose tolerance test is conducted by giving a fasted individual a dose of glucose, and determining the time taken for the elevated blood glucose level (due to the dose of glucose) to return to normal. With impaired glucose tolerance, the time taken for blood glucose to return to normal is prolonged, because of insulin insufficiency or insulin resistance.

7. Equine metabolic syndrome refers to a disorder in horses that resembles human metabolic syndrome. Affected animals are obese, have insulin resistance and chronic laminitis. The condition seems to be provoked by a diet high in soluble carbohydrates (high glycaemic diets). Affected horses should not be given access to grain or pasture, and should be fed grass hay with a low sugar content (which must be assessed by a feed analysis). High glycaemic diets promote insulin resistance, a key factor in equine metabolic syndrome.

8. Fructose metabolism has some key differences from that of glucose. Fructose is catabolized in the liver by phosphorylation of the 1-position, which bypasses the rate-limiting phosphofructokinase step. Thus there is no 'brake' on fructose metabolism as there is for glucose. Fructose metabolism stimulates lipogenesis, including synthesis of glycerol and fatty acids. Fructose does not stimulate insulin secretion.

9. The glucose tolerance factor is a complex that contains chromium, niacin and amino acids. It participates in the uptake of glucose by cells.

10. It has been known for many years that caloric restriction of animals increases longevity, while 'supernutrition' tends to reduce lifespan. The relevance of this to the current American diet is that supernutrition prevails, with caloric intakes exceeding caloric requirements by a wide margin. This causes obesity and may reduce lifespan. It is commonly said that the current generation of young Americans may be the first to have a shorter lifespan than their parents.

11. Three of the enzymes involved in activation and metabolism of thyroid hormones contain selenium.

Chapter 17

1. Moose kept in zoos are highly susceptible to chronic wasting disease. This is related to the fact that they are concentrate selectors (in Hofmann's scheme). Thus they are very susceptible to omasal compaction from consumption of coarse roughage.

2. Traditionally the four major taste responses have been considered to be sweet, salty, sour and bitter. A fifth taste sensation, umami, has been recognized, and is the taste representative of protein.

3. Specialist feeders (besides thousands of species of insects) include the koala, giant panda and the pygmy rabbit.

4. A 'sweet tooth' is an adaptation to attract animals to foods high in energy, such as fruit. Carnivores do not have a sweet tooth, because their prey animals do not contain sugar. It would be of no survival value to a carnivore to have a sweet tooth.

5. Other terms for plant secondary compounds are plant chemical defences or plant toxins. They are secondary to the primary processes of cellular metabolism of plants.

6. Deer have salivary tannin-binding proteins, which bind tannins and prevent them from exerting negative effects on palatability and protein digestion.

7. Plant chemicals are involved in population cycles of small herbivores. With increasing herbivory pressure, plants synthesize higher concentrations of defensive chemicals. In the case of Arctic vegetation and snowshoe hares, high populations of the hares cause the vegetation to become unpalatable and indigestible, such that it can no longer support hare survival and the population crashes.

8. As is the case with snowshoe hares, trees subjected to beaver herbivory synthesize higher concentrations of defensive chemicals, causing the beavers to abandon the area, allowing the trees to regenerate.

9. Specialist feeders adapt to specific plant chemicals and evolve efficient detoxification strategies for those particular chemicals. Generalist feeders develop a broad array of feeding strategies and detoxifying enzymes that allow them to cope with many different plant toxins.

10. The term 'talking trees' refers to phenomenon in which herbivory of one tree results in increased formation of defensive chemicals in adjacent trees. The information is apparently transmitted by ethylene gas, a well-known plant hormone.

11. The concept of 'nutritional wisdom' implies that animals innately know what's good for them, and select feed sources to balance their nutrient needs. An example discussed in the chapter is that of band-tailed pigeons, which actively seek out a source of sodium to balance the high potassium contents of their diets.

12. In non-ruminants, feed intake is correlated with energy requirements. Animals eat sufficient feed to meet their energy requirements, except if the dietary energy content is so low that they cannot eat enough because gut capacity becomes limiting. The blood glucose concentration is the mediator of feed intake regulation in non-ruminants. In ruminants, blood concentrations of VFAs perform a similar function. However, ruminants are much more likely than non-ruminants to consume a low energy diet, resulting in feed intake being limited by gut capacity. When fed concentrate-type diets, ruminants display chemostatic regulation of feed intake.

13. For both sheep and cattle, the NDF intake was highest with C4 grasses, because C4 grasses (tropical grasses) have a much higher NDF content than temperate forages.

14. Halophytes are plants which can grow in alkali soils and accumulate high concentrations of sodium. Some desert animals such as the kangaroo rat have highly specialized kidneys that are able to excrete high concentrations of sodium. They also are able to selectively remove accumulated salt on the exterior of plant leaves.

15. The 'skyscraper theory' is a good analogy for visualizing the effect of NDF on feed intake. The effective volume of a skyscraper is changed only by smashing it apart. Similarly, the effective volume of forage in the rumen is reduced only when the plant cell walls have been torn apart by the action of microbial enzymes.

16. The zone of thermal neutrality is the 'comfort zone' or range of environmental temperature in which an animal displays minimal regulation of body temperature. Above and especially below the comfort zone, an increase in metabolic rate is necessary to maintain body temperature.

17. Wild ruminants display seasonal variation in feed intake. Feed intake is highest in the summer, resulting in the deposition of large quantities of adipose tissue which is mobilized during the winter to meet energy needs.

18. The feed intake of pregnant ewes decreases in late gestation because the increasing size of the fetus(es) takes up an increasing amount of the volume of the abdominal cavity, reducing rumen volume.

19. Metabolic size is defined as the body weight raised to the 0.75 power. As body weight increases, metabolic rate (and therefore feed intake) increases at a lower rate. The smallest mammal, the shrew, has a very high metabolic rate and must consume its body weight in food each day to stay alive. Obviously, a 70 kg human or 450 kg horse does not consume its body weight in feed each day. But on a metabolic size basis, the shrew, human and horse consume about the same amount.

20. (i) Daily caloric intake:
   Diet 1 = 2700 kcal dietary energy/kg
   Diet 2 = 3800 kcal dietary energy/kg
   Daily caloric intake = 6460 kcal dietary energy

Daily feed intake:
   Diet 1 = 6460 kcal/2700 kcal/kg = 2.39 kg
   Diet 2 = 6460 kcal/3800 kcal/kg = 1.70 kg

(ii) Optimal percentage of protein:
Diet 1
   Need 285 g crude protein (CP)/day, in 2.39 kg of feed
   2.39 kg feed has 285 g CP
   1 kg feed has 285 g/2.39 kg = 119.25 g/kg = 11.93% CP
Diet 2
   Need 285 g CP in 1.70 kg feed
   1.70 kg feed has 285 g CP
   1 kg feed has 285/1.70 = 167.65 g/kg = 16.77% CP

Optimal percentage of lysine:
Diet 1
   Need 14.3 g lysine in 2.39 kg feed
   2.39 kg feed has 14.3 g lysine
   1 kg feed has 14.3/2.39 = 5.98 g/kg = 0.598% lysine
Diet 2
   1.70 kg feed has 14.3 g lysine
   1 kg feed has 14.3/1.70 = 8.41 g/kg = 0.841% lysine

(iii) Optimal protein/kcal ratio:
Diet 1
   Per kg diet: 2700 kcal dietary energy
   119.25 g CP = 119250 mg CP
   Protein/kcal = 119250 mg CP/2700 kcal dietary energy = 44.17 mg CP/kcal
Diet 2
   Protein/kcal = 167650 mg CP/3800 kcal = 44.1 mg CP/kcal

Optimal lysine/kcal:
   Diet 1: 5980 mg lysine/2700 kcal = 2.215 mg lysine/kcal
   Diet 2: 8410 mg lysine/3800 kcal = 2.213 mg lysine/kcal

These calculations show the value of expressing nutrient requirements on a per unit of energy basis.

Since animals eat to meet their energy requirements, when they have eaten enough feed to do this, they will have automatically consumed the correct amount of other nutrients. In this example, a diet with 11.9% protein and one with 16.8% protein each provided the same amount of protein intake per day. If the diets had been formulated on a percentage basis, Diet 1 would have had a great excess of protein if formulated to provide 16.8% protein, while Diet 2 would have been markedly deficient if it had contained 11.9% protein. These diets are more extreme in energy content than most practical diets, but serve to illustrate the significance of nutrient/kcal ratios. The energy to protein ratio is sometimes calculated. Hopefully the above answer illustrates why it is the protein to energy ratio which is useful.

21. The highest energy concentration of any feedstuff is pure fat, at 9000 kcal/kg. It is impossible to formulate a diet with a dietary energy content higher than this. Pure fat is of course not a balanced diet, so the practical limit would be somewhat lower than 9000 kcal/kg.

22. As the protein/kcal ratio increases from 30 to 75 mg crude protein/kcal, the lipid content of the carcasses decreased. This is because the lower protein/kcal diets are deficient in protein, but the animals still consume an amount of feed sufficient to meet their energy requirements. Because protein is deficient, they cannot utilize all of the consumed energy to support growth, so they deposit the excess as body fat.

As caloric density (kcal/kg) increased, the percentage of carcass fat increased. The author (Wood, 1964) explained the results of this study as follows:

> The results given in this table confirm certain basic nutritional facts. If the animal is presented with an excess of energy in relation to protein, the extra energy above that required for growth can only be deposited as body fat. Hence the rats receiving 30 mg of protein per kcal deposited more body fat with each increase in energy level in the ration. The provision of extra protein in a low calorie ration leads to more rapid growth and hence a leaner carcass since the energy is used to a maximum for the additional growth permitted by the extra protein. These results re-emphasize the fact that growth rate, body composition and, ultimately, carcass quality are markedly influenced by the nutritive intake.

Chapter 18

1. Rickets is a disorder of growing animals characterized by spongy, poorly mineralized misshapen

bones. It is caused by deficiencies of calcium, phosphorus and/or vitamin D. In adults, lack of these nutrients causes osteomalacia (adult rickets). Osteoporosis refers to the loss of bone mass.

2. Parathyroid hormone (PTH) stimulates the mobilization of bone mineral. In dairy cattle, the onset of lactation necessitates the mobilization of bone calcium, which is stimulated by PTH. If this mobilization is inadequate, serum calcium decreases (hypocalcaemia), causing the symptoms of milk fever.

3. When serum calcium declines, the parathyroid gland is stimulated to increase PTH secretion. PTH stimulates mobilization of bone calcium and also stimulates the activation of vitamin D to produce the active form of the vitamin, calcitriol. Calcitriol stimulates calcium absorption. Increased calcium absorption and mobilization of bone calcium help to restore the serum calcium concentration to normal.

4. Vitamin D is a steroid. It is a hormone because it is produced in a gland (the kidney) and transported by the blood to the target tissue (the intestine). Its formation and secretion are controlled by a feedback mechanism (blood calcium concentration).

5. Aflatoxin causes liver damage, which reduces bile acid formation and secretion. Bile acids are necessary for the emulsification and absorption of lipids, including the fat-soluble vitamins. Reduced absorption of vitamin D as a result can lead to rickets. In addition, the hepatoxic effects of aflatoxin may impair the formation of 25-OHD$_3$ in the liver, further aggravating a vitamin D deficiency.

6. In the African mole rat, calcium is absorbed in an efficient non-vitamin-D-dependent process, so these animals do not require vitamin D.

7. Rabbits are very efficient in absorbing calcium and excrete the excess in the urine as calcium carbonate, which causes the urine to appear white or creamy, with an orange-red pigmentation.

8. Bone remodelling refers to the Schoenheimer concept of the dynamic state of body constituents (see Chapter 1). Bone is in a continuous state of formation and mobilization. Continual renewal of bone is called remodelling.

9. The growing bone is mineralized in the region of the proliferative zone of cartilage, at the junction of the epiphysis and the diaphysis.

10. Vitamin K functions in the creation of calcium-binding sites on glutamic acid by forming gamma-carboxyglutamic acid (GLA). Bone contains GLA-containing proteins, such as osteocalcin, whose formation requires vitamin K.

11. Vitamin C is required for the activity of enzymes involved in the crosslinking of collagen fibres. In vitamin C deficiency, collagen formation is impaired, causing skeletal deformities.

12. Cage layer fatigue is a disorder of laying hens kept in battery cages. It is a type of osteoporosis caused by the mobilization of leg bone calcium to support the calcium needs of eggshell formation. The birds may have broken bones as a result. This is an animal welfare issue.

13. Bone development disorders are often associated with excessive growth rates, leading to a body weight greater than what the skeletal system, especially the legs, can support.

14. Several species of tropical grasses contain high concentrations of oxalic acid, which impairs calcium absorption by forming insoluble calcium oxalate in the gut. This effectively creates an excess of absorbed phosphorus. Bone mineral is mobilized to provide calcium to prevent hypocalcaemia. Prolonged mobilization of bone mineral results in the bones becoming demineralized and fibrotic. In horses, bones in the head and legs are the first affected; the enlarged bones cause 'big head' and lameness.

Chapter 19

1. Achromatrichia is lack of hair pigmentation. Deficiencies of iron, copper, biotin and pantothenic acid may cause achromatrichia. Iron and copper are cofactors for tyrosinase, an enzyme that converts tyrosine to melanin. The roles of biotin and pantothenic acid in hair pigmentation are unknown.

2. Trimethylamine oxide (TMAO) is a component of raw fish of the cod family. Fish contain amines (responsible for 'fishy' odour). Trimethylamine in fish is oxidized to TMAO. TMAO can bind with iron and prevent its absorption. Mink fed raw fish of the cod family may become iron deficient, with anaemia and lack of hair pigmentation (cotton fur syndrome).

3. It is difficult to relate the metabolic role of biotin (decarboxylation reactions) to its effects in improving hoof health. One possible explanation is that biotin has a role in maintaining cell division. Fast-growing tissues, such as those of the skin and related structures, would presumably be those most affected by impaired cell division.

4. Fructans are polymers of fructose. Animals do not secrete fructanase, so fructans in the horse are fermented in the large intestine, contributing to production of lactic acid and bacterial endotoxins. These substances have roles in inducing laminitis.

5. Ponies have a high susceptibility to laminitis. Ponies originated in harsh environments with meagre feed resources, such as the Shetland Islands in Scotland. It is postulated that they have 'thrifty genes', meaning that in rare times when food is abundant in their natural habitat, they have a great capacity to store excess energy for mobilization during lean times. When raised in an environment with continual availability of abundant feed, they are likely to develop insulin resistance (Chapter 16) which seems to enhance metabolic disturbances such as laminitis.

6. Intracellular fluids have high concentrations of K^+, Mg^{++} and PO_4^- while extracellular fluids are high in Na^+, Ca^{++} and Cl^-.

7. Cholesterol has numerous essential functions in animals. Perhaps its most critical function is as a component of cell membranes. Therefore all animal tissues contain cholesterol. Meat, being muscle tissue, is no exception, and contains cholesterol in the muscle cell membranes. Adipose tissue has a lower cholesterol content than lean tissue. This is because per unit of volume, lean tissue has more membranes than adipose tissue. Fat cells are large, so the membranes constitute a smaller proportion of the total than is the case with smaller cells. An analogy is that a basket filled with marbles will have more surface area than the same sized basket filled with golf balls.

8. The extracellular matrix is also known as connective tissue. It is composed primarily of the protein collagen.

9. Collagen is the most abundant protein in the body.

10. A proteoglycan is a protein that contains glycosaminoglycans. These are carbohydrates containing repeating units of disaccharides, one of which is an amino sugar such as glucosamine. The other sugar in the disaccharide-repeating unit is a uronic acid, such as glucuronic acid. Examples of glycosaminoglycans are hyaluronic acid, chondroitin sulfate and heparin.

11. The major collagens of skin, bone and cartilage are collagens I and II.

12. Carotenoid pigments are either carotenes or xanthophylls. Xanthophylls contain oxygen, as alcohol, keto or ester groups on the terminal rings.

13. Wild salmon eat crustaceans such as shrimp and krill, as well as other fish that have consumed these crustaceans. Crustaceans contain pink pigments such as astaxanthin, which they obtain from consuming phytoplankton which synthesize carotenoids. Salmon deposit these pigments, obtained from their natural food, in their flesh. Farmed salmon are either fed crustaceans (e.g. krill meal) or have synthetic xanthophylls such as astaxanthin and canthaxanthin added to their diets.

14. The blue pigmentation of feathers is a structural feature, arising from the orientation of the keratin proteins in the feather. Structural blue of feathers results from light scattering.

15. At least one species of vulture, the Egyptian vulture, owes its colourful head to carotenoid pigments in cattle dung, which the birds consume. North American vultures also consume cattle dung, which might account for their pigmented heads.

16. Lycopene is a red carotenoid found in tomatoes and other red or orange fruits. Lycopene consumption has been linked to reduced incidence of prostate and gastrointestinal cancer in humans. Ketchup (tomato paste) is a better source of lycopene than fresh tomatoes, because the tomato solids are concentrated (water is removed) in the manufacture of ketchup. Also, cooking increases the bioavailability of lycopene.

17. Cattle consuming grass may deposit carotenoid pigments such as β-carotene in their body fat. There are breed differences among cattle in their capacity to metabolize carotenoids. Jersey and Guernsey breeds have a low capacity to metabolize carotenes and therefore have a high incidence of yellow milk and yellow body fat.

18. Retinol is an alcohol (containing an hydroxyl group) while in retinal the hydroxyl group has been oxidized to an aldehyde structure. So retinol is vitamin A alcohol and retinal is vitamin A aldehyde.

19. Rhodopsin is a light-sensitive protein in the eye, and has an essential role in the visual process.

20. Vitamin A deficiency causes night blindness because there is insufficient 11-*cis* retinal produced.

21. Polar bears and dogs accumulate high liver concentrations of vitamin A in specialized liver cells. Consumption of their livers by humans may induce vitamin A toxicity.

Chapter 20

1. Metabolic water is water that is produced when carbohydrates, lipids and amino acids are catabolized to carbon dioxide and water.

2. The kangaroo rat has a number of water-conserving adaptations, such as producing very concentrated urine, and a low transpiration rate of water via the lungs. The pack rat has a high water requirement, but it has behavioural adaptations that allow it to consume succulent desert vegetation such as cactus.

3. Marine mammals such as seals, sea lions and whales obtain their water from their food. For example, fish-eating species such as seals obtain their water needs from water in the flesh of the fish they consume.

4. High protein diets increase the requirements for water, because water is required to dilute nitrogenous end products such as urea in the urine.

5. In grazers such as cattle, the volume capacity of the colon is restricted in the abdominal cavity because of the high rumen volume. Therefore they have a reduced capacity for water absorption from the colon, so the faeces have a relatively high water content (pies versus pellets).

6. Oryx are well adapted to survival in desert conditions (except for survival against poachers). They have a very low rate of evaporative water loss. Another desert antelope, the addax, can store large amounts of water in the rumen.

Chapter 21

1. The major protein in blood is serum albumin. Its major function is to maintain osmotic balance between the blood plasma and tissue fluids.

2. Vitamin K functions in the creation of a calcium-binding site of the blood protein prothrombin, allowing it to be activated by calcium to the enzyme thrombin. Vitamin K functions in the carboxylation of glutamic acid residues in prothrombin to produce calcium-binding sites (two adjacent carboxyl groups).

3. Iron is absorbed most efficiently as haem iron, the form in which it occurs in haemoglobin and myoglobin in meat. Iron in haem is in the Fe^{2+} (ferrous) state, which is absorbed more efficiently than ferric iron.

4. Vitamin C reduces ferric iron (Fe^{3+}) to ferrous iron (Fe^{2+}). Ferrous iron is absorbed more efficiently than ferric iron.

5. Ferritin is an iron-containing protein in the intestinal mucosa. It can function in iron storage. Transferrin is the plasma protein which transports iron in the blood. Haemosiderin is an iron-storage protein in the liver, bone marrow and spleen.

6. Ceruloplasmin is a copper-containing blood protein. Also known as ferroxidase, it oxidizes Fe^{2+} to Fe^{3+} in transferrin. This is necessary for the mobilization of stored iron. Ceruloplasmin also is the major form in which copper is transported in the blood.

7. Molybdenum and inorganic sulfate react in the rumen to produce thiomolybdates. Thiomolybdates react with copper, making it non-absorbable. High dietary molybdenum intensifies copper deficiencies and may even induce a copper deficiency even though dietary copper is in the normal range.

8. Copper deficiency can cause anaemia, because copper is necessary for haemoglobin formation. Ataxia in copper-deficient animals is attributed to a deficiency of cytochrome oxidase (which contains copper) in the motor neurons of the central nervous system. Lack of hair pigmentation is because copper and iron are cofactors of tyrosinase, the enzyme involved in melanin biosynthesis. Skeletal deformity occurs because of the role of copper as an activator of lysyloxidase, an enzyme involved in collagen synthesis. Collagen forms the cartilaginous matrix of bone. Infertility results from impaired steroid hormone synthesis. The severe diarrhoea seen in copper deficiency is a malabsorption syndrome caused by diminished cytochrome oxidase activity in mucosal cells, producing villi atrophy.

9. Pernicious anaemia is caused by vitamin B_{12} deficiency. It occurs in individuals who lack the intrinsic factor, a small glycoprotein secreted by the gastric mucosa. The intrinsic factor is essential for vitamin B_{12} absorption. Vitamin B_{12} functions in the metabolism of folic acid, a vitamin required for haemoglobin synthesis. Thus a vitamin B_{12} deficiency, as well as folic acid deficiency, cause anaemia.

10. Excretion of arsenic involves the folate-dependent methylation of inorganic arsenic to methylated arsenic acids. Supplementation of arsenic-intoxicated people with folic acid thus increases urinary arsenic excretion.

11. Vitamin E is a lipid antioxidant that is a constituent of cell membranes, including the red blood cell membrane. In vitamin E deficiency, the red blood cell membrane is very susceptible to oxidant damage and rupture, causing the red blood cells to rupture.

12. Selenium provides a second line of defence, after vitamin E, in preventing red blood cell haemolysis. Selenium is a component of glutathione peroxidase,

an enzyme which reduces (provides hydrogen to) oxidants by reacting them with reduced glutathione (GSH). Glucose catabolism via the pentose shunt is necessary to provide the hydrogens necessary to maintain a supply of GSH.

13. Various plants contain oxidants that can cause red blood cell haemolysis. These include fava beans, *Brassica* species (plants in the cabbage family), onions and red maple leaves.

14. The North Ronaldsay breed of sheep has adapted to a diet of seaweed on the Scottish island of North Ronaldsay. Seaweed has a very low copper content. Thus this breed has adapted to a low copper diet by developing efficient copper uptake and retention mechanisms. As a consequence, they are very susceptible to copper toxicity, which they develop on diets with normal copper levels for other breeds of sheep.

15. Herbivores commonly have a hunger for salt. This is because plants in general have much higher contents of potassium than of sodium. Animals seek out sources of sodium to balance their high potassium intakes.

16. Dietary electrolyte balance can affect calcium metabolism in dairy cows. Diets that are acidic favour calcium absorption, while those with excess cations may reduce calcium availability. High cation prepartum diets, especially those high in potassium and sodium, can cause milk fever in cows by inducing metabolic alkalosis that impairs the cow's ability to maintain calcium homeostasis at the onset of lactation. High cation diets also impair calcium mobilization from bone.

17. Hypomagnesaemia can cause a downer cow situation (grass tetany) because magnesium functions at the neuromuscular junction in transmission of nerve impulses to muscle tissue. As such, magnesium deficiency can be a contributory factor to the hypocalcaemia-induced downer cow condition (milk fever).

Chapter 22

1. Phosphorus deficiency is a common cause of impaired reproduction in cattle. Phosphorus is very important in energy metabolism. Glucose and its metabolites (e.g. glucose-6-phosphate) are phosphorylated compounds in the pathways of carbohydrate metabolism. ATP, the major cellular energy source, is a phosphorylated substance. Thus phosphorus deficiency can result in impaired energy metabolism, which in turn has adverse effects on

reproduction. It is an adaptive strategy of animals to put reproduction 'on hold' if the animal is experiencing an energy shortage. It is not a good strategy to initiate reproduction if an energy shortage is on the horizon.

2. 6-MBOA is a substance produced in early spring growth of grass. It is postulated that it acts as a dietary cue for initiating spring reproduction in small herbivores (e.g. meadow voles).

3. Vitamin E has only one known function, as a tissue antioxidant. Its reproductive effects are due to its prevention of damage to the reproductive tissues and fetuses by oxidants.

4. Vitamin A is essential for male and female fertility and for fetal development. Vitamin A functions in biosynthesis of steroid hormones such as progesterone, and regulates cell differentiation and proliferation. Vitamin A deficiency can result in fetal resorption or abortion.

5. Endophytes are microscopic fungi that grow in plant tissues. Endophyte-infected tall fescue contains ergot alkaloids that adversely affect reproduction in horses. Tall fescue grass that does not contain endophytes (endophyte-free tall fescue) does not cause reproductive problems or any other adverse effects.

6. Phyto-oestrogens commonly occur in plants of the legume family, such as lucerne, clovers and soybeans. Clovers and soybeans contain a type of phyto-oestrogen with an isoflavone structure. Lucerne phyto-oestrogens are of a type called coumestans.

7. DDT affects only certain types of birds – mainly raptors (e.g. hawks, eagles) and waterfowl. The primary effect is eggshell thinning and breakage, preventing successful embryo development. DDT affects the activity of hepatic cytochrome P_{450} enzymes that metabolize steroid hormones including vitamin D. Disturbances in vitamin D activation in the liver by DDT adversely affect calcium absorption, causing reduced eggshell thickness. These effects are not seen with domestic poultry such as chickens and quail.

Chapter 23

1. Innate immunity is the antigen-non-specific defence mechanisms of the immune system that is activated very quickly after exposure to an antigen. It is the first line of defence against pathogens. Acquired immunity is the part of the immune system for the production of antibodies against

specific antigens that have been previously encountered, so the body has 'acquired' a mechanism to defend against them.

2. Cells of the innate immune system recognize invading pathogens by their presentation of distinct 'pathogen-associated molecular patterns'. Pathogens contain molecules not found in mammalian cells, which can be recognized by the immune system as foreign entities.

3. IgM and IgG are the first immunoglobulins to be produced by the immune system in response to an infection. They have relatively low affinity against antigens. Their major limitation as a measure of immune status is that the fetal IgM or IgG fraction represents the combined titre against all antigens to which an organism has been exposed. Thus testing for IgM and IgG lacks specificity.

4. The induction of a fever increases energy requirements by 10–15% for every degree of body temperature increase associated with an immune response. This is a result of the increased catabolism necessary to generate heat.

5. When the immune response is generated, there is increased production of oxidants (reactive oxygen species, ROS). Oxidants kill pathogens, but in addition cause damage to cellular membranes. Thus there is an increased demand for antioxidants to prevent this damage. Nutrients with antioxidant activity are vitamin E, selenium and vitamin C.

6. As discussed in Chapter 16, chromium is a component of the glucose tolerance factor which potentiates the action of insulin in the uptake of glucose by cells. The favourable effects of chromium on immune responses in the presence of stress may reflect enhanced glucose utilization via chromium involvement in the glucose tolerance factor.

Chapter 24

1. The inflammatory response is the production of chemical defences (proinflammatory cytokines) in response to invasion by pathogens. Cytokines include interleukins, tumour necrosis factor, interferons, histamine, kinins and acute phase proteins.

2. Cytokines function in cell signalling to direct immune cells such as T cells and macrophages to sites of infection. They cause nutrients to be partitioned away from normal metabolic processes to pathways that specifically target pathogens.

3. NFκB is nuclear transcription factor kappa B. It is a transcription factor which stimulates the synthesis of acute phase proteins. It also functions in the expression of cytokines.

4. Sickness behaviour characterizes the non-specific symptoms of infection and inflammation that include weakness, malaise, listlessness, inability to concentrate, depression, lethargy and anorexia. These are characteristic symptoms of influenza in humans, for example.

5. ω-3 and ω-6 fatty acids are precursors of eicosanoids, including prostaglandins, thromboxanes and leukotrienes. The ω-6 fatty acids produce eicosanoids that have inflammatory properties, while the ω-3 fatty acids produce eicosanoids with anti-inflammatory activity.

6. In segregated early weaning, pigs are weaned at as young age as possible, to avoid activating the immune system by exposure to pathogens. Activation of the immune system diverts nutrients away from growth to the production of cytokines, thus reducing growth rate.

7. GALT is gut-associated lymphoid tissue. It is the largest component of the immune system in the body. The gut is the largest interface of an animal with its environment, and a major site of entry of foreign antigens.

8. Antibiotics may suppress intestinal microbes which produce immunogens that stimulate an immune response. Responding to immunogens diverts nutrients away from growth towards cytokine synthesis.

9. Sub-therapeutic means a concentration lower than that required to kill pathogens. Growth-promoting antibiotics are not used to treat disease. A new theory suggests that dietary antibiotics exert their effects via anti-inflammatory activity in the intestinal mucosa.

Index

Page numbers with suffix 'n' refer to Notes, those in *italics* refer to figures and tables.

antioxidants (*Continued*)
    polyphenolic 154
    selenium 150–151
    synthetic 153, *154*
    vitamin C 153
    vitamin E 146–147, 150, 278
antiperistalsis 18
antler growth 232–233
aortic rupture, copper deficiency 265
apolipoproteins 133
appetite 189
arachidonic acid 124, 294
Arctic animals, vitamin A liver concentrations 245, 247
arginine 68, 77
arid environments, water metabolism strategies *253*, 257–260
arsenic poisoning 268
arteriovenous anastomoses (AVAs), dilated 234, 237
ascites 71
ascorbic acid *see* vitamin C
aspartate 77
ataxia 265
atherosclerosis *115*
autoenzymatic digesters 11–20
    avian species 18–20
    digestive tract 11–12
    small intestine 16
    stomach 12–15
autoenzymatic digestion
    classification of animals *12, 13*
    protein 56
aversive conditioning 201
avian species *see* birds
avidin 232

B cells 291, 292
bacteria
    amylolytic 100, 102, 112
    cell wall amino acid 59
    cellulolytic 32, 98–99, 101, 112
    pathogenic 32
    rumen 100, 142
    saccharolytic 100
    stomach 14, 15
basal metabolic rate (BMR) 201, *202*
    imported livestock 200
bears, hibernation 165
beavers 191
Bergmann's rule 203
betaine 70–71
bile
    entero-hepatic recycling 126
    lipid emulsification 149
    pigments 126–127
    salts 126

bile acids 6
    ruminant 131
    synthesis 126, *127*
biochemical individuality 9
biohydrogenation theory 142, *143*
biotin 137, 233
biotin deficiency 232, 233
birds
    autoenzymatic digesters 18–20
    bone growth disorders 219–221
    caecal fermenters 37
    carbohydrate digestion 95–96
    digestion 18–20
    feather pigmentation 230
    foregut fermenters 33, *34, 35*
    uric acid metabolism 69
    water requirements 255, *256*
    see also feathers
biuret 56, 58, 61
black walnut toxicosis 235, 237
blindness, vitamin A deficiency 219, *220*
blood 262–270
    clotting 262–263
    diet-induced anaemias 268–270
    haemoglobin formation 263–268
blood urea nitrogen (BUN) 57–58
blue-green algae 257
boar taint 73
body size
    feed intake 201, *202*, 203
    foregut fermenters 23, 24, 38–39
    hindgut fermenters 35, 37, 38–39
    nutritional animal models 39
bomb calorimeter 163, *164*
bone
    metabolism 218–219
    remodelling 218
    growth 218–219
        disorders 219–222
bovine hyperexcitability 88
bovine spongiform encephalopathy (BSE) 272
branch-chain fatty acids (BCFA) 131, 142
Brassica 269, 270
brown adipose tissue 170
browning reactions
    enzymatic 78
    non-enzymatic 78–79
browsers
    tannin intake 149
    see also concentrate selectors
brush border 16, *17*
bulk eaters *see* grazers
butylated hydroxyanisole (BHA) 145, 153, *154*
butylated hydroxytoluene (BHT) 145, 153, *154*
butyrate 100–101, 110
butyric acid 117
bypass protein 195–196

feed intake (*continued*)
    pregnancy 200–201
    regulation 193–195
    seasonal variation 199
feeding
    behaviour 187–188
    strategies in classification of animals 11, *12*, *13*
feet 233–235, *236*, *237*
felinine 72–73
fetal resorption in rabbits *275*, 286–287
fish
    feeding mink 231, *232*
    marine mammal diet 255
    nitrogen excretion 69–70
    reproduction 287
    thiaminases 106
    water requirements 255
    see also trimethylamine oxide (TMAO)
fish oils 123, 124
fluoroacetate 109
flushing 285–286
folic acid 70, 265–267
folivores, arboreal 33
food
    heat increment 200
    human 171–173
    preference 189
    processing 173
    refining 173
    water-holding capacity 198
    see also feed feeding
food plants, coevolution with herbivores 190
foot-pad dermatitis 233
forage
    carbohydrate content 93
    composition 197–198
    nutritional value 93
    physicomechanical characteristics 26, 27
    potassium levels 271
    structural carbohydrate characteristics 92–93
    water content 198
foregut fermenters 22–35
    body size 23, 24, 38–39
    evolution 40
    hindgut fermentation comparison 38–39
    non-ruminant 33–35
    ruminant 22–33
formaldehyde
    iron absorption inhibition 263
    protein treatment 60
formononetin 280, *281*, *282*, *283*
free fatty acids (FFA) 128, 131, 133
free radicals 145
    scavenging 147
fructans 90, 235
fructose 85, 86, *86*, 104–105
    metabolic syndrome 180

obesity association 181
fumonisin 121, 267–268
fungi
    anaerobic in rumen 32, *33*
    rumen 99
    white-rot 100
    see also mycotoxins
fur animals 228

galactose 105–106
gamma-carboxyglutamic acid (GLA) 219
gastric inhibitory polypeptides (GIP) 13
gastric secretion control 13
gastrin 13
gazelle 258
generalist feeders 189, 191
ghrelin 194
giraffes
    browsing 191–193
    wasting disease 24
gizzard/gizzard teeth 18, *19*
global warming 100
globulins 52
glucagon 168
β-glucans 90, 96–97
gluconeogenesis 168
glucose 4, 85, *86*, 87
    blood levels 177, 194
    carbohydrate digestion 95
    carbon/hydrogen/oxygen content *137*
    catabolism 104
    metabolism 8, 268
    pentose phosphate pathway 109
    ruminant blood levels 111
    spike 179
    tolerance 179, 181
        factor 181
        test 168, *169*
glucose-6-phosphate dehydrogenase deficiency 268–269
glucuronosyltransferase 157
glutamate 77
glutamic acid 64, 65, 67
glutamine 65
glutathione 65, 76, 77
    reduced 109
glutathione peroxidase 109, 145, *146*, 150, 268
glutathione-S-transferase 156–157
glutelins 52
glycaemic index 179
glycine conjugates 76
glycocalyx 16, *17*
glycocholic acid 126, *127*
glycogen 8, 90, 168
glycogenolysis 168
glycolipids 91, 121
glycolysis 7, 104–106